2010
# YEAR BOOK OF MEDICINE®

# The 2010 Year Book Series

**Year Book of Anesthesiology and Pain Management™:** Drs Chestnut, Abram, Black, Gravlee, Lien, Mathru, and Roizen

**Year Book of Cardiology®:** Drs Gersh, Cheitlin, Elliott, Gold, Graham, and Suri

**Year Book of Critical Care Medicine®:** Drs Dellinger, Parrillo, Balk, Dorman, Dries, and Zanotti-Cavazzoni

**Year Book of Dermatology and Dermatologic Surgery™:** Dr Del Rosso

**Year Book of Diagnostic Radiology®:** Drs Osborn, Abbara, Birdwell, Elster, Manaster, Oestreich, Offiah, Rosado de Christenson, and Walker

**Year Book of Emergency Medicine®:** Drs Hamilton, Bruno, Handly, Mullin, Quintana, and Ramoska

**Year Book of Endocrinology®:** Drs Schott, Apovian, Clarke, Eugster, Ludlam, Meikle, Ovalle, Schinner, Schteingart, and Toth

**Year Book of Gastroenterology™:** Drs Talley, Ambikaipaker, Bollipo, DeVault, Harnois, Pearson, Picco, Rombeau, Scolapio, and Smith

**Year Book of Hand and Upper Limb Surgery®:** Drs Yao and Steinmann

**Year Book of Medicine®:** Drs Barker, Garrick, Gersh, Khardori, LeRoith, Seo, Talley, and Thigpen

**Year Book of Neonatal and Perinatal Medicine®:** Drs Fanaroff, Benitz, Donn, Neu, and Papile

**Year Book of Neurology and Neurosurgery®:** Drs Klimo and Rabinstein

**Year Book of Obstetrics, Gynecology, and Women's Health®:** Drs Dungan and Shulman

**Year Book of Oncology®:** Drs Arceci, Bauer, Gordon, Lawton, and Thigpen

**Year Book of Ophthalmology®:** Drs Rapuano, Cohen, Flanders, Hammersmith, Milman, Myers, Nelson, Penne, Pyfer, Sergott, Shields, and Vander

**Year Book of Orthopedics®:** Drs Morrey, Beauchamp, Huddleston, Swiontkowski, and Trigg

**Year Book of Otolaryngology-Head and Neck Surgery®:** Drs Sindwani, Balough, Franco, Gapany, and Mitchell

**Year Book of Pathology and Laboratory Medicine®:** Drs Raab, Parwani, Bejarano, and Bissell

**Year Book of Pediatrics®:** Dr Stockman

**Year Book of Plastic and Aesthetic Surgery™:** Drs Miller, Gosain, Gurtner, Gutowski, Ruberg, Salisbury, and Smith

**Year Book of Psychiatry and Applied Mental Health®:** Drs Talbott, Ballenger, Buckley, Frances, Krupnick, and Mack

**Year Book of Pulmonary Disease®:** Drs Barker, Jones, Maurer, Raza, Tanoue, and Willsie

**Year Book of Sports Medicine®:** Drs Shephard, Cantu, Feldman, Jankowski, Khan, Lebrun, Nieman, Pierrynowski, and Rowland

**Year Book of Surgery®:** Drs Copeland, Behrns, Daly, Eberlein, Fahey, Huber, Jones, Mozingo, and Pruett

**Year Book of Urology®:** Drs Andriole and Coplen

**Year Book of Vascular Surgery®:** Drs Moneta, Gillespie, Starnes, and Watkins

2010

# The Year Book of MEDICINE®

Editors
**James A. Barker**
**Renee Garrick**
**Bernard J. Gersh**
**Nancy M. Khardori**
**Derek LeRoith**
**Philip Seo**
**Nicholas J. Talley**
**James Tate Thigpen**

ELSEVIER
MOSBY

ELSEVIER
MOSBY

*Vice President, Continuity:* Kimberly Murphy
*Developmental Editor:* Rachel A. Glover
*Production Supervisor:* Donna M. Skelton
*Electronic Article Manager:* Jennifer C. Pitts
*Illustrations and Permissions Coordinator:* Dawn Vohsen

**2010 EDITION**


Printed in the United States of America
Composition by TNQ Books and Journals Pvt Ltd, India
Printing/binding by Sheridan Books, Inc.

Editorial Office:
Elsevier
Suite 1800
1600 John F. Kennedy Blvd
Philadelphia, PA 19103-2899

International Standard Serial Number: 0084-3873
International Standard Book Number: 978-0-323-06833-8

# Editorial Board

# Table of Contents

# Journals Represented

Journals represented in this YEAR BOOK are listed below.

American Heart Journal
American Journal of Cardiology
American Journal of Clinical Pathology
American Journal of Gastroenterology
American Journal of Hypertension
American Journal of Infection Control
American Journal of Kidney Diseases
American Journal of Medicine
American Journal of Obstetrics and Gynecology
American Journal of Respiratory and Critical Care Medicine
American Surgeon
Anaesthesia
Annals of Allergy, Asthma & Immunology
Annals of Internal Medicine
Annals of Neurology
Annals of Otology Rhinology & Laryngology
Annals of the Rheumatic Diseases
Annals of Thoracic Surgery
Archives of Internal Medicine
Arthritis Care & Research (Hoboken)
Arthritis Research & Therapy
Arthritis & Rheumatism
British Journal of Cancer
British Medical Journal
Cancer Epidemiology, Biomarkers & Prevention
Chest
Circulation
Clinical Cancer Research
Clinical Endocrinology
Clinical & Experimental Rheumatology
Clinical Infectious Diseases
Clinical Journal of the American Society of Nephrology
Critical Care Medicine
Cochrane Database of Systematic Reviews
Diabetes
Diabetes Care
Digestive Diseases and Sciences
Diseases of the Colon and Rectum
Endocrine Practice
European Heart Journal
European Journal of Cancer
European Journal of Echocardiography
European Journal of Radiology
European Respiratory Journal
FASEB Journal
Fertility and Sterility
Gastroenterology

Gynecologic Oncology
Heart
Heart Rhythm
Hepatology
Hypertension
International Journal of Radiation Oncology Biology Physics
JACC Cardiovascular Interventions
Journal of Burn Care & Research
Journal of Bone Mineral Research
Journal of Clinical Endocrinology & Metabolism
Journal of Clinical Microbiology
Journal of Clinical Oncology
Journal of Clinical Pathology
Journal of Emergency Medicine
Journal of Heart and Lung Transplantation
Journal of Hypertension
Journal of Immunology
Journal of Infectious Diseases
Journal of Neurology Neurosurgery and Psychiatry
Journal of Pediatric Gastroenterology and Nutrition
Journal of Pediatric Surgery
Journal of Rheumatology
Journal of the American College of Cardiology
Journal of the American College of Surgeons
Journal of the American Medical Association
Journal of the American Society of Nephrology
Journal of the National Cancer Institute
Journal of Thoracic and Cardiovascular Surgery
Journal of Urology
Kidney International
Lancet
Mayo Clinic Proceedings
Medicine
Medicine (Baltimore)
Muscle & Nerve
Nephrology Dialysis Transplantation
Neurology
New England Journal of Medicine
Oncology
Osteoarthritis and cartilage
Otolaryngology-Head and Neck Surgery
Pediatric Infectious Disease Journal
Pediatrics
PloS One
Proceedings of the National Academy of Sciences of the United States of America

Radiology
Rheumatology (Oxford)
Seminars in Radiation Oncology
Sleep
Surgery

## Standard Abbreviations

The following terms are abbreviated in this edition: acquired immunodeficiency syndrome (AIDS), cardiopulmonary resuscitation (CPR), central nervous system (CNS), cerebrospinal fluid (CSF), computed tomography (CT), deoxyribonucleic acid (DNA), electrocardiography (ECG), health maintenance organization (HMO), human immunodeficiency virus (HIV), intensive care unit (ICU), intramuscular (IM), intravenous (IV), magnetic resonance (MR) imaging (MRI), ribonucleic acid (RNA), and ultrasound (US).

## Note

The Year Book of Medicine is a literature survey service providing abstracts of articles published in the professional literature. Every effort is made to assure the accuracy of the information presented in these pages. Neither the editors nor the publisher of the Year Book of Medicine can be responsible for errors in the original materials. The editors' comments are their own opinions. Mention of specific products within this publication does not constitute endorsement.

To facilitate the use of the Year Book of Medicine as a reference tool, all illustrations and tables included in this publication are now identified as they appear in the original article. This change is meant to help the reader recognize that any illustration or table appearing in the Year Book of Medicine may be only one of many in the original article. For this reason, figure and table numbers will often appear to be out of sequence within the Year Book of Medicine.

PART ONE

# RHEUMATOLOGY

PHILIP SEO, MD, MHS

# 1 Osteoarthritis

**Association between radiographic features of knee osteoarthritis and pain: results from two cohort studies**

Neogi T, Felson D, Niu J, et al (Univ School of Medicine, Boston, MA; et al)

*BMJ* 339:b2844, 2009

*Objective.*—To examine the relation of radiographic features of osteoarthritis to knee pain in people with knees discordant for knee pain in two cohorts.

*Design.*—Within person, knee matched, case-control study.

*Setting and Participants.*—Participants in the Multicenter Osteoarthritis (MOST) and Framingham Osteoarthritis studies who had knee radiographs and assessments of knee pain.

*Main Outcome Measures.*—Association of each pain measure (frequency, consistency, and severity) with radiographic osteoarthritis, as assessed by Kellgren and Lawrence grade (0-4) and osteophyte and joint space narrowing grades (0-3) among matched sets of two knees within individual participants whose knees were discordant for pain status.

*Results.*—696 people from MOST and 336 people from Framingham were included. Kellgren and Lawrence grades were strongly associated with frequent knee pain—for example, for Kellgren and Lawrence grade 4 *v* grade 0 the odds ratio for pain was 151 (95% confidence interval 43 to 526) in MOST and 73 (16 to 331) in Framingham (both P<0.001 for trend). Similar results were also seen for the relation of Kellgren and Lawrence scores to consistency and severity of knee pain. Joint space narrowing was more strongly associated with each pain measure than were osteophytes.

*Conclusions.*—Using a method that minimises between person confounding, this study found that radiographic osteoarthritis and individual radiographic features of osteoarthritis were strongly associated with knee pain.

▶ Despite the fact that pain is the most prominent symptom of knee osteoarthritis (OA) and the major reason for seeking surgical intervention, very little is known about the pathogenetic mechanisms of pain in knee OA. A major impairment in the study of pain mechanisms is the apparent lack of a correlation between radiographical changes in the knee and joint pain. This study is the first to analyze the relation of radiographic OA changes to knee pain in patients who had knees that were discordant for pain (ie, one knee was painful, and the other one was not), thus eliminating confounders at the level of the participants (such as genetic, psychological, and sociodemographic factors). Grade of radiographic OA, osteophytes, and joint space narrowing were compared between the paired knees. This led to the finding that strong structure-symptom association exists in OA of the knee, particularly for joint space narrowing (more than for osteophytes). An accompanying editorial points out legitimate limitations to the study.[1] However, this important study supports a causative role for structural changes in the joint in knee pain and will pave the way for a better understanding of the causes of OA pain.

**A-M. Malfait, MD**

*Reference*

1. Pincus T, Block JA. Pain and radiographic damage in osteoarthritis. *BMJ*. 2009; 339:b2802.

---

**Diet-induced obesity differentially regulates behavioral, biomechanical, and molecular risk factors for osteoarthritis in mice**

Griffin TM, Fermor B, Huebner JL, et al (Duke Univ Med Ctr, Durham, NC; et al)

*Arthritis Res Ther* 12:R130, 2010

---

*Introduction.*—Obesity is a major risk factor for the development of osteoarthritis in both weight-bearing and nonweight-bearing joints. The mechanisms by which obesity influences the structural or symptomatic features of osteoarthritis are not well understood, but may include systemic inflammation associated with increased adiposity. In this study, we examined biomechanical, neurobehavioral, inflammatory, and osteoarthritic changes in C57BL/6J mice fed a high-fat diet.

*Methods.*—Female C57BL/6J mice were fed either a 10% kcal fat or a 45% kcal fat diet from 9 to 54 weeks of age. Longitudinal changes in musculoskeletal function and inflammation were compared with endpoint neurobehavioral and osteoarthritic disease states. Bivariate and multivariate analyses were conducted to determine independent associations with diet, percentage body fat, and knee osteoarthritis severity. We also examined healthy porcine cartilage explants treated with physiologic doses of leptin, alone or in combination with IL-1$\alpha$ and palmitic and oleic fatty acids, to determine the effects of leptin on cartilage extracellular matrix homeostasis.

*Results.*—High susceptibility to dietary obesity was associated with increased osteoarthritic changes in the knee and impaired musculoskeletal force generation and motor function compared with controls. A high-fat diet also induced symptomatic characteristics of osteoarthritis, including hyperalgesia and anxiety-like behaviors. Controlling for the effects of diet and percentage body fat with a multivariate model revealed a significant association between knee osteoarthritis severity and serum levels of leptin, adiponectin, and IL-1α. Physiologic doses of leptin, in the presence or absence of IL-1α and fatty acids, did not substantially alter extracellular matrix homeostasis in healthy cartilage explants.

*Conclusions.*—These results indicate that diet-induced obesity increases the risk of symptomatic features of osteoarthritis through changes in musculoskeletal function and pain-related behaviors. Furthermore, the independent association of systemic adipokine levels with knee osteoarthritis severity supports a role for adipose-associated inflammation in the molecular pathogenesis of obesity-induced osteoarthritis. Physiologic levels of leptin do not alter extracellular matrix homeostasis in healthy cartilage, suggesting that leptin may be a secondary mediator of osteoarthritis pathogenesis.

▶ This is a detailed study of the effects of feeding a high-fat diet (HFD) to female C57BL/6 mice for 45 weeks on body mass, body fat, and visceral fat, in relationship to (1) longitudinal measurements of musculoskeletal function (as determined by grip strength, gait, and spontaneous activity), (2) longitudinal measurements of serum cytokine and adipokine levels, (3) end point assessment of pain sensitivity (hot plate and tail-flick test) and anxiety behavioral traits (measured in an elevated zero maze), and (4) end point assessment of osteoarthritic changes in the knee joints (assessed by histology and biomechanical measurements of cartilage compressive material properties).

The authors make a few very interesting points. First, the differences observed between the 2 different responder groups to HFD: the group that had significantly greater body mass than the controls after 4 weeks of HFD feeding (high gainer [HG]) and the group that did not develop significantly greater body mass until after 38 weeks of HFD (low gainer [LG]). The HG had a significantly higher incidence of knee osteoarthritis (OA) (mainly because of accelerated loss of proteoglycan from the cartilage, as determined by safranin-O staining) compared with controls, whereas the LGs were markedly protected from proteoglycan loss compared with controls (in spite of the weight gain). Next, HFD also resulted in hyperalgesia and anxiety-like behavior, which may be indicative of changes in pain-sensing and coping strategies. Importantly, these symptoms were present in both the HG and LG, indicating that they are the consequence of the HFD, more than of the degree of diet-induced obesity. Next, musculoskeletal strength, locomotor speed, and motor coordination, but not spontaneous locomotor activity, were significantly impaired by HFD. Importantly, reduction in grip strength occurred much earlier than changes in motor coordination and gait, indicating that the neuromuscular deficits associated with muscular force generation are an initiating factor in the pathogenesis of obesity-induced murine OA. Finally, the effects of prolonged HFD on systemic cytokine levels were minimal, but systemic levels of leptin, adiponectin, and IL-1α were predictive of knee OA severity.

Obesity is one of the most important risk factors for OA at weight-bearing and nonbearing joints. This thorough study supports the use of HFD-induced obesity in C57BL/6 mice as a model optimally suited to analyze the complex relationships between body fat, joint structural changes, and symptoms in

OA. This model will allow researchers to study systemic mechanisms in the pathogenesis of symptomatic OA.

**A-M. Malfait, MD**

---

**Different risk factors are involved in clinically severe large joint osteoarthritis according to the presence of hand interphalangeal nodes**

Valdes AM, McWilliams D, Arden NK, et al (King's College London, UK)

*Arthritis Rheum* 2010 [Epub ahead of print]

---

*Objective.*—To quantify the differences in the risk factors influencing total hip replacement (THR) and total knee replacement (TKR) depending on the presence of multiple finger interphalangeal nodes in two or more rays of each hand.

*Methods.*—3800 total joint replacement (TJR) cases (1201 having the nodal phenotype) and 1906 controls from two case-control studies and a population based cohort in the UK were studied. Odds ratios (OR) and 95% confidence intervals (CI) were calculated for age, gender, body mass index (BMI), height, and prevalence of the "T" allele in the GDF5 rs143383 polymorphism. ORs were compared between nodal and non-nodal cases and between TKR and THR.

*Results.*—Age, gender and BMI had significantly different ORs in nodal than in non-nodal cases. The GDF5 polymorphism was significantly associated with THR for nodal but not non-nodal cases, and height was a risk factor for non-nodal THR only. Female gender was a protective risk factor for non-nodal TKR (OR=0.60, 95% CI 0.52-0.70) but predisposing for the nodal form (OR=1.83 95% CI 1.49-2.26). Nodal status determined a significantly higher risk of having both a THR and TKR (OR=1.45 95%CI 1.09-1.94) and of bilateral TKR (OR=1.70 95% CI 1.37-2.11) but was paradoxically associated with a lower risk of bilateral THR (OR=0.71 95% CI 0.55-0.91).

*Conclusions.*—Nodal and non-nodal forms of large joint OA have significantly different risk factors and outcomes, indicating a different etiology for the two forms of OA. For THR, this appears to be at least in part genetically determined.

▶ Many genetic associations with osteoarthritis (OA) have been reported, although few have been consistently validated and reported in different populations. An issue with genetic studies in OA, as with OA biomarker studies, has been incomplete disease phenotyping. The authors of this study included nodal status (presence of Heberden's and/or Bouchard's nodes) in addition to knee and hip outcomes to determine whether the presence of nodes affected associations with one of the more promising genetic markers, a single nucleotide polymorphism in the promoter region of the growth differentiation factor (GDF5) gene. They used data from 3 studies: The Nottingham OA and Genetics of OA and Lifestyle case-control studies, of individuals undergoing hip or knee replacement and asymptomatic controls from the same hospitals, all of whom had assessment of nodal status, and additional controls from the Hertfordshire cohort study without radiographic knee OA (no nodal assessment). This sample included 2142 cases of knee replacement (total knee replacement [TKR]) and 1879 of hip replacement (total hip replacement [THR]), about one-third of which were nodal, and 1906 controls. About two-thirds of the overall sample had the risk (T) allele of the GDF5 polymorphism. The results showed that body mass index and age were risk factors for joint replacement in both nodal and nonnodal cases. However, female gender was a significant predictor of joint replacement only in nodal cases. Presence of the GDF5 T allele was positively associated with TKR for both nodal and nonnodal cases but only in nodal cases for THR. T-allele carriage was not associated with nodal status in the controls in which nodal assessments were available. Individuals with nodes were at higher risk of having both a knee and hip replacement, or having bilateral TKR, but were less likely to have bilateral THR. Therefore, while nodal and nonnodal cases of severe hip OA appear to have different genetic profiles (based on GDF5 status), knee OA risk profiles were similar between individuals with and without nodes. This study is an advance in the understanding of the importance of phenotypic characterization of the whole body burden of OA in genetic studies, although it remains limited by less complete phenotyping of the controls compared with the cases. An important point is that even restricting OA case definitions to severe large joint involvement (joint replacement) leaves a great deal of heterogeneity in case definition and contributing risk factors to be considered in future genetic studies.

**A. E. Nelson, MD**

---

**A statistical model of shape and density of the proximal femur in relation to radiological and clinical OA of the hip**

Waarsing JH, Rozendaal RM, Verhaar JAN, et al (Erasmus MC, Rotterdam, The Netherlands)

*Osteoarthritis Cartilage* 18:787-794, 2010

---

*Objective.*—Common radiological measures of osteoarthritis (OA) relate poorly to symptoms as experienced by patients. We created a statistical model of shape and density to see if Dual Energy X-ray (DXA) images of the hip contain symptom-related information that is not captured by common radiological measures.

*Methods.*—DXA images of the hip were made in a prospective study of patients that met the American College of Rheumatology (ACR) criteria for hip OA. From the DXA scans, we constructed a statistical model of the appearance (shape combined with density) of the proximal femur of left and right side. The model yields a number of independent descriptors of the appearance (modes) which we related to various measures of radiological and clinical OA. These outcome measures were defined using Joint Space Width (JSW), Kellgren and Lawrence (K–L) scores, Visual Analogue Scale (VAS) and Western Ontario MacMaster Universities (WOMAC) pain scores and a self-reported global assessment score.

*Results.*—Various modes showed significant relations with measures of OA. Interestingly, the modes that related well with radiological OA did not relate to clinical OA and *vice-versa*. Moreover, the modes were predictors of status and progression of clinical OA, independent from JSW and K–L.

*Conclusion.*—Statistical modeling of the appearance captures the patterns of variation in projected femoral morphology as visible on DXA images. We showed that these descriptors of subtle aspects of shape and density of the hip contain information about clinical status which common radiological measures do not. The presented results warrant further careful study of the method as a monitoring tool in clinical trials.

▶ This study expands on previous work in hip osteoarthritis (HOA) by using both bone density and active shape modeling on hip Dual Energy X-ray (DXA) scans to determine associations with presence and progression of HOA by clinical and radiographic definitions. This represents a novel line of research aiming to better understand the effects of combined hip shape and density on the incidence and progression of HOA. The authors used data from 218 individuals meeting American College of Rheumatology criteria for HOA with mild symptoms, enrolled in a clinical trial of glucosamine. Participants had baseline and 24-month follow-up anteroposterior pelvis radiographs (read for Kellgren-Lawrence [KL] grade and minimal Joint Space Width [JSW]) and DXA scans. Participants also completed Western Ontario MacMaster Universities (WOMAC) questionnaires and a visual analogue scale (VAS) for pain as well as a global assessment of improvement. Active shape statistical appearance models were created by placing 23 points around the proximal femur to the level of the lesser trochanter. Modes of variation were determined by principal components analysis. Radiographic HOA was defined as a KL score > 1 and JSW < 1.5 mm; progression of radiographic HOA was defined as a decrease in JSW of more than 20%. Clinical outcomes were defined by WOMAC, pain VAS scores, and global assessments. The results showed that 30 modes of variation were needed to describe 95% of the total variation in appearance, ranging from 23% described by mode 1 to 0.2% by mode 30. Most modes showed only a modest relation with the OA measures. Interestingly, the modes associated with radiographic HOA were not associated with clinical HOA and vice versa. Recalling that the reported appearance modes are reflective not only of shape but also of density distribution within that shape, the data presented in this study suggest that differences in hip biomechanics, reflected by alterations in bone density, in addition to variations in femoral head and neck morphology, may contribute to HOA. Also, based on these results, it appears that the alterations in shape and density associated with radiographic HOA differ from those associated with clinical HOA measures. This type of analysis, including the shape of the entire femoral head along with information about density from DXA, provides a more complete view of HOA compared with 2D geometric measures and may lead to a better overall understanding of factors that predispose an individual to developing HOA.

**A. E. Nelson, MD**

**First Qualification Study of Serum Biomarkers as Indicators of Total Body Burden of Osteoarthritis**

Kraus VB, Kepler TB, Stabler T, et al (Duke Univ Med Ctr, Durham, NC; et al)
*PLoS One* 5:e9739, 2010

*Background.*—Osteoarthritis (OA) is a debilitating chronic multijoint disease of global proportions. OA presence and severity is usually documented by x-ray imaging but whole body imaging is impractical due to radiation exposure, time and cost. Systemic (serum or urine) biomarkers offer a potential alternative method of quantifying total body burden of disease but no OA-related biomarker has ever been stringently qualified to determine the feasibility of this approach. The goal of this study was to evaluate the ability of three OA-related biomarkers to predict various forms or subspecies of OA and total body burden of disease.

*Methodology/Principal Findings.*—Female participants (461) with clinical hand OA underwent radiography of hands, hips, knees and lumbar spine; x-rays were comprehensively scored for OA features of osteophyte and joint space narrowing. Three OA-related biomarkers, serum hyaluronan (*s*HA), cartilage oligomeric matrix protein (*s*COMP), and urinary Ctelopeptide of type II collagen (*u*CTX2), were measured by ELISA. *s*HA, *s*COMP and *u*CTX2 correlated positively with total osteophyte burden in models accounting for demographics (age, weight, height): $R^2 = 0.60$, $R^2 = 0.47$, $R^2 = 0.51$ (all $p<10^{-6}$); *s*COMP correlated negatively with total joint space narrowing burden: $R^2 = 0.69$ ($p<10^{-6}$). Biomarkers and demographics predicted 35–38% of variance in total burden of OA (total joint space narrowing or osteophyte). Joint size did not determine the contribution to the systemic biomarker concentration. Biomarker correlation with disease in the lumbar spine resembled that in the rest of the skeleton.

*Conclusions/Significance.*—We have suspected that the correlation of systemic biomarkers with disease has been hampered by the inability to fully phenotype the burden of OA in a patient. These results confirm the hypothesis, revealed upon adequate patient phenotyping, that systemic joint tissue concentrations of several biomarkers can be quantitative indicators of specific subspecies of OA and of total body burden of disease.

► A major difficulty of biomarker studies in osteoarthritis is the frequent reliance upon disease status in a single joint without any accounting for whole body osteoarthritis burden, despite the fact that biomarkers are measured systemically and therefore are necessarily reflective of the entire body burden of disease. Kraus and colleagues present a novel approach to address the idea of whole body osteoarthritis burden, by utilizing radiographic information from multiple joint sites and joint surfaces, in conjunction with biomarker data. They analyzed data from the Genetics of Generalized Osteoarthritis study, in which siblings with clinical hand osteoarthritis were recruited along with affected and unaffected family members. Biomarker data (serum hyaluronan [sHA], urinary C-telopeptide fragment of type II collagen [uCTX2], and serum cartilage oligomeric matrix protein [sCOMP]) were available on 461 of 840 women in the cohort. Radiographs of the hands, knees, hips, and lumbar spine were scored for global Kellgren-Lawrence (KL) grade as well as osteophytes and joint space narrowing (disc space narrowing in the lumbar spine was considered a joint space narrowing equivalent). Summary scores of the total number of joint faces with osteophytes and the total number of joints with joint space narrowing were calculated, as was a sum score for the number of joints with KL >1. Serum HA and uCTX2 were strongly positively correlated with the latter sum score, while sCOMP demonstrated a negative correlation. All 3 markers had a positive association with the number of joint faces affected by osteophytes (regardless of the affected joint). A positive association between sHA and uCTX2 for joint space narrowing was observed, but this was not seen after adjustment for osteophytes; however, the negative association between sCOMP and joint space narrowing was persistent even with adjustment for osteophyte score. Certain joints, such as the carpometacarpal joints of the thumbs and the knee, contributed more to the associations than did other joints (clearly not related to joint size). An exhaustive analysis of all potential predictors, including joint space narrowing and osteophytes in all joint sites (>130 000 models) showed that individual biomarkers are more or less affected by specific joint characteristics (ie, sHA and uCTX2 with knee and hip osteophytes), in previously unknown patterns (Table 1 in the original article). Lastly, they found that the addition of biomarkers to models containing traditional covariates increased the proportion of variance (in % maximum osteophyte and joint space narrowing burden) explained by those models, such that a model containing all 3 biomarkers plus age, weight, and height explained 35% to 38% of the variance in the joint space narrowing or osteophyte burden, compared with 26% to 28% explained in models without biomarkers. This study, by using data from multiple joints and a set of 3 biomarkers, shows that a more comprehensive explanation of phenotypes in osteoarthritis can improve the predictive capability of biomarkers.

**A. E. Nelson, MD**

**Region of interest analysis: by selecting regions with denuded areas can we detect greater amounts of change?**

Hunter DJ, for the OAI Investigators (New England Baptist Hosp, Boston, MA; et al)

*Osteoarthritis Cartilage* 18:175-183, 2010

*Introduction.*—Based on recent analyses, the measures of short-term responsiveness of magnetic resonance imaging (MRI) derived cartilage morphometry may not be as large as earlier studies had suggested. We examined if by selecting regions of interest with denuded cartilage, the remaining cartilage within this region of interest was susceptible to greater rates of cartilage loss.

*Methods.*—Subjects included for this analysis are a subset of the approximately 4700 participants in the Osteoarthritis Initiative (OAI) Study. Bilateral radiographs and 3 T MRI (Siemens Trio) of the knees and clinical data are obtained at baseline and annually in all participants. Hundred and fifty subjects from the OAI progression subcohort all of whom had both frequent symptoms and, in the same knee, radiographic osteoarthritis (ROA defined as definite tibio-femoral osteophytes on X-ray) based on a screening reading done at the OAI clinics. One knee from each subject was selected for analysis. Using sagittal 3D DESSwe MR images from the baseline and 12-month follow-up visit, a segmentation algorithm was applied to the cartilage plates of the index knee to compute the cartilage volume, normalized cartilage volume (volume normalized to bone surface interface area), and percent denuded area (Total Cartilage Bone Interface area denuded of cartilage). Summary statistics of the changes (absolute and percentage) from baseline at 1 year and the standardized response mean (SRM), i.e., mean change divided by the standard deviation (SD) of that change were calculated. Analyses are stratified into three groups according to baseline assessment of denuded area: those with no denuded area in the region of interest at baseline, and then two groups (intermediate denuded area (≤median) and severe (≥median) denuded area) of equal sample size.

*Results.*—On average the subjects were 60.9 years of age and obese with a mean body mass index (BMI) of 30.3 kg/m$^2$. For the combined central medial femur and tibia the mean volume change for the whole sample was −48.2 (SD 159.8) mm$^3$, which gives an SRM of −0.30. In the subsample of knees with no denuded area the SRM was −0.25, in the knees with intermediate denuded area the SRM was −0.30, and in knees with severe denuded area the SRM was −1.00. For normalized volume of the central medial femur in the subsample of knees with no denuded area the SRM was −0.22, in the knees with intermediate denuded area the SRM was −0.26, and in knees with severe denuded area (n = 23) the SRM was −0.71. The magnitude of the SRMs was generally smaller in participants with no denuded area. In contrast, the SRMs in participants with denuded area were larger.

*Conclusion.*—By selecting participants with the presence of cartilage regions with denuded area the ability to demonstrate change in cartilage loss in that specific location is markedly improved compared to persons without a full thickness lesion in that cartilage plate. This option for screening during recruitment in clinical trials could facilitate the detection of participants at greater risk of subsequent cartilage loss.

▶ The authors present a novel way to demonstrate short-term changes in cartilage loss by following participants with knee osteoarthritis and denuded areas of cartilage. This analysis used radiographic and MRI data, at baseline and a 12-month follow-up visit, for 150 single knees from individuals in the progression cohort of the Osteoarthritis Initiative. Cartilage segmentation was performed using proprietary software, allowing assessment of cartilage volume and denuded area (reflective of a full-thickness cartilage defect). By stratifying into 3 groups according to baseline denuded area, the authors were able to determine that the mean change in cartilage volume after 12 months was higher in knees with more severely denuded areas of cartilage at baseline. This is best appreciated by looking at the standardized response means (SRMs) (mean change divided by the standard deviation of the change), which can be thought of as a way to quantify responsiveness of a measure (here cartilage volume by MRI) to change. By SRMs, the responsiveness was greatest in knees with severely denuded areas in the central medial femur and tibia. These data help to explain the lack of responsiveness when measuring larger cartilage areas, which may include not only denuded areas but also areas of swelling/edema, leading to an averaging effect and inability to detect progression. The overall small rates of change in this study are consistent with others, but the authors were still able to demonstrate progression by selecting areas at high risk for cartilage loss because of existing defects. This suggests that selection of individuals with denuded areas for inclusion in clinical trials may increase the chances of detecting differences and that benefit could offset any costs associated with an initial screening MRI. It remains unclear, however, if knees with an existing cartilage defect will actually be amenable to a given therapeutic intervention and would likely depend on the nature of the specific intervention.

**A. E. Nelson, MD**

---

**Effect of Glucosamine on Pain-Related Disability in Patients With Chronic Low Back Pain and Degenerative Lumbar Osteoarthritis: A Randomized Controlled Trial**

Wilkens P, Scheel IB, Grundnes O, et al (Univ of Oslo, Norway; SINTEF Health Res, Oslo, Norway)

*JAMA* 304:45-52, 2010

---

*Context.*—Chronic low back pain (LBP) with degenerative lumbar osteoarthritis (OA) is widespread in the adult population. Although glucosamine is increasingly used by patients with chronic LBP, little is known about its effect in this setting.

*Objective.*—To investigate the effect of glucosamine in patients with chronic LBP and degenerative lumbar OA.

*Design, Setting, and Participants.*—A double-blind, randomized, placebo-controlled trial conducted at Oslo University Hospital Outpatient Clinic, Oslo, Norway, with 250 patients older than 25 years of age with chronic LBP (>6 months) and degenerative lumbar OA.

*Interventions.*—Daily intake of 1500 mg of oral glucosamine (n=125) or placebo (n=125) for 6 months, with assessment of effect after the 6-month intervention period and at 1 year (6 months postintervention).

*Main Outcome Measures.*—The primary outcome was pain-related disability measured with the Roland Morris Disability Questionnaire (RMDQ). Secondary outcomes were numerical scores from pain-rating scales of patients at rest and during activity, and the quality-of-life EuroQol-5 Dimensions (EQ-5D) instrument. Data collection occurred during the intervention period at baseline, 6 weeks, 3 and 6 months, and again 6 months following the intervention at 1 year. Group differences were analyzed using linear mixed models analysis.

*Results.*—At baseline, mean RMDQ scores were 9.2 (95% confidence interval [CI], 8.4-10.0) for glucosamine and 9.7 (95% CI, 8.9-10.5) for the placebo group (*P*=.37). At 6 months, the mean RMDQ score was the same for the glucosamine and placebo groups (5.0; 95% CI, 4.2-5.8). At 1 year, the mean RMDQ scores were 4.8 (95% CI, 3.9-5.6) for glucosamine and 5.5 (95% CI, 4.7-6.4) for the placebo group. No statistically significant difference in change between groups was found when assessed after the 6-month intervention period and at 1 year:RMDQ (*P*=.72), LBP at rest (*P*=.91), LBP during activity (*P*=.97), and quality-of-life EQ-5D (*P*=.20). Mild adverse events were reported in 40 patients in the glucosamine group and 46 in the placebo group (*P*=.48).

*Conclusions.*—Among patients with chronic LBP and degenerative lumbar OA, 6-month treatment with oral glucosamine compared with placebo did not result in reduced pain related disability after the 6-month intervention and after 1-year follow-up.

*Trial Registration.*—clinicaltrials.gov Identifier: NCT00404079.

▶ This large and rigorous long-term study convincingly shows that glucosamine sulfate failed to benefit the observed patient population. The trial data on glucosamine are, of course, notoriously confusing. Some studies suggest it to be effective for controlling osteoarthritis (OA) pain in weight-bearing joints, but others fail to do so. The reasons for the contradictions could be manifold and relate to the type of preparation, use, the dose, or the particulars of the patient studied.

The negative result of this trial could be because of similar reasons. Or could it be that glucosamine does not affect small vertebral joints? Or that these joints are not the origin of pain-related disability in patients suffering from chronic low back pain? Perhaps the negative result indicates that OA and chronic low back pain are less closely related than the authors of this trial had assumed.

Whatever the answers may be, glucosamine is taken by many back pain sufferers at considerable expense. The results of this study indicate that there is little good evidence for doing so and that the money might be spent more wisely on other therapeutic options.

**E. Ernst, MD, PhD**

**A randomized controlled trial of acupuncture for osteoarthritis of the knee: effects of patient-provider communication**

Suarez-Almazor ME, Looney C, Liu Y, et al (Univ of Texas M.D. Anderson Cancer Ctr)

*Arthritis Care Res (Hoboken)* 2010 [Epub ahead of print]

*Objectives.*—There is conflicting evidence on the efficacy of Traditional Chinese Acupuncture (TCA), and the role of placebo effects elicited by acupuncturists' behavior has not been elucidated. We conducted a 3-month randomized clinical trial in patients with knee osteoarthritis to compare the efficacy of TCA to sham acupuncture, and examine the effects of acupuncturists' communication style.

*Methods.*—Acupuncturists were trained to interact in one of two communication styles: 'high' or 'neutral' expectations. Patients were randomized to one of 3 groups: waiting list, 'high' or 'neutral', and nested within style, TCA or sham acupuncture over 6 weeks. Sham acupuncture was performed in non-meridian points, with shallow needles and minimal stimulation. Primary outcome measures were: Joint-specific Multidimensional Assessment of Pain (J-MAP), Western Ontario McMaster Osteoarthritis Index (WOMAC), and satisfaction.

*Results.*—455 patients who received treatment (TCA or sham) and 72 controls were included. No statistically significant differences were observed between TCA or sham acupuncture, but both groups had significant reductions in J-MAP and WOMAC pain compared to the waiting group (−1.1, −1.0, and −0.1, $p<0.001$; −13.7, −14, −1.7, $p<0.001$). Statistically significant differences were observed in J-MAP pain reduction and satisfaction, favoring the 'high' expectations group. Fifty-two percent and 43% in the TCA and sham groups thought they had received TCA (kappa=0.05), suggesting successful blinding.

*Conclusion.*—TCA was not superior to sham acupuncture. However, acupuncturists' style had significant effects on pain reduction and satisfaction, suggesting that the analgesic benefits of acupuncture can be partially mediated through placebo effects related to the acupuncturist's behavior.

▶ This study uses an elegant trial design in an attempt to answer several important research questions. Firstly, it tests whether real acupuncture is superior to sham acupuncture for osteoarthritis of the knee. Several previous randomized control trials had suggested that acupuncture does generate symptom relief. Yet, most of these studies failed to rigorously control for nonspecific effects. This new trial suggests that the benefit of acupuncture is because of a placebo response.

Secondly, the study tests whether the communication style of the clinician can influence the outcome. Some of the acupuncturists in the trial were trained to generate high expectations in their patients. They turned out to be more successful in controlling symptoms than those who behaved neutrally.

This finding seems important as it might explain some of the contradictions that had emerged in previous studies. One might expect that acupuncturists are frequently enthusiastic about their treatment. According to the results of this trial, this attitude would significantly determine the clinical outcome. In clinical routine, this may be a desired effect; in clinical research, however, it represents an important confounder, which can distort the results of a trial. It follows that, in the future, trialists should control for communication style.

**E. Ernst, MD, PhD**

# 2 Rheumatoid Arthritis

**Well controlled, double-blind, placebo-controlled trials of classical Ayurvedic treatment are possible in rheumatoid arthritis**

Furst DE, Venkatraman MM, Krishna Swamy BG, et al (Univ of California, Los Angeles; Univ of Washington, Seattle; The Ayurvedic Trust, Coimbatore, India)

*Ann Rheum Dis* 2010 [Epub ahead of print]

*Background.*—One of the concerns of practitioners of Ayurvedic and other complementary and alternative medicine (CAM) methods is the ability to individualize treatment to the patient when participating in well-controlled, double-blind, placebo-controlled trials. The feasibility and effectiveness of multiple placebos to tailor treatments to patients were evaluated in an evaluation of classical Ayurveda to manage rheumatoid arthritis.

*Methods.*—Forty-six patients age 18 years or older with active rheumatoid arthritis were randomly assigned to three groups for outpatient treatment. Groups received methotrexate+placebo Ayurveda, Ayurveda+ placebo methotrexate, or methotrexate+Ayurveda. The practitioner of Ayurveda chose from 148 formulations in six traditional dosage forms: decoctions, herbal powders, pills, herbal wines, herbal jams, and herb-infused oils. The six placebos developed represented dosage forms as well. Visits with allopathic and Ayurvedic doctors were scheduled every 2 weeks for 36 weeks and included physical examinations, rheumatoid arthritis assessments, and studies of safety and efficacy. Allopathic doctors performed all the assessments of efficacy and toxicity. The patients and doctors were questioned separately at the end of treatment about which regimen the patient had undergone.

*Results.*—The actual treatment received and the speculations of the patients and doctors showed a relationship. The double-blind procedure was successful, with blinding maintained throughout the study. The use of six placebos and permitting doctors to individualize treatment proved to be an effective approach.

*Conclusions.*—Clinical research on Ayurveda can move forward based on this study because it shows that one can successfully develop and use placebos for multiple dosage forms in a randomized placebo-controlled, double-blind trial. This approach may also permit clinical investigation of other CAM systems.

▶ This is a pilot study with rather clever design features. Much of alternative medicine is individualized and the various options do not come as 1 item. Ayurvedic herbal medicine is such a treatment. An Ayurvedic doctor would insist that, for optimal results, he must be able to prescribe herbal decoctions, powders, pills, or oils tailor-made to the patient's needs, conditions, and symptoms. This renders placebo controls and successful blinding a true obstacle. The authors of this trial have demonstrated that the obstacle is surmountable. The results show that the need for individualization can be incorporated in an otherwise standard randomized controlled trial design and that blinding can be successful if more than one placebo preparations are used. The study might therefore be used as a blueprint for testing the efficacy on interventions that present similar problems.

**E. Ernst, MD, PhD**

# 3 Genetics

## A genome-wide association study identifies an osteoarthritis susceptibility locus on chromosome 7q22

Kerkhof HJ, Lories RJ, Meulenbelt I, et al (Erasmus Med Centre, Rotterdam, The Netherlands)

*Arthritis Rheum* 62:499-510, 2010

*Objective.*—To identify novel genes involved in osteoarthritis (OA), by means of a genome-wide association study.

*Methods.*—We tested 500,510 single-nucleotide polymorphisms (SNPs) in 1,341 Dutch Caucasian OA cases and 3,496 Dutch Caucasian controls. SNPs associated with at least 2 OA phenotypes were analyzed in 14,938 OA cases and approximately 39,000 controls. Meta-analyses were performed using the program Comprehensive Meta-analysis, with *P* values $<1 \times 10^{-7}$ considered genome-wide significant.

*Results.*—The C allele of rs3815148 on chromosome 7q22 (minor allele frequency 23%; intron 12 of the COG5 gene) was associated with a 1.14-fold increased risk (95% confidence interval 1.09-1.19) of knee and/or hand OA ($P = 8 \times 10^{-8}$) and also with a 30% increased risk of knee OA progression (95% confidence interval 1.03-1.64) ($P = 0.03$). This SNP is in almost complete linkage disequilibrium with rs3757713 (68 kb upstream of GPR22), which is associated with GPR22 expression levels in lymphoblast cell lines ($P = 4 \times 10^{-12}$). Immunohistochemistry experiments revealed that G protein-coupled receptor protein 22 (GPR22) was absent in normal mouse articular cartilage or synovium. However, GPR22-positive chondrocytes were found in the upper layers of the articular cartilage of mouse knee joints that were challenged with in vivo papain treatment or methylated bovine serum albumin treatment. GPR22-positive chondrocyte-like cells were also found in osteophytes in instability-induced OA.

*Conclusion.*—Our findings identify a novel common variant on chromosome 7q22 that influences susceptibility to prevalence and progression of OA. Since the GPR22 gene encodes a G protein-coupled receptor, this is potentially an interesting therapeutic target.

▶ Osteoarthritis (OA) has a substantial genetic component. The largest genome-wide association scan (GWAS) published to date was carried out by a Dutch-led European consortium. Having tested 14 938 OA cases and 39 000 controls in total (discovery plus replication), the study found a strong significant association with knee and/or hand OA in individuals of European descent with a linkage disequilibrium (LD) block mapping to a˜300 kilobase region in chromosome 7. An LD block is a DNA segment that contains markers that are in significant LD with each other, which implies that genetic variation in this region is highly or even totally correlated. A number of potential causative genes are located within this LD block in chromosome 7q22. Gene expression and immunohistochemistry studies suggested that the G protein-coupled receptor protein 22 (*GPR22*) might be the causative locus. GPR22 is present in cartilage and osteophytes in mouse OA models and absent in normal cartilage. The protein encoded by *GPR22* is an orphan receptor whose function and role in OA pathogenesis is unknown as yet. The results from this GWAS indicate that the genetic architecture of OA is likely to be polygenic with multiple variants along the spectrum of allele frequencies contributing modest and small effects. This is typical of common complex diseases that require very large sample sizes for their detection. In fact, future studies aiming to unravel the genetic determinants of OA will almost certainly require large numbers of cases and controls and therefore considerable collaborative efforts. On the other hand, this study clearly illustrates the ability of the GWAS approach to identify novel genes of unknown function, which will help increase our understanding of the disease pathogenesis.

**A. M. Valdes, PhD**

---

**Pain perception is altered by a nucleotide polymorphism in *SCN9A***

Reimann F, Cox JJ, Belfer I, et al (Addenbrooke's Hosp, Cambridge, UK; Univ of Pittsburgh, PA; et al)

*Proc Natl Acad Sci U S A* 107:5148-5153, 2010

---

The gene *SCN9A* is responsible for three human pain disorders. Nonsense mutations cause a complete absence of pain, whereas activating mutations cause severe episodic pain in paroxysmal extreme pain disorder and primary erythermalgia. This led us to investigate whether single nucleotide polymorphisms (SNPs) in *SCN9A* were associated with differing pain perception in the general population. We first genotyped 27 *SCN9A* SNPs in 578 individuals with a radiographic diagnosis of osteoarthritis and a pain score assessment. A significant association was found between pain score and SNP rs6746030; the rarer A allele was associated with increased pain scores compared to the commoner G allele ($P = 0.016$). This SNP was then further genotyped in 195 pain-assessed people with sciatica, 100 amputees with phantom pain, 179 individuals after lumbar discectomy, and 205 individuals with pancreatitis. The combined $P$ value for increased A allele pain was 0.0001 in the five cohorts tested (1277 people in total). The two alleles of the SNP rs6746030 alter the coding sequence of the sodium channel Nav1.7. Each was separately transfected into HEK293 cells and electrophysiologically assessed by patch-clamping. The two alleles showed a difference in the voltage-dependent slow inactivation ($P = 0.042$)

where the A allele would be predicted to increase Nav1.7 activity. Finally, we genotyped 186 healthy females characterized by their responses to a diverse set of noxious stimuli. The A allele of rs6746030 was associated with an altered pain threshold and the effect mediated through C-fiber activation. We conclude that individuals experience differing amounts of pain, per nociceptive stimulus, on the basis of their SCN9A rs6746030 genotype.

▶ Pain, not cartilage degradation, is the main clinical outcome of severe osteoarthritis (OA). However, some patients with very severe radiographic joint damage present little or no pain, whereas there are patients with fairly modest joint damage who have extreme pain and disability, even to the extent of requiring total joint arthroplasty. The study by Reimann and coworkers is the first one to look for the role of genetic variants in a gene involved in pain perception in the severity of symptoms of patients with either knee or hip OA. The variant identified in this study associated with worse pain scores in OA cases encodes an R1150W amino acid change and is also significantly associated with other forms of pain (sciatica, postdiscectomy, and postamputation pain) and with altered pain thresholds. Importantly, compounds to target the molecule in question (Nav1.7) are under development and have potent analgesic/antihyperalgesic effects in rat models of neuropathic pain.[1] Understanding the molecular pathways involved in OA pain can have direct clinical significance for the choice of pharmacotherapy used to treat OA. Therefore, this area of genetics has the potential of determining which pain-related molecules are implicated in OA pain. In addition, this type of research should help resolve the disconnection between OA pain and joint damage as measured by imaging methods.

**A. M. Valdes, PhD**

*Reference*

1. Ghelardini C, Desaphy JF, Muraglia M, et al. Effects of a new potent analog of tocainide on hNav1.7 sodium channels and in vivo neuropathic pain models. *Neuroscience*. 2010;169:863-873.

# 4 Myopathies

---

**Cancer-associated myositis and anti-p155 autoantibody in a series of 85 patients with idiopathic inflammatory myopathy**

Trallero-Araguás E, Labrador-Horrillo M, Selva-O'Callaghan A, et al (Vall d'Hebron General Hosp, Barcelona, Spain)

*Medicine (Baltimore)* 89:47-52, 2010

---

A new autoantibody against a 155-kDa protein has been described in patients with myositis. We conducted a study to determine the occurrence and types of cancer occurring in a cohort of patients with polymyositis (PM) or dermatomyositis (DM) and analyzed the value of this autoantibody as a serologic marker of cancer-associated myositis (CAM). Serum samples from all patients were examined by protein immunoprecipitation assays with HeLa cells to determine the presence of a 155-kDa protein band. HLA-DRB1 and DQA1 typing was performed by polymerase chain reaction-reverse sequence specific oligonucleotide. Statistical analyses were carried out with the Mann Whitney U and Fisher exact tests. Associations were determined using odds ratios (ORs) with 95% confidence intervals (CI). Eighty-five patients with myositis (20 PM and 65 DM) were included. CAM was detected in 16 patients (19%), 14 with DM. The shawl sign rash was significantly more frequent in patients with CAM than in those without ($p < 0.01$). Adenocarcinoma was the most frequent type of cancer (87.5%). Anti-p155 autoantibody was found in 1 of the 20 (5%) patients with PM and in 15 of the 65 (23%) patients with DM. A relationship between anti-p155 and CAM was found in DM patients (OR, 23; 95% CI, 5.23-101.2). The HLA-DQA1*0102 allele was not found in any of the anti-p155-positive patients. The prevalence of CAM in our cohort was 19%. Autoantibody against p155 was highly related to CAM and could be a reliable marker of cancer in patients with DM.

▶ It is becoming increasingly clearer that there are tight autoantibody-phenotypic associations in many rheumatic diseases. The idiopathic inflammatory myopathies are an excellent example of how myositis-specific autoantibodies help to predict the phenotype.

Both Targoff and colleagues[1] and Kaji and colleagues[2] described 2 new and similar myositis-specific autoantibodies reactive with a 155-kDa nuclear protein and with two 155/140-kDa nuclear proteins, respectively, that showed a significant association with cancer-associated myositis (CAM). It is broadly assumed that these autoantibodies are, in fact, the same.

The study by Trallero-Araguas was conducted in adult myositis patients to determine the occurrence and types of cancer that occur in a cohort of patients with polymyositis (PM) or dermatomyositis (DM) and to analyze the value of the presence of this newly described anti-p155 autoantibody as a serologic marker of CAM. Human leukocyte antigen (HLA)-DRB1 and DQA1 typing was also performed. This study's conclusion that the finding of the autoantibody against p155 was highly related to CAM and could be a reliable marker of cancer in patients with DM carries great significance as a potential predictive cancer marker.

Several investigators have tried to uncover pathologic findings on skin or muscle biopsy or clinical findings that are enhanced in those myositis patients with malignancy or those who are likely to develop one. This particular study also assessed this by comparing clinical and laboratory characteristics of patients with CAM to the group with no-CAM. No significant difference in sex distribution was found between the CAM group (women: 75%) and no-CAM group (women: 75.3%) ($P = 1$). Median age at time of myositis onset was higher in the CAM group (63 years) than in the no-CAM group (51 years) when both PM and DM patients were analyzed together, but the difference was not statistically significant ($P = .18$). Similarly, no statistical association was found when the analysis was performed in the DM group alone. In DM patients, the shawl sign was the only clinical characteristic seen more often in patients with CAM than in those without ($P < .01$). There were no statistical associations in either the overall group or in the separate idiopathic inflammatory myopathies (DM and PM) between the CAM and no-CAM groups when other signs and symptoms were analyzed. In contrast, the anti-p155 autoantibody was enhanced in DM patients with malignancy.

The new anti-p155 autoantibody, when available in routine clinical testing, may provide an excellent marker for malignancy in such patients, allowing us to be hypervigilant in malignancy screening in this select population. An additional finding noted was the presence of Mi-2 autoantibodies in 4 of the 24 patients with cancer who were negative for the anti-p155 autoantibody. The authors do not comment on the significance of this; however, Mi-2 is traditionally regarded as a good prognostic myositis-specific autoantibody with typical DM cutaneous disease and little clinical muscle involvement.

We cannot become complacent about good response to treatment in such patients, assuming little chance of malignancy, as clearly malignancy is possible in spite of the presence of these antibodies. It is unclear if these particular patients were uncharacteristically difficult to treat in this patient cohort.

Of note, the investigators did not find the previously reported association[1] between DQA1*0301 and presence of anti-p155 in their population, although a similar trend was observed: 16.7% of anti-p155 autoantibody-positive patients presented the DQA1*0301 allele compared with 8.3% of anti-p155-negative patients. Because routine HLA testing is not routinely performed in the context of clinical care, this information is not applicable in general clinical practice.

**L. Christopher-Stine, MD, MPH**

*References*

1. Targoff IN, Mamyrova G, Trieu EP, et al. A novel autoantibody to a 155-kd protein is associated with dermatomyositis. *Arthritis Rheum.* 2006;54:3682-3689.
2. Kaji K, Fujimoto M, Hasegawa M, et al. Identification of a novel autoantibody reactive with 155 and 140 kDa nuclear proteins in patients with dermatomyositis: an association with malignancy. *Rheumatology (Oxford).* 2007;46:25-28.

## Clinical and serologic characterization of an Argentine pediatric myositis cohort: identification of a novel autoantibody (anti-MJ) to a 142-kDa protein

Espada G, Maldonado Cocco JA, Fertig N, et al (Univ of Buenos Aires, Argentina)

*J Rheumatol* 36:2547-2551, 2009

*Objective.*—Autoantibodies are frequently found in adult patients with polymyositis (PM), dermato-myositis (DM), and overlap myositis disorders. They are less common in pediatric patients with myositis. We investigated the autoantibody pattern in a pediatric Argentine Caucasian cohort to characterize novel autoantibodies.

*Methods.*—Sera from children that satisfied published criteria for idiopathic inflammatory myopathy were analyzed for autoantibodies by RNA and protein immunoprecipitation and immunoblotting techniques. Routine myositis-specific and myositis-associated autoantibodies as well as autoantibody specificities were determined.

*Results.*—We tested sera from 64 consecutive pediatric myositis patients, including 40 with juvenile DM, 7 with juvenile PM, and 17 with overlap myositis syndromes. Sixteen (25%) patients were found to have anti-MJ autoantibody exclusively, which appears to identify a subset of pediatric myositis patients with severe disease characterized by muscle contractures and atrophy and significant compromise of functional status. Fourteen (22%) patients were found to have an antibody targeting 2 proteins of 155 and 140 kDa. Other myositis-specific autoantibodies were uncommon in this pediatric cohort.

*Conclusion.*—A newly recognized autoantibody, anti-MJ, was the most common antibody found in this Argentine pediatric cohort. The clinical features indicated that this antibody is distinct from other reported antibodies in pediatric patients with myositis.

▶ While the tight autoantibody-phenotype connection is well understood in adult idiopathic inflammatory myopathy (IIM) patients, these autoantibodies are less common in pediatric patients and their significance of helping to predict clinical characteristics is largely unknown. The fact that these investigators explored their own local Argentine Caucasian cohort for the presence of novel autoantibodies and found, upon retrospective review, the novel MJ autoantibody, which precipitated at 142 kDa in 14 of 64 patients with various forms of juvenile myositis who had been referred for routine clinical care over a 10-year period, suggests that there are numerous myositis autoantibodies that remain undiscovered. Interestingly, known myositis-associated and myositis-specific autoantibodies were rarely detected. Like previously described autoantibodies found in patients with myositis, the MJ autoantibody had a severe clinical phenotype with associated muscle contractures and atrophy. It is unlikely that these autoantibodies are found only in Argentinians, but it does suggest that there may be autoantibodies such as this one found preferentially in childhood-onset IIM. With regard to other noted autoantibodies, patients with anti-Mi-2 had a more benign course. Anti-MJ–positive patients had more severe disease as evidenced by their disease course consisting of functional status and more persistent disease activity, while p155/140 children generally had a more benign disease course and no evidence of cancer, in contrast to adults.

Further exploration in well-defined myositis cohorts in other children and adults is likely to reveal more novel autoantibodies that may provide, at least, good clinical characterizations and tighter phenotypes and, at best, a better understanding into the potential pathogenic mechanism of these autoantibodies. It is possible, as evidenced by the fact that children with the anti-155/140 autoantibody do not appear to have an increased risk of malignancy like their adult counterparts with this autoantibody, that clinical manifestations associated with specific autoantibodies may differ between children and adults with myositis.

**L. Christopher-Stine, MD, MPH**

---

**Conventional Cancer Screening versus PET/CT in Dermatomyositis/ Polymyositis**

Selva-O'Callaghan A, Grau JM, Gámez-Cenzano C, et al (Universitat Autonoma Barcelona, Spain; Universitat de Barcelona, Spain; Bellvitge Hosp, Barcelona, Spain)

*Am J Med* 123:558-562, 2010

---

*Objective.*—To determine the value of whole-body [$^{18}$F] fluorodeoxyglucose positron emission tomography/computed tomography (FDG-PET/CT) for diagnosing occult malignant disease in patients with myositis compared with broad conventional cancer screening.

*Methods.*—We prospectively studied 55 consecutive patients with a recent diagnosis of myositis in 3 teaching hospitals over a 3-year period by whole-body FDG-PET/CT and compared the results with those of conventional cancer screening, which included thoracoabdominal CT, mammography, gynecologic examination, ultrasonography, and tumor marker analysis. Comparisons were made using predictive values and their 95% confidence intervals.

TABLE 1.—Diagnostic Performance of the Two Cancer Detection Approaches

| | FDG-PET/CT | Conventional Screening |
|---|---|---|
| PPV | 85.7 (42.1-99.6) | 77.8 (40.0-97.2) |
| NPV | 93.8 (82.8-98.7) | 95.7 (85.2-99.5) |
| OPV | 92.7 (82.4-98.0) | 92.7 (82.4-98.0) |
| Sensitivity | 66.7 (29.9-92.5) | 77.8 (40-97.2) |
| Specificity | 97.8 (88.5-99.4) | 95.7 (85.2-99.5) |

FDG-PET/CT = [$^{18}$F] fluorodeoxyglucose positron emission tomography/computed tomography; NPV = negative predictive value; OPV = overall predictive value: PPV = positive predictive value. Results are expressed as percentages with 95% confidence interval.

*Results.*—A total of 9 of 55 patients were diagnosed with paraneoplastic myositis. FDG uptake was positive in 7 patients (1 false-positive), negative in 44 patients (3 false-negative), and inconclusive in 4 patients. Positive and negative predictive values of FDG-PET/CT for the diagnosis of cancer were 85.7% and 93.8%, respectively. Conventional screening was cancer-positive in 9 patients (2 false-positive) and negative in the remaining 46 patients (2 false-negative). Positive and negative predictive values were 77.8% and 95.7%, respectively. The overall predictive value of broad conventional screening was the same as that of FDG-PET/CT (92.7 vs 92.7).

*Conclusion.*—The performance of FDG-PET/CT, a single imaging study, for diagnosing occult malignant disease in patients with myositis was comparable to that of broad conventional screening, which includes multiple tests (Table 1).

▶ An association between cancer and inflammatory myopathies (cancer-associated myositis or CAM), mainly dermatomyositis and, to a lesser extent, polymyositis, is well known.[1,2] How to routinely assess for malignancy in patients with a known diagnosis of dermatomyositis or polymyositis is unknown and widely debated. Pan-CT scans (chest/abdomen/pelvis) are one way to assess for solid tumors; however, the amount of radiation may be unjustified in light of these patients already being predisposed to malignancy based on their underlying disease as well as the risks from immunosuppressive medications used. Although novel autoantibodies may predict those at highest risk for malignancy, exactly who will develop malignancy and which type they will develop has not been predictable.

As newer imaging techniques develop, it is reasonable to compare their utility to the conventional studies that are being used. In this study, 9 of 55 consecutive myositis patients (16%) over a 3-year period were diagnosed with paraneoplastic myositis. The authors appropriately note that the incidence of CAM may be underestimated in this study because the median follow-up was less than 3 years.

Positron emission tomography (PET)/CT findings were scored from 1 to 5 by visual interpretation from definitely malignant to definitely benign. Three categories were arbitrarily established: positive (score 1 or 2), when abnormal uptake or pathologic findings were detected; negative (score 4 or 5), with physiologic uptake without pathologic findings; and inconclusive or nonspecific findings (score 3). To simplify the analysis, equivocal results were considered negative. The number of additional tests to rule out cancer was similar with the 2 approaches (2 vs 2; P = not significant).

The overall predictive value of broad conventional screening was the same as that of [$^{18}$F] fluorodeoxyglucose (FDG)-PET/CT (92.7 vs 92.7) (Table 1).

The authors state that PET/CT has the added advantage of a single imaging test that is more convenient for both the patient and the physician. A comparison of radiation exposure as well as a cost-effective comparison between the 2 studies (CT for the chest/abdomen/pelvis compared with PET/CT) would be helpful in determining the most appropriate testing. This is the first head-to-head comparison of 2 similar malignancy screening methods. Perhaps the incorporation of known anti-155/140 autoantibody status into our imaging repertoire can help to enhance our diagnostic accuracy of CAM.

**L. Christopher-Stine, MD, MPH**

*References*

1. Dalakas MC, Hohlfeld R. Polymyositis and dermatomyositis. *Lancet.* 2003;362: 971-982.
2. Buchbinder R, Forbes A, Hall S, Dennett X, Giles G. Incidence of malignant disease in biopsy-proven inflammatory myopathy. A population-based cohort study. *Ann Intern Med.* 2001;134:1087-1095.

---

**Immune-mediated necrotizing myopathy associated with statins**

Grable-Esposito P, Katzberg HD, Greenberg SA, et al (Brigham and Women's Hosp, Boston, MA)

*Muscle Nerve* 41:185-190, 2010

---

We report patients from two neuromuscular centers who were evaluated between the years 2000 and 2008 and met the following criteria: (1) proximal muscle weakness occurring during or after treatment with statins; (2) elevated serum creatine kinase (CK); (3) persistence of weakness and elevated CK despite discontinuation of the statin; (4) improvement with immunosuppressive agents; and (5) muscle biopsy showing necrotizing myopathy without significant inflammation. Twenty-five patients fulfilled our inclusion criteria. Twenty-four patients required multiple immunosuppressive agents. Fifteen patients relapsed after being tapered off immunosuppressive therapy. Exposure to statins prior to onset was significantly higher in patients with necrotizing myopathy (82%) as compared to those with dermatomyositis (18%), polymyositis (24%), and inclusion-body myositis (38%) seen in the same time period. The lack of improvement following discontinuation of statins, the need for immunosuppressive therapy, and frequent relapse when treatment was tapered suggest an immune-mediated etiology for this rare, statin-associated necrotizing myopathy.

▶ This intriguing report from 2 neuromuscular centers between years 2000 and 2008 was the second of 2 recent articles to report a statin-associated seemingly immune-mediated myopathy progressive in spite of statin cessation and responsive to immunosuppressive therapy.[1] With clinical features similar to polymyositis, the histologic findings were suggestive of a necrotizing myopathy with little to no inflammation. The disease frequently relapsed when immuosuppression was tapered. This newly described entity is of paramount importance among myopathies, as it adds to our ever-growing understanding of new and distinct autoimmune inflammatory myopathy subsets. While somewhat confusing in nomenclature, this type of inflammatory myopathy is one not mediated by primary infiltration of lymphocytes against normal muscle cells, but rather, myophagocytosis leading to necrosis and muscle edema as seen on MRI.

This entity is probably best described as an autoimmune necrotizing myopathy and expands our current understanding of statin myopathies. Unlike the typical statin myopathy that is thought to result when the statin acts as a direct myotoxin and ceases when the statin is stopped, this new myopathy seems to be either propagated or perpetuated by statins and appears to progress despite stopping stain therapy. It is an important entity for not only rheumatologists and neurologists to recognize but also for primary care physician and cardiologists who are likely to prescribe the statin to the patient initially. Our own observations in our clinical practice lead me to believe that this is an entity underappreciated among statin-prescribing physicians. This can have devastating consequences when this disease is not recognized, as the autoimmune process has the potential to become more aggressive and more difficult to treat if we fail to recognize it as a potentially immunosuppressive therapy-responsive myopathy and therefore withhold this treatment for extended periods of time.

**L. Christopher-Stine, MD, MPH**

*Reference*

1. Needham M, Fabian V, Knezevic W, Panegyres P, Zilko P, Mastaglia FL. Progressive myopathy with up-regulation of MHC-I associated with statin therapy. *Neuromuscul Disord.* 2007;17:194-200.

# 5 Vasculitis

---

**Cancer Preceding Giant Cell Arteritis: A Case–Control Study**

Kermani TA, Schäfer VS, Crowson CS, et al (Mayo Clinic, Rochester, MN)

*Arthritis Rheum* 62:1763-1769, 2010

---

*Objective.*—To study the association between previous cancer and giant cell arteritis (GCA).

*Methods.*—Using the resources of the Rochester Epidemiology Project, we identified incident cases of GCA diagnosed between January 1, 1950 and December 31, 2004. Each GCA patient was matched for age, sex, and length of medical history to 2 subjects without GCA from the same population. Medical records were reviewed. Diagnosis of cancer was confirmed by histopathologic analysis.

*Results.*—We identified 204 GCA cases and 407 controls. The GCA group included 163 women (80%) and 41 men (20%). Their mean ± SD age was 76.0 ± 8.2 years. The non-GCA group consisted of 325 women (80%) and 82 men (20%). Their mean ± SD age was 75.6 ± 8.4 years. At the index date, 45 GCA patients (22%) and 125 non-GCA patients (31%) had had a previous cancer. The odds ratio (OR) for previous cancer in cases compared with controls, adjusted for age, sex, and calendar year, was 0.63, and the 95% confidence interval (95% CI) was 0.42–0.94 ($P = 0.022$). The mean age at diagnosis of the first cancer before the index date was similar in the cases (67.5 ± 11.9 years) and the controls (64.9 ± 13.2 years) ($P = 0.32$). The mean ± SD duration from the first cancer to the index date was 9.8 ± 9.9 years in the cases and 11.7 ± 10.8 years in the controls ($P = 0.31$). Cancer types were similar in both groups, but fewer gynecologic malignancies were noted in GCA patients (OR 0.39 [95% CI 0.13–1.15], $P = 0.09$). Colon cancer also appeared less commonly in the cases compared with the controls (OR 0.22 [95% CI 0.03–1.74], $P = 0.15$).

*Conclusion.*—The findings of this population-based case–control study indicate that GCA patients had significantly fewer malignancies prior to the index date as compared with controls.

▶ This article describes a population-based case-control study evaluating previous cancer in 204 cases of giant cell arteritis (GCA) compared with 407 randomly selected controls matched for age, sex, and length of medical history. Adjustment for smoking status was also performed. The authors found that patients with GCA actually had significantly fewer malignancies before the index date (date of diagnosis of GCA) than controls. To evaluate whether their findings could be related to an excess of nonmelanoma skin cancers in the controls, the authors analyzed their data without nonmelanoma skin cancers and found that the reduced risk of cancer preceding GCA was more pronounced. While there were fewer gynecological and colon cancers in the GCA cases, this did not reach statistical significance, and the types of malignancies were generally similar in GCA cases and controls. Although women with GCA had significantly fewer cancers than women without GCA, this was not true of the men and, overall, there was no difference between women and men. Lastly, the authors also analyzed the rate of malignancy in the year immediately before the index date to explore the possibility of a paraneoplastic phenomenon and no significant difference was noted between GCA cases and controls.

Whether or not GCA may be associated with malignancy has been controversial. As GCA is a disease of the elderly and generally presents with a markedly elevated erythrocyte sedimentation rate and often with constitutional symptoms, cancer is commonly in the differential diagnosis. While it is prudent to exclude malignancy at presentation, particularly in atypical or biopsy-negative cases, a perceived possible association with malignancy might otherwise lead to an unnecessary extensive search for cancer. This study helps to put perspective on a reasonable approach to the patient suspected of having GCA. One potential limitation of this study is that not all cases were biopsy proven (clinical diagnosis, fulfilling 1990 classification criteria for GCA); a previous study by Haga et al reported an increased risk of developing cancer in the subset of their patients with GCA who had a positive biopsy.[1] However, the findings in this study are supported by another study reported this year by Hill et al, which did not demonstrate any increased risk of malignancy in patients with biopsy-proven GCA.[2]

In addition to the clinical utility, this study has potential implications in considering the pathogenesis of GCA and/or malignancy. Because the patients with GCA in Kermani's study had significantly fewer malignancies before the diagnosis than controls, the authors of this thought-provoking study raise the possibility that some of the immunologic factors that predispose individuals to GCA may play a protective role in the development of malignancy.

**E. Belilos, MD**

*References*

1. Haga HJ, Eide GE, Brun J, Johansen A, Langmark F. Cancer in association with polymyalgia rheumatica and temporal arteritis. *J Rheumatol.* 1993;20:1335-1339.
2. Hill CL, Cole A, Rischmueller M, et al. Risk of cancer in patients with biopsy-proven giant cell arteritis. *Rheumatology (Oxford).* 2010;49:756-759.

**Malignancy risk in patients with giant cell arteritis: a population-based cohort study**

Kermani TA, Schäfer VS, Crowson CS, et al (Mayo Clinic, Rochester, MN)

*Arthritis Care Res (Hoboken)* 62:149-154, 2010

*Objective.*—To determine the incidence of cancer in a population-based cohort of patients with giant cell arteritis (GCA) compared with age- and sex-matched referent subjects.

*Methods.*—Using the resources of the Rochester Epidemiology Project, all incident cases of GCA diagnosed between January 1, 1950 and December 31, 2004 were identified. For each GCA patient, 2 subjects without GCA of the same sex and similar age and length of medical history were selected. Diagnosis of malignancy was made by histopathology. Patients were followed until death, last contact, or December 31, 2006.

*Results.*—Our study included 204 GCA patients and 407 non-GCA subjects. The GCA cohort had 163 (79%) women and 41 (21%) men, a mean ± SD age of 76.0 ± 8.2 years, and a median followup of 7.7 years. The non-GCA cohort consisted of 325 (80%) women and 82 (20%) men, a mean ± SD age of 75.6 ± 8.4 years, and a median followup of 8.1 years. During followup, 46 GCA patients and 76 non-GCA subjects developed cancer (hazard ratio [HR] 1.26, 95% confidence interval [95% CI] 0.87-1.83). Adjustment for smoking did not alter the results. The 1-, 10-, and 20-year cumulative incidences of any malignancy were 5.9%, 33.6%, and 50.0% among GCA patients and 2.6%, 27.0%, and 47.0% among non-GCA patients, respectively. There were no differences in hematologic or solid malignancies between both groups. Colon cancer appeared more commonly in the GCA group ($P = 0.07$). Mortality following cancer was similar in both cohorts (HR 0.80, 95% CI 0.52-1.24).

*Conclusion.*—GCA patients are not at an increased risk of first cancer after diagnosis.

▶ This population-based cohort study examines the incidence of cancer following the diagnosis of giant cell arteritis (GCA) in cases and controls from the Rochester Epidemiologic Project. The authors found that patients with GCA are not at an increased risk of first cancer following the diagnosis of GCA. There was no increased risk of malignancy whether the data were analyzed including or excluding patients with prevalent malignancy or nonmelanoma skin cancer. Adjustment for smoking did not significantly alter these results. Overall, there were no differences in the types of cancer seen in the 2 groups, although there was a nonsignificant trend toward an increase in colon cancer in the GCA group. The authors report that there may be a slight increased risk of cancer in the first year after the diagnosis of GCA, but this difference was not statistically significant in their study, and they comment that this could have been influenced by surveillance bias. In this study, there was no increased incidence of malignancy in the subset of patients with GCA who were biopsy positive.

Similar to their study on the prevalence of cancer before the diagnosis of GCA, this study helps to address how far to take the search for underlying malignancy in newly diagnosed patients with GCA. The risk of cancer in the first year following GCA diagnosis may need to be further studied in a larger population; this may have significant implications in considering trials of newer therapies, particularly biologic agents. Currently, corticosteroids, and all their attendant long-term complications, remain the only definitive treatment option for GCA. Despite the initial disappointment with tumor necrosis factor inhibition in GCA, it is likely that additional biologic or immunosuppressive agents will be considered for clinical trials, making it imperative to understand the baseline risk for malignancy in these patients.

**E. Belilos, MD**

---

**Clinical relevance of persistently elevated circulating cytokines (tumor necrosis factor α and interleukin-6) in the long-term followup of patients with giant cell arteritis**

García-Martínez A, Hernández-Rodríguez J, Espígol-Frigolé G, et al (Univ of Barcelona, Spain)

*Arthritis Care Res (Hoboken)* 62:835-841, 2010

---

*Objective.*—To assess the clinical relevance of increased circulating cytokines in patients with giant cell arteritis (GCA) after long-term followup.

*Methods.*—We performed a cross-sectional evaluation of 54 patients with biopsy-proven GCA prospectively followed for a median of 5.4 years (range 4-10.5 years). GCA-related complications, vascular events, relapses, current prednisone dose, time required to achieve a maintenance prednisone dosage <10 mg/day, cumulated prednisone at that point, and adverse effects during followup were recorded. Serum interleukin-6 (IL-6) and tumor necrosis factor α (TNFα) were determined by immunoassay.

*Results.*—All patients were in clinical remission. Both cytokines were significantly higher in patients than in controls (mean ± SD 21 ± 35 versus 5 ± 11 pg/ml; $P < 0.001$ for IL-6 and mean ± SD 32 ± 14 versus 16 ± 9 pg/ml; $P < 0.001$ for TNFα). No differences were found in patients with or without GCA-related complications or vascular events during followup. Circulating cytokines were significantly higher in patients who had experienced relapses (mean ± SD 25 ± 39 versus 10 ± 11 pg/ml; $P = 0.04$ for IL-6 and mean ± SD 34 ± 15 versus 25 ± 11 pg/ml; $P = 0.042$ for TNFα). IL-6 was significantly higher in patients still requiring prednisone (mean ± SD 29 ± 45 versus 13 ± 17 pg/ml; $P = 0.008$), and TNFα correlated with cumulated prednisone dose ($r = 0.292$, $P = 0.04$). No significant relationship was found between elevated cytokines and prednisone adverse effects or patients' quality of life.

*Conclusion.*—Circulating TNFα and IL-6 may persist elevated in GCA patients after long-term followup and remain higher in patients who have experienced more relapsing disease. However, in this patient cohort, elevated circulating cytokines were not associated with increased frequency of GCA complications, vascular events, or treatment-related side effects.

► Giant cell arteritis is the most common form of systemic vasculitis in North America and can be associated with potentially devastating results, including blindness. Many patients with giant cell arteritis will experience disease relapse after treatment; however, there is currently no way to differentiate such patients from others who may not require prolonged immunosuppression. This study tests the interesting hypothesis that serum cytokines associated with inflammation might provide an important clue to help clinicians differentiate these 2 phenotypes. Although preliminary, the results of this study imply that patients with elevated levels of tumor necrosis factor α and interleukin-6 may require prolonged glucocorticoid therapy; conversely, patients who have normal levels of these proinflammatory cytokines may be treated with a less aggressive approach, potentially saving them all of the side effects associated with prolonged glucocorticoid exposure. It is interesting that patients with these proinflammatory cytokines did not also have a higher rate of disease- or treatment-related morbidity, although this presumably reflects the small number of subjects included in this study.

**P. Seo, MD, MHS**

**Interferon-alpha for maintenance of remission in Churg-Strauss syndrome: a long-term observational study**

Metzler C, Csernok E, Gross WL, et al (Krankenhaus der Barmherzigen Brüder Regensburg, Germany)

*Clin Exp Rheumatol* 28:24-30, 2010

*Background.*—Interferon-alpha has been successfully used for induction of remission in patients with Churg-Strauss syndrome, but data on its ability to prevent relapses and its safety during long-term use are lacking.

*Objectives.*—To examine the safety and efficacy of interferon-alpha for maintenance of remission in Churg-Strauss syndrome.

*Patients and Methods.*—In a prospective open-label long-term observational study, 13 patients with CSS in stable remission received interferon-alpha (3 × 3 Mio. I.U/week s.c.) for maintenance of remission. Primary end point was the incidence of relapses. Secondary end points were the doses of concomitant prednisolone and the frequency adverse events.

*Results.*—After a median follow up of 64 month three patients were still on treatment with interferon-alpha all with a dose of 9 million units/week. In nine patients, interferon-alpha was discontinued for lack of efficacy (n=5), due to adverse events (n=2), or both (n=2) after median of 63 months (15-153) of therapy. A total of 3 major and 18 minor relapses occurred in 10 of the 13 patients with a median time to first relapse of 17 months (range 5-46). Sera of relapsing patients did not contain antibodies against interferon-alpha. In 6 relapsing patients treatment was switched to cyclophosphamide (n=4) or methotrexate (n=2). Four episodes of worsened asthmatic symptoms associated with a mild rise of blood eosinophils occurred in 3 patients and resolved following a transient increase of the oral prednisolone dosage. After 49 months one patient died probably due to a relapse. IFN-alpha was ceased prematurely, because of autoimmune-thyreoiditis in one, depression in another and cerebral leukoencephalopathy in two patients. Overall, 18 infectious episodes with need of antimicrobial treatment were observed.

*Conclusions.*—Recombinant interferon-alpha appears to be partially effective in the prevention of major relapses in patients with Churg-Strauss syndrome. Due to numerous side effects and infections during long-term administration its use should be restricted to patients with contraindications against conventional immunosuppressive therapies.

▶ The Churg-Strauss syndrome is classified as an antineutrophil cytoplasmic antibody-associated vasculitis, although patients with this disorder are often quite distinct from those who have Wegener granulomatosis or microscopic polyangiitis. The Churg-Strauss syndrome is characterized by the presence of adult-onset asthma and hypereosinophilia, each of which presents its own unique challenges for management. Although classically, it is said that the asthmatic component of this disease burns out with time, this is often not the case, and bronchospasm may be the most challenging aspect of this disease to treat. Although patients with this disease almost always respond to high-dose glucocorticoids, experience with other treatments has been mixed. When this group first reported their experience with interferon-α, their early results were quite encouraging. This study highlights the importance of long-term follow-up to determine the true effectiveness of any new treatment. From their experience, it seems that most patients treated with interferon-α had to stop either because of intolerance or lack of effect. Although sobering, these results push us to examine other potential alternate therapies such as mepolizumab and rituximab, both of which have been used in small groups of patients with some success.

**P. Seo, MD, MHS**

**Rituximab versus Cyclophosphamide for ANCA-Associated Vasculitis**

Stone JH, for the RAVE–ITN Research Group (Massachusetts General Hosp, Boston, MA; et al)

*N Engl J Med* 363:221-232, 2010

*Background.*—Cyclophosphamide and glucocorticoids have been the cornerstone of remission-induction therapy for severe antineutrophil cytoplasmic antibody (ANCA)–associated vasculitis for 40 years. Uncontrolled studies suggest that rituximab is effective and may be safer than a cyclophosphamide-based regimen.

*Methods.*—We conducted a multicenter, randomized, double-blind, double-dummy, noninferiority trial of rituximab (375 mg per square meter of body-surface area per week for 4 weeks) as compared with cyclophosphamide (2 mg per kilogram of body weight per day) for remission induction. Glucocorticoids were tapered off; the primary end point was remission of disease without the use of prednisone at 6 months.

*Results.*—Nine centers enrolled 197 ANCA-positive patients with either Wegener's granulomatosis or microscopic polyangiitis. Baseline disease activity, organ involvement, and the proportion of patients with relapsing disease were similar in the two treatment groups. Sixty-three patients in the rituximab group (64%) reached the primary end point, as compared with 52 patients in the control group (53%), a result that met the criterion for noninferiority ($P<0.001$). The rituximab-based regimen was more efficacious than the cyclophosphamide-based regimen for inducing remission of relapsing disease; 34 of 51 patients in the rituximab group (67%) as compared with 21 of 50 patients in the control group (42%) reached the primary end point ($P=0.01$). Rituximab was also as effective as cyclophosphamide in the treatment of patients with major renal disease or alveolar hemorrhage. There were no significant differences between the treatment groups with respect to rates of adverse events.

*Conclusions.*—Rituximab therapy was not inferior to daily cyclophosphamide treatment for induction of remission in severe ANCA-associated vasculitis and may be superior in relapsing disease. (Funded by the National Institutes of Allergy and Infectious Diseases, Genentech, and Biogen; ClinicalTrials.gov number, NCT00104299.)

► Wegener's granulomatosis and microscopic polyangiitis are the 2 major forms of the so-called antineutrophil cytoplasmic antibody (ANCA)-associated vasculitides, a family of diseases characterized by the presence of small-vessel and medium-vessel vasculitis and the presence of circulating ANCA. Without treatment, these diseases can be life threatening; unfortunately, the standard treatment regimen, which includes the use of cyclophosphamide and high-dose glucocorticoids, is also fraught; patients managed with these drugs are at increased risk of a large number of untoward effects, including infection, hemorrhagic cystitis, malignancy, and glucocorticoid-induced osteoporosis. Rituximab may represent the first significant advance in the treatment of microscopic polyangiitis and severe Wegener's granulomatosis and in this study seems to be at least as effective as standard cytotoxic therapies. This trial further demonstrated that rituximab might be even more effective for the treatment of patients with disease that has previously failed treatment with cyclophosphamide. Enthusiasm for this agent, however, must be tempered by the relatively short follow-up (ie, 6 months), which is inadequate to judge the long-term effects associated with rituximab therapy for the treatment of these diseases.

**P. Seo, MD, MHS**

---

**Rituximab versus Cyclophosphamide in ANCA-Associated Renal Vasculitis**

Jones RB, for the European Vasculitis Study Group (Addenbrooke's Hosp, Cambridge, UK; et al)

*N Engl J Med* 363:211-220, 2010

---

*Background.*—Cyclophosphamide induction regimens for antineutrophil cytoplasmic antibody (ANCA)–associated vasculitis are effective in 70 to 90% of patients, but they are associated with high rates of death and adverse events. Treatment with rituximab has led to remission rates of 80 to 90% among patients with refractory ANCA-associated vasculitis and may be safer than cyclophosphamide regimens.

*Methods.*—We compared rituximab with cyclophosphamide as induction therapy in ANCA-associated vasculitis. We randomly assigned, in a 3:1 ratio, 44 patients with newly diagnosed ANCA-associated vasculitis and renal involvement to a standard glucocorticoid regimen plus either rituximab at a dose of 375 mg per square meter of body-surface area per week for 4 weeks, with two intravenous cyclophosphamide pulses (33 patients, the rituximab group), or intravenous cyclophosphamide for 3 to 6 months followed by azathioprine (11 patients, the control group). Primary end points were sustained remission rates at 12 months and severe adverse events.

*Results.*—The median age was 68 years, and the glomerular filtration rate (GFR) was 18 ml per minute per 1.73 $m^2$ of body-surface area. A total of 25 patients in the rituximab group (76%) and 9 patients in the control group (82%) had a sustained remission (P=0.68). Severe adverse events occurred in 14 patients in the rituximab group (42%) and 4 patients in the control group (36%) (P=0.77). Six of the 33 patients in the rituximab group (18%) and 2 of the 11 patients in the control group (18%) died (P=1.00). The median increase in the GFR between 0 and 12 months was 19 ml per minute in the rituximab group and 15 ml per minute in the control group (P=0.14).

*Conclusions.*—A rituximab-based regimen was not superior to standard intravenous cyclophosphamide for severe ANCA-associated vasculitis. Sustained-remission rates were high in both groups, and the rituximab-based regimen was not associated with reductions in early severe adverse events. (Funded by Cambridge University Hospitals National Health

Service Foundation Trust and F. Hoffmann–La Roche; Current Controlled Trials number, ISRCTN28528813.)

▶ Like the preceding article, this study also examined the use of rituximab for the treatment of patients with antineutrophil cytoplasmic antibody (ANCA)-associated vasculitis. It is important to note, however, the significant differences in study design. First, this study only included patients with glomerulonephritis due to Wegener granulomatosis, microscopic polyangiitis, or renal-limited vasculitis. Second, patients randomized to receive treatment with rituximab also received treatment with cyclophosphamide during the first month of therapy. Finally, this trial only included 44 patients, as compared with the 197 patients enrolled in the Rituximab in ANCA-Associated Vasculitis (RAVE) trial. Given the high mortality observed among patients with renal failure due to ANCA-associated glomerulonephritis, the high number of deaths observed in both arms is not completely unexpected and may have more to do with the specific population studied rather than the toxicities of the specific therapies. This trial and the RAVE trial are unable to answer questions regarding long-term outcomes among patients with ANCA-associated vasculitis treated with rituximab. In particular, concern has been raised regarding the association between rituximab and progressive focal leukoencephalopathy, an opportunistic infection caused by the JC virus that can be fatal. Although this seems to occur only rarely among patients with rheumatic disease who are treated with rituximab, this, and questions regarding the long-term risk of relapse among patients with rituximab, will have to be answered in later years.

**P. Seo, MD, MHS**

---

**Treatment of Polyarteritis Nodosa and Microscopic Polyangiitis Without Poor-Prognosis Factors: A Prospective Randomized Study of One Hundred Twenty-Four Patients**

Ribi C, for the French Vasculitis Study Group (Hôpital Cantonal Universitaire, Geneva, Switzerland; et al)

*Arthritis Rheum* 62:1186-1197, 2010

---

*Objective.*—To assess the efficacy of systemic corticosteroids alone as first-line treatment of polyarteritis nodosa (PAN) and microscopic polyangiitis (MPA) without poor-prognosis factors as defined by the Five-Factors Score (FFS), and to compare the efficacy and safety of azathioprine versus pulse cyclophosphamide as adjunctive immunosuppressive therapy for patients experiencing treatment failure or relapse.

*Methods.*—This prospective, multicenter, therapeutic trial included 124 patients with newly diagnosed PAN or MPA (FFS of 0) treated with corticosteroids alone. At the time of treatment failure or disease relapse, patients were randomized to receive 6 months of therapy with oral azathioprine or 6 pulses of cyclophosphamide. Analyses was performed according to an intent-to-treat strategy.

*Results.*—The mean ± SD followup period was 62 ± 33 months. Treatment with corticosteroids alone induced remission in 98 patients; 50 (40%) of these patients had sustained disease remission, 46 (37%) experienced a relapse, and 2 became corticosteroid dependent (daily prednisone dose ≥20 mg). In 26 patients (21%), treatment with corticosteroids alone failed, and 49 patients (40%) required additional immunosuppression. Among the 39 patients randomized, 13 of 19 achieved remission with cyclophosphamide pulses, and 14 of 20 achieved remission with azathioprine. Among all patients, the 1-year and 5-year survival rates were 99% and 92%, respectively. Six deaths occurred in the cyclophosphamide-treated group compared with 2 deaths in the azathioprine-treated group. Disease-free survival was significantly lower for patients with MPA than for those with PAN ($P = 0.046$).

*Conclusion.*—For patients with PAN or MPA with an FFS of 0, overall 5-year survival was good, but first-line corticosteroid treatment was able to achieve and maintain remission in only about half of the patients, and 40% of the patients required additional immunosuppressive therapy. Azathioprine or pulse cyclophosphamide was fairly effective for treating corticosteroid-resistant disease or major relapses.

► Although polyarteritis nodosa is the first well-described form of primary systemic vasculitis, it has become progressively rare, making studies such as this, which take advantage of a large catchment area, even more important than they might have been a generation ago. The Five-Factor Score is a prognostic index developed by the French Vasculitis Study Group. Using the Five-Factor Score, this study essentially indicates that patients with microscopic polyangiitis or polyarteritis nodosa who are aged 65 years or younger and lack gastrointestinal, cardiac, or renal dysfunction can be safely treated with glucocorticoids alone. Unfortunately, as with other forms of primary systemic vasculitis, relapse in the absence of steroid-sparing agents is quite common. It is interesting to note that patients who had glucocorticoid-resistant disease responded well to treatment with azathioprine since this is not a standard remission induction drug for microscopic polyangiitis in the United States. This study also demonstrates that relapse is not uncommon among patients with microscopic polyangiitis, and these patients should continue to be followed carefully, even after remission has been achieved.

**P. Seo, MD, MHS**

# 6 Sjögren's Syndrome

**Effectiveness of Rituximab Treatment in Primary Sjögren's Syndrome: A Randomized, Double-Blind, Placebo-Controlled Trial**

Meijer JM, Meiners PM, Vissink A, et al (Univ of Groningen, The Netherlands)

*Arthritis Rheum* 62:960-968, 2010

*Objective.*—To study the efficacy and safety of B cell depletion with rituximab, a chimeric murine/human anti-CD20 monoclonal antibody, in patients with primary Sjögren's syndrome (SS) in a double-blind, randomized, placebo-controlled trial.

*Methods.*—Patients with active primary SS, as determined by the revised American–European Consensus Group criteria, and a rate of stimulated whole saliva secretion of ≥0.15 ml/minute were treated with either rituximab (1,000 mg) or placebo infusions on days 1 and 15. Patients were assigned randomly to a treatment group in a ratio of 2:1 (rituximab: placebo). Followup was conducted at 5, 12, 24, 36, and 48 weeks. The primary end point was the stimulated whole saliva flow rate, while secondary end points included functional, laboratory, and subjective variables.

*Results.*—Thirty patients with primary SS (29 female) were randomly allocated to a treatment group. The mean ± SD age of the patients receiving rituximab was 43 ± 11 years and the disease duration was 63 ± 50 months, while patients in the placebo group were age 43 ± 17 years and had a disease duration of 67 ± 63 months. In the rituximab group, significant improvements, in terms of the mean change from baseline compared with that in the placebo group, were found for the primary end point of the stimulated whole saliva flow rate ($P = 0.038$ versus placebo) and also for various laboratory parameters (B cell and rheumatoid factor [RF] levels), subjective parameters (Multidimensional Fatigue Inventory [MFI] scores and visual analog scale [VAS] scores for sicca symptoms), and extraglandular manifestations. Moreover, in comparison with baseline values, rituximab treatment significantly improved the stimulated whole saliva flow rate ($P = 0.004$) and several other variables (e.g., B cell and RF levels, unstimulated whole saliva flow rate, lacrimal gland function on the lissamine green test, MFI scores, Short Form 36 health survey scores, and VAS scores for sicca symptoms). One patient in the rituximab group developed mild serum sickness–like disease.

*Conclusion.*—These results indicate that rituximab is an effective and safe treatment strategy for patients with primary SS.

▶ Meijer and colleagues at the University of Groningen conducted a single-center, randomized, double-blind trial of rituximab for the treatment of primary Sjögren's syndrome (SS). The study included 48 weeks of follow-up. Improvement in all major manifestations of the disease was demonstrated, including oral dryness, ocular dryness, fatigue, and extraglandular manifestations. Improvement in the primary end point, a significant increase in stimulated salivary flow, was achieved within 5 weeks. Unstimulated salivary flow, a secondary end point, was also significantly increased. However, only 1 of 3 secondary end points related to lacrimal function (reduction in corneal staining using lissamine green) was achieved. One patient receiving rituximab experienced a serum sickness-like reaction. Approximately one-half of subjects who received rituximab developed an infection; none resulted in hospitalization.

Despite significant successes in the targeted biological therapy of autoimmune rheumatic disease, demonstration of benefit for the glandular manifestations of SS has, to date, been elusive. Tumor necrosis factor alpha inhibitors have, in particular, been disappointing for the treatment of primary SS. Following reports of initial benefit for glandular and systemic features of SS in uncontrolled pilot trials, a randomized, multicenter, double-blind controlled trial of infliximab failed to demonstrate significant improvement.[1] B cell depletion using rituximab has previously shown promise in SS in case reports and small series. Despite having a relatively small scope (30 patients studied, 20 randomized to rituximab), the study by Meijer et al is quite important in that it is a well-conducted, double-blind, controlled trial that demonstrates improvement in the glandular manifestations of SS as well as in extraglandular manifestations and laboratory parameters. Although exocrine glandular infiltrates in SS generally exhibit T-cell predominance, the robust polyclonal autoantibody response and the enhanced risk for B cell non-Hodgkin's lymphoma suggest a significant role for B cells in the pathogenesis of this disease. The report of Meijer et al not only further supports a role for B cells in the pathogenesis of hyposalivation in SS but also takes a further step toward the establishment of B cell depletion therapy as an important option for its management. Patients in this study tended to be somewhat younger (43 years) than the average SS patient, had a relatively brief disease duration (~5 years), and were all seropositive for Anti-Ro/SSA (compared with the ~70% usually reported). Multicenter trials involving larger patient numbers will help determine the future scope of B cell depletion therapy for SS.

**S. E. Carsons, MD**

*Reference*

1. Mariette X, Ravaud P, Steinfeld S, et al. Inefficacy of infliximab in primary Sjögren's syndrome: results of the randomized, controlled Trial of Remicade in Primary Sjögren's Syndrome (TRIPSS). *Arthritis Rheum.* 2004;50:1270-1276.

### Treatment of Primary Sjögren Syndrome: A Systematic Review

Ramos-Casals M, Tzioufas AG, Stone JH, et al (Hosp Clínic, Barcelona, Spain; Univ of Athens, Greece; Massachusetts General Hosp, Boston; et al)
*JAMA* 304:452-460, 2010

*Context.*—A variety of topical and systemic drugs are available to treat primary Sjögren syndrome, although no evidence-based therapeutic guidelines are currently available.

*Objective.*—To summarize evidence on primary Sjögren syndrome drug therapy from randomized controlled trials.

*Data Sources.*—We searched MEDLINE and EMBASE for articles on drug therapy for primary Sjögren syndrome published between January 1, 1986, and April 30, 2010.

*Study Selection.*—Controlled trials of topical and systemic drugs including adult patients with primary Sjögren syndrome were selected as the primary information source.

*Results.*—The search strategy yielded 37 trials. A placebo-controlled trial found significant improvement in the Schirmer and corneal staining scores, blurred vision, and artificial tear use in patients treated with topical ocular 0.05% cyclosporine. Three placebo-controlled trials found that pilocarpine was associated with improvements in dry mouth (61%-70% vs 24%-31% in the placebo group) and dry eye (42%-53% vs 26%). Two placebo-controlled trials found that cevimeline was associated with improvement in dry mouth (66%-76% vs 35%-37% in the placebo group) and dry eye (39%-72% vs 24%-30%). Small trials (<20 patients) found no significant improvement in sicca outcomes for oral prednisone or hydroxychloroquine and limited benefits for immunosuppressive agents (azathioprine and cyclosporine). A large trial found limited benefits for oral interferon alfa-2a. Two placebo-controlled trials of infliximab and etanercept did not achieve the primary outcome (a composite visual analog scale measuring joint pain, fatigue, and dryness); neither did 2 small trials (<30 patients) testing rituximab, although significant results were observed in some secondary outcomes and improvement compared with baseline.

*Conclusions.*—In primary Sjögren syndrome, evidence from controlled trials suggests benefits for pilocarpine and cevimeline for sicca features and topical cyclosporine for moderate or severe dry eye. Anti–tumor necrosis factor agents have not shown clinical efficacy, and larger controlled trials are needed to establish the efficacy of rituximab.

▶ No treatment modifies the evolution of primary Sjögren's syndrome (SS). In the last 3 decades, therapeutic approaches in primary SS have been based on the use of substitute agents for sicca features and glucocorticoids and immunosuppressive agents for systemic involvement. Unhappily, one of the main problems in reviewing therapies and offering solid therapeutic recommendations in primary SS is the limited level of reported evidence, together with the lack of consensual end points for evaluating outcomes. This article is the first to systematically review the scientific evidence available on drug therapy in primary SS and shows that the body of evidence for most drugs relies predominantly on uncontrolled studies and small randomized controlled trials (generally including no more than 20 to 30 patients in each arm), with fewer than 10% of these studies being designed to compare different drugs in the same clinical scenario. In summary, evidence from controlled trials suggests benefits for pilocarpine and cevimeline for sicca features, topical cyclosporine for moderate or severe dry eye, and no benefit for antitumor necrosis factor therapies such as infliximab and etanercept. Although 2 small trials testing rituximab did not achieve the primary outcomes, significant results were observed in some secondary outcomes and there was improvement compared with baseline. It seems reasonable to suppose that, in the future, B cell-targeted therapies may play a role in modifying the etiopathogenesis of primary SS, a disease characterized by B cell hyperactivity.

Advances in our knowledge of the molecular mechanisms involved in the etiopathogenesis of primary SS should allow the development of new, more effective, highly selective therapies without the adverse effects often associated with standard less selective drugs. However, there are no current evidence-based therapeutic guidelines for the management of primary SS, and there is even less scientific evidence available for patients who do not respond to first-line therapies. In this context, it is not surprising that therapeutic decision making continues to be based on clinical experience and expert opinion.

**M. Ramos-Casals, MD, PhD**

---

**EULAR Sjögren's syndrome disease activity index: development of a consensus systemic disease activity index for primary Sjögren's syndrome**

Seror R, on behalf of the EULAR Sjögren's Task Force (Hôpital Bichat, Paris, France; et al)

*Ann Rheum Dis* 69:1103-1109, 2010

---

*Objective.*—To develop a disease activity index for patients with primary Sjögren's syndrome (SS): the European League Against Rheumatism (EULAR) Sjögren's syndrome disease activity index (ESSDAI).

*Methods.*—Thirty-nine SS experts participated in an international collaboration, promoted by EULAR, to develop the ESSDAI. Experts identified 12 organ-specific 'domains' contributing to disease activity. For each domain, features of disease activity were classified in three or four levels according to their severity. Data abstracted from 96 patients with systemic complications of primary SS were used to generate 702 realistic vignettes for which all possible systemic complications were represented. Using the 0–10 physician global assessment (PhGA) scale, each expert scored the disease activity of five patient profiles and 20 realistic vignettes. Multiple regression modelling, with PhGA used as the dependent variable, was used to estimate the weight of each domain.

*Results.*—All 12 domains were significantly associated with disease activity in the multivariate model, domain weights ranged from 1 to 6. The ESSDAI scores varied from 2 to 47 and were significantly correlated with PhGA for both real patient profiles and realistic vignettes ($r=0.61$ and $r=0.58$, respectively, $p<0.001$). Compared with 57 (59.4%) of the real patient profiles, 468 (66.7%) of the realistic vignettes were considered likely or very likely to be true.

*Conclusion.*—The ESSDAI is a clinical index designed to measure disease activity in patients with primary SS. Once validated, such a standardised evaluation of primary SS should facilitate clinical research and be helpful as an outcome measure in clinical trials.

▶ The development of a standardized measurement of disease activity and outcomes should be considered essential for the design of controlled clinical trials in primary Sjögren's syndrome (SS), as occurs in other autoimmune diseases, such as rheumatoid arthritis and systemic lupus erythematosus. Unfortunately, the development of specific indexes for primary SS has begun recently by groups from Italy and the United Kingdom, resulting in 2 proposed disease activity indexes: the SS Disease Activity Index (SSDAI) and the Sjögren's Systemic Clinical Activity Index (SCAI). However, both these indexes have been developed and applied in only 1 country and are not accepted internationally yet.

The European collaborative project presented in this article by Seror et al aims to develop a consensual index. In this project, the EULAR (European League Against Rheumatism) has promoted and supported an international collaborative study with the aim of developing and validating an international consensus index for evaluating disease activity in primary SS. The steering committee of the project, with the approval of nearly 100 experts included in the EULAR SS Task Force, proposed the design of 2 indexes: (1) the EULAR Sjögren's Syndrome Patient Reported Index (ESSPRI), which consists of a patient-administered questionnaire to assess patient symptoms and (2) the EULAR Sjögren's Syndrome Disease Activity Index (ESSDAI), which evaluates systemic SS involvement. For the ESSDAI, 39 international SS experts identified 12 types of organ involvement (domains), which contribute to disease activity. For each domain, features of disease activity were classified in 3 or 4 levels (items) according to severity. Seror et al found that all 12 proposed domains were significantly associated with disease activity and that the global ESSDAI score correlated well with disease activity. Analyses of sensitivity to change revealed no significant differences with respect to the SCAI and SSDAI, although the ESSDAI was the most robust in detecting changes in disease activity, especially in stable patients. In summary, the ESSDAI is an international consensual scoring system that may detect changes in disease activity accurately, offering a standard tool for evaluating systemic involvement in primary SS. This new index will play a key role in the development of future epidemiological and therapeutic controlled studies in primary SS, leading to more accurate evaluation of disease activity in both large cohorts and individual patients.

**M. Ramos-Casals, MD, PhD**

## Articular manifestations in primary Sjögren's syndrome: clinical significance and prognosis of 188 patients

Fauchais AL, Ouattara B, Gondran G, et al (Limoges Univ Hosp, France; et al)
*Rheumatology (Oxford)* 49:1164-1172, 2010

*Objectives.*—Articular manifestations (AMs) occurred in ~30-60% of patients with primary SS (pSS). We conducted the current study to describe clinical presentation, specific treatment and to report clinical outcome of pSS patients with AM in a large bicentric French cohort.

*Methods.*—Clinical, biological and immunological features of 419 consecutive patients with pSS were recorded in order to describe the clinical and immunological course of pSS AM and to point out the impact of those rheumatological features on pSS evolution.

*Results.*—A total of 188 patients with pSS (172 women, 16 men) exhibited AM. They preceded sicca symptoms in 32, were simultaneous to pSS diagnosis in 98 and followed diagnosis in 59 patients. Clinical presentation was polyarticular and concerned mostly peripheral joints (synovitis, $n = 66$). Symptoms responded readily to symptomatic treatment in 45 cases (24%). DMARDs or immunosuppressive treatments were introduced in 133 patients: HCQ ($n = 111$), corticosteroid ($n = 53$), MTX ($n = 12$), SSZ ($n = 6$), AZA ($n = 3$), LEF (n = 1), etanercept ($n = 1$) and allochrysine ($n = 1$). Only one case of RA was diagnosed during the evolution. Statistical analysis identified clinical and biological factors associated with AM ($P \leq 0.05$): RP, muscular manifestations, renal involvement, peripheral neuropathy, cutaneous vasculitis, and positivity of RF, anti-SSB antibodies and cryoglobulinaemia. Patients with AM at diagnosis were characterized by a multisystemic involvement at the end of the follow-up period ($P < 0.001$).

*Conclusion.*—Although AMs are frequent and usually mild in pSS, these manifestations are associated with a pluri-systemic involvement of pSS.

► In patients with primary Sjögren's syndrome (SS), joint involvement is the most frequent extraglandular manifestation. Generalized arthralgias are reported in 25% to 75% of patients. Less frequently, joint disease presents as an intermittent symmetric arthritis primarily affecting small joints. Joint deformity and mild erosions are rare, except for some cases that may evolve to an associated rheumatoid arthritis (RA), while asymmetrical swollen joint suggests a non-autoimmune origin, such as crystalline or infectious arthropathy. However, no study has specifically analyzed and characterized articular involvement in large series of patients with primary SS.

The study by Fauchais et al is the first to evaluate articular involvement in a cohort of 419 patients fulfilling the 2002 criteria. Articular involvement was defined as arthralgia and/or nonerosive arthritis characterized by tenderness, swelling, or effusion involving one or more peripheral joints. Of the 419 patients, 188 (45%) had articular involvement. Arthralgia was polyarticular in 88% of cases and oligoarticular in the remaining 12%, while 35% of patients had symmetrical synovitis. Only 4% of patients presented with monoarthritis. The radiographic features showed erosive disease in only 3 patients who tested positive for anticyclic citrullinated peptide antibodies. In 29% of cases, symptoms were mild and responded rapidly to short therapy with nonsteroidal anti-inflammatory drugs (NSAIDs); corticosteroids were added in 25% of cases; only 3 cases were classified as having a corticodependent arthritis. Hydroxychloroquine was used in nearly 60% of cases and methotrexate in only 6%. Multivariate analysis identified Raynaud phenomenon, vasculitis, neuropathy, renal involvement, and cryoglobulins as variables associated with articular involvement.

In summary, articular involvement was found in nearly half the patients with primary SS, with synovitis being found in 30% of cases, a higher percentage than that found in other large series. The arthritis of primary SS is characterized by short-lived episodes of joint inflammation that remit spontaneously, usually within days or after a short course of NSAIDs. This clinical course is milder than in other systemic autoimmune diseases such as systemic lupus erythematosus and especially RA, in which arthritis is rapidly progressive, erosive, and often can lead to hand deformities. In primary SS, only 25% of patients with articular involvement require pharmacological treatment.

**M. Ramos-Casals, MD, PhD**

---

**Assessment of patients with primary Sjögren's syndrome—outcome over 10 years using the Sjögren's Syndrome Damage Index**

Krylova L, Isenberg D (Univ College London Hosp, UK)

*Rheumatology (Oxford)* 49:1559-1562, 2010

---

*Objective.*—To evaluate the long-term outcome in a cohort of patients with primary SS (PSS) using the recently proposed Sjogren's Syndrome Damage Index.

*Methods.*—We reviewed the clinical records of 60 patients attending our Sjögren's clinic at University College London Hospital, who strictly fulfilled the American-European Consensus Group criteria and on whom we had a minimum of 10 years of follow-up (or until death) during this decade. However, we could not retrospectively identify damage in the oral domain as this had not been recorded reliably.

*Results.*—Fifty-five per cent of patients in this study had no damage after 10 years of disease—a lower figure than our comparative group of patients with SLE (32.4%). Damage accrual was mostly in the ocular domain, parotid swelling and malignancy categories. There was a 6-fold increase in the 'malignancy damage' compared with the 2-fold increase in the total damage score in PSS.

*Conclusions.*—Unlike patients with SLE, it is clear that fewer patients with SS develop permanent damage, even after 10 years of follow-up. These data are thus encouraging but clearly larger numbers of patients need to be assessed.

▶ The few studies that have prospectively analyzed outcomes in patients with primary Sjögren's syndrome (SS) show that the disease usually progresses very slowly, with no rapid deterioration in salivary function or dramatic changes in sicca symptoms. The main exceptions to this benign course are the development of extraglandular manifestations and the high incidence of lymphoma. With respect to extraglandular involvement, patients with SS may be divided into 2 groups with a different prognosis. A more stable, chronic SS course is usually found in patients with predominantly periepithelial lesions (such as interstitial nephritis and liver or lung disease), while those with predominantly extraepithelial expression (glomerulonephritis, polyneuropathy, and vasculitis) present higher morbidity and mortality. Cryoglobulinemia probably plays a central etiopathogenic role in this latter group of patients, contributing to the development of the main extraepithelial manifestations.

The study by Krylova and Isenberg is the first to assess cumulative permanent damage in various organs and systems in patients with primary SS, using the Sjögren's Syndrome Damage Index (SSDI) developed by the British Sjögren's Group, in which damage items are grouped in 3 domains (ocular, oral, and systemic domains). The SSDI is based on a similar index for systemic lupus erythematosus (SLE) (Systemic Lupus International Collaborating Clinics/ American College of Rheumatology Disease Damage Index). The systemic domain is subclassified into 7 subdomains (neurological, renal, pulmonary, cardiovascular, gastrointestinal, musculoskeletal, endocrine, and malignancy). There are 27 items in total, with a maximum score of 1 for each item if present. Krylova and Isenberg included 60 patients with a minimum of 10 years of follow-up who were retrospectively assessed. At the end of the follow-up, less than half the patients had developed damage, and no patient accrued a damage score >3 during the entire period of follow-up. The main items contributing to cumulative damage were the ocular domain, parotid swelling, and malignancy, and the percentage of patients with damage increased from 28% in the first year to 37% after 5 years and 45% at 10 years.

This study confirms the completely different evolution of primary SS in terms of cumulative internal organ damage with respect to other autoimmune diseases such as SLE, systemic vasculitis, or rheumatoid arthritis. Damage levels are clearly lower than those observed in patients with SLE, who are much younger and at higher risk of developing chronic damage to vital organs, such as the kidneys or the central nervous system.

**M. Ramos-Casals, MD, PhD**

**Functional impairment of the arterial wall in primary Sjögren's syndrome: combined action of immunologic and inflammatory factors**

Gerli R, Vaudo G, Bocci EB, et al (Univ of Perugia, Italy)

*Arthritis Care Res (Hoboken)* 62:712-718, 2010

*Objective.*—Primary Sjögren's syndrome (SS) shares clinical and serologic features with rheumatoid arthritis and systemic lupus erythematosus, 2 diseases characterized by acceleration of atherosclerosis. Signs of precocious atherosclerosis have also been shown in SS, although the pathogenic basis of early arterial damage is unclear. The arterial wall was functionally evaluated in SS subjects with analysis of the role played by disease-related factors.

*Methods.*—Endothelium-dependent flow-mediated vasodilation (FMV) and endothelium-independent nitrate-mediated vasodilation (NMV) were evaluated in 45 women with SS and 59 age-matched female controls. In addition, serum soluble intercellular adhesion molecule 1, soluble vascular cell adhesion molecule 1 (VCAM-1), and nitrotyrosine were detected.

*Results.*—Although patient FMV values did not differ from those of control subjects (mean ± SD 7.4 ± 3.6 versus 7.7 ± 1.9; not significant), NMV was lower in SS patients than in controls (mean ± SD 8.1 ± 3.5 versus 10.3 ± 2.1; $P \leq 0.001$). Patient NMV was inversely correlated with soluble VCAM-1 levels ($r = -0.38$, $P = 0.001$) and directly correlated with leukocyte count ($r = 0.26$, $P = 0.03$). An NMV decrease was confirmed in SS patient subsets with evidence of leukopenia, rheumatoid factor, anti-SSB antibodies, and joint involvement. However, patients with joint involvement or parotid enlargement, 2 of the sites mainly affected by chronic inflammation in SS, had an FMV lower than controls and patients without these clinical features.

*Conclusion.*—Our results suggest that a functional impairment of the arterial wall may sustain early phases of atherosclerotic damage in SS. A combined effect of disease-related chronic inflammatory and immunologic factors appears to support dysfunction of endothelium and vascular smooth muscle cells, respectively.

▶ Cardiovascular events have emerged as major causes of morbidity and mortality in patients with autoimmune diseases, such as systemic lupus erythematosus and rheumatoid arthritis, and are associated with both traditional cardiovascular risk factors and autoimmune diseases themselves. However, the clinical significance of cardiovascular disease in patients with primary Sjögren's syndrome (SS) is little studied, even though SS predominantly affects a specific epidemiological subset (postmenopausal women), which has a higher risk of cardiovascular complications. In late 2005, two small case-control studies suggested that primary SS may be associated with a higher frequency of cardiovascular and metabolic abnormalities, while, more recently, a large series found a 2-fold higher prevalence of diabetes mellitus and a 1.5-fold higher prevalence of hypertriglyceridemia in patients with primary SS in comparison with primary care patients without autoimmune diseases, with corticosteroid use being closely associated with cardiovascular risk factors. These results suggest that cardiovascular risk factors should be taken into account in the management of patients with primary SS and show the importance of recognizing and controlling both traditional and SS-related modifiable risk factors.

Gerli et al evaluated functional impairment of the arterial wall by studying endothelium-dependent flow-mediated vasodilation (FMV) and endothelium-independent nitrate-mediated vasodilation (NMV) in 45 women with SS and 59 age-matched healthy controls. Although FMV values did not differ between patients and controls, NMV values were significantly lower in SS patients, especially those with articular involvement, leukopenia, and positive immunological markers (rheumatoid factor and anti-La/SSB antibodies). The authors suggest the existence of pathophysiologic mechanisms involving the smooth muscle cells of large arterial vessels in patients with primary SS. However, the epidemiological profile of the studied cohort is far from that considered standard for primary SS (median age 42 years, only 20% postmenopausal) and may be considered as a cohort of patients with early disease. The link between functional impairment of the arterial wall and cardiovascular disease (subclinical atheromatosis and cardiovascular events) should be demonstrated in prospective studies, including patients with primary SS with a more standard epidemiological profile.

**M. Ramos-Casals, MD, PhD**

# 7 Miscellaneous

---

**Combined chiropractic interventions for low-back pain**

Walker BF, French SD, Grant W, et al (Murdoch Univ, Australia)

*Cochrane Database Syst Rev* 4:CD005427, 2010

---

*Background.*—Chiropractors commonly use a combination of interventions to treat people with low back pain (LBP).

*Objectives.*—To determine the effects of combined chiropractic interventions (that is, a combination of therapies, other than spinal manipulation alone) on pain, disability, back-related function, overall improvement, and patient satisfaction in adults with LBP, aged 18 and older.

*Search Strategy.*—We searched: The Cochrane Back Review Group Trials Register (May 2009), CENTRAL (The Cochrane Library 2009, Issue 2), and MEDLINE (from January 1966), EMBASE (from January 1980), CINAHL (from January 1982), MANTIS (from Inception) and the Index to Chiropractic Literature (from Inception) to May 2009. We also screened references of identified articles and contacted chiropractic researchers.

*Selection Criteria.*—All randomised trials comparing the use of combined chiropractic interventions (rather than spinal manipulation alone) with no treatment or other therapies.

*Data Collection and Analysis.*—At least two review authors selected studies, assessed the risk of bias, and extracted the data using standardised forms. Both descriptive synthesis and meta-analyses were performed.

*Main Results.*—We included 12 studies involving 2887 participants with LBP. Three studies had low risk of bias. Included studies evaluated a range of chiropractic procedures in a variety of sub-populations of people with LBP. No trials were located of combined chiropractic interventions compared to no treatment. For acute and subacute LBP, chiropractic interventions improved short- and medium-term pain (SMD −0.25 (95% CI −0.46 to −0.04) and MD −0.89 (95%CI −1.60 to −0.18)) compared to other treatments, but there was no significant difference in long-term pain (MD −0.46 (95% CI −1.18 to 0.26)). Short-term improvement in disability was greater in the chiropractic group compared to other therapies (SMD −0.36 (95% CI −0.70 to −0.02)). However, the effect was small and all studies contributing to these results had high risk of bias. There was no difference in medium- and long-term disability. No difference was demonstrated for combined chiropractic interventions for chronic LBP and for studies that had a mixed population of LBP.

*Authors' Conclusions.*—Combined chiropractic interventions slightly improved pain and disability in the short-term and pain in the medium-term for acute and subacute LBP. However, there is currently no evidence that supports or refutes that these interventions provide a clinically meaningful difference for pain or disability in people with LBP when compared to other interventions. Future research is very likely to change the estimate of effect and our confidence in the results.

▶ Establishing the evidence for or against chiropractic treatments can be a tricky business. The hallmark treatment of chiropractors is spinal manipulation. If the evaluation of spinal manipulation fails to show what chiropractors had hoped for, the argument usually is that chiropractors combine a wide range of modalities, for example, manipulation, mobilization, massage, exercise, heat, etc. Thus, it might not be fair to judge the value of chiropractic treatments solely by the effectiveness of spinal manipulation.

This Cochrane Review is an attempt to overcome this pitfall. Its results show that, even for the most prevalent indication for chiropractic treatments, that is, low back pain (LBP), very few studies are available. Those that do exist are often seriously flawed. For acute and subacute LBP, chiropractic treatments seem to be marginally better than conventional treatments. I recommend, however, taking these results with a pinch of salt and believe that we require independent replication through high-quality studies, which also account for the risks and costs associated with chiropractic treatments. For chronic LBP, chiropractic treatments do not seem to be better than conventional treatments.

All in all, this review serves as a poignant reminder that chiropractic treatments are not as soundly based on evidence, as it often is made out to be.

**E. Ernst, MD, PhD**

**PART TWO**

# INFECTIOUS DISEASES

NANCY M. KHARDORI, MD

# Introduction

My introduction to the Infectious Diseases section of the 2008 YEAR BOOK OF MEDICINE ended with a quote from Hans Zinsser: "Infectious disease is one of the great tragedies of living things—the struggle for existence between different forms of life... Incessantly the pitiless war goes on, without quarter or armistice—a nationalism of species against species." This year, this quote's validity even today is exemplified by one of the selections for the 2010 YEAR BOOK. The study concludes that infections continue to make a major (20%) contribution to deaths in children in England and Wales. These geographic areas are among the developed parts of the world. The significance of this selection is in the fact that the data are not from areas of the world where infectious diseases are known to be major contributors to overall morbidity and mortality. Of the bacterial causes of death, 46% were caused by meningococci and pneumococci, both vaccine-preventable infections. Another selection gives an insight into the variables involved in host-pathogen interactions and the role of genetic susceptibility to major infectious diseases. A selection on influenza contains an extensive discussion of clinical aspects of 2009 pandemic influenza caused by influenza A ($H_1N_1$) virus of swine origin. Emergence of resistance to oseltamivir and also a new neuraminidase inhibitor, peramivir, is concerning. As noted in another selection on pandemic influenza, inhaled zanamivir is still effective and intravenous zanamivir is now available for critically ill patients, especially those on mechanical ventilation. Tuberculosis remains a challenge worldwide. The diagnosis of *Tuberculous meningitis* especially is often delayed, causing further increases in mortality. The first selection on tuberculosis this year helps improve the yield of early diagnostic tests for *Tuberculous meningitis,* and the second gives a rationale for less than optimal efficacy of BCG vaccine.

Natural and acquired resistance of bacteria to the currently available antibiotics is the single most significant contributor to infection-related mortality in critically ill patients. The selections include clinically relevant studies on the role, clinical factors, and emerging resistance relating to common pathogens, including *Staphylococcus aureus*. The role of disseminated Herpes simplex virus infections in immunocompromised patients, in this instance a patient with severe burn injury, is highlighted. The other selection raises the issues of acyclovir resistance in Herpes simplex virus infection, even in patients who have not received acyclovir previously. I have included a study on antifungal susceptibility of Candida isolates and the significance of bacterial coinfections in patients with paranasal sinus fungus balls in the chapter on fungal infections. Two other clinically relevant articles in this chapter deal with the role of invasive fungal infections among organ transplant recipients and in culture negative early prosthetic valve endocarditis. There are 6 selections on *Clostridium difficile,* 3 on clinical issues including predictors of death, 1 on the in vitro efficacy of rifaximin, a new agent approved for treatment of Traveler's Diarrhea,

1 on the most exciting data on treatment with monoclonal antibodies against C. *difficile* toxins, and the last deals with.the airborne dispersal of *C difficile* for patients with *Clostridium difficile* infection (CDI). This year *C difficile* has taken over as the No. 1 cause of nosocomial infection in the United States. These selected papers on *C difficile* should be helpful to the readers in understanding clinical management as well as prevention aspects of CDI. The selection on pathogenesis of infectious diseases covers a number of areas, including infectious complications of COPD, associations of recurrent furunculosis with PVL leukocidin of *S aureus*, toxin-targeting in the management of PVL leukocidin producing *S aureus*, genetic marker of *Candida albicans* that confer resistance to neutrophil killing, synergistic activity of human phagocytes, and antifungal agents against *C albicans* biofilms, *S aureus* biofilm eradication in infection control, and the role of complement activation in patients with severe sepsis. The 4 miscellaneous selections discuss the utility of blood cultures in patients with febrile urinary tract infection, the probability of elevation in creatinine phosphokinase during daptomycin therapy, and current management of pyogenic liver abscess. The last chapter on vaccines covers vaccine dose sparing by alternate routes of administration, asymptomatic polio virus infection among vaccinated children, need for improved immunity strategies to protect young infants against pertussis, and new vaccines against Japanese encephalitis and *Neisseria meningitides*. The selection on human papilloma virus (HPV) implicates infections in cancer biology. The study showed significantly better survival of patients with oropharyngeal cancer if the tumors are positive for HPV. The majority of the HPV types implicated in this cancer (type16 and 18) are present in the 2 vaccines already available for prevention of cervical cancer. This gives me an optimistic note to end this discussion. After all, an ounce of prevention is worth tons of cure.

**Nancy M. Khardori, MD**

# 8 Bacterial Infections

**Continuing Impact of Infectious Diseases on Childhood Deaths in England and Wales, 2003–2005**

Ladhani S, Pebody RG, Ramsay ME, et al (Health Protection Agency, London, UK; et al)

*Pediatr Infect Dis J* 29:310-313, 2010

*Background.*—Data on the contribution of specific infections to childhood deaths in developed countries are limited.

*Methods.*—Infection-related deaths in children aged 28 days to 14 years who died in England and Wales between 2003 and 2005 were identified from routine anonymized death certificate dataset provided by the Office for National Statistics to the Health Protection Agency, using predefined International Classification of Diseases codes for infection.

*Results.*—There were 1368 infection-related deaths documented, constituting 20% of all childhood deaths. An underlying medical condition was recorded in 50% (676 cases), the most common being prematurity in infants (322/660, 52%), cerebral palsy in 1 to 4 year olds (46/190, 24%), and malignancy (46/163, 28%) in 5 to 14 year olds. Of the 837 deaths where a pathogen was coded, 494 (59%) specified bacterial infection, 256 (31%) viral infection, and 69 (8%) fungal infection. Among deaths with recorded bacterial infections, a lower proportion of meningococcal and pneumococcal infections (14% [22/155] vs. 60% [205/339], $P < 0.0001$) and a higher proportion of Gram-negative enteric bacilli (78/155 cases [50%] vs. 17/339 cases [5%], $P < 0.0001$) were reported in children with and without documented underlying medical conditions, respectively.

*Conclusions.*—Infections continue to make a major contribution to deaths in children, particularly among those with underlying conditions. Identification of the pathogens associated with childhood deaths should help prioritize the development of intervention strategies for reducing pediatric mortality. Linkage of death registrations to national infectious disease surveillance systems should be undertaken to strengthen monitoring of infectious deaths and evaluate the effect of interventions.

▶ Globally, infectious diseases remain the most common cause of death in children. Although the public health infrastructure and industrialization of North America and Western Europe have reduced the impact of communicable disease in these regions, the globalization of travel, trade, and tourism has created the opportunities for microbes to travel fast among continents. From a microbiological point of view, an infectious agent anywhere in the world is an infectious disease everywhere in the world.

A recent survey in the United Kingdom, Confidential Enquiry into Maternal and Child Health (CEMACH) reported infection to be the largest single cause of death in children dying of an acute physical illness.[1]

In this original study, the authors present data on the contribution of infectious disease to childhood (28 days to 14 years) deaths in a developed part of the world, that is, England and Wales (2003-2005). Infection-related deaths constituted 20% of all deaths in this age group. The strong point in this study is the data on specific pathogens causing death. In both of these databases, because of a multitude of limitations, this number was considered a minimum. Underlying medical conditions, for example prematurity in infants, cerebral palsy in 1 to 4 year olds, and malignancy in 5 to 14 year olds, were recorded in 50% of the children. Specific pathogen or pathogens were identified in 837 (62%) out of 1356 deaths.

The pathogens included bacteria (61%), viruses (31%), fungi (8%), and others (0.6%). Microbiological documentation of the infection was more likely for deaths in previously healthy children (6.9%) compared with 50% in children with underlying illnesses. Meningococcal infection was responsible for more deaths in previously healthy children compared with those with underlying medical conditions. All pertussis-related deaths (9) occurred in previously healthy infants younger than 4 months of age, of whom 6 were younger than 2 months. Viral causes of infection were equal in previously healthy children and those with underlying medical conditions. Respiratory syncytial virus (16%), adenovirus (12%), influenza virus (12%), and cytomegalovirus (10%) were responsible for more than 50% of the viral causes of death.

Common Bacterial Causes of Death

| *Previously healthy children* | *Children with underlying medical conditions* |
|---|---|
| All bacteria 50% | All bacteria 23% |
| Meningococci 28% | Gram-negative enteric bacilli 52% |
| Pneumonococci 18% | Staphylococci + enterococci 20% |
| Group A streptococci 3.2% | |
| Group B streptococci 5% | |
| Other streptococci 13% | |
| Gram-negative bacilli 5% | |

Although similar data from other European countries are lacking, it is logical to assume comparable figures for infection-related deaths. The 2 most common bacterial causes of death (and pertussis) and third most common viral cause of death reported in this study are vaccine preventable. Early recognition, faster and improved diagnosis methods, and aggressive (appropriate) antibiotic use will reduce these early life deaths. Primary immunization of children and regular boosters as needed remain the first-line defense. The CEMACH report identified that both in outpatient and hospital settings, health care professionals had difficulty in recognizing serious infections and failed to implement national guidelines.

**N. M. Khardori, MD**

*Reference*

1. Pearson GA, ed. Why Children Die: A Pilot Study 2006; England (South West, North East and West Midlands), Wales and Northern Ireland. London: Confidential Enquiry into Maternal and Child health (CEMACH); 2008.

## *CISH* and Susceptibility to Infectious Diseases

Khor CC, Vannberg FO, Chapman SJ, et al (Univ of Oxford, UK; et al)
*N Engl J Med* 362:2092-2101, 2010

*Background.*—The interleukin-2–mediated immune response is critical for host defense against infectious pathogens. Cytokine-inducible SRC homology 2 (SH2) domain protein (CISH), a suppressor of cytokine signaling, controls interleukin-2 signaling.

*Methods.*—Using a case–control design, we tested for an association between *CISH* polymorphisms and susceptibility to major infectious diseases (bacteremia, tuberculosis, and severe malaria) in blood samples from 8402 persons in Gambia, Hong Kong, Kenya, Malawi, and Vietnam. We had previously tested 20 other immune-related genes in one or more of these sample collections.

*Results.*—We observed associations between variant alleles of multiple *CISH* polymorphisms and increased susceptibility to each infectious disease in each of the study populations. When all five single-nucleotide polymorphisms (SNPs) (at positions −639, −292, −163, +1320, and +3415 [all relative to *CISH*]) within the CISH-associated locus were considered together in a multiple-SNP score, we found an association between *CISH* genetic variants and susceptibility to bacteremia, malaria, and tuberculosis ($P = 3.8 \times 10^{-11}$ for all comparisons), with −292 accounting for most of the association signal ($P = 4.58 \times 10^{-7}$). Peripheral-blood mononuclear cells obtained from adult subjects carrying the −292 variant, as compared with wild-type cells, showed a muted response to the stimulation of interleukin-2 production — that is, 25 to 40% less *CISH* expression.

*Conclusions.*—Variants of CISH are associated with susceptibility to diseases caused by diverse infectious pathogens, suggesting that negative regulators of cytokine signaling have a role in immunity against various infectious diseases. The overall risk of one of these infectious diseases was increased by at least 18% among persons carrying the variant *CISH* alleles.

▶ The outcomes of host-pathogen interactions are determined by a number of variables, including genetic associations and acquired immune responses. Interleukin-2 is controlled by a suppressor of cytokine signaling called cytokine-inducible SRC homology 2 domain protein (C1SH). The control of cytokine signaling in humans is partly mediated by negative feedback from the suppressor of cytokine signaling (SOCS) family of proteins.[1] An association was observed between variant alleles of multiple *CISH* polymorphisms and increased susceptibility to major infectious diseases. The subjects included patients with bacteremia, tuberculosis, and severe malaria from 5 different countries with geographically matched controls. The association seen in each of the study populations to each of the infectious diseases studied suggests the role of *CISH* polymorphism in inflammatory response in general and infectious disease host response in particular.[2] CISH was the first member of the SOCS family to be described and is the gene most consistently upregulated by interleukin-2 stimulation in humans.[3]

The risk of disease increased significantly with an increase in the number of risk alleles carried in each population. The implication of CISH in multiple-pathogen susceptibility raises the possibility that pharmacologic manipulation of the SOCS pathway may be useful in treating multiple diverse infectious diseases.

**N. M. Khardori, MD**

*References*

1. Jin P, Wang E, Provenzano M, et al. Molecular signatures induced by interleukin-2 on peripheral blood mononuclear cells and T cell subsets. *J Transl Med.* 2006;4: 26.
2. Tishkoff SA, Varkonyi R, Cahinhinan N, et al. Haplotype diversity and linkage disequilibrium at human G6PD: recent origin of alleles that confer malarial resistance. *Science.* 2001;293:455-462.
3. Yoshimura A, Ohkubo T, Kiguchi T, et al. A novel cytokine-inducible gene CIS encodes an SH2-containing protein that binds to tyrosine-phosphorylated interleukin 3 and erythropoietin receptors. *EMBO J.* 1995;14:2816-2826.

## Antibiotic Therapy and Treatment Failure in Patients Hospitalized for Acute Exacerbations of Chronic Obstructive Pulmonary Disease

Rothberg MB, Pekow PS, Lahti M, et al (Baystate Med Ctr, Springfield, MA; Univ of Massachusetts School of Public Health, Amherst)
*JAMA* 303:2035-2042, 2010

*Context.*—Guidelines recommend antibiotic therapy for acute exacerbations of chronic obstructive pulmonary disease (COPD), but the evidence is based on small, heterogeneous trials, few of which include hospitalized patients.

*Objective.*—To compare the outcomes of patients treated with antibiotics in the first 2 hospital days with those treated later or not at all.

*Design, Setting, and Patients.*—Retrospective cohort of patients aged 40 years or older who were hospitalized from January 1, 2006, through December 31, 2007, for acute exacerbations of COPD at 413 acute care facilities throughout the United States.

*Main Outcome Measures.*—A composite measure of treatment failure, defined as the initiation of mechanical ventilation after the second hospital day, inpatient mortality, or readmission for acute exacerbations of COPD within 30 days of discharge; length of stay, and hospital costs.

*Results.*—Of 84 621 patients, 79% received at least 2 consecutive days of antibiotic treatment. Treated patients were less likely than nontreated patients to receive mechanical ventilation after the second hospital day (1.07%; 95% confidence interval [Cl], 1.06%-1.08% vs 1.80%; 95% Cl, 1.78%-1.82%), had lower rates of inpatient mortality (1.04%; 95% Cl, 1.03%-1.05% vs 1.59%; 95% Cl, 1.57%-1.61%), and had lower rates of readmission for acute exacerbations of COPD (7.91%; 95% Cl, 7.89%-7.94% vs 8.79%; 95% Cl, 8.74%-8.83%). Patients treated with antibiotic agents had a higher rate of readmissions for *Clostridium difficile* (0.19%; 95% Cl, 0.187%-0.193%) than those who were not treated (0.09%; 95% Cl, 0.086%-0.094%). After multivariable adjustment, including the propensity for antibiotic treatment, the risk of treatment failure was lower in antibiotic-treated patients (odds ratio, 0.87; 95% Cl, 0.82-0.92). A grouped treatment approach and hierarchical modeling to account for potential confounding of hospital effects yielded similar results. Analysis stratified by risk of treatment failure found similar magnitudes of benefit across all subgroups.

*Conclusion.*—Early antibiotic administration was associated with improved outcomes among patients hospitalized for acute exacerbations of COPD regardless of the risk of treatment failure.

▶ Respiratory infections are the most frequent cause of acute exacerbations of chronic obstructive pulmonary disease (COPD).[1] Most of these may be viral in origin. The recommendations for antibacterial therapy are based on changes in symptomatology, that is, purulent sputum, increased sputum production, and worsening of dyspnea. Evidence from small, heterogeneous trials demonstrates that antibacterials can reduce short-term mortality and treatment failure.[2] The benefit appears to be more in patients with severe disease, especially those requiring mechanical ventilation.

In this retrospective study, outcomes in hospitalized patients with COPD who received antibacterials in the first 2 hospital days were compared with those not receiving them at all or those receiving them later during the course. Defined criteria of initiation of mechanical ventilation after the second hospital day, inpatient mortality, length of stay, hospital costs, and readmission for acute exacerbation of COPD within 3 days of discharge were used to measure outcomes. In a large patient cohort (84 621), antibacterial administration was associated with a 13% decrease in the risk of treatment failure, decrease in inpatient mortality, and late mechanical ventilation. Until more objective and rapid laboratory tests became available to document a bacterial etiology of acute exacerbation in patients with COPD, the routine use of antibacterials will remain a part of the management. However, attention needs to be paid to optimization by maintaining previous antibiotic use and respiratory culture records, basing presumptive choices on local antibiograms, and following a microbiological diagnosis as vigorously as possible.

**N. M. Khardori, MD**

*References*


1. Snow V, Lascher S, Mottur-Pilson C. Evidence base for management of acute exacerbations of chronic obstructive pulmonary disease. *Ann Intern Med.* 2001;134: 595-599.
2. Ram FS, Rodriguez-Roisin R, Granadeo-Navarrete A, Garcia-Aymerich J, Barnes NC. Antibiotics for exacerbation of chronic obstructive pulmonary disease. *Cochrane Database Syst Rev.* 2006;CD004403.


## Association of Recurrent Furunculosis with Panton-Valentine Leukocidin and the Genetic Background of *Staphylococcus aureus*

Masiuk H, Kopron K, Grumann D, et al (Pomeranian Med Univ, Szczecin, Poland; Univ of Greifswald, Germany; Universitätsklinikum Tübingen, Germany)

*J Clin Microbiol* 48:1527-1535, 2010

*Staphylococcus aureus* is a major cause of skin and soft tissue infections, such as furuncles, carbuncles, and abscesses, but it also frequently colonizes the human skin and mucosa without causing clinical symptoms. Panton-Valentine leukocidin (PVL) is a pore-forming toxin that has been associated with soft tissue infections and necrotizing pneumonia. We have compared the genotypes, virulence gene repertoires, and phage patterns of 74 furunculosis isolates with those of 108 control strains from healthy nasal carriers. The large majority of furunculosis strains were methicillin sensitive. Clonal cluster (CC) 121 (CC121) and CC22 accounted for 70% of the furunculosis strains but for only 8% of the nasal isolates. The PVL-encoding genes *luk-PV* were detected in 85% of furunculosis strains, while their prevalence among colonizing *S. aureus* strains was below 1%. *luk-PV* genes were distributed over several lineages (CCs 5, 8, 22, 30, and 121 and sequence type 59). Even within the same lineages, *luk-PV*-positive phages characterized furunculosis strains, while their *luk-PV*-negative variants were frequent among nasal strains. The very tight epidemiological linkage between *luk-PV* and furunculosis, which could be separated from the genetic background of the *S. aureus* strain as well as from the gene makeup of the *luk-PV*-transducing phage, lends support to the notion of an important role for PVL in human furunculosis. These results make a case for the determination of *luk-PV* in recurrent soft tissue infections with methicillin-sensitive as well as methicillin-resistant *S. aureus*.

▶ Patients suffering from chronic/recurrent furuncles are usually persistent nasal carriers of *Staphylococcus aureus*.[1] In addition to progression of furunculosis to deeper soft tissue infections, bacteremia and invasive *S aureus* disease can occur from these sources. The *S aureus* population structure is highly clonal with 10 major and many minor clonal clusters (CCs). Fifteen percent of the *S aureus* genome is comprised of mobile genetic elements, which can readily spread horizontally among *S aureus* strains of the same CC. Because they contain a variety of virulence and resistance genes, their spread leads to further increase in morbidity and mortality associated with *S aureus* infection.

In this study from Germany, the genotype, virulence gene repertoires, and phage pattern of 74 furunculosis isolates were compared with 108 control strains from healthy nasal carriers. Most of the furunculosis strains were methicillin susceptible. CC121 and CC22 accounted for 70% of furunculosis strains but only 8% of nasal isolates. Panton-Valentine leukocidin (PVL), a pore forming toxin, has been associated with soft tissue infections and necrotizing pneumonia. Genes encoding for PVL were detected in 85% of furunculosis strains compared with 1% of colonizing strains. Irrespective of antimicrobial susceptibility, skin and soft tissue infections are characterized by PVL toxin, and PVL-associated symptoms are not unique to community-associated methicillin-resistant *S aureus*. The PVL test has the potential of offering rapid diagnosis of *S aureus* infection. Because 87% to 100% of patients with recurrent furunculosis are nasal carriers of their infecting *S aureus* strain,[2] the eradication of the strain from the whole body and the patient's environment should be a part of management.

**N. M. Khardori, MD**

*References*

1. El-Gilany AH, Fathy H. Risk factors of recurrent furunculosis. *Dermatol Online J.* 2009;15:16.
2. Durupt F, Mayor L, Bes M, et al. Prevalence of *Staphylococcus aureus* toxins and nasal carriage in furuncles and impetigo. *Br J. Dermatol.* 2007;157:1161-1167.

## Clinical Outbreak of Linezolid-Resistant *Staphylococcus aureus* in an Intensive Care Unit

García MS, De La Torre MÁ, Morales G, et al (Universidad Complutense, Madrid, Spain)

*JAMA* 303:2260-2264, 2010

*Context.*—Linezolid resistance is extremely uncommon in *Staphylococcus aureus.*

*Objective.*—To report an outbreak with linezolid and methicillin-resistant *S aureus* (LRSA) in an intensive care department and the effective control measures taken.

*Design, Setting, and Patients.*—Outbreak study of consecutive critically ill patients colonized and/or infected with LRSA at an intensive care department of a 1000-bed tertiary care university teaching hospital in Madrid, Spain. Patients were placed under strict contact isolation. Daily updates of outbreak data and recommendations for the use of linezolid were issued. Extensive environmental sampling and screening of the hands of health care workers were performed.

*Main Outcome Measures.*—Linezolid use and clinical and epidemiological characteristics and outcomes using minimal inhibitory concentrations, pulsed-field gel electrophoresis, and polymerase chain reaction of LRSA isolates.

*Results.*—Between April 13 and June 26, 2008, 12 patients with LRSA were identified. In 6 patients, LRSA caused ventilator-associated pneumonia and in 3 patients it caused bacteremia. Isolates were susceptible to trimethoprim-sulfamethoxazole, glycopeptides, tigecycline, and daptomycin. Genotyping identified 1 predominant clone and 3 other types. *Cfr*-mediated linezolid resistance was demonstrated in all isolates. Potential hospital staff carriers and environmental samples were negative except for one. Six patients died, 5 of them in the intensive care unit, with 1 death attributed to LRSA infection. Linezolid use decreased from 202 defined daily doses in April 2008 to 25 defined daily doses in July 2008. Between July 2008 and April 2010, no new cases have been identified in the weekly surveillance cultures or diagnostic samples.

*Conclusions.*—The first clinical outbreak, to our knowledge, with LRSA mediated by the *cfr* gene developed at our center, was associated with nosocomial transmission and extensive usage of linezolid. Reduction of linezolid use and infection-control measures were associated with the termination of the outbreak.

▶ Linezolid, an oxazolidinone, is now 1 of the 4 (quinupristin-dalfopristin, linezolid, daptomycin, and tigecycline) agents available for treatment of infection by methicillin-resistant *Staphylococcus aureus* and other multiresistant gram-positive bacteria. The mechanism of action is inhibition of bacterial protein synthesis. The mechanism of resistance, the G2576T point mutation, has been documented in *S aureus, S epidermidis, Enterococcus faecalis,* and *E faecium*. The *cfr* gene, resides in a potentially mobile genetic element, has recently been shown to confer resistance to linezolid in *S aureus* and *S epidermidis*.

The report describes the first outbreak with linezolid and methicillin-resistant *S aureus* (LRSA) in a 1000-bed tertiary care hospital in Madrid, Spain. The linezolid resistance was mediated by the *cfr* gene and associated with extensive use of linezolid and nosocomial transmission.

Of the 12 patients with LRSA between April 13 and June 26, 2008, 6 had ventilator-associated pneumonia and 3 had pneumonia. LRSA isolates were susceptible to trimethoprim/sulfamethoxazole, glycopeptides (vancomycin and teicoplanin), tigecycline, and daptomycin. Hospital staff and environmental samples were negative expect for one. Linezolid usage was reduced as part of the outbreak management. Between July 2008 and April 2010, no new cases have been identified in the weekly surveillance cultures or diagnostic specimens. This well-described outbreak highlights the role of excessive use of antibiotics in creating resistant pathogens, which is reversible by early reduction in the use of the offending agent and institution of infection control measures.

**N. M. Khardori, MD**

## Clinical Utility of an Automated Instrument for Gram Staining Single Slides

Baron EJ, Mix S, Moradi W (Stanford Univ Med Ctr, CA; Willamette Univ, Salem, OR; Univ of California Davis)

*J Clin Microbiol* 48:2014-2015, 2010

Gram stains of 87 different clinical samples were prepared by the laboratory's conventional methods (automated or manual) and by a new single-slide-type automated staining instrument, GG&B AGS-1000. Gram stains from either heat- or methanol-fixed slides stained with the new instrument were easy to interpret, and results were essentially the same as those from the methanol-fixed slides prepared as a part of the routine workflow. This instrument is well suited to a rapid-response laboratory where Gram stain requests are commonly received on a stat basis.

▶ The Gram staining of clinical specimens can be a rapid and sensitive method for early diagnosis of infections. However, variables like appropriate specimen collection, time for transit to microbiology laboratory, time of the day it is processed, and the expertise of the personnel at that time, make this investigation more a routine than of practical use. Commercial automated instruments have now become available to expedite the process, and studies have demonstrated that an automated Gram stain could enhance the consistency of the staining process and save technologists time. AGS-1000, one of the Gram staining instruments, has been validated only for use with heat-fixed slides. This study compared methanol-fixed slides by AGS-1000 and manual methods.

Automated method showed results equivalent to those of standard manual laboratory method. However, the automated method produced more uniform results, required less hands-on time, and conserved reagents. The instrument would be useful in rapid-response laboratories, busy clinical laboratories, and in laboratories where nonmicrobiologist clinical laboratory scientists perform Gram stains on all 3 shifts.

**N. M. Khardori, MD**

## Colectomy for Fulminant *Clostridium difficile* Colitis: Predictors of Mortality

Perera AD, Akbari RP, Cowher MS, et al (Western Pennsylvania Hosp, Pittsburgh; Allegheny General Hosp, Pittsburgh, PA; et al)
*Am Surg* 76:418-421, 2010

The purpose of this study was to define clinical and radiographic variables associated with postoperative mortality after urgent colectomy for fulminant *Clostridium difficile* colitis. Data were obtained regarding patients undergoing colectomy for fulminant *C. difficile* colitis at two institutions (1997–2005). Univariate analysis of factors predicting 30-day mortality was performed using $\chi^2$ and Student's *t* tests. Multivariable logistic regression was done to include all variables whose *P* value was < 0.20. Clinical variables analyzed included: age, gender, recent operation, comorbidities, preoperative multisystem organ failure, vasopressors, symptom duration, time to surgery, serum albumin, change in serum albumin, serum creatinine, white blood cell count, and extent of colectomy. Computed tomography variables included: ascites, megacolon, and extent of colitis. Thirty-five patients (mean age 70 years, 46% male) underwent urgent colectomy for *C. difficile* colitis. The 30-day mortality rate was 45.7 per cent (16/35). The only clinical variable associated with mortality was preoperative multisystem organ failure (non-survivors 9/16 *vs* survivors: 4/19; $P = 0.037$). None of the three patients undergoing partial colectomy survived, although the difference in survival *versus* those undergoing subtotal colectomy was not significant. Patients with fulminant *C. difficile* colitis undergoing colectomy have a high mortality rate. Preoperative presence of multisystem organ failure was independently predictive of mortality.

► With recent significant increase in *Clostridium difficile* infection (CDI) and progression to fulminant disease in some patients, colectomy is considered an option to cure this otherwise fatal complication.[1] The rates of fulminant colitis among patients who develop CDI are reported to be 9% to 19%.[2] Commonly accepted indications for surgery in fulminant colitis are failure of optimal medical therapy, toxic megacolon, uncontrolled sepsis, multisystem organ failure (MSOF), and the presence of an acute abdomen. The published mortality rates for colectomy performed for these indications vary from 37% to 80%.[3]

This retrospective review of patients undergoing colectomy for fulminant *C difficile* colitis between 1997 and 2005 has looked at predictors of mortality in these patients. Inclusion criteria were met in 35 of the 50 potential patients identified by coding data. Partial colectomy was done in 3 patients, and all 3 died.

The rate of MSOF was higher among nonsurvivors (9/16) than the survivors (4/19) ($P = .03$). CT evidence of megacolon was seen in 7/18 survivors compared with 3/16 nonsurvivors ($P = .20$). Other variables did not show statistically significant difference between the 2 groups.

Although a prospective trial with intent-to-treat analysis is needed to further validate these observations, the data point to close observation of patients with severe CDI and surgical benefit before MSOF or toxic megacolon is established.

**N. M. Khardori, MD**

*References*

1. Muto CA, Pokrywka M, Shutt K. A large outbreak of *Clostridium difficile*-associated disease with an unexpected proportion of death and colectomies at a teaching hospital following increased fluoroquinolone use. *Infect Control Hosp Epidemiol.* 2005;26:273-280.
2. Warny M, Pepin J, Fang A, et al. Toxin production by an emerging strain of *Clostridium difficile* associated with outbreaks of severe disease in North America and Europe. *Lancet.* 2005;366:1079-1084.
3. Koss K, Clark MA, Sanders DS, Morton D, Keighley MR, Goh J. The outcome of surgery in fulminant *Clostridium difficile* colitis. *Colorectal Dis.* 2006;8:149-154.

## Control of methicillin-resistant *Staphylococcus aureus* in planktonic form and biofilms: A biocidal efficacy study of nonthermal dielectric-barrier discharge plasma

Joshi SG, Paff M, Friedman G, et al (Drexel Univ, Philadelphia, PA)
*Am J Infect Control* 38:293-301, 2010

*Background.*—Bacterial contamination of surfaces with methicillin-resistant *Staphylococcus aureus* (MRSA) is a serious problem in the hospital environment and is responsible for significant nosocomial infections. The pathogenic contaminants form biofilms, which are difficult to treat with routine biocides. Thus, a continuous search for novel disinfection methods is essential for effective infection control measures. This demonstration of a novel technique for the control of virulent pathogens in planktonic form as well as in established biofilms may provide a progressive alternative to standard methodology.

*Methods.*—We evaluated a novel technique of normal atmospheric nonthermal plasma known as *floating-electrode dielectric-barrier discharge* (FE-DBD) plasma against a control of planktonic and biofilm forms of *Escherichia coli, S aureus*, multidrug-resistant methicillin-resistant *S aureus* (MRSA) -95 (clinical isolate), -USA300, and -USA400, using widely accepted techniques such as colony count assay, LIVE/DEAD BacLight Bacterial Viability assay, and XTT (2,3-Bis(2-methoxy-4-nitro-5-sulfophenyl)-2H-tetrazolium-5-carboxanilide) assay.

*Results.*—Exposure of free living planktonic forms of *E coli, S aureus*, and MRSA were rapidly inactivated by DBD plasma. Approximately $10^7$ bacterial cells were completely (100%) killed, whereas $10^8$ and $10^9$ were reduced by approximately 90% to 95% and 40% to 45%, respectively, in less than 60 seconds (7.8 J/cm$^2$) and completely disinfected in $\leq$120 seconds. In established biofilms, the susceptibility of MRSA

USA400 was comparable with USA300 but less susceptible than MRSA95 (clinical isolate), *S aureus*, and *E coli* ($P < .05$) to FE-DBD plasma, and plasma was able to kill MRSA more than 60% within 15 seconds (1.95 J/cm$^2$). The killing responses were plasma exposure-time dependent, and cell density dependent. The plasma was able disinfect surfaces in a less than 120 seconds.

*Conclusion.*—Application of DBD plasma can be a valuable decontamination technique for the removal of planktonic and biofilm-embedded bacteria such as MRSA -USA 300, -USA 400, methicillin-sensitive *S aureus* (MSSA), and *E coli*, the more common hospital contaminants. Of interest, *E coli* was more resistant than *S aureus* phenotypes.

▶ The preferred mode of growth for most bacteria is sessile, resulting in adherence to tissues and surfaces and biofilm formation. The Centers for Disease Control and Prevention and the National Institutes of Health estimate that anywhere between 65% and 80% of bacterial infections involve biofilm growth.[1] The vast use of implanted medical devices provides an ideal attachment site for many common bacteria. Pieces of biofilm detach from tissues or device surfaces by a quorum sensing mechanism and lead to invasion of the blood stream. When treated with antibiotics that kill the free-floating or planktonic bacteria, they tend to recur because of lack of efficacy of antibiotics on the sessile or adherent bacteria. Device removal and debridement of tissues become necessary in most cases.

Importantly, the adherence of bacteria to surfaces and equipment in the hospitals is the most significant factor involved in hospital-acquired infection. In this setting, it is the drop-off and pick-up of bacteria to and from these sources by the health care providers that leads to transmission of bacteria, including those with multiple drug resistance. Like most antibiotics, routine biocides are not effective against the biofilm bacteria.

This article presents data on a novel method of removing both planktonic (free) and sessile (adherent) bacteria. The authors use nonthermal dielectric-barrier discharge plasma generating probe designed at the Drexel Plasma Institute.[2] This methodology has been shown earlier to have no significant toxicity when tested through a series of in vitro cell culture experiments as well as in vivo mouse and rat skin experiments. Both direct and indirect plasma treatments are novel and easy to apply to various surfaces. Bacterial growth of methicillin-resistant *Staphylococcus aureus*, methicillin-sensitive *S aureus*, and *Escherichia coli* was significantly reduced or completely eliminated (depending on the inoculum size) in less than 60 seconds.

The plasma was able to disinfect surfaces in less than 120 seconds. In addition to environmental infection control, this technique will be potentially useful for management of infected wounds and perhaps skin decontamination before surgery and invasive procedures.

**N. M. Khardori, MD**

*References*

1. Harriott MM, Noverr MC. Candida albicans and *Staphylococcus aureus* form polymicrobial biofilms: effects on antimicrobial resistance. *Antimicrob Agents Chemother.* 2009;53:3914-3922.
2. Lauderdale KJ, Malone CL, Boles BR, Morcuende J, Horswill AR. Biofilm dispersal of community-associated methicillin-resistance *Staphylococcus aureus* on orthopedic implant material. *J Orthop Res.* 2010;28:55-61.

---

**Daptomycin Exposure and the Probability of Elevations in the Creatine Phosphokinase Level: Data from a Randomized Trial of Patients with Bacteremia and Endocarditis**

Bhavnani SM, Rubino CM, Ambrose PG, et al (Ordway Res Inst, Albany, NY)
*Clin Infect Dis* 50:1568-1574, 2010

---

*Background.*—The objective of this analysis was to evaluate the relationship between daptomycin exposure and the probability of an elevation in the creatine phosphokinase (CPK) level (hereafter, "CPK elevation") in patients with *Staphylococcus aureus* bacteremia with or without infective endocarditis.

*Methods.*—Phase 3 data for patients with *S. aureus* bacteremia, with or without infective endocarditis, who received intravenous daptomycin (6 mg/kg daily) and in whom pharmacokinetic data were collected were evaluated. On the basis of univariate logistic regression, the relationship between Bayesian post hoc exposure estimates and the probability of a CPK elevation was evaluated. Time to CPK elevation was examined with Kaplan-Meier analysis and Cox proportional hazards regression.

*Results.*—Significant relationships between the minimum concentration of drug ($C_{min}$) and area under the plasma concentration time curve and probability of CPK elevation were observed in 108 evaluable patients. Of the 108 patients evaluated, 6 (5.56%) demonstrated a defined CPK elevation, regardless of treatment relationship. $C_{min}$ (breakpoint of 24.3 mg/L) was most significantly associated with CPK elevation ($P = .002$). The probabilities of a CPK elevation with a $C_{min}$ ≥24.3 mg/L and <24.3 mg/L were 0.5 and 0.029, respectively. Increases in $C_{min}$, evaluated as a continuous variable, were also significantly associated with CPK elevation ($P = .01$). Stratified Kaplan-Meier analysis and Cox proportional hazards regression demonstrated $C_{min}$ to be a significant predictor of time to a CPK elevation ($P \leq .003$). The probability of a CPK elevation was 0 and 0.01 after 7 days of treatment in patients with a $C_{min}$ ≥24.3 mg/L or <24.3 mg/L, respectively. After 14 days, the probabilities were 0.5 and 0.025, respectively.

*Conclusions.*—This analysis demonstrated that a daptomycin $C_{min}$ ≥24.3 mg/L was associated with an increased probability of a CPK elevation.

*Clinical Trials Registration.*—Clinicaltrials.gov NCT00093067.

▶ Early during its development, daptomycin, a cyclic lipopeptide with activity against gram-positive bacteria, including methicillin-resistant *Staphylococcus aureus*, showed adverse skeletal muscle events. The drug was used every 12 hours at 4 mg/kg daily. Subsequent animal studies in dogs showed decreased skeletal myopathy and creatine phosphokinase (CPK) elevation when the drug was administered once a day. Daptomycin was subsequently approved by the Food and Drug Administration in doses of 4 mg/kg to 6 mg/kg every 24 hours for the treatment of complicated skin and skin structure infection, bacteremia, and endocarditis caused by gram-positive organisms.

This study provides analysis of CPK elevation on a subset of data from a phase 3 bacteremia and endocarditis study.[1] CPK elevation does not always correlate with muscle weakness and pain but may serve as an early indicator. Of the 108 patients analyzed, 5.5% demonstrated a defined CPK elevation. The minimum concentration of drug ($C_{min}$ > 24.3 mg/L) showed a significant relationship with the probability of CPK elevation, and the probability increased significantly after 14 days compared with 7 days of treatment. Overall, CPK elevation during daptomycin therapy was infrequent, manifested at 2 weeks (when the $C_{min}$ values were > 24.3 mg/L), and was not always associated with adverse musculoskeletal effects.

**N. M. Khardori, MD**

*Reference*

1. Fowler VG Jr, Boucher HW, Corey GR, et al. Daptomycin versus standard therapy for bacteremia and endocarditis caused by *Staphylococcus aureus*. *N Engl J Med*. 2007;355:653-665.

---

**Eschar with cellulitis as a clinical predictor in community-acquired methicillin-resistant *Staphylococcus aureus* (MRSA) skin abscess**

Busch BA, Ahern MT, Topinka M, et al (Doctors Hosp, Columbus, OH; et al)
*J Emerg Med* 38:563-566, 2010

---

This study was designed to determine the validity of a central eschar with surrounding cellulitis as a clinical predictor for CA-MRSA infection. In this 10-month prospective observational study, patients with a chief complaint or clinical findings of skin infection with abscess had study data sheets placed on their chart. All abscesses were treated with incision and drainage, and wound cultures were obtained. Exclusionary criteria included patient age under 18 years, recently incarcerated within 14 days, and hospitalized or in a nursing home within 10 days. Correlation of wound culture results with recorded physical examination determined the sensitivity, specificity, and positive/negative predictive values. A total of 224 patients with abscesses were enrolled; 18 patients met exclusion criteria. An additional 78 patients were excluded because no wound cultures had been obtained, study data form was incomplete, or there was no evidence of wound cellulitis. Of the 128 remaining patients, 91 wound cultures grew MRSA (71% prevalence). Of these 91 cases, 50 tested positive for central black eschar, yielding a sensitivity of 55% (95% confidence interval [CI] 0.45–0.65). Thirty-seven patients had abscesses that grew non-MRSA bacteria. Three of these were positive for central black eschar, yielding a specificity of 92% (95% CI 0.83–1.01). The positive predictive value was 94% (95% CI 0.88–1.01) and the negative predictive value was 45% (95% CI 0.32–0.59). A central black eschar with cellulitis has good specificity and high positive predictive value in diagnosing CA-MRSA infection.

► In the outpatient setting including emergency departments, it is difficult to differentiate noninfections from infectious skin lesions, especially those caused by methicillin-resistant *Staphylococcus aureus* (MRSA). Having been bitten by a spider or another insect is a common presenting complaint. Predicting community-acquired methicillin-resistant *Staphylococcus aureus* (CA-MRSA) infection would allow appropriate targeted antimicrobial therapy and decision to drain as needed.

The authors of this study used clinical experience to consider an abscess with black eschar and surrounding cellulitis as a possible CA-MRSA infection. In the 10-month prospective observational period, 224 patients with a chief complaint or clinical findings of skin infection with abscess were enrolled. All abscesses were drained. Of the 128 evaluable patients, 91 (71%) wound cultures grew MRSA. Of these, black eschar had been noted on initial examination for 55 patients. Of the 37 patients with non-MRSA abscesses, only 3 had recorded central black eschar.

Presence of a central black eschar is a simple clinical tool to suspect skin infection caused by CA-MRSA. Given the current high prevalence of these infections in young healthy adults, such validated criteria are useful in selecting presumptive antibiotic therapy.

**N. M. Khardori, MD**

---

**In vitro susceptibility of *Clostridium difficile* to rifaximin and rifampin in 359 consecutive isolates at a university hospital in Houston, Texas**

Jiang Z-D, DuPont HL, La Rocco M, et al (Univ of Texas School of Public Health, Houston; St Luke's Episcopal Hosp, Houston, TX)

*J Clin Pathol* 63:355-358, 2010

---

*Aim.*—This was an in vitro study to analyse the susceptibility of *Clostridium difficile* isolates to rifampin and rifaximin.

*Methods.*—Stool samples from patients who had nosocomial diarrhoea and *C difficile* toxin B at a university hospital between August 2006 and

December 2007 were cultured for C *difficile*. Susceptibility of C *difficile* isolates to rifaximin and rifampin was determined by agar dilution and E strips, respectively. C *difficile* isolates were analysed via PCR for genes encoding toxins A and B, for binary toxin (BT), and for partial deletions of the *tcdC* gene (*tcdC*-del).

*Results.*—Rifaximin exhibited high-level activity against 359 C *difficile* isolates, with $MIC_{50}$ <0.01 μg/ml and $MIC_{90}$ 0.25 μg/ml; rifampin had $MIC_{50}$ <0.002 μg/ml and $MIC_{90}$ 4 μg/ml. Among isolates analysed, 55 (15%) were positive for BT and *tcdC*-del. 28 (8% of 359) isolates were resistant to rifampin (≥32 μg/ml), of which 6 (2% of 359) were resistant to rifaximin and rifampin with MIC values ≥32 μg/ml. 2 of the 28 isolates resistant to rifampin were $A^+/B^+/BT^+/$*tcdC*-$del^+$, 5 were $A^+/B^+/BT^-/$*tcdC*-$del^+$, 4 were $A^+/B^+/BT^+/$*tcdC*-$del^-$, 13 were $A^+/B^+/BT^-/$*tcdC*-$del^-$, and 4 had no detectable toxin genes. Of the 11 isolates resistant to rifaximin alone, 1 was $A^+/B^+/BT^-/$*tcdC*-$del^+$, 2 were $A^+/B^+/BT^+/$*tcdC*-$del^-$, 6 were $A^+/B^+/BT^-/$*tcdC*-$del^-$, and 2 had no detectable toxin genes.

*Conclusions.*—The study demonstrates that rifaximin has high-level activity against C *difficile* in vitro.

Determination of resistance to rifampin by E strip did not predict rifaximin resistance.

▶ The severity and incidence of *Clostridium difficile* infection (CDI) have been on the rise since the mid-1990s.[1] One of the known reasons for this change is the emergence of previously uncommon hypervirulent strains of the organism (eg, BI/NAP1/027), which have been reported to be implicated in CDI outbreaks in the United States, Canada, and Europe. These hypervirulent strains have frequently been positive for toxins A and B and binary toxin.[2] The increased severity of disease by these strains is associated with resistance to some previously effective antibiotics and increased production of toxins A and B. Standard antibiotic therapy for CDI has been metronidazole or vancomycin. CDI is unresponsive to these 2 agents about 25% of the time, and recurrence has been reported in up to 28% of patients after successful initial treatment with one of these agents. Vancomycin resistance in *C difficile* has been documented in 3% to 8% of isolates. The need for new therapies is urgent.

This article reports on the in vitro susceptibility of *C difficile* to rifampin and rifaximin. Stool samples from patients with diarrhea and *C difficile* toxin B between August 2006 and December 2007 were cultured for *C difficile*. A total of 359 isolates were cultured. Rifaximin demonstrated low minimum inhibitory concentration levels (MIC90 0.25 μg/mL) compared with rifampin (MIC90 4 μg/mL). Rifaximin leads to high levels of the drug in the intestine and has no significant systemic absorption. Although this study does not provide correlation with clinical response, findings support the clinical use of rifaximin in CDI, including that caused by the hypervirulent strains. Small clinical studies have reported the efficacy of rifaximin in CDI. Another new agent, nitazoxanide, has been shown to be more effective than vancomycin in a randomized trial of 50 patients.[3]

**N. M. Khardori, MD**

*References*

1. McFarland LV, Beneda HW, Clarridge JE, Raugi GJ. Implication of the changing face of *Clostridium difficile* diseases for health car practitioner. *Am J Infect Control.* 2007;35:237-253.
2. Loo VG, Poirer L, Miller MA, et al. A predominantly clonal multi-institutional outbreak of *Clostridium difficile*-associated diarrhea with high morbidity and mortality. *N Engl J Med.* 2005;353:2442-2449.
3. Voelker R. Increased *Clostridium difficile* virulence demands new treatment approach. *JAMA.* 2010;303:2017-2019.

**Postoperative *Clostridium difficile*-associated diarrhea**

Southern WN, Rahmani R, Aroniadis O, et al (Albert Einstein College of Medicine, Bronx, NY)

*Surgery* 148:24-30, 2010

*Background.*—Abdominal surgery is thought to be a risk factor for *Clostridium difficile*-associated diarrhea (CDAD). The aims of this study were to discern pre-operative factors associated with postoperative CDAD, examine outcomes after postoperative CDAD, and compare outcomes of postoperative versus medical CDAD.

*Methods.*—Data from 3904 patients who had abdominal operations at Montefiore Medical Center were extracted from Montefiore's clinical information system. Cases of 30-day postoperative CDAD were identified. Pre-operative factors associated with developing postoperative CDAD were identified using logistic regression. Medical patients and surgical patients with postoperative CDAD were compared for demographic and clinical characteristics, CDAD recurrence, and 90-day postinfection mortality.

*Results.*—The rate of 30-day postoperative CDAD was 1.2%. After adjustment for age and comorbidities, factors significantly associated with postoperative CDAD were: antibiotic use (OR: 1.94), proton pump inhibitor (PPI) use (OR: 2.32), prior hospitalization (OR: 2.27), and low serum albumin (OR: 2.05). In comparison with medical patients with CDAD, postoperative patients with CDAD were significantly more likely to have received antibiotics (98% vs 85%), less likely to have received a PPI (39% vs 58%), or to have had a prior hospitalization (43% vs 67%). Postoperative patients with CDAD had decreased risk of mortality when compared with medical patients with CDAD (HR 0.36).

*Conclusion.*—CDAD is an infrequent complication after abdominal operations. Several avoidable pre-operative exposures (eg, antibiotic and PPI use) were identified that increase the risk of postoperative CDAD. Postoperative CDAD is associated with decreased risk of mortality when compared with CDAD on the medical service.

▶ A significant increase in the incidence and severity of infections caused by *Clostridium difficile* persists in US hospitals.[1] Abdominal surgery is considered among the risk factors for *C difficile* infection (CDI). The reported rates of postoperative CDI are 0.2% to 8% depending on the surgical population studied and types of operations performed.

This study compares postoperative CDI with CDI in medical patients to define risk factors and outcomes. The postoperative group contained all patients who underwent an inpatient abdominal surgical procedure within 30 days of admission between January 2006 and February 2008. The rate of CDI during the 30-day postoperative period was 1.2%. Prior hospitalization (OR 2.27), proton pump inhibitor (PPI) use (OR 2.32), low serum albumin (OR 2.05), and antibiotic use (OR 1.94) showed significant association with postoperative CDI. The prophylactic dose of antibiotics within 2 hours of the procedure was excluded. Compared with the medical patients, postoperative patients with CDI were more likely to have received antibiotics, less likely to have received a PPI, and less likely to have had a prior hospitalization. The 90-day mortality rate in postoperative patients was 19% compared with 36% in medical patients.

CDI is an infrequent complication after abdominal surgery, and the risk is increased by avoidable factors like PPI and antibiotic use.

**N. M. Khardori, MD**

*Reference*

1. Zilberberg MD, Shorr AF, Kollef MH. Increase in adult *Clostridium difficile*-related hospitalizations and case-fatality rate, United States, 2000-2005. *Emerg Infect Dis*. 2008;14:929-931.

---

**Predictors of Death after *Clostridium difficile* Infection: A Report on 128 Strain-Typed Cases from a Teaching Hospital in the United Kingdom**

Wilson V, Cheek L, Satta G, et al (Brighton and Sussex Univ Hosps Natl Health Service Trust, UK; Univ of Brighton, Falmer, UK; et al)

*Clin Infect Dis* 50:e77-e81, 2010

---

We assessed the relationship between strain type, clinical factors, and outcome in 128 patients with *Clostridium difficile* infection. Strain type was not associated with any outcome measure. On multivariate analysis, ischemic heart disease and hypoalbuminemia predicted death. Metronidazole treatment in severe disease was associated with a higher rate of treatment failure and death.

▶ The relationship between BI/027 strains of *Clostridium difficile* and enhanced virulence has emerged from settings with rapid emergence of these strains. More severity of disease and higher mortality rates have not been observed in settings where BI/027 strains are endemic.[1]

This is a prospective cohort study to establish the role of strain type and clinical and management factors in the outcome of *C difficile* infection (CDI).

The strain types among the 128 isolates were restriction endonuclease (REA) group DH (ribotype 106) 40%, REA group B1 (ribotype 027) 26%, and others 34%. CDI was related to death in 22 patients of the 46 patients who died < 30 days after diagnosis. Early treatment failure after specific treatment for CDI occurred in 50% of patients. There was no association between BI/027 infection and severe disease, early treatment failure, relapse, attributable mortality, or excess mortality. The major predictors of death among patients in this study were comorbid conditions, especially ischemic heart disease and severity of illness at presentation manifested by hypoalbuminemia and renal impairment. Overall mortality was not affected by metronidazole treatment. Among the subgroup of 78 patients with severe disease who received specific treatment, metronidazole was associated with a higher risk of death and a higher rate of early treatment failure compared with treatment with oral vancomycin.

This study provides data to take the focus off from hypervirulent B1/027 strains with regard to outcomes in CDI. Instead, efforts to improve outcomes in CDI should focus on assessment of risk, including comorbid conditions, severity of disease, and optimization of treatment.

**N. M. Khardori, MD**

*Reference*

1. Cloud J, Noddin L, Pressman A, Hu M, Kelly C. *Clostridium difficile* strain NAP-1 is not associated with sever disease in a nonepidemic setting. *Clin Gastroenterol Hepatol.* 2009;7:868-873.

---

## Prompt and Successful Toxin-Targeting Treatment of Three Patients with Necrotizing Pneumonia Due to *Staphylococcus aureus* Strains Carrying the Panton-Valentine Leukocidin Genes

Rouzic N, Janvier F, Libert N, et al (Université de Lyon, France; Hôpital d'Instruction des Armées du Val de Grâce et Ecole du Val de Grâce, Paris, France; et al)

*J Clin Microbiol* 48:1952-1955, 2010

---

Three patients with extensive necrotizing pneumonia due to Panton-Valentine leukocidin-positive *Staphylococcus aureus* strains and with aggravating factors (leukopenia count of less than $3 \times 10^9$/liter in all three cases and hemoptysis in two cases) were successfully treated with toxin-suppressing agents introduced rapidly after hospital admission.

► Necrotizing pneumonia caused by Panton-Valentine leukocidin (PVL)-positive *Staphylococcus aureus* strains is fatal in 50% to 75% of cases.[1] It mainly affects children and young adults and leads to rapid death after a median time of only 4 days. PVL is overexpressed in the presence of cell wall-active antistaphylococcal agents. It can be blocked by adding a toxin-suppressing agent (eg, clindamycin, linezolid, or rifampin) to the cell wall-active agents.[2]

The lytic effect of PVL on polymorphonuclear cells in vitro has shown to be blocked by intravenous immunoglobulin (IVIG).[3] The first case in this report, a 6-month-old boy received vancomycin, clindamycin, and ceftriaxone initially followed by clindamycin plus rifampin for a PVL-positive methicillin-resistant *S aureus* necrotizing pneumonia. He was discharged home on hospital day 28.

The second patient, a 38-year-old man, was admitted for an influenza-like syndrome. He deteriorated on ceftriaxone, amikacin, and levofloxacin. During intubation, tracheal aspiration yielded hemorrhagic fluid containing gram-positive cocci in clusters. Antibiotics were switched to vancomycin and gentamicin. When *S aureus* (methicillin-susceptible *S aureus*) was grown in culture, the patient was switched to clindamycin and linezolid plus IVIG (1 gm/kg body weight per day on 2 consecutive days). The patient improved. Subsequently, antibiotics were changed to vancomycin and rifampin because of suspected clindamycin-induced colitis. Influenza infection was documented by serological tests. Patient was discharged home on day 39.

The third patient, a previously healthy 35-year-old man was admitted for fever and chest pain. He was started on ofloxacin and amoxicillin-clavulanate. Patient developed acute respiratory distress and lactic acidosis. Chest CT scan showed bilateral pneumonia with disseminated necrotizing lesions. *S aureus* susceptible to methicillin and clindamycin was cultured from bronchoalveolar lavage. *PVL* gene was detected in the isolate. Antibiotics were changed to linezolid, clindamycin, and ofloxacin. IVIG was added. Patient improved and discharged on day 23.

All 3 patients showed a rapid fall in leukocyte count, indicating the possibility of PVL-producing *S aureus* prior to the availability of culture results. The management and outcomes of these 3 patients suggest that rapid addition of treatment targeted at the PVL toxin either by inhibiting it (clindamycin/linezolid) or by blocking its lytic effect on polymorphonuclear leukocytes (IVIG) should be considered in patients with necrotizing pneumonia, especially when a rapid fall in leukocyte count is observed.

**N. M. Khardori, MD**

*References*

1. Gillet Y, Vanhems P, Lina G, et al. Factors predicting mortality in necrotizing community-acquired pneumonia caused by *Staphylococcus aureus* containing Panton-Valentine leukocidin. *Clin Infect Dis*. 2007;45:315-321.
2. Stevens DL, Ma Y, Salmi DB, McIndoo E, Wallace RJ, Bryant AE. Impact of antibiotics on expression of virulence-associated exotoxin genes in methicillin-sensitive and methicillin-resistant *Staphylococcus aureus*. *J Infect Dis*. 2007;195:202-211.
3. Gauduchon V, Cozon G, Vandenesch F, et al. Neutralization of *Staphylococcus aureus* Panton Valentine leukocidin by intravenous immunoglobulin in vitro. *J Infect Dis*. 2004;189:346-353.

**Resistant Pathogens in Nonnosocomial Pneumonia and Respiratory Failure: Is It Time To Refine the Definition of Health-care-Associated Pneumonia?**

Schreiber MP, Chan CM, Shorr AF (Washington Hosp Ctr, DC)

*Chest* 137:1283-1288, 2010

*Background.*—The concept of health-care-associated pneumonia (HCAP) exists to identify patients infected with highly resistant pathogens. It is unclear how precise this concept is and how well it performs as a screening tool for resistance.

*Methods.*—We retrospectively identified patients presenting to the hospital with pneumonia complicated by respiratory failure. We examined the microbiology of these infections based on pneumonia type and determined the sensitivity and specificity of HCAP as a screen for resistance. Through logistic regression and modeling, we created a scoring tool for determining who may be infected with resistant pathogens.

*Results.*—The cohort included 190 subjects (37% with ARDS) and we noted resistant pathogens in 33%. Resistance was more common in HCAP (78% vs 44%, $P = .001$). HCAP alone performed poorly as a screening test (sensitivity and specificity 78.3% and 56.2%, respectively). Variables independently associated with a resistant organism included immunosuppression (adjusted odds ratio [AOR] 4.85, $P < .001$), long-term care admission (AOR 2.36, $P = .029$), and prior antibiotics (AOR 2.12, $P = .099$). A decision rule based only on these factors performed moderately well at identifying resistant infections. The presence of HCAP itself, based on meeting defined criteria, was not independently associated with resistance using logistic regression to control for covariates.

*Conclusions.*—HCAP is common in patients presenting to the hospital with pneumonia leading to respiratory failure. The HCAP concept does not correlate well with the presence of infection due to a resistant pathogen. A simpler clinical decision rule based on select HCAP criteria performs as well as the HCAP concept for potentially guiding antibiotic decision making (Table 1).

▶ Pneumonia remains the sixth most common cause of death and the most common cause of infection-related death in the United States. Historically, the microbiological spectrum of pneumonia in patients from the community requiring hospitalization has been thought to be *Streptococcus pneumoniae* and *Legionella* species. For pneumonias acquired in the hospital, methicillin-resistant *Staphylococcus aureus* (MRSA) and *Pseudomonas aeruginosa* are thought to be the common bacterial pathogens. Nosocomial pneumonias have generally been linked to highly resistant pathogens. This retrospective study identified patients presenting to the hospital with pneumonia complicated by respiratory failure. The goal was to study the role of resistant bacteria in non-nosocomial health care-associated pneumonia (HCAP). HCAP was considered in the presence of at least one of the following: recent hospitalization (last 90 days), transfer from a long-term care facility, chronic hemodialysis

TABLE 1.—Pathogens by Pneumonia Type

| Pathogen | HCAP (n = 94) | CAP (n = 96) | *P* Value |
|---|---|---|---|
| Resistant organisms | | | |
| MRSA | 22.3 | 14.6 | .193 |
| PA | 23.4 | 3.1 | .001 |
| ESBL-producing organisms | 2.1 | 0.0 | .001 |
| Nonresistant organisms | | | |
| *Streptococcus pneumoniae* | 6.4 | 21.9 | .003 |
| *Streptococcus viridans* | 10.6 | 29.2 | .002 |
| Methicillin-susceptible *Staphylococcus aureus* | 10.6 | 14.6 | .514 |
| *Escherichia coli* | 12.8 | 4.2 | .038 |
| *Klebsiella pneumoniae* | 10.6 | 4.2 | .102 |
| *Legionella* species | 3.2 | 2.1 | .681 |

Data are given as percentages. CAP = community-acquired pneumonia; ESBL = extended-spectrum β-lactamase; HCAP = health-care-associated pneumonia; MRSA = methicillin-resistant *Staphylococcus aureus;* PA = *Pseudomonas aeruginosa.*

or wound care, immunosuppressive and/or recent (last 30 days) use of broad spectrum antimicrobial agents. Immunosuppressed patients included patients on corticosteroids, that is, 10-mg prednisone or equivalent daily for at least 30 days. Resistant pathogens were noted in 33% of the 190-subject cohort (Table 1).

The sensitivity and specificity of HCAP alone as a screening test for resistant pathogens were 78% and 56%, respectively. Immunosuppression (odds ratio [OR] 4.8), long-term care admission (OR 2.3), and prior antibiotics (OR 2.10) were independently associated with a resistant organism. Patients with HCAP were more likely to be infected with MRSA, *P aeruginosa*, and extended-spectrum β-lactamase-producing organisms. However, patients with community-associated pneumonia needing mechanical ventilation may also be infected with such pathogens as shown by results in this study.

**N. M. Khardori, MD**

## Risk Factors for Bacteremia with Uropathogen Not Cultured from Urine in Adults with Febrile Urinary Tract Infection

van Nieuwkoop C, Bonten TN, van't Wout JW, et al (Leiden Univ Med Ctr, the Netherlands; et al)
*Clin Infect Dis* 50:e69-e72, 2010

In a prospective study involving 642 patients with febrile urinary tract infection (UTI), we found antimicrobial pretreatment (odds ratio [OR], 3.3), an indwelling urinary catheter (OR, 2.8), and malignancy (OR, 2.7) to be independent risk factors for bacteremia with a uropathogen that was not cultured or recognized in the urine. Although the diagnostic

TABLE 2.—Uropathogens Isolated from Blood and Urine Cultures from 583 Patients with Febrile Urinary Tract Infection

| Uropathogen(s) Recovered from Urine Culture | Uropathogen(s) Recovered from Blood Culture, No. (%) of Isolates | | | | | | |
|---|---|---|---|---|---|---|---|
| | *Escherichia coli* | *Klebsiella* species | *Proteus* species | *Enterococcus* species | Other | None or Contaminated | No. (%) of Isolates from Urine Culture |
| *E. coli* | 91 | 0 | 0 | 0 | 1[a] | 240 | 332 (56.9)[b] |
| *Klebsiella* species | 1[a] | 5 | 0 | 0 | 1[a] | 20 | 27 (4.6) |
| *Proteus* species | 0 | 0 | 5 | 0 | 0 | 8 | 13 (2.2) |
| *Enterococcus* species | 0 | 0 | 0 | 1 | 0 | 9 | 10 (1.7) |
| Other | 1[a] | 1[a] | 0 | 0 | 5[c] | 43 | 50 (8.6) |
| None or contaminated | 18[a] | 0 | 1[a] | 1[a] | 4[a] | 127 | 151 (25.9) |
| Isolates from blood culture, no (%) of total | 111 (19.0)[d] | 6 (1.0) | 6 (1.0) | 2 (0.3) | 11 (1.9) | 447 (76.7) | 583 (100) |

[a]Discordant culture results.
[b]This is 76.9% of the 432 urine cultures with positive results.
[c]Of the 5 cultures categorized as other, *Pseudomonas aeruginosa* ($n = 3$), *Staphylococcus aureus* ($n = 1$), and *Aerococcus urinae* ($n = 1$) were isolated. None of these cultures were discordant.
[d]This is 81.6% of the 136 isolates recovered from blood cultures.

value of blood cultures has been questioned in UTI, we advocate performing blood cultures for patients with these risk factors (Table 2).

▶ The mortality rate of patients with acute pyelonephritis and concomitant bacteremia has been reported to be as high as 7% to 30%, compared with the overall mortality of 0.3% in acute pyelonephritis.[1] Because conventional uropathogens can be detected in urine specimens, routine use of blood cultures in febrile urinary tract infection (UTI) or acute pyelonephritis has been debatable.[2] However, the studies that have presented this debate have not led to changes in clinical practice, and the use of blood cultures is increasing.

The objective of this study was to evaluate risk factors for bacteremia due to uropathogens that could not be cultured from urine in patients with community onset febrile UTI. This is a prospective, observational, multicenter cohort study from 8 emergency departments of 7 hospitals and 35 affiliated primary health centers serving a single area of the Netherlands. Uropathogens isolated from blood and urine from 582 patients with febrile UTI are shown in Table 2.

The independent risk factors for bacteremia with a uropathogen that was not cultured or recognized in the urine were prior antibiotic treatment (OR 3.3), presence of an indwelling urinary catheter (OR 2.8), and malignancy (OR 2.7). The rate of discordant results between blood and urine cultures was 5% (higher than in previous retrospective studies). However, the low proportion of discordant culture results still supports previous findings that the performance of blood cultures for all patients with febrile UTI is of limited additional diagnostic value. Bacteremia has not been shown to be a risk factor for complicated outcome in patients with febrile UTI[3] and based on this study does not have a prognostic value. The discordance rate in the subgroup of patients with a urinary catheter or malignancy or recent antibiotic failure for UTI was 8%. However, the discordant culture results were associated with a 4-fold higher mortality risk over a 90-day follow-up period, providing a justification for blood cultures in this group of patients.

**N. M. Khardori, MD**

*References*

1. Brown P, Ki M, Foxman B. Acute pyelonephritis among adults: cost of illness and considerations for the economic evaluation of therapy. *Pharmacoeconomics*. 2005;23:1123-1142.
2. Chen Y, Nitizan O, Saliba W, Chazan B, Colodner R, Raz R. Are blood cultures necessary in the management of women with complicated pyelonephritis? *J Infect*. 2006;53:235-240.
3. van Nieuwkoop C, van't Wout JW, Spelt IC, et al. Prospective cohort study of acute pyelonephritis in adults: safety of triage towards home based oral antimicrobial treatment. *J Infect*. 2010;60:114-121.

**_Staphylococcus aureus_ Meningitis Case Series and Literature Review**

Aguilar J, Urday-Cornejo V, Donabedian S, et al (Henry Ford Hosp, Detroit, MI)

*Medicine* 89:117-125, 2010

*Staphylococcus aureus* meningitis is a challenging disease and little is known about its epidemiology. There are no established management guidelines. We retrospectively reviewed the clinical information, bacteriologic data, and outcomes of all 33 patients with cerebrospinal fluid (CSF) cultures positive for *S aureus* seen at a single urban teaching hospital from 1999 to 2008. Pulsed-field gel electrophoresis (PFGE) and polymerase chain reaction for staphylococcal cassette chromosome mec (SCCmec), accessory gene regulator (agr) typing, and Panton-Valentine leukocidin (PVL) loci were done on methicillin-resistant *S aureus* (MRSA) CSF isolates starting in 2005.

*S aureus* caused 12 (36%) cases of postoperative and 21 (64%) cases of hematogenous meningitis. MRSA isolates were found in 6 (50%) cases of postoperative and 10 (48%) cases of hematogenous meningitis. Twelve (75%) of the 16 MRSA infections occurred in the last 5 years of the study. Hematogenous meningitis was associated with older age ($p = 0.04$), injection drug use ($p < 0.01$), community-acquired infection ($p < 0.01$), underlying disease ($p = 0.01$), staphylococcal infection outside the central nervous system ($p = 0.01$), altered mental status ($p = 0.02$), fever ($p = 0.01$), septic shock ($p = 0.03$), and bacteremia ($p < 0.01$). The analysis of the 9 MRSA isolates showed 3 PFGE types: 3 USA100 (33%), 5 USA300 (56%), and 1 USAnot100-1100 (11%). For SCCmec typing, there were 2 (22%) type II and 7 (78%) type IV. All USA300 strains were SCCmec IVa. For agr typing, there were 5 (56%) type I and 4 (44%) type II. Three isolates (33%) were positive for the PVL gene and were USA300 strains. Most patients received nafcillin or vancomycin with or without rifampin or trimethoprim/ sulfamethoxazole for a mean period of 17 days (range, 1–42 d). Overall mortality was 36%, and it was associated with community-acquired infection ($p = 0.02$).

Postoperative and hematogenous *S aureus* meningitis are distinct clinical syndromes. *S aureus* hematogenous meningitis has devastating clinical consequences and elevated mortality rates, especially if it is acquired in the community. The incidence of MRSA meningitis increased over the last 5 years of the study. Treatment of choice is nafcillin for methicillin-sensitive strains and vancomycin for MRSA strains. The addition of trimethoprim/ sulfamethoxazole or rifampin, to vancomycin is recommended in severe cases and community-acquired MRSA infections. Linezolid is also a good option due to its good CSF penetration and favorable case reports. The mortality rate is higher in infections acquired in the community.

▶ *Staphylococcus aureus* accounts for 1% to 3% of cases of meningitis in the United States and is associated with a mortality of about 50% in adults.[1]

Worldwide, *S aureus* carries 0.3% to 8.8% of all cases of bacterial meningitis.[2] The incidence of *S aureus* meningitis, especially that caused by community-associated methicillin-resistant strains of *S aureus* (CA-MRSA), is increasing. There are 2 distinct pathogenic mechanisms for *S aureus* meningitis. Postoperative meningitis is caused by *S aureus* introduced during trauma, neurosurgical procedures, cerebrospinal fluid (CSF) shunt device placement, or spread from a contiguous focus of infection. In hematogenous or spontaneous meningitis, *S aureus* disseminates to the central nervous system (CNS) because of systemic infection from a focus outside the CNS. Conventional antimicrobial therapy of *S aureus* meningitis is nafcillin/oxacillin for methicillin susceptible strains and vancomycin with or without rifampin or trimethoprim/sulfamethoxazole for methicillin resistant strains. Newer antistaphylococcal agents (eg, linezolid and daptomycin) have been used with good outcomes.[3,4]

This case series and literature review provides a comprehensive resource for *S aureus* meningitis. In their case series between January 1999 and December 2008, 12 (36%) cases of postoperative and 21 (64%) cases of hematogenous meningitis in adults are discussed. Methicillin-resistant isolates were found in 50% of postoperative and 48% of hematogenous meningitis with 75% of 16 methicillin-resistant *S aureus* (MRSA) infections occurring in the last 5 years. Overall mortality rate was 36%, 43% in hematogenous meningitis, and 25% in postoperative meningitis. Community-acquired infections had a higher mortality rate than those acquired in the hospital. Postoperative meningitis was usually associated with CSF shunt devices and is clinically less severe. Except for 1 patient with a strain of *S aureus* with intermediate resistance to vancomycin (VISA) treated with linezolid, others received nafcillin/oxacillin, vancomycin, or trimethoprim/sulfamethoxazole. The mean length of treatment was 17 days (1-42 days) and was based on the type of primary infection. Intrathecal antimicrobial therapy or corticosteroids were not used in any patients in this series. In 9 patients with ventriculoperitoneal shunts, all components of the shunt were eventually removed. Antibiotics of choice are nafcillin for methicillin-susceptible *S aureus* strains and vancomycin for MRSA strains. The addition of trimethoprim/sulfamethoxazole or rifampin to vancomycin should be considered for infections caused by CA-MRSA and in severe cases. Linezolid has good CNS penetration and has shown favorable response in case reports. One of the highlights in this review is that the mortality rate is higher in infections acquired in the community than in nosocomial infections.

**N. M. Khardori, MD**

*References*

1. Pizon AF, Bonner MR, Wang HE, Kaplan RM. Ten years of clinical experience with adult meningitis at an urban academic medical center. *J Emerg Med.* 2006; 30:367-370.
2. Dzupova O, Rozspal H, Prochazka B, Benes J. Acute bacterial meningitis in adult: predictors of outcome. *Scand J Infect Dis.* 2009;41:348-354.
3. Kessler AT, Kourtis AP. Treatment of meningitis caused by methicillin-resistant *Staphylococcus aureus* with linezolid. *Infection.* 2007;35:271-274.
4. Lee DH, Palermo B, Chowdhury M. Successful treatment of methicillin–resistant *Staphylococcus* aureus meningitis with daptomycin. *Clin Infect Dis.* 2008;47: 588-590.

# 9 Viral Infections

---

**Clinical Aspects of Pandemic 2009 Influenza A (H1N1) Virus Infection**

Writing Committee of the WHO Consultation on Clinical Aspects of Pandemic (H1N1) 2009 Influenza (Natl Inst of Respiratory Diseases, Mexico City; Queen Sirikit Natl Inst of Child Health, Bangkok, Thailand; Peking Univ, People's Hosp, Beijing; et al)

*N Engl J Med* 362:1708-1719, 2010

---

As of March 2010, illness caused by the 2009 H1N1 virus had occurred in almost all countries, with more than 16,000 deaths from laboratory-confirmed cases reported to the World Health Organization (WHO). The United States saw an estimated 59 million pandemic H1N1 illnesses, 265,000 hospitalizations, and 12,000 deaths. This review by WHO experts summarizes the virologic, epidemiologic, and clinical data on the 2009 H1N1 virus and assesses future directions.

▶ The 2009 pandemic caused by a novel influenza A (H1N1) virus of swine origin started in Mexico during the spring. After the initial spread to the United States and Canada, the virus spread globally. As of March 2010, more than 17 700 deaths among laboratory-confirmed cases had been reported to the World Health Organization. To date, reassortment of this virus with human influenza viruses has not occurred. The pandemic strain does not carry mutations that are associated with increased pathogenicity in other influenza viruses. Most illnesses were acute and self-limited. The highest attack rates occurred among children and young adults. This is assumed to be because of cross-protective antibodies in adults older than 60 years from infections due to related viruses earlier in life. Household transmission was also lowest among adults older than 50 years.

The mechanisms of transmission, including person-to-person, were similar to those of seasonal influenza. The risk factors for complications due to underlying conditions were similar to that of seasonal influenza. About 25% to 50% of patients with 2009 pandemic influenza leading to hospitalization or death had no reported coexisting medical conditions. Risk of hospitalization among pregnant patients increased by a factor of 4 to 7 compared with age-matched control. Pregnant women were at the highest risk during the third trimester of pregnancy. As compared with seasonal influenza viruses, 2009 H1N1 virus shows higher replication in human bronchial epithelium at 33°C and also in human lung tissue. This observation may explain the ability of the virus to cause severe pneumonitis in humans.

The 2009 H1N1 virus is susceptible to the neuraminidase inhibitors (oseltamivir and zanamivir) but resistant to amantadine and rimantadine. Oseltamivir resistance has been shown to emerge in 96 cases globally. These strains remain susceptible to zanamivir. Intravenous formulation of zanamivir and an investigational neuraminidase inhibitor peramivir are options for critically ill patients, especially those on mechanical ventilation. Peramivir is less active by a factor of at least 80 for oseltamivir-resistant viruses carrying the H275Y mutation than for oseltamivir-susceptible viruses. This knowledge makes intravenous zanamivir the preferred option for patients with suspected or documented oseltamivir-resistant H1N1 influenza virus. A recent report of rapid selection of oseltamivir- and peramivir-resistant pandemic H1N1 virus during therapy is of further concern in this regard.[1]

**N. M. Khardori, MD**

*Reference*

1. Memoli MJ, Hrabal RJ, Hassantoufighi A, Eichelberger MC, Taubenberger JK. Rapid selection of oseltamivir- and peramivir-resistant pandemic H1N1 virus during therapy in 2 immunocompromised Hosts. *Clin Infect Dis*. 2010;50: 1252-1255.

---

## Intravenous Zanamivir for Patients with Pneumonitis due to Pandemic (H1N1) 2009 Influenza Virus

Härter G, Zimmermann O, Maier L, et al (Univ Hosp Ulm Pharmacy, Germany)
*Clin Infect Dis* 50:1249-1251, 2010

We report on 2 critically ill patients with pneumonitis and acute respiratory distress syndrome due to pandemic (H1N1) 2009 influenza A virus who were treated with intravenous zanamivir and had favorable clinical outcomes. Zanamivir given intravenously may be a therapeutic option in patients with critical illness and mechanical ventilation.

► The main causes of death attributable to the H1N1 2009 influenza A pandemic were pneumonitis, respiratory failure, and acute respiratory distress syndrome. Antiviral treatment with neuraminidase inhibitors (oseltamivir or zanamavir) is recommended for patients at higher risk of complications.[1] Oseltamivir is available in oral formulation and zanamavir in inhaled form, both of which may not deliver sufficient drug to critically ill patients on mechanical ventilation. Also H275Y mutation in H1N1 2009 pandemic influenza virus induces oseltamivir resistance. Oseltamivir resistance has been documented in 96 cases so far. Such strains remain susceptible to zanamavir.

The intravenous formulation of zanamavir is in development. This report discusses 2 critically ill patients with pneumonitis and adult respiratory distress syndrome due to H1N1 pandemic influenza A infection. A favorable clinical response was observed in both patients after the compassionate use of intravenous formulation of zanamavir. There were no adverse events from the use of intravenous zanamavir.

Peramivir, a new neuraminidase inhibitor, can be used in adult and pediatric patients after an emergency use authorization by the Food and Drug Administration.[2]

**N. M. Khardori, MD**

*References*

1. Dominguez-Cherit G, Lapinsky SE, Macias AE, et al. Critically ill patients with 2009 influenza A(H1N1) in Mexico. *JAMA*. 2009;302:1880-1887.
2. Birnkrant D, Cox E. The emergency use authorization of peramivir for treatment of 2009 H1N1 influenza. *N Engl J Med*. 2009;361:2204-2207.

---

**Overwhelming Disseminated Herpes Simplex Virus Type 2 Infection in a Patient With Severe Burn Injury: Case Report and Literature Review**

Peppercorn A, Veit L, Sigel C, et al (Univ of North Carolina, Chapel Hill; Memorial Sloan Kettering Cancer Ctr, NY)

*J Burn Care Res* 31:492-498, 2010

---

Viral-mediated organ disease is an infrequent but recognized complication of severe burn injury. This occurs primarily because of herpes family viruses such as cytomegalovirus, herpes simplex virus (HSV), and Epstein-Barr virus given their ability to establish lifelong latency after primary infection and reactivate in the setting of altered immune function. In this report, we describe a severely burned patient who succumbed to fulminant HSV-2 pneumonitis and hepatitis, and summarize the existing literature on HSV infections in this unique patient population. To our knowledge, this is the first report of disseminated visceral HSV-2 infection in a burn patient in the medical literature.

▶ Patients with significant burn wounds experience multiple immune defects, including loss of skin and mucosal barriers. In addition, they suffer from reduced innate, humoral, and cell-mediated immune responses. Bacterial and fungal pathogens are well documented to cause significant morbidity and mortality in burn patients. The role of viral pathogens to morbidity and mortality in this patient population has not been studied. Serious infections caused by herpes simplex virus (HSV) are known to occur in this patient population based on clinical experience and small case studies.

This article reports a severely burned patient who died from fulminant HSV-2 pneumonitis and hepatitis and summarizes the existing literature on HSV infections in burn patients. The incidence of HSV infection in burn patients is surprisingly high—40% in adults and 8% to 25% in pediatric burn patients.[1,2] Most cases occur in patients with extensive burns (mean TBSA burns, 36%). Skin of face and neck are involved in more than 85% of cases consistent with reactivation of latent HSV-1. HSV infection in burn patients was shown to have a significant correlation with patient age >50 years, facial burn, smoke inhalation, full-thickness burn, intubation, and more than 3 weeks of hospital stay.[1] The manifestations of HSV infection in burn patients range from asymptomatic shedding to typical oral vesicular lesions, burn wound infection (including graft, perigrafts, and native skin regions), and infrequent cases of visceral dissemination. Herpetic skin lesion in areas of burn injury may not demonstrate the typical grouped vesicular pattern. They can present as hemorrhagic, purpuric, papulovesicular, pustular, or ulcerative lesions. Prolonged unexplained fever can be an early indication of HSV skin infection before the herpetic lesions erupt. The most common manifestation of HSV organ infection is the involvement of respiratory tract, including larynx, tracheobronchial tree, and lungs.

HSV infection is often either not considered or remains undetected in this patient population and, therefore, remains untreated. HSV pneumonitis and hepatitis are both associated with significant mortality in immunocompromised patients including patients with extensive burns.

The patient in this case report had a long prodrome of unexplained fevers with negative bacterial and fungal cultures until he became infected with a multidrug resistant strain of *Enterobacter cloacae*. Toward the end, he had rapid deterioration with coagulopathy and hypotension indicative of herpetic hepatitis as diagnosed at autopsy. In high-risk burn patients, viral infections, especially due to HSV, should be considered in the differential diagnosis of infectious complication. Presumptive therapy with acyclovir should be considered in patients with a high index of suspicion while waiting for culture and polymerase chain reaction results.

**N. M. Khardori, MD**

*References*

1. Kagan RJ, Naraqi S, Matsuda T, Jonasson OM. Herpes simplex virus and cytomegalovirus infections in burned patients. *J Trauma.* 1985;25:40-45.
2. Linnemann CC Jr, MacMillan BG. Viral infections in pediatric burn patients. *Am J Dis Child.* 1981;135:750-753.

## Acyclovir Resistance in Herpes Simplex Encephalitis

Schulte EC, Sauerbrei A, Hoffmann D, et al (Technische Universität München, Munich; Friedrich Schiller Univ, Jena, Germany)

*Ann Neurol* 67:830-833, 2010

Herpes simplex virus type 1 is a common cause of severe sporadic encephalitis. Treatment with acyclovir is highly effective in this disease. We report the case of a 27-year-old, immunocompetent woman with acyclovir-resistant herpes simplex encephalitis. Although she had not been treated before, herpes simplex virus type 1 DNA from the cerebrospinal fluid showed a non-synonymous mutation in the thymidine kinase gene, which is likely to have caused resistance to acyclovir. Herpes simplex encephalitis resolved after treatment with foscarnet. To our knowledge, this is the first report of acyclovir-resistant herpes simplex virus encephalitis in an immunocompetent, previously therapy-naive adult.

▶ The mortality associated with herpes simplex virus encephalitis has reduced from >70% to 20% by effective antiviral therapy with acyclovir. Resistance to antivirals is uncommon among herpes simplex virus type 1 (HSV-1) in immunocompetent patients and patients not previously treated with acyclovir. The estimated overall prevalence of resistance to acyclovir in HSV-1 is 0.3%.[1]

This article reports an immunocompetent, 27-year-old lady with encephalitis caused by HSV-1 resistance to acyclovir. She had not received acyclovir before. HSV-1 DNA from the cerebrospinal fluid showed a mutation in the thymidine kinase gene, which is known to confer resistance to the antivirals that need intracellular activation by the viral thymidine kinase. This includes acyclovir, valacyclovir, penciclovir, famciclovir, and ganciclovir. The patient in this report responded to foscarnet.

This case report, first of its kind, highlights the possibility of primary acyclovir resistance in HSV-1. Patients not improving after 5 to 6 days of acyclovir therapy should receive a nonnucleoside analog antiviral agent.

**N. M. Khardori, MD**

*Reference*

1. Puchhammer-Stöckl E, Presterl E, Croÿ C, et al. Screening for possible failure of herpes simplex virus PCR in cerebrospinal fluid for the diagnosis of herpes simplex encephalitis. *J Med Virol.* 2001;64:531-536.

# 10 Tuberculosis

## Antigen Load Governs the Differential Priming of CD8 T Cells in Response to the Bacille Calmette Guérin Vaccine or *Mycobacterium tuberculosis* Infection

Ryan AA, Nambiar JK, Wozniak TM, et al (Univ of Sydney, Australia)
*J Immunol* 182:7172-7177, 2009

One reason proposed for the failure of *Mycobacterium bovis* bacille Calmette Guérin (BCG) vaccination to adequately control the spread of tuberculosis is a limited ability of the vaccine to induce effective CD8 T cell responses. However, the relative capacity of the BCG vaccine and virulent *Mycobacterium tuberculosis* to induce activation of CD8 T cells, and the factors that govern the initial priming of these cells after mycobacterial infection, are poorly characterized. Using a TCR transgenic CD8 T cell transfer model, we demonstrate significant activation of Ag-specific CD8 T cells by BCG, but responses were delayed and of reduced magnitude compared with those following infection with *M. tuberculosis*. The degree of CD8 T cell activation was critically dependent on the level of antigenic stimulation, as modifying the infectious dose to achieve comparable numbers of BCG or *M. tuberculosis* in draining lymph nodes led to the same pattern of CD8 T cell responses to both strains. Factors specific to *M. tuberculosis* infection did not influence the priming of CD8 T cells, as codelivery of *M. tuberculosis* with BCG did not alter the magnitude of BCG-induced T cell activation. Following transfer to RAG-1$^{-/-}$ recipients, BCG and *M. tuberculosis*-induced CD8 T cells conferred equivalent levels of protection against *M. tuberculosis* infection. These findings demonstrate that BCG is able to prime functional CD8 T cells, and suggest that effective delivery of Ag to sites of T cell activation by vaccines may be a key requirement for optimal CD8 T cell responses to control mycobacterial infection.

► Cell-mediated immunity mediated by CD4 T cells is known to play a central role in protection against *Mycobacterium tuberculosis*.[1] More recently, CD8 T cells have also been shown to be important in antimycobacterial immunity.[2] Vaccines with mycobacterial antigens encoded by viral vectors induce high levels of protective immunity against experimental tuberculosis. Transfer of apoptotic vesicles from infected macrophages to bystander dendritic cells can stimulate CD8 T cell responses. Mycobacterial antigens from *M tuberculosis* and *M leprae* in the cytosol of dendritic cells allow antigens to be directly presented as MHC class 1 molecules with CD8 T cell activation, a property not shared by the BCG vaccine strain. This could be one reason for its limited protective efficacy.

This study reports on the ability of BCG to prime functional CD8 cells if effective delivery of antigen to sites of T cell activation by the vaccine is achieved. This was accomplished by using a TCR transgenic CD8 T cell transfer model. The Ag-specific CD8 T cell activation by BCG was significant but delayed and of reduced magnitude compared with those following *M tuberculosis* infection. The reduced response by BCG was associated with reduced bacterial load in the draining lymph nodes at the time of T cell priming. The delivery of equivalent number of BCG and *M tuberculosis* to the draining lymph nodes resulted in equivalent CD8 T cell responses leading to the conclusion that antigen load is the key determinant of CD8 T cell activation after mycobacterial infection. BCG and *M tuberculosis*–induced CD8 T cells conferred equivalent levels of protection to mice against *M tuberculosis* challenge. These data suggest that vaccine strategies to enhance the delivery of protective antigens to processing sites would lead to better efficacy and protection.

**N. M. Khardori, MD**

*References*

1. Mogues T, Goodrich ME, Ryan L, La Course R, North RJ. The relative importance of T cell subsets in immunity and immunopathology of airborne *Mycobacterium tuberculosis* infection in mice. *J Exp Med.* 2001;193:271-280.
2. McShane HA, Pathan A, Sander CR, et al. Recombinant modified vaccinia virus Ankara expressing antigen 85A boosts BCG-primed and naturally acquired antimycobacterial immunity in humans. *Nat Med.* 2004;10:1240-1244.

---

## Rapid Diagnosis of Tuberculous Meningitis by T Cell–Based Assays on Peripheral Blood and Cerebrospinal Fluid Mononuclear Cells

Kim S-H, Cho O-H, Park S-J, et al (Univ of Ulsan College of Medicine, Seoul, Republic of Korea)
*Clin Infect Dis* 50:1349-1358, 2010

---

*Background.*—The role of the new *Myocbacterium tuberculosis*–specific enzyme-linked immunosorbent spot (ELISPOT) assay for diagnosis of tuberculous meningitis (TBM) has not yet been fully assessed. Here, we conducted a prospective, blinded, observational study to evaluate the diagnostic accuracy of this assay, compared with the conventional tests, for diagnosing TBM.

*Methods.*—All adult patients with suspected TBM were enrolled at a tertiary care hospital (Seoul, South Korea) during a 12-month period. ELISPOT assays were performed on peripheral mononuclear cells and mononuclear cells from cerebrospinal fluid (CSF).

*Results.*—Eighty-nine patients with suspected TBM were enrolled. Of these, 31 (35%) were classified as having TBM (10 confirmed, 6 highly probable, and 15 probable cases), and 55 (62%) were classified as not having active tuberculosis. The remaining 3 (3%) with possible TBM were excluded from the final analysis. The sensitivities and specificities,

TABLE 5.—Diagnostic Accuracy of Diagnosis of Tuberculosis (TB) Meningitis in 86 Patients with Suspected TB Meningitis

| Population, Assay | Sensitivity[a] Proportion | Sensitivity[a] Percentage (95% CI) | Specificity[b] Proportion | Specificity[b] Percentage (95% CI) | PPV, % (95% CI) | NPV, % (95% CI) | Positive Likelihood Ratio (95% CI) | Negative Likelihood Ratio (95% CI) |
|---|---|---|---|---|---|---|---|---|
| All patients ($n = 86$) | | | | | | | | |
| Tuberculin skin test result ≥10 mm | 7/31 | 23 (10–41) | 39/45 | 87 (73–95) | 54 (25–81) | 62 (49–74) | 1.69 (0.63–4.56) | 0.90 (0.72–1.12) |
| PBMC ELISPOT ≥6 spots | 22/31 | 71 (51–86) | 30/53 | 57 (42–70) | 49 (34–64) | 77 (61–89) | 1.64 (1.12–2.39) | 0.51 (0.28–0.93) |
| CSF-MC ELISPOT ≥6 spots | 13/22 | 59 (36–79 | 25/28 | 89 (72–98) | 81 (54–96) | 74 (56–87) | 5.52 (1.79–16.98) | 0.46 (0.27–0.77) |
| CSF ADA level >5.8 IU/L | 23/26 | 89 (69–98) | 37/51 | 73 (58–84) | 62 (45–78) | 93 (79–98) | 3.22 (2.02–5.14) | 0.16 (0.05–0.47) |
| CSF/serum glucose ratio ≤0.44 | 20/27 | 74 (54–89) | 35/51 | 69 (54–81) | 56 (38–72) | 83 (69–93) | 2.36 (1.49–3.75) | 0.38 (0.19–0.73) |
| PBMC ELISPOT or CSF ADA >5.8 IU/L | 29/31 | 94 (79–99) | 25/55 | 46 (32–59) | 49 (36–63) | 93 (76–99) | 1.72 (1.32–2.22) | 0.14 (0.03–0.55) |
| CSF-MC ELISPOT assay performed ($n = 50$) | | | | | | | | |
| Tuberculin skin test result ≥10 mm | 2/22 | 9 (1–29) | 21/23 | 91 (72–99) | 50 (7–67) | 51 (35–67) | 1.05 (0.16–6.79) | 0.99 (0.82–1.19) |
| PBMC ELISPOT ≥6 spots | 15/22 | 68 (45–86) | 17/26 | 65 (44–83) | 63 (41–81) | 71 (49–87) | 1.97 (1.08–3.59) | 0.48 (0.24–0.95) |
| CSF-MC ELISPOT ≥6 spots | 13/22 | 59 (39–79) | 25/28 | 89 (72–98) | 81 (54–96) | 74 (56–87) | 5.52 (1.79–16.98) | 0.46 (0.27–0.77) |
| CSF ADA >5.8 IU/L | 19/21 | 91 (69–99) | 16/27 | 59 (39–78) | 63 (44–80) | 89 (65–99) | 2.22 (1.38–3.57) | 0.16 (0.04–0.62) |
| CSF/serum glucose ratio ≤0.44 | 17/22 | 77 (55–92) | 17/27 | 63 (42–81) | 63 (42–81) | 77 (55–92) | 2.09 (1.21–3.59) | 0.36 (0.16–0.82) |
| PBMC ELISPOT or CSF ADA level >5.8 IU/L | 21/22 | 96 (77–99) | 14/28 | 50 (31–69) | 60 (42–76) | 93 (68–99) | 1.91 (1.30–2.79) | 0.09 (0.01–0.64) |
| Only PBMC ELISPOT assay performed ($n = 36$) | | | | | | | | |
| Tuberculin skin test results ≥10 mm | 5/9 | 56 (21–86) | 18/22 | 82 (59–95) | 56 (21–86) | 82 (59–95) | 3.06 (1.06–8.83) | 0.54 (0.25–1.16) |
| PBMC ELISPOT ≥6 spots | 7/9 | 78 (39–97) | 13/27 | 48 (29–68) | 33 (15–57) | 87 (59–98) | 1.50 (0.91–2.48) | 0.46 (0.12–1.67) |
| CSF ADA >5.8 level IU/L | 4/5 | 80 (28–99) | 21/24 | 88 (68–97) | 57 (18–90) | 95 (77–99) | 6.40 (2.04–20.12) | 0.23 (0.04–1.33) |
| CSF/serum glucose ratio ≤0.44 | 3/5 | 60 (15–95) | 18/24 | 75 (53–90) | 33 (7–70) | 90 (68–99) | 2.40 (0.89–6.49) | 0.53 (0.17–1.59) |
| PBMC ELISPOT or CSF ADA level >5.8 IU/L | 8/9 | 89 (52–99) | 11/27 | 41 (22–61) | 33 (16–99) | 92 (61–99) | 1.50 (1.02–2.21) | 0.27 (0.04–1.82) |

NOTE. ADA, adenosine deaminase; CI, confidence interval; CSF, cerebrospinal fluid; CSF-MC, cerebrospinal fluid-mononuclear cell; ELISPOT, enzyme-linked immunosorbent spot; NPV, negative predictive value; PBMC, peripheral blood mononuclear cell; PPV, positive predictive value; TB, tuberculosis.

[a]Sensitivity is determined by dividing the no of patients with a positive test result by the no of patients tested.

[b]Specificity is determined by dividing the no of patients with a negative test result by the no of patients tested.

respectively, of the tested methods for diagnosing TBM were as follows: CSF adenosine deaminase level >5.8 U/L, 89% (95% confidence interval [CI], 69%–98%) and 73% (95% CI, 58%–84%); peripheral mononuclear cells ELISPOT, 71% (95% CI, 51%–86%) and 57% (95% CI, 42%–70%); and CSF mononuclear cells ELISPOT assay, 59% (95% CI, 36%–79%) and 89% (95% CI, 72%–98%). The combined sensitivity of an adenosine deaminase level >5.8 U/L or a positive peripheral mononuclear cells ELISPOT assay result was 94% (95% CI, 79%–99%), conferring a negative likelihood ratio of 0.14 (95% CI, 0.03–0.55) when both test results were negative.

*Conclusion.*—ELISPOT assays using peripheral mononuclear cells and CSF mononuclear cells are useful adjuncts to the current tests for diagnosing TBM, particularly when used in combination with the assessment, of adenosine deaminase level in CSF (Table 5).

▶ The initiation of antituberculous therapy in tuberculous meningitis (TBM) is often delayed and has been associated with high mortality rates.[1] The results of routine analysis of cerebrospinal fluid (CSF) are usually not helpful in suspecting TBM, and the conventional diagnostic tests are relatively insensitive and time consuming. A new generation of diagnostic assays using *Mycobacterium tuberculosis*-specific antigens encoded by genes located in the region of difference 1 has shown promising results in the diagnosis of latent TB infection and active pulmonary or extrapulmonary TB disease.[2] Most of the studies have used peripheral blood mononuclear cells (PBMCs) for these assays. Mononuclear cells that are compartmentalized at the sites of infection (eg, pleural fluid, bronchoalveolar fluid, and CSF) have higher interferon-γ response rates compared to PBMCs.

In this study, there were 89 adult patients with suspected TBM. Of these, 31 patients were subsequently classified as having TBM (10 confirmed, 6 highly probable, and 15 probable cases). Enzyme-linked immunosorbent spot (ELISPOT) assays were performed on PBMCs and mononuclear cells from CSF. Diagnostic accuracy of various tests is shown in Table 5. The sensitivity of CSF adenosine deaminase (> 5.8 U/L), PBMC ELISPOT, and CSF mononuclear cell ELISPOT was 89%, 71%, and 59%, respectively. The sensitivity of the combination of CSF adenosine deaminase (> 5.8 U/L) or a positive PBMC ELISPOT assay was 94% with a negative likelihood ratio of 0.14 when both results are negative. The results indicate that ELISPOT assays of PBMC and CSF mononuclear cells are useful adjuncts for the diagnosis of TBM, especially in combination with adenosine deaminase levels in CSF.

**N. M. Khardori, MD**

*References*

1. Thwaites G, Fisher M, Hemingway C, et al. British Infection Society guidelines for the diagnosis and treatment of tuberculosis of the central nerve system in adults and children. *J Infect*. 2009;59:167-187.
2. Pai M, Riley LW, Colford JM Jr. Interferon-gamma assays in the immunodiagnosis of tuberculosis: a systematic review. *Lancet Infect Dis*. 2004;4:761-776.

# 11 Fungal Infections

**Antifungal Susceptibility Testing of *Candida* Isolates from the Candida Surveillance Study**

Lyon GM, Karatela S, Sunay S, et al (Emory Univ School of Medicine, Atlanta, GA)

*J Clin Microbiol* 48:1270-1275, 2010

*Candida* species are a common cause of nosocomial bloodstream infections. Recent surveillance has shown an increase in the relative proportion of infections caused by *Candida glabrata*, which has reduced susceptibility to fluconazole. We undertook sentinel surveillance with antifungal susceptibility testing to monitor the trends in the proportions of various *Candida* species causing invasive disease. Forty-one institutions participated in the Candida Surveillance Study. All isolates were submitted to a central laboratory for identification and susceptibility testing. Susceptibility testing was performed in compliance with CLSI guidelines using a custom, broth dilution, microtiter system. There were 5,900 isolates submitted for identification and antifungal susceptibility testing. The distribution of species was as follows: *C. albicans*, 2,567 (43.5%) isolates; *C. glabrata*, 1,464 (24.8%) isolates; *C. parapsilosis*, 1,048 (17.8%) isolates; *C. tropicalis*, 527 (8.9%) isolates; *C. krusei*, 109 (1.9%) isolates; *C. lusitaniae*, 76 (1.3%) isolates; and other *Candida* species, 109 (1.9%) isolates. Resistance to fluconazole occurred in 1.2% of *C. albicans* isolates, 5.9% of *C. glabrata* isolates, 0.3% of *C. parapsilosis* isolates, and 0.4% of *C. tropicalis* isolates. Resistance to fluconazole was highly predictive of resistance to voriconazole. Resistance to echinocandins was rarely found, occurring in only 0.2% of all isolates. The rate of fluconazole susceptibility increased significantly from 87.5% in 2005 to 97.4% in 2007. The proportion of cases of disease caused by various *Candida* species did not change appreciably between 2004 and 2007, and the rate of antifungal susceptibility was high.

▶ *Candida albicans* and other species of *Candida* have become important nosocomial pathogens in the past 2 decades.[1] A shift of *C albicans* toward *Candida glabrata* infections has also been shown in a number of studies. This has clinical relevance because of the fact that *C glabrata* is less susceptible to fluconazole.

This is a sentinel surveillance study looking at changing trends in the species distribution and antifungal susceptibility of *Candida* species from invasive infections. *C albicans* comprised 43% and *C glabrata* 25% of the isolates

(Fig 1 in the original article). Fluconazole resistance was demonstrated in 1.2% of *C albicans* isolates and 5.9% of *C glabrata* isolates, which was also highly predictive of voriconazole resistance. Only 0.2% of all isolates were resistant to echinocandins. Because *C glabrata* and *C krusei* are more likely to be resistant to fluconazole, the authors recommend the initial use of echinocandins in institutions with high proportion of cases of invasive candidiasis carried by these 2 species. Once the species is known, therapy can be changed to fluconazole for *C albicans, C parapsilosis*, and *C tropicalis*.

**N. M. Khardori, MD**

*Reference*

1. Trick WE, Fridkin SK, Edwards JR, Hajjeh RA, Gaynes RP. Secular trend of hospital acquired candidemia among intensive care unit patients in the United States during 1989–1999. *Clin Infect Dis*. 2002;35:627-630.

## Bacterial Coinfection and Antimicrobial Resistance in Patients With Paranasal Sinus Fungus Balls

Wang JH, Lee B-J, Jang YJ (Univ of Ulsan College of Medicine, Seoul, Korea)
*Ann Otol Rhinol Laryngol* 119:406-411, 2010

*Objectives.*—The aim of this study was to investigate the incidence of bacterial coinfection and antimicrobial resistance in cases of fungus balls of the paranasal sinuses.

*Methods.*—Between December 1991 and August 2008, 229 patients underwent endoscopic sinus surgery or the Caldwell-Luc procedure for paranasal sinus fungus ball treatment. From 123 of these patients, a total of 124 specimens were obtained for aerobic and anaerobic culture. Antimicrobial susceptibility tests were performed.

*Results.*—Ninety-one cultures (73.4%) were positive for bacteria, and 33 showed no bacterial growth. A total of 134 bacterial organisms were isolated: 65 gram-positive, 55 gram-negative, and 14 anaerobic. The most frequently isolated organisms were coagulase-negative *Staphylococcus* (14.9%), *Staphylococcus aureus* (12.7%), *Enterobacter aerogenes* (12.7%), viridans-group streptococci (8.9%), and *Pseudomonas aeruginosa* (8.2%). Among the gram-positive cocci, 12.2% were resistant to ciprofloxacin, 27.6% to clindamycin, 30% to oxacillin, 35.8% to erythromycin, 35.9% to trimethoprim-sulfamethoxazole, 56.5% to penicillin, 56.8% to gentamicin, and 0% to teicoplanin and vancomycin. Among the gram-negative rods, fewer than 10% were resistant to imipenem, piperacillin-tazobactam, amikacin, gentamicin, ceftazidime, cefepime, and tobramycin, whereas more than 80% showed resistance to ampicillin and cefazolin. When we compared the data from the periods 1991 to 2000 and 2001 to 2008, there were no significant differences in the isolation rates of particular bacterial species and no significant differences in resistance rates except for clindamycin-resistant gram-positive cocci and cefazolin-resistant gram-negative rods.

*Conclusions.*—Bacterial coinfections were identified in more than two thirds of patients with fungus balls and purulent secretions. This finding suggests that bacterial infection may influence the development and persistence of clinical symptoms in a substantial portion of fungus ball cases.

▶ Noninvasive form of fungal sinusitis due to fungus balls causes long-lasting nonspecific symptoms similar to those of chronic rhinosinusitis (CRS).[1] *Aspergillus fumigatus* is the most common organism seen in fungus balls. Current treatment of choice is removal of the fungus ball by endoscopic surgery. Incomplete removal of the fungal load seems to be the major cause of recurrence. The investigators in this study found purulent secretions similar to those in bacterial rhinosinusitis in the paranasal sinuses of patients with fungus balls. They investigated the incidence of bacterial coinfection and antimicrobial resistance among bacterial isolates from purulent secretions in patients with fungus balls. Of the 124 specimens, 91 (73.4%) grew bacteria. Of the 134 bacteria isolated, 65 were gram positive, 55 were gram negative, and 14 were anaerobic (Table 2 in the original article). Antibiotic resistance was common among both gram-positive and gram-negative isolates. In comparison to similar data on CRS from 1991 to 2000, the results from 2001 to 2008 did not show significant difference in the isolation rates of particular bacterial species and their antimicrobial susceptibility patterns except for clindamycin-resistant gram-positive cocci and cefazolin resistant gram-negative bacilli.

Concomitant bacterial infection may explain the persistence of symptoms in large numbers of patients with fungus balls. In addition to known pathogens, the isolation of coagulase-negative staphylococci (CNS) in 15% of cultures and their resistance to multiple antibiotics may need to be considered in managing these patients. CNS have been suggested as a true pathogen in chronic sinusitis.[2] This study does not address the issue of antibacterial therapy before or after surgical removal of the fungus ball.

**N. M. Khardori, MD**

*References*

1. deShazo RD, Chapin K, Swain RE. Fungal sinusitis. *N Engl J Med.* 1997;337: 254-259.
2. Nadel DM, Lanza DC, Kennedy DW. Endoscopically guided cultures in chronic sinusitis. *Am J Rhinol.* 1998;12:233-241.

## Invasive Fungal Infections among Organ Transplant Recipients: Results of the Transplant-Associated Infection Surveillance Network (TRANSNET)

Pappas PG, Alexander BD, Andes DR, et al (Univ of Alabama at Birmingham Med Ctr; Duke Univ Med Ctr, Durham, NC; Univ of Wisconsin, Madison; et al)
*Clin Infect Dis* 50:1101-1111, 2010

*Background.*—Invasive fungal infections (IFIs) are a major cause of morbidity and mortality among organ transplant recipients. Multicenter prospective surveillance data to determine disease burden and secular trends are lacking.

*Methods.*—The Transplant-Associated Infection Surveillance Network (TRANSNET) is a consortium of 23 US transplant centers, including 15 that contributed to the organ transplant recipient dataset. We prospectively identified IFIs among organ transplant recipients from March, 2001 through March, 2006 at these sites. To explore trends, we calculated the 12-month cumulative incidence among 9 sequential cohorts.

*Results.*—During the surveillance period, 1208 IFIs were identified among 1063 organ transplant recipients. The most common IFIs were invasive candidiasis (53%), invasive aspergillosis (19%), cryptococcosis (8%), non-*Aspergillus* molds (8%), endemic fungi (5%), and zygomycosis (2%). Median time to onset of candidiasis, aspergillosis, and cryptococcosis was 103, 184, and 575 days, respectively. Among a cohort of 16,808 patients who underwent transplantation between March 2001 and September 2005 and were followed through March 2006, a total of 729 IFIs were reported among 633 persons. One-year cumulative incidences of the first IFI were 11.6%, 8.6%, 4.7%, 4.0%, 3.4%, and 1.3% for small bowel, lung, liver, heart, pancreas, and kidney transplant recipients, respectively. One-year incidence was highest for invasive candidiasis (1.95%) and aspergillosis (0.65%). Trend analysis showed a slight increase in cumulative incidence from 2002 to 2005.

*Conclusions.*—We detected a slight increase in IFIs during the surveillance period. These data provide important insights into the timing and incidence of IFIs among organ transplant recipients, which can help to focus effective prevention and treatment strategies (Table 2).

▶ Post-transplantation infections, especially invasive fungal infections (IFIs), remain a significant cause for morbidity and mortality in organ transplant recipients. The most common fungal organisms in this setting are *Candida* species, *Cryptococcus neoformans*, *Aspergillus* species, and Zygomycetes.[1] Compared with patients with bone marrow transplantation, the in-depth understanding of the overall burden of IFIs in this population is lacking.

The Transplant-Associated Infection Surveillance network was established in 2001 as a consortium of 23 US transplant centers. This multicenter prospective data is collected from 15 of these centers.

During a 5-year (2001-2006) surveillance period, 1208 IFIs were identified among 1063 organ transplant recipients (Table 2). Small bowel and lung transplant recipients showed the highest 1-year incidence of IFIs, the most common

TABLE 2.—No. (%) of Invasive Fungal Infection (IFI) Cases in the Surveillance Cohort, by Transplant Type

| IFI Type | Kidney ($n = 332$) | Liver ($n = 378$) | Pancreas ($n = 128$) | Lung ($n = 248$) | Heart ($n = 99$) | Small Bowel ($n = 22$) |
|---|---|---|---|---|---|---|
| Candidiasis | 164 (49) | 255 (68) | 97 (76) | 56 (23) | 48 (49) | 19 (85) |
| Aspergillosis | 47 (14) | 42 (11) | 6 (5) | 109 (44) | 23 (23) | 0 (0) |
| Zygomycosis | 8 (2) | 9 (2) | 0 (0) | 8 (3) | 3 (3) | 0 (0) |
| Other mold | 10 (3.0) | 9 (2.4) | 4 (3.1) | 49 (19.8) | 7 (7.1) | 0 (0.0) |
| Unspecified mold | 7 (2.1) | 8 (2.1) | 0 (0.0) | 7 (2.8) | 2 (2.0) | 0 (0.0) |
| Cryptococcosis | 49 (15) | 24 (6) | 6 (5) | 6 (2) | 10 (10) | 1 (5) |
| Endemic mycoses | 33 (10) | 17 (5) | 8 (6) | 3 (1) | 3 (3) | 0 (0) |
| Pneumocystosis | 5 (1) | 0 (0) | 1 (1) | 4 (2) | 3 (3) | 0 (0) |
| Other yeast | 6 (1.8) | 9 (2.4) | 5 (3.9) | 0 (0.0) | 0 (0.0) | 1 (5) |
| Unspecified yeast | 3 (0.9) | 5 (1.3) | 1 (0.8) | 6 (2.4) | 0 (0.0) | 1 (5) |

being invasive candidiasis. IFIs typically occurred > 3 months after transplantation: a large number occurred > 1 year after transplantation, and 25% of IFIs developed > 3 years after transplantation. Overall, invasive candidiasis was the most common IFIs in all, except lung transplant patients. *Candida albicans* and *Candida glabrata* were the dominant species in patients with invasive candidiasis.

This first study to evaluate secular trends of IFIs among organ transplant recipients using cumulative incidence provides much needed information in this area.

The data have significant implications for future studies and for strategies toward the early diagnosis and prevention of IFIs in this diverse, growing, and highly immunocompromised patient population.

**N. M. Khardori, MD**

*Reference*

1. Singh N. Fungal infections in the recipients of solid organ transplantation. *Infect Dis Clin North Am*. 2003;17:113-134.

**Investigation of blood culture-negative early prosthetic valve endocarditis reveals high prevalence of fungi**

Thuny F, Fournier P-E, Casalta J-P, et al (Université de la Méditerranée, Marseille, France; Hôpital de la Timone, Marseille, France)

*Heart* 96:743-747, 2010

*Context.*—Early prosthetic valve endocarditis is a deadly disease and blood cultures remain negative in 14–30% of cases.

*Objectives.*—To analyse the clinical and microbiological profile of patients with blood culture-negative (BCN) early prosthetic valve endocarditis (PVE) in order to define the most appropriate empiric treatment.

*Design, Setting and Participants.*—From June 2001 to February 2009, a prospective multimodal strategy incorporating serological, molecular and histopathological assays was performed in all the samples referred to the laboratory for a suspicion of blood culture-negative endocarditis (BCNE) from France and abroad (n=718). A total of 31 patients with BCN early PVE was identified. Their microbiological profile was compared with that of 22 patients with blood culture-positive (BCP) early PVE and 628 patients with community-acquired BCNE identified during the same period.

*Results.*—A pathogen was identified in 10 patients (32%) with BCN early PVE. Fungi were the most common pathogens identified, being found in 16% versus 4.5% in the case of PBC early PVE and 0.5% in community-acquired BCNE (p<0.001). The global microbiological profile of BCN early PVE differed strongly from that of PBC early PVE and community-acquired BCNE. A higher rate of microbiological diagnosis was obtained in patients who underwent surgery (9/21 (43%) vs 1/10 (10%), p=0.07) and an increased rate of recurrences was observed when a pathogen could not be identified (9/21 (43%) vs 1/10 (10%), p=0.07).

*Conclusions.*—BCN early PVE exhibits specific aetiologies as fungi are the most frequent pathogens identified. Therefore, fungi should be investigated particularly by molecular methods on surgical specimens and an antifungal drug might be added to the empiric treatment (Table 3).

► The incidence of prosthetic valve endocarditis (PVE) is reported to be 0.3% to 1% per patient year[1] and represents more than 20% of all infective endocarditis. Early postoperative endocarditis occurs within the first year following valve surgery. The most frequent organisms grown in the blood are

**TABLE 3.**—Comparison of Microbiological Profile According to the Type of Infective Endocarditis

| | BCN Early PVE n=31 | BCP Early PVE* n=22 | Community-Acquired BCNE* n=628 | p Value† |
|---|---|---|---|---|
| Staphylococci | 0 (0%) | 12 (54.5%) | 13 (2%) | <0.0001 |
| Streptococci | 3 (10%) | 3 (14%) | 28 (4.5%) | 0.07 |
| Enterococci | 0 (0%) | 3 (14%) | 0 (0%) | <0.0001 |
| Fungi | 5 (16%) | 1 (4.5%) | 3 (0.5%) | <0.0001 |
| *Coxiella burnetii* | 0 (0%) | 0 (0%) | 229 (36.5%) | <0.0001 |
| *Bartonella* spp | 0 (0%) | 0 (0%) | 86 (14%) | 0.002 |
| *Legionella* spp | 1 (3%) | 0 (0%) | 1 (0.2%) | 0.008 |
| *Tropheryma whipplei* | 0 (0%) | 0 (0%) | 12 (2%) | 0.60 |
| Others | 1 (3%) | 3 (14%) | 29 (5%) | 0.14 |
| No diagnosis | 21 (68%) | NA | 227 (36%) | 0.0004 |

BCP, blood culture-positive; NA, not available.

*Data only from the Department of Cardiology (Timone Hospital, Marseille, France) during the same period.

†All the comparisons were made between the three groups but for the 'no diagnosis' variable in which only blood culture-negative (BCN) early prosthetic valve endocarditis (PVE) and community-acquired blood culture-negative endocarditis (BCNE) groups were compared.

staphylococci, gram-negative bacilli, enterococci, and fungi. Recent series showed that blood cultures remain negative in 14% to 30% of cases. Most guidelines recommend empiric antibiotic selection based on the pathogens in culture-positive PVE. The American Heart Association guidelines recommend a combination of vancomycin, gentamicin, and cefepime.[2]

This study analyses the clinical and microbiological profile of patients with culture-negative early PVE using a prospective multimodal strategy. Serological, histopathological, and molecular assays were performed on all samples referred to the laboratory between 2001 and 2009. Extensive workups led to identification of a pathogen in 10 patients (32%), with blood culture-negative early PVE (Table 3).

Fungi were the most common pathogens identified (16%). This study showed that pathogens found in blood culture-negative early PVE do not mirror those of blood culture-positive early PVE. The addition of antifungal therapy in patients not responding to empiric antibacterial therapy should be considered, especially given the fact that fungi are the second most frequently identified pathogen in all early PVEs.[3]

**N. M. Khardori, MD**

*References*

1. Wang A, Athan E, Pappas PA, et al. Contemporary clinical profile and outcome of prosthetic valve endocarditis. *JAMA*. 2007;297:1354-1361.
2. Baddour LM, Wilson WR, Bayer AS, et al. Infective endocarditis: diagnosis, antimicrobial therapy, and management of complications: a statement for healthcare professionals from the Committee on Rheumatic Fever, Endocarditis, and Kawasaki Disease, Council on Cardiovascular Disease in the Young, and the councils on Clinical Cardiology, Stroke, and Cardiovascular Surgery and Anesthesia, American Heart Association: endorsed by the Infectious Disease Society of America. *Circulation*. 2005;111:e394-e434.
3. López J, Revilla A, Vilacosta L, et al. Definition, clinical profile, microbiological spectrum, and prognostic factors of early-onset prosthetic valve endocarditis. *Eur Heart J*. 2007;28:760-765.

## Current Management of Pyogenic Liver Abscess: Surgery is Now Second-Line Treatment

Mezhir JJ, Fong Y, Jacks LM, et al (Memorial Sloan-Kettering Cancer Ctr, NY)
*J Am Coll Surg* 210:975-983, 2010

*Background.*—The objective of this study was to examine the current treatment for liver abscess and to assess the factors associated with failure of percutaneous drainage.

*Study Design.*—Records of 58 patients with pyogenic hepatic abscess, from 1998 to 2009, were examined. Clinicopathologic variables were analyzed as predictors of failure of percutaneous drainage using multivariable logistic regression. The results of surgical intervention after failure of percutaneous treatment were also examined.

*Results.*—Fifty-one patients (88%) had a history of malignancy including pancreas (36%), cholangiocarcinoma (17%), colon (12%), and gallbladder (10%). Recent hepatic artery embolization or radiofrequency ablation preceded development of abscess in 13 patients (22%). Fifteen patients (26%) had evidence of biliary tract communication, and 14 of 15 (93%) of these patients had concomitant biliary tract obstruction. Percutaneous drainage was successful in 38 patients (66%) with a median drain dwell time of 26 days (range 3 to 319 days). Five patients (9%) required operative intervention and 2 of these patients (3% overall) died postoperatively from septic complications. Fifteen patients (26%) died with percutaneous drains in place; 9 (60%) of these patients died of cancer progression without evidence of sepsis. Independent predictors of failure of percutaneous drainage included abscesses containing yeast ($p = 0.003$) and communication of the abscess cavity with the biliary tree ($p = 0.02$).

*Conclusions.*—Pyogenic hepatic abscess was treated successfully in the majority of patients with advanced malignancy, although mortality remained high. The presence of yeast and communication with an untreated obstructed biliary tree were associated with failure of percutaneous drainage. The need for surgical salvage was associated with a high mortality.

▶ The etiological spectrum and the management of pyogenic liver abscess (PLA) have both seen a shift in recent years. The overall incidence of PLA has decreased, and the most common cause has shifted from portal seeding from appendicitis and diverticulitis to malignant biliary disease. Use of percutaneous drainage is now the preferred first-line management in addition to antibiotics. Abscesses related to benign disease, especially larger and multiloculated abscesses have been shown to have better clinical outcomes with early operative intervention.[1]

This is a retrospective study of 58 patients with PLAs (1998-2009). A history of pancreatic, biliary tract, and gall bladder malignancy was present in 88% of the patients. Percutaneous drainage of abscesses was successful in 66% of the patients, 5 patients (9%) required surgical intervention and 2 of these patients died postoperatively from septic complications.

The presence of yeast in the abscess and communication with an unresolved biliary obstruction were associated with failure of percutaneous drainage. The authors conclude that percutaneous drainage is a safe and effective first-line treatment for the management of PLA patients with biliary tract communication, and concomitant biliary obstruction should have biliary drainage in addition to percutaneous abscess drainage. Operative intervention as a second-line treatment should be considered when clinically indicated and for abscesses that grow yeast.

**N. M. Khardori, MD**

*Reference*

1. Tan YM, Chung AY, Chow PK, et al. An appraisal of surgical and percutaneous drainage for pyogenic liver abscesses larger than 5 cm. *Ann Surg*. 2005;241: 485-490.

## ***Candida albicans*** **Hyr1p Confers Resistance to Neutrophil Killing and Is a Potential Vaccine Target**

Luo G, Ibrahim AS, Spellberg B, et al (Los Angeles Biomed Res Inst at Harber-UCLA Med Ctr Torrance, CA; et al)
*J Infect Dis* 201:1718-1728, 2010

*Candida albicans* is the most common cause of invasive fungal infections in humans. It is unclear how *C. albicans* escapes from phagocytic attack and survives in the hostile blood environment during life-threatening systemic infections. Using a conditional overexpression or suppression genetic strategy, we discovered that *HYR1* gene reduced phagocytic killing activity of *C. albicans* in vitro and increased tissue fungal burden in vivo. Concordant with its positive regulation by the transcription factor Bcr1p, autonomous expression of *HYR1* complemented the hypersusceptibility to phagocyte-mediated killing of a *bcr1* null mutant of *C. albicans* in vitro. As for *C. albicans*, heterologous expression of *HYR1* in *Candida glabrata* rendered the organism more resistant to neutrophil killing activity. Vaccination with a recombinant Hyr1p significantly protected mice against hematogenously disseminated candidiasis ($P = .001$). Finally, anti-rHyr1p polyclonal antibodies enhanced mouse neutrophil killing activity by directly neutralizing rHyr1p effects in vitro. Thus, Hyr1 is an important virulence factor for *C. albicans*, mediating resistance to phagocyte killing. Hyr1p is a promising target for vaccine or other immunological or small molecule intervention to improve the outcomes of disseminated candidiasis.

► The first-line host defense against invasive infections by *Candida albicans* is the phagocytic activity of neutrophils and the monocyte-macrophage system.[1,2] Quantitative and/or qualitative defects in phagocytic activity is a major risk factor for disseminated candidiasis. Resistance of *C albicans* to phagocytic killing is a significant virulence factor of the organism.

The critical interface between *C albicans* and host defense mechanisms is the cell surface glycosyl phosphatidylinositol (GPI)-anchored proteins. Their involvement in resistance to phagocytosis is likely. In this study, the investigators screened for conditional overexpression or suppression system focusing on GPI-anchored proteins in *C albicans*. They found that *HYR1* (a hyphae coexpressed gene) reduced phagocytic killing of *C albicans* in vitro and increased fungal burden of tissues in vivo, defining this protein as a virulence factor. Heterogeneous expression of *HYR1* in *Candida glabrata* rendered the organism more resistant to phagocytic killing. To explore the vaccine potential of this protein, recombinant Hyr1p (rHyr1p) was shown to protect mice against experimental disseminated candidiasis. Antibodies against rHyr1p enhanced the neutrophils' killing activity by directly neutralizing the effects of rHyr1p in vitro. The data are significant in opening the field for studies of such proteins as vaccines or small molecule therapeutic agents.

**N. M. Khardori, MD**

*References*

1. Spellberg BJ, Filler SG, Edwards JE Jr. Current treatment strategies for disseminated candidiasis. *Clin Infect Dis*. 2006;42:244-251.
2. Stone HH. Studies in the pathogenesis, diagnosis and treatment of Candida sepsis in children. *J Pediatr Surg*. 1974;9:127-133.

---

## Interactions between Human Phagocytes and *Candida albicans* Biofilms Alone and in Combination with Antifungal Agents

Katragkou A, Kruhlak MJ, Simitsopoulou M, et al (Aristotle Univ Med School, Thessaloniki, Greece; Natl Cancer Inst, Bethesda, MD; et al)
*J Infect Dis* 201:1941-1949, 2010

---

*Background.*—Biofilm formation is an important component of vascular catheter infections caused by *Candida albicans*. Little is known about the interactions between human phagocytes, antifungal agents, and *Candida* biofilms.

*Methods.*—The interactions between *C. albicans* biofilms and human phagocytes alone and in combination with anidulafungin or voriconazole were investigated and compared with their corresponding planktonic counterparts by means of an in vitro biofilm model with clinical intravascular and green fluorescent protein (GFP)–expressing strains. Phagocyte-mediated and antifungal agent–mediated damages were determined by 2,3-bis[2-methoxy-4nitro-5-sulfophenyl]2H- tetrazolium-5-carboxanilide assay, and structural effects were visualized by confocal microscopy. Oxidative burst was evaluated by flow cytometric measurement of dihydrorhodamine 123 oxidation, and cytokine release was measured by enzyme-linked immunosorbent assay.

*Results.*—Phagocytes alone and in combination with antifungal agents induced less damage against biofilms compared with planktonic cells. However, additive effects occurred between phagocytes and anidulafungin against *Candida* biofilms. Confocal microscopy demonstrated the absence of phagocytosis within biofilms but marked destruction caused by anidulafungin and phagocytes. Anidulafungin but not voriconazole elicited tumor necrosis factor $\alpha$ release from phagocytes compared with that from untreated biofilms.

*Conclusions.*—*C. albicans* within biofilms are more resistant to phagocytic host defenses but are susceptible to additive effects between phagocytes and an echinocandin.

▶ Biofilm formation by bacteria and fungi on tissues and devices is a major contributor to initiation and persistence of infections. The persistent focus and the sessile (adherent) made of growth within biofilms renders host defense mechanisms and antimicrobial agents much less effective.

The fully established biofilms of *Candida* consist of a dense network of yeasts, hyphae, and pseudohyphae embedded in a matrix of polysaccharides, proteins, etc.[1] *Candida* biofilms are particularly resistant to amphotericin B and azoles compared with the planktonic (free floating) organism. Within the biofilms, *Candida albicans* is more resistant to phagocyte host defenses.

The authors in the study investigated the interactions between *C albicans* biofilms and polymorphonuclear leukocytes (PMNs) and monocytes alone and in combination with voriconazole (an azole antifungal agent) or anidulafungin (an echinocandin cell wall inhibitor). The experimental model mimicked the condition of vascular catheter infection. The data show that anidulafungin, unlike voriconazole, acts with immune cells in an additive mode against *Candida* biofilms. This additive interaction resulted in a differential release of the proinflammatory cytokine TNF-$\alpha$ and the chemokine IL-8.

The echinocandins may offer an advantage over azoles and amphotericin B in the treatment of biofilm-mediated *Candida* infections, especially in patients with adequate neutrophil counts. The differential release of TNF-$\alpha$ and IL-8 during the interaction between PMN cells, *Candida* species, and echinocandins introduces the potential role of targeting of biological response modifiers as a therapeutic option.

**N. M. Khardori, MD**

*Reference*

1. Nett J, Andes D. *Candida albicans* biofilm development, modeling a host-pathogen interaction. *Curr Opin Microbiolo.* 2006;9:340-345.

# 12 Nosocomial Infections

**The Potential for Airborne Dispersal of *Clostridium difficile* from Symptomatic Patients**

Best EL, Fawley WN, Parnell P, et al (Leeds Teaching Hosps Natl Health Service Trust, UK)

*Clin Infect Dis* 50:1450-1457, 2010

*Background.*—The high transmissibility and widespread environmental contamination by *Clostridium difficile* suggests the possibility of airborne dissemination of spores. We measured airborne and environmental *C. difficile* adjacent to patients with symptomatic *C. difficile* infection (CDI).

*Methods.*—We conducted air sampling adjacent to 63 patients with CDI for 180 h in total and for 101 h in control settings. Environmental samples were obtained from surfaces adjacent to the patient and from communal areas of the ward. *C. difficile* isolates were characterized by ribotyping and multilocus variable-number tandem-repeat analysis to determine relatedness.

*Results.*—Of the first 50 patients examined (each for 1 h), only 12% had positive air samples, most frequently those with active symptoms of CDI (10%, vs 2% for those with no symptoms). We intensively sampled the air around 10 patients with CDI symptoms, each for 10 h over 2 days, as well as a total of 346 surface sites. *C. difficile* was isolated from the air in the majority of these cases (7 of 10 patients tested) and from the surfaces around 9 of the patients; 60% of patients had both air and surface environments that were positive for *C. difficile*. Molecular characterization confirmed an epidemiological link between airborne dispersal, environmental contamination, and CDI cases.

*Conclusions.*—Aerosolization of *C. difficile* occurs commonly but sporadically in patients with symptomatic CDI. This may explain the widespread dissemination of epidemic strains. Our results emphasize the importance of single-room isolation as soon as possible after the onset of diarrhea to limit the dissemination of *C. difficile*.

▶ Environmental contamination and airborne transmission of *Clostridium difficile* was first suspected in hamster experiments.[1] A patient with *C difficile* infection (CDI) can excrete $1 \times 10^4$ to $1 \times 10^7$ *C difficile* per gram of feces.[2]

The spores of *C difficile* can survive for months or years on contaminated surfaces and may be resistant to disinfectants. In spite of cleaning, environmental contamination with *C difficile* spores occurs at 35% to 58% of sites. If the environment is heavily contaminated with the bacterium, the hands of health care workers are significantly more likely to be positive for *C difficile*. The potential for airborne transmission of *C difficile* has been alluded to in a number of studies.[3] The aim of this study was to determine the extent of *C difficile* contamination in ward environments by sampling air and environmental surfaces in the immediate vicinity of patients with symptomatic CDI.

Environmental samples were obtained from communal areas of the ward and from surfaces adjacent to the patients. Of the 10 patients studied intensively, *C difficile* was commonly but sporadically present in the air close to symptomatic patients with CDI. *C difficile* was cultured from surfaces around 9 of the patients. Both air and surface environments were positive for *C difficile* in 60% of patients. The strains of *C difficile* in the environment, air, and patients' fecal specimens were indistinguishable or highly related. The epidemiological link between airborne dispersal, environmental contamination, and CDI cases was confirmed by molecular characterization. These findings underscore the importance of early isolation of patients at the onset of diarrhea even before laboratory diagnosis of CDI is confirmed.

**N. M. Khardori, MD**

*References*

1. Larson HE. The experimental pathogenesis of antibiotic related colitis. *Scand J Infect Dis Suppl.* 1980;22:7-10.
2. Mulligan ME, Rolfe RD, Finegold SM, et al. Contamination of a hospital environment by *Clostridium difficile. Curr Microbiol Infect.* 2008;14:2-20.
3. Roberts K, Smith CF, Snelling AM, et al. Aerial dissemination of *Clostridium difficile* spores. *BMC Infect Dis.* 2008;8:7.

---

### Treatment with Monoclonal Antibodies against *Clostridium difficile* Toxins

Lowy I, Molrine DC, Leav BA, et al (Medarex, Princeton, NJ; Univ of Massachusetts Med School, Boston; et al)

*N Engl J Med* 362:197-205, 2010

---

*Background.*—New therapies are needed to manage the increasing incidence, severity, and high rate of recurrence of *Clostridium difficile* infection.

*Methods.*—We performed a randomized, double-blind, placebo-controlled study of two neutralizing, fully human monoclonal antibodies against *C. difficile* toxins A (CDA1) and B (CDB1). The antibodies were administered together as a single infusion, each at a dose of 10 mg per kilogram of body weight, in patients with symptomatic *C. difficile* infection who were receiving either metronidazole or vancomycin. The primary outcome was laboratory-documented recurrence of infection during the 84 days after the administration of monoclonal antibodies or placebo.

*Results.*—Among the 200 patients who were enrolled (101 in the antibody group and 99 in the placebo group), the rate of recurrence of *C. difficile* infection was lower among patients treated with monoclonal antibodies (7% vs. 25%; 95% confidence interval, 7 to 29; $P<0.001$). The recurrence rates among patients with the epidemic BI/NAP1/027 strain were 8% for the antibody group and 32% for the placebo group ($P=0.06$); among patients with more than one previous episode of *C. difficile* infection, recurrence rates were 7% and 38%, respectively ($P=0.006$). The mean duration of the initial hospitalization for inpatients did not differ significantly between the antibody and placebo groups (9.5 and 9.4 days, respectively). At least one serious adverse event was reported by 18 patients in the antibody group and by 28 patients in the placebo group ($P=0.09$).

*Conclusions.*—The addition of monoclonal antibodies against *C. difficile* toxins to antibiotic agents significantly reduced the recurrence of *C. difficile* infection. (ClinicalTrials.gov number, NCT00350298.) (Fig 1).

► Given the increase in prevalence of *Clostridium difficile* infection (CDI) and the paucity of effective antimicrobial agents, other therapeutics approaches are being studied. Probiotic use in the form of drinks and supplements is acceptable but probably ineffective.[1] Fecal transplantation, probably effective, is less acceptable aesthetically.[2] Pooled human intravenous immunoglobulin has been used for passive immunotherapy, but efficacy and pharmacokinetic data

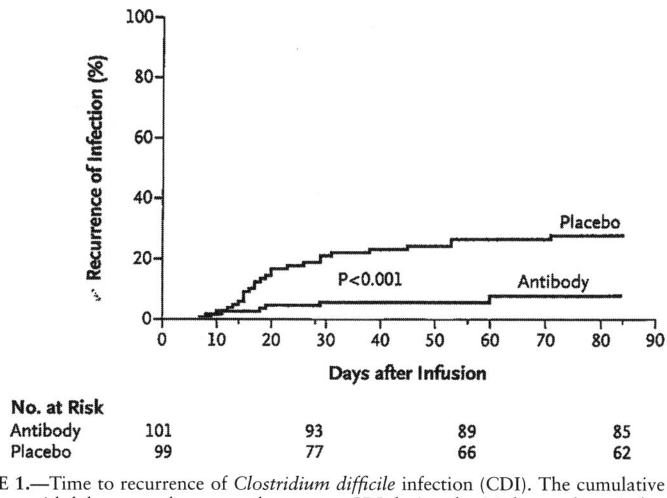


FIGURE 1.—Time to recurrence of *Clostridium difficile* infection (CDI). The cumulative percentages of 32 patients with laboratory-documented recurrent CDI during the 84-day study period are shown for the two study groups: 7% in the antibody group and 25% in the placebo group. Five patients had a second episode of CDI recurrence: two in the antibody group and three in the placebo group. The P value was calculated by means of the log-rank test. (Reprinted from Lowy I, Molrine DC, Leav BA, et al. Treatment with monoclonal antibodies against *Clostridium difficile* toxins. *N Engl J Med.* 2010;362:197-205. Copyright 2010 Massachusetts Medical Society. All rights reserved.)

are not available. *C difficile* toxin for active immunization is currently in phase 2 of a randomized secondary prevention trial.

This study presents the results of a multicenter, randomized, double-blind, placebo-controlled trial of 2 fully human monoclonal antibodies against toxins A and B of *C difficile* for secondary prevention of CDI. The 2 antibodies were administered together in patients with CDI receiving either metronidazole or vancomycin. A total of 101 patients (out of 200) were randomized to the antibody group. The recurrence rate of CDI was 7% in patients treated with monoclonal antibodies compared with 25% placebo recipients showing a relative reduction of 72%. The relative reduction was higher (82%) in patients with more than 1 prior recurrence. The recurrence rate among patients with CDI due to the epidemic B1/NAP1/027 was 8% for the antibody group compared with 32% for the placebo group. The adverse event profile was similar between antibody and placebo groups, and the monoclonal antibodies were not immunogenic.

**N. M. Khardori, MD**

*References*

1. Kyne L. *Clostridium difficile*–beyond antibiotics. *N Engl J Med.* 2010;362: 264-265.
2. van Nood E, Speelman P, Kuijper EJ, Keller JJ. Struggling with recurrent *Clostridium difficile* infections: is donor faeces the solution? *Euro Surveill.* 2009;14: 19316.

# 13 Vaccines

**Randomized Controlled Clinical Trial of Fractional Doses of Inactivated Poliovirus Vaccine Administered Intradermally by Needle-Free Device in Cuba**

Resik S, Tejeda A, Lago PM, et al (Pedro Kouri Inst, Havana, Cuba; Provincial Health Office, Camagüey, Cuba; et al)

*J Infect Dis* 201:1344-1352, 2010

*Background.*—As part of an evaluation of strategies to make inactivated poliovirus vaccine (IPV) affordable for developing countries, we conducted a clinical trial of fractional doses of IPV in Cuba.

*Methods.*—We compared the immunogenicity and reactogenicity of fractional-dose IPV (0.1 mL, or 1/5 of a full dose) given intradermally using a needle-free jet injector device compared with full doses given intramuscularly. Subjects were randomized at birth to receive IPV at 6, 10, and 14 weeks.

*Results.*—A total of 471 subjects were randomized to the 2 study groups, and 364 subjects fulfilled the study requirements. No significant differences at baseline were detected. Thirty days after completing the 3-dose schedule of IPV, 52.9%, 85.0%, and 69.0% of subjects in the fractional-dose IPV arm seroconverted for poliovirus types 1, 2, and 3, respectively, whereas 89.3%, 95.5%, and 98.9% of subjects in the full-dose IPV arm seroconverted for poliovirus types 1, 2, and 3, respectively (all comparisons, $P < .001$). The median titers of each poliovirus serotype were significantly lower in the intradermal arm than in the intramuscular arm ($P < .001$). Only minor local adverse effects and no moderate or serious adverse events were reported.

*Conclusions.*—This large-scale evaluation demonstrates the feasibility of fractional doses of IPV given intradermally as an antigen-sparing strategy but also shows that IPV given to infants at 6, 10, and 14 weeks of age results in suboptimal immunogenicity (especially for the fractional-dose arm).

▶ The World Health Assembly called for global eradication of poliomyelitis by the year 2000. The current world poliomyelitis scene is a clearance of cases by >99%, eradication of 1 serotype, and persistence of serotypes 1 and 3 in 4 countries (India, Pakistan, Afghanistan, and Nigeria) compared with >125 polio-endemic countries in 1988. The discontinuation of the use of live oral poliovirus vaccine was formally endorsed in 2005 by the Advisory Committee on Poliomyelitis Eradication.[1] The availability of an "affordable inactivated poliovirus vaccine (IPV)" appropriate for use in developing countries is one of the prerequisites for the change. A number of strategies are under evaluation to achieve this prerequisite, including adjuvant use and dose/schedule reduction.

This study describes the finding of a randomized controlled clinical trial of fractional doses of inactivated poliovirus vaccine(IPV) administered intradermally by a needle-free device in Cuba. The findings demonstrate that fractional dose of IPV (one-fifth of the full dose) given intradermally results in significantly lower seroconversion rates than full-dose IPV given intramuscularly for all poliovirus serotypes. Because this was not a dose-finding study, the question of a higher antigen dose giving a better immune response cannot be answered. And because an arm with intramuscular route was not studied, the impact of the route of administration also cannot be determined. The vaccine was well tolerated by both routes. The vaccine doses were given at 6, 10, and 14 weeks. It would have provided further insight into the feasibility of this approach if a fourth fractional dose of IPV was administered at 9 months of age to determine if any of the nonseroconverting children had been primed and would have responded with a booster dose. Even a 4-dose fractional schedule would require less antigen than 1 full dose of IPV. The other strategy would be to administer the first dose at 2 months of age based on a 28-day half-life of maternally derived antibody. Subsequent doses would then be given at intervals of 2 months.

**N. M. Khardori, MD**

*Reference*

1. World Health Organization. Conclusions and recommendations of the Ad Hoc Advisory Committee on Poliomyelitis Eradication, Geneva, 21–22 September 2005. *Wkly Epidemiol Rec.* 2005;47:410-416.

## Immunogenicity and Safety of Intradermal Influenza Vaccination in Healthy Older Adults

Chi R-C, Rock MT, Neuzil KM (Univ of Washington; Vanderbilt Univ Med Ctr, Nashville, TN)

*Clin Infect Dis* 50:1331-1338, 2010

*Background.*—Influenza vaccine immunogenicity is suboptimal in older persons. Intradermal (ID) vaccination may be a promising alternative to intramuscular (IM) vaccination.

*Methods.*—This randomized trial compared the immunogenicity of 60% dose ID influenza vaccination to standard IM vaccination of full-dose or 60% dose vaccine. Pre- and postvaccination measurements in the hemagglutination inhibition antibody titer were compared. Participants who received reduced-dose vaccine were revaccinated with full-dose IM vaccine.

*Results.*—257 healthy adults aged ≥65 years received 1 of the following trivalent inactivated influenza vaccines: standard-dose (15 μg each of 3 hemagglutinin vaccine antigens in 0.5 mL) IM injection, reduced-dose (9 μg, 0.3 mL) IM injection, reduced-dose (9 μg, 0.3 mL) ID injection, or 2 reduced-dose (4.5 μg, 0.15 mL) ID injections. Respective seroprotection rates were 65.6%, 57.8%, 68.9%, and 67.2% against A/H1N1; 76.6%, 75.0%, 75.4%, and 75.0% against A/H3N2; and 26.6%, 17.2%, 16.4%, and 25.0% against influenza B. Subsequent full-dose IM vaccination of participants randomized to reduced-dose vaccine by either IM or ID routes did not improve seroprotection rates. Local reactions of redness, swelling, and itching were significantly more frequent among recipients of ID injections.

*Conclusion.*—Influenza vaccine at 60% dose by either IM or ID route elicited antibody responses generally similar to full-dose IM vaccination among healthy elderly persons (ClinicalTrials.gov identifier: NCT00504231).

▶ The efficacy of influenza vaccine in preventing laboratory-confirmed influenza illness among healthy elderly aged 60 to 69 years was 59% in the only randomized controlled efficacy trial.[1] This correlates with lower influenza antibody levels in older adults compared to younger persons. Despite yearly influenza vaccination, a significant number of older adults remain susceptible to influenza and its complications.

Because of the presence of large numbers of dendritic cells in the skin and their role as potent antigen-presenting cells, intradermal (ID) injection of influenza vaccine may induce a better immune response.

This randomized trial compared 2 doses and 2 routes of vaccination in 257 healthy adults over 65 years of age. Influenza vaccine at the standard dose of 15 μg and reduced dose of 9 μg was administered intramuscularly (IM). The other 2 groups received reduced dose (9 μg) or 2 reduced doses (4.5 μg each) side by side (3 mm apart) intradermally (ID). At 4 weeks postimmunization, antibody titers were determined, and those assigned to reduced dose IM or ID vaccination received full-dose IM influenza vaccination. Influenza antibody titers were repeated at 8 weeks. At 14 days postvaccination, T-cell assays to study cell-mediated immune response were studied in a nonrandomized subset of vaccines.

The results show that a 60% (9 μg) dose by either IM or ID routes yielded antibody titers and seroprotection rates comparable to conventional full-dose influenza vaccination in the elderly subjects. A follow-up full-dose IM vaccination of those randomized to reduced dose vaccine by either IM or ID routes did not improve seroprotection rates. ID injection led to significantly more local reactions of redness, swelling, and itching (ie, indicators of a local immune response). The severity of these local reactions was mild, and they were well tolerated by the subjects. Systemic symptoms and pain were comparable to IM injections. Reduced dose influenza vaccination by either ID or IM routes may be reasonable for healthy older adults during times of influenza vaccine shortage.

**N. M. Khardori, MD**

*Reference*

1. Govaert TM, Thijs CT, Masurel N, Sprenger MJ, Dinant GJ, Knottnerus JA. The efficacy of influenza vaccination in elderly individuals: a randomized double-blind placebo-controlled trial. *JAMA*. 1994;272:1661-1665.

## Asymptomatic Wild-Type Poliovirus Infection in India among Children with Previous Oral Poliovirus Vaccination

Grassly NC, Jafari H, Bahl S, et al (Imperial College London, UK; World Health Organization–Government of India, New Delhi; et al)
*J Infect Dis* 201:1535-1543, 2010

*Background.*—Mucosal immunity induced by oral poliovirus vaccine (OPV) is imperfect and potentially allows immunized individuals to participate in asymptomatic wild-type poliovirus transmission in settings with efficient fecal-oral transmission of infection.

*Methods.*—We examined the extent of asymptomatic wild-type poliovirus transmission in India by measuring the prevalence of virus in stool samples obtained from 14,005 healthy children who were in contact with 2761 individuals with suspected poliomyelitis reported during the period 2003–2008.

*Results.*—Wild-type poliovirus serotypes 1 and 3 were isolated from the stool samples of 103 (0.74%) and 104 (0.74%) healthy contacts, respectively. Among contacts of individuals with laboratory-confirmed poliomyelitis, 27 (12.7%) of 213 and 29 (13.9%) of 209 had serotypes 1 and 3, respectively, isolated from their stool samples. The odds ratio of excreting serotype 1 wild-type poliovirus was 0.13 (95% confidence interval, 0.02–0.87) among healthy children reporting ≥6 doses of OPV, compared with children reporting 0–2 doses. However, two-thirds of healthy children who excreted this virus reported ≥6 doses, and the prevalence of this virus did not decrease with age over the sampled range.

*Conclusions.*—Although OPV is protective against infection with poliovirus, the majority of healthy contacts who excreted wild-type poliovirus were well vaccinated. This is consistent with a potential role for OPV-vaccinated children in continued wild-type poliovirus transmission and requires further study.

▶ Oral polio vaccine (OPV) has been used exclusively in the Global Polio Eradication Initiative (GPEI). The use of OPV in routine and mass vaccination activities has led to global eradication of serotype 2 wild poliovirus. In 2009, only 4 countries (India, Afghanistan, Pakistan, and Nigeria) reported indigenous transmission of serotypes 1 and 3. This has led to the reintroduction of infection and polio outbreaks in a number of African and Asian countries.[1] Children immunized with OPV may be infected and excrete poliovirus as the mucosal immunity wanes over time.[2]

This investigation examines the extent of asymptomatic wild-type poliovirus transmission in India. Stool samples from 14 005 healthy children who were in contact with 2761 individuals with suspected poliomyelitis were studied during 2003-2008. Wild-type serotypes 1 and 3 were isolated from 0.74% and 0.74% of stool samples from healthy children compared with 2.6% and 2.2% from children suspected to have poliomyelitis. Vaccine poliovirus serotypes 1, 2, and 3 were recovered from 3.4%, 1.7%, and 3.1% of healthy contacts, respectively. Most healthy contacts who excreted the wild-type polioviruses were well vaccinated. Forty percent and 38% of individuals with laboratory-confirmed serotype 1 and serotype 3 poliomyelitis, respectively, had 1 or more healthy contacts with wild-type poliovirus in the stool. The data indicate that OPV is protective against symptomatic infection with wild-type poliovirus in India. However, the protection is incomplete and results in continued excretions of wild-type poliovirus among older, OPV-vaccinated children with potential for continued transmission. Strategies to boost mucosal immunity to polioviruses in northern India may be needed to remove this particular obstacle from the path of global poliomyelitis eradication.

**N. M. Khardori, MD**

*References*

1. World Health Organization. Progress towards interrupting wild poliovirus transmission worldwide, January 2007–April 2008. *Wkly epidemiol Rec.* 2008;83: 170-177.
2. Laassri M, Lottenback K, Belshe R, et al. Effect of different vaccination schedules on excretion or oral poliovirus vaccine strains. *J Infect Dis.* 2005;192:2092-2098.

---

**Pertussis Disease Burden in the Household: How to Protect Young Infants**

de Greeff SC, Mooi FR, Westerhof A, et al (Natl Inst for Public Health and the Environment, Bilthoven, the Netherlands; et al)

*Clin Infect Dis* 50:1339-1345, 2010

---

*Background.*—We conducted a population-based, nation-wide, prospective study to identify who introduced pertussis into the household of infants aged ≤6 months admitted to the hospital for pertussis in the Netherlands.

*Methods.*—During the period 2006–2008, a total of 560 household contacts of 164 hospitalized infants were tested by polymerase chain reaction, culture, and serological examination to establish *Bordetella pertussis* infection. Clinical symptoms and vaccination history were obtained by a questionnaire submitted during sample collection and 4–6 weeks afterwards.

*Results.*—Overall, 299 household contacts (53%) had laboratory-confirmed pertussis; 159 (53%) had symptoms compatible with typical pertussis infection, and 42 (14%) had no symptoms. Among children vaccinated with a whole-cell vaccine, 17 (46%) of 37 had typical pertussis 1–3 years after completion of the primary series, compared with 9 (29%) of 31 children who had been completely vaccinated with an acellular vaccine. For 96 households (60%), the most likely source of infection of the infant was established, being a sibling (41%), mother (38%), or father (17%).

*Conclusions.*—If immunity to pertussis in parents is maintained or boosted, 35%–55% of infant, cases could be prevented. Furthermore, we found that, 1–3 years after vaccination with whole-cell or acellular vaccine, a significant percentage of children are again susceptible for typical pertussis. In the long term, pertussis vaccines and vaccination strategies should be improved to provide longer protection and prevent transmission.

▶ In the past decade, a resurgence of pertussis has been observed in many countries, including those in developed parts of the world.[1] The increase has been attributed to waning immunity, pathogen adaptation, and increased awareness. The circulation of pertussis and atypical presentations in previously vaccinated young adults puts infants who have not been completely vaccinated at risk. Morbidity and mortality related to pertussis are highest in this group. Studies based mostly on clinical diagnosis have demonstrated that adults play an important role in the transmission of pertussis to children because of high attack rates after household exposure.[2] Two small recent multinational studies concluded that parents, especially mothers, were the source for most infants. Vaccination of parents would substantially reduce the burden of infant pertussis.

This is a population-based, nationwide (the Netherlands) prospective study to identify the household members who introduced pertussis to an infant hospitalized for pertussis. Both clinical and laboratory diagnoses (culture, serological testing, and polymerase chain reaction) were used to identify infected household sources of infection. Of the household contacts with onset of symptoms at least 1 week before onset in the index infant, 41% were siblings, 38% were mothers, and 17% were fathers. The larger role of siblings in the transmission of pertussis in the Netherlands may be a result of using a less effective whole-cell vaccine in the 1990s. More than 70% of siblings in this study had not received the preschool acellular vaccine booster introduced in 2001. Young children introduce pertussis into a household most often in areas with low vaccine coverage. In high-coverage areas, adolescents and adults play a larger role in transmission. The attack rate of symptomatic pertussis in vaccinated household contacts was 46%. Only 39% of infected household contacts consulted a physician, 20% were tested, and only 9% were treated with antibiotics prior to the onset of symptoms in the index infant. Pertussis vaccination at birth (if proven safe), infant vaccination starting at age 6 weeks, vaccination of mothers during pregnancy, selective vaccination of new parents, and improved rates of overall adult vaccination are potential methods to protect young infants against pertussis. If immunity to pertussis in parents is maintained or boosted, 35% to 55% of infant cases can be prevented. Improved vaccines and vaccination strategies against pertussis will maintain protection in children and adults and prevent transmission to infants.

**N. M. Khardori, MD**

*References*

1. Roush SW, Murphy TV. Historical comparison of morbidity and mortality for vaccine preventable disease in the United States. *JAMA*. 2007;298:2155-2163.
2. Bisgard KM, Pascua FB, Eresmann KR, et al. Infant pertussis: who was the source. *Pediatr Infect Dis J*. 2004;23:985-989.

---

### Japanese Encephalitis: New Options for Active Immunization

Halstead SB, Thomas SJ (Pediatric Dengue Vaccine Initiative, Rockville, MD; US Army Med Component–Armed Forces Res Inst of Med Sciences, Bangkok, Thailand)
*Clin Infect Dis* 50:1155-1164, 2010

---

Japanese encephalitis (JE) is a mosquito-borne flavivirus infection responsible for significant morbidity and mortality across Asia. Indigenous populations and those who undertake short- and long-term travel to endemic regions are at risk of infection and development of neuroinvasive disease. Effective mouse brain–derived vaccines have been available in select countries, including the United States, for decades. Limited access in Asia and safety concerns with regard to mouse brain products prompted the Chinese to develop a live, attenuated virus vaccine (SA14-14-2; Chengdu Institute of Biological Products), which has proven to be safe and efficacious following administration of >300 million doses. Recently, the portfolio of JE vaccines increased again with licensure in the United States, Europe, and Australia of a purified, inactivated virus JE vaccine (IC51; Intercell AG) and filing for licensure in Thailand and Australia of a Yellow fever–JE chimeric vaccine (ChimeriVax-JE; Sanofi Pasteur). JE is a vaccine-preventable disease with numerous options now available for active immunization. Aggressive and responsible vaccination programs should greatly diminish the burden of disease.

▶ Japanese encephalitis (JE) is caused by a flavivirus that is transmitted by the *Culex* species of mosquito. It is the leading cause of viral encephalitis in Asia. The candidates for vaccination against JE include residents in endemic areas and travelers from other parts of the world to these areas. An inactivated JE vaccine made from infected mouse brain proved to have an unacceptable adverse event profile.

This article reviews the recent advances in the JE vaccine availability. A safe and effective live-attenuated vaccine developed in China has become available to many Asian countries. It is a convenient single-dose vaccine. The integration of JE vaccine into routine vaccination programs has had a significant impact on the disease burden.[1]

For travelers to endemic areas, inactivated JE vaccine is now available in Europe, Australia, and the United States. The vaccine construct was developed at the Walter Reed Army Institute of Research. Early studies established the safety and immunogenicity of the vaccine. Subsequent studies demonstrated high seroconversion rates (83%) 1 year following vaccination. Another second-generation vaccine against JE is close to licensure. This is a Yellow fever-JE chimeric vaccine candidate.

The Advisory Committee on Immunization Practices published provisional recommendations for use of the JE vaccine. Travel to known endemic areas during the rainy season, residence in rural or agricultural areas, residence near pig farms, or long duration visits increase the risk for JE. Travel to an endemic area without a defined destination is also an indication for the vaccine.

The authors in this review recommend that JE vaccines (now safe and effective) should be administered to all who live in or visit areas where JE is endemic.

**N. M. Khardori, MD**

*Reference*

1. Halstead S, Jacobson J. Japanese encephalitis vaccine. In: Plotkin S, Orenstein W, Offit P, eds. *Vaccines*. 5th ed. Philadelphia, PA: Elsevier; 2008:311–352.

---

**Advances in the Development of Vaccines against *Neisseria meningitidis***

Tan LKK, Carlone GM, Borrow R (Imperial College London, UK; Ctrs for Disease Control and Prevention, Atlanta, GA; Manchester Royal Infirmary, UK)
*N Engl J Med* 362:1511-1520, 2010

---

Although two centuries have passed since Vieusseux described epidemic meningococcal disease, *Neisseria meningitidis* remains a leading cause of meningitis and sepsis. Overwhelming meningococcal disease can develop rapidly and is associated with mortality rates exceeding 20%. Thus, efforts to control the disease have focused on vaccination. In the past, vaccines against meningococcal disease have failed to provide immunogenicity and long-term protection in infants, who are at greatest risk. Although recent vaccines have improved coverage for this age group, there is still no broadly effective vaccine against *N. meningitidis* group B (NMB), now the predominant disease-causing isolate in industrialized countries.

Developments during the past decade have renewed hopes for solving this seemingly intractable problem. Knowledge of the meningococcal genome has led to the identification of novel antigens that have been incorporated into the NMB vaccines now being studied in clinical trials. However, it remains unclear whether these vaccines will provide sufficient immunogenicity in infants as well as wide-ranging coverage. This review highlights the evolution of meningococcal vaccines in general and discusses strategies being used to overcome the barriers to developing vaccines against NMB.

▶ Meningococcus, like smallpox virus, is a pathogen only in humans and hence amenable to eradication. There are an estimated 1.2 million cases of invasive meningococcal disease and 135 000 related deaths annually.[1] According to the World Health Organization, only 6 capsular groups (A, B, C, W-135, X, and Y) are associated with invasive disease. The first successful capsular polysaccharide vaccines were developed against groups A and C in the 1960s followed by a vaccine against groups W-135 and Y. Since 1981 a quadrivalent meningococcal polysaccharide vaccine (A, C, W-135, and Y) has been licensed in the United States, giving over 85% efficacy against the A and C in older children and adults. These T-cell independent polysaccharide vaccines are poorly immunogenic in children less than 2 years, have no memory response, and require dosing every 3 to 5 years.

Covalent binding (conjugation) of polysaccharides to a protein carrier results in T cell-dependent immunity and a memory response.[2] This is the technology that was used on the meningococcal group C polysaccharide-protein conjugate vaccine that was introduced into schedules for routine infant immunization. Since its introduction in 1999 the vaccine led to 95% effectiveness at 1 year and has been shown to provide herd immunity. Between 1997 and 2002, 37% of all cases of meningococcal disease in the United States were caused by group Y. This led to the licensure of a quadrivalent (A, C, W-135, and Y) vaccine conjugated to diphtheria toxoid for persons 2 to 55 years. Its immunogenicity in infants is poor.

A conjugate vaccine is being introduced against the epidemic disease caused by group A in Africa and India based on safety and immunogenicity in phase 2 and 3 trials. This vaccine does not offer protection against serogroups, W-135 and X, which have emerged in Africa.

The development of a vaccine against group B has been impeded by the structural identity between group B polysaccharide and fetal brain cell adhesion molecules. Concern about possible autoimmunity has led to the study of noncapsular outer membrane structures as vaccines. Such vaccines have been used in Chile, Cuba, Brazil, and Norway with variable results. Because these vaccines generate a largely strain-specific immune response, they are effective in epidemics caused by a single strain but not against the diverse strains seen in endemic settings. The combinations of outer membrane vesicles from different strains are currently being studied. The potential of antigenic shift or gene deletion would render outer membrane vesicle vaccines ineffective. This concern has led to finding conserved antigens for a universal group B vaccine. Using the technique of reverse vaccinology (Fig 1 in the original article), 350 genes from *Neisseria meningitidis* genome encoding potential surface-exposed protein antigens were shown to induce bactericidal antibodies against 78% of selected group B strains. Two such vaccines containing factor H-binding protein (rMenB and rLP2086) are undergoing further evaluation.

Although a lot of progress has been made in the study of meningococcal vaccines, invasive meningococcal disease continues to be a global public health challenge.

**N. M. Khardori, MD**

*References*

1. Epidemics of meningococcal disease. African meningitis belt, 2001. *Wkly epidem-iol Rec.* 2001;76:282-288.
2. Bilukha OO, Rosenstein N. Prevention and control of meningococcal disease: recommendations of the Advisory Committee on Immunization Practices (ACIP). *MMWR Recomm Rep.* 2005;54:1-21.

**Human Papillomavirus and Survival of Patients with Oropharyngeal Cancer**

Ang KK, Harris J, Wheeler R, et al (Univ of Texas MD Anderson Cancer Ctr, Houston; Thomas Jefferson Univ Hosp, Philadelphia, PA; Huntsman Cancer Inst, Salt Lake City, UT; et al)

*N Engl J Med* 363:24-35, 2010

*Background.*—Oropharyngeal squamous-cell carcinomas caused by human papillomavirus (HPV) are associated with favorable survival, but the independent prognostic significance of tumor HPV status remains unknown.

*Methods.*—We performed a retrospective analysis of the association between tumor HPV status and survival among patients with stage III or IV oropharyngeal squamous-cell carcinoma who were enrolled in a randomized trial comparing accelerated-fractionation radiotherapy (with acceleration by means of concomitant boost radiotherapy) with standard-fractionation radiotherapy, each combined with cisplatin therapy, in patients with squamous-cell carcinoma of the head and neck. Proportional-hazards models were used to compare the risk of death among patients with HPV-positive cancer and those with HPV-negative cancer.

*Results.*—The median follow-up period was 4.8 years. The 3-year rate of overall survival was similar in the group receiving accelerated-fractionation radiotherapy and the group receiving standard-fractionation radiotherapy (70.3% vs. 64.3%; P=0.18; hazard ratio for death with accelerated-fractionation radiotherapy, 0.90; 95% confidence interval [CI], 0.72 to 1.13), as were the rates of high-grade acute and late toxic events. A total of 63.8% of patients with oropharyngeal cancer (206 of 323) had HPV-positive tumors; these patients had better 3-year rates of overall survival (82.4%, vs. 57.1% among patients with HPV-negative tumors; P<0.001 by the log-rank test) and, after adjustment for age, race, tumor and nodal stage, tobacco exposure, and treatment assignment, had a 58% reduction in the risk of death (hazard ratio, 0.42; 95% CI, 0.27 to 0.66). The risk of death significantly increased with each additional pack-year of

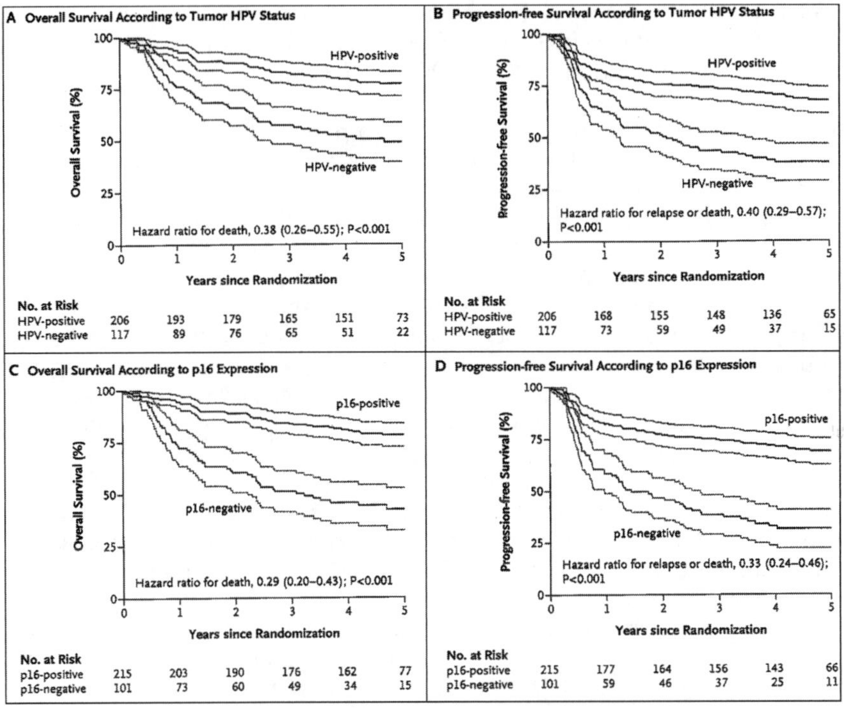


FIGURE 1.—Kaplan–Meier estimates of survival among the study patients with oropharyngeal cancer, according to tumor HPV Status or p16-expression status. Data on overall survival and progression-free survival are shown according to stratification on the basis of tumor HPV status (Panels A and B, respectively) or p16-expression status (Panels C and D, respectively). The Kaplan–Meier curves are shown in black, and the associated 95% confidence intervals in gray. Patients with HPV-positive tumors had significantly better overall survival and progression-free survival than did patients with HPV-negative tumors (P<0.001 for both comparisons by the two-sided log-rank test). The 3-year rates of overall survival were 82.4% (95% CI, 77.2 to 87.6) in the HPV-positive subgroup and 57.1% (95% CI, 48.1 to 66.1) in the HPV-negative subgroup (Panel A), and the 3-year rates of progression-free survival were 73.7% (95% CI, 67.7 to 79.8) and 43.4% (95% CI, 34.4 to 52.4), respectively (Panel B). The 3-year absolute benefit of HPV-positive status for overall survival was 25 percentage points (95% CI, 11 to 40), and the absolute benefit for progression-free survival was 30 percentage points (95% CI, 15 to 45). The results were similar with stratification according to p16-expression status. The 3-year rates of overall survival were 83.6% (95% CI, 78.7 to 88.6) in the subgroup that was positive for p16 expression and 51.3% (95% CI, 41.5 to 61.0) in the subgroup that was negative for p16 expression (P<0.001) (Panel C), and the 3-year rates of progression-free survival were 74.4% (95% CI, 68.5 to 80.2) and 38.4% (95% CI, 28.9 to 47.9), respectively (P<0.001) (Panel D). (Reprinted from Ang KK, Harris J, Wheeler R, et al. Human papillomavirus and survival of patients with oropharyngeal cancer. *N Engl J Med*. 2010;363:24-35. Copyright 2010 Massachusetts Medical Society. All rights reserved.)

tobacco smoking. Using recursive-partitioning analysis, we classified our patients as having a low, intermediate, or high risk of death on the basis of four factors: HPV status, pack-years of tobacco smoking, tumor stage, and nodal stage.

*Conclusions.*—Tumor HPV status is a strong and independent prognostic factor for survival among patients with oropharyngeal cancer. (ClinicalTrials.gov number, NCT00047008.) (Fig 1).

▶ Human papillomaviruses (HPV) cause an enormous disease burden in the form of genital warts in both genders; cervical, vaginal, and vulvar cancers in females; anogenital cancers in males; and oropharyngeal cancers in both genders. With the now-established protective efficacy of HPV vaccines in cervical cancer, the potential of preventing other HPV-related cancers has become real. A prerequisite for future interventional strategies is to establish the clinicopathological profile of HPV-related cancers. Oropharyngeal squamous cell carcinoma is the most common of cancers other than cervical cancer with HPV as the etiologic agent.[1] HPV type 16 is present in approximately 90% of HPV-positive oropharyngeal squamous cell cancers, and another 5% contain HPV 18. Both currently approved HPV vaccines contain types 16 and 18.

This article reports a retrospective analysis of the association between tumor HPV status and survival among patients with stage III or IV oropharyngeal squamous cell carcinoma. The data are derived from patients enrolled in a randomized trial to compare 2 different types of radiotherapy combined with cisplatin therapy in patients with squamous cell carcinoma of the head and neck. Of the 323 patients with oropharyngeal cancer, 206 (64%) had HPV-positive tumors. HPV status, pack years of tobacco smoking, tumor stage, and nodal stage were used to classify the patients as having low, intermediate, or high risk of death. The 3-year survival rate was 82% for patients with HPV-positive tumors compared with 57% among patients with HPV-negative tumors. There was 58% reduction in the risk of death after adjustment for age, race, tumor, and nodal stage, treatment assignment, and tobacco exposure. Each additional pack year of tobacco smoking increased the risk of death significantly. The use of vaccination before exposure to HPV might prevent a large number of HPV-positive cases of oropharyngeal squamous cell carcinoma. At this time, it is not known if vaccines can prevent oropharyngeal HPV infection. The vaccines do prevent persistent genital infections with HPV types 16, 18, 6, and 8. Further studies focusing on HPV-positive oropharyngeal cancers will provide this much-needed information.

**N. M. Khardori, MD**

*Reference*

1. Chaturvedi AK. Beyond cervical cancer: burden of other HPV-related cancers among men and women. *J Adolesc Health*. 2010;46:S20-S26.

PART THREE

# HEMATOLOGY AND ONCOLOGY

JAMES TATE THIGPEN, MD

# 14 Breast Cancer

**Breast Cancer after Use of Estrogen plus Progestin in Postmenopausal Women**

Chlebowski RT, Kuller LH, Prentice RL, et al (Los Angeles Biomedical Res Inst at Harbor–UCLA Med Ctr, Torrance, CA; Univ of Pittsburgh; Fred Hutchinson Cancer Res Ctr, Seattle; et al)

*N Engl J Med* 360:573-587, 2009

*Background.*—Following the release of the 2002 report of the Women's Health Initiative (WHI) trial of estrogen plus progestin, the use of menopausal hormone therapy in the United States decreased substantially. Subsequently, the incidence of breast cancer also dropped, suggesting a cause-and-effect relation between hormone treatment and breast cancer. However, the cause of this decrease remains controversial.

*Methods.*—We analyzed the results of the WHI randomized clinical trial — in which one study group received 0.625 mg of conjugated equine estrogens plus 2.5 mg of medroxyprogesterone acetate daily and another group received placebo — and examined temporal trends in breast-cancer diagnoses in the WHI observational-study cohort. Risk factors for breast cancer, frequency of mammography, and time-specific incidence of breast cancer were assessed in relation to combined hormone use.

*Results.*—In the clinical trial, there were fewer breast-cancer diagnoses in the group receiving estrogen plus progestin than in the placebo group in the initial 2 years of the study, but the number of diagnoses increased over the course of the 5.6-year intervention period. The elevated risk decreased rapidly after both groups stopped taking the study pills, despite a similar frequency of mammography. In the observational study, the incidence of breast cancer was initially about two times as high in the group receiving menopausal hormones as in the placebo group, but this difference in incidence decreased rapidly in about 2 years, coinciding with year-to-year reductions in combined hormone use. During this period, differences in the frequency of mammography between the two groups were unchanged.

*Conclusions.*—The increased risk of breast cancer associated with the use of estrogen plus progestin declined markedly soon after discontinuation of combined hormone therapy and was unrelated to changes in frequency of mammography.

▶ Concerns related to breast cancer risk in postmenopausal women who take supplemental estrogen and progestin have been a topic of debate for over 2 decades. The results of the Women's Health Initiative (WHI) published in

2002[1] raised significant concerns about what appeared to be a clear relationship with use of hormone supplements and increased breast cancer risk. Thus, following the 2002 WHI report, supplemental hormone use in this population decreased in the United States. Yet many women struggle daily with debilitating physical and emotional effects of menopause.

This study is a follow-up to the initial WHI. It has shown that while there is an increase in a risk of breast cancer seen after 5 years of hormone supplement compared with placebo, this increased risk does quickly decrease after approximately 2 years with cessation of hormone therapy. Thus, one message for women who simply cannot deal with the effects of menopause without hormone supplement is that they can take the supplements for as short a period of time as possible and can be comforted that within 2 years of cessation of the hormone supplements, their increased risk of breast cancer will come back down.

**C. A. Lawton, MD**

*Reference*

1. Rossouw JE, Anderson GL, Prentice RL, et al. Risks and benefits of estrogen plus progestin in healthy postmenopausal women: principle results from the Women's Health Initiative randomized controlled trial. *JAMA*. 2002;288:321-333.

---

## Breast Cancer Surveillance Practices Among Women Previously Treated With Chest Radiation for a Childhood Cancer

Oeffinger KC, Ford JS, Moskowitz CS, et al (Memorial Sloan-Kettering Cancer Ctr, NY; et al)

*JAMA* 301:401-414, 2009

---

*Context.*—Women treated with chest radiation for a pediatric malignancy have a significantly increased risk of breast cancer at a young age and are recommended to have an annual screening mammogram starting at age 25 years or 8 years after radiation, whichever occurs last.

*Objective.*—To characterize the breast cancer surveillance practices among female pediatric cancer survivors who were treated with chest radiation and identify correlates of screening.

*Design, Setting, and Participants.*—Between June 2005 and August 2006, a 114-item questionnaire was administered to a random sample of 625 women aged 25 through 50 years who had survived pediatric cancer, who had been treated with chest radiation, and who were participating in the Childhood Cancer Survivor Study (CCSS), a North American cohort of long-term survivors diagnosed from 1970-1986. Comparisons were made with similarly aged pediatric cancer survivors not treated with chest radiation (n = 639) and the CCSS siblings cohort (n = 712).

*Main Outcome Measure.*—Screening mammogram within the previous 2 years.

*Results.*—Of 1976 cancer survivors and siblings who were contacted, 87.9% participated. Among the 551 women with a history of chest radiation, 55% reported a screening mammogram in the past 2 years (ages 25-39 years, 36.5%; 95% confidence interval [CI], 31.0%-42.0%; ages 40-50 years, 76.5%; 95% CI, 71.3%-81.7%). In comparison, 40.5% of survivors without chest radiation and 37.0% of CCSS siblings reported a screening mammogram in the same time interval. Notably, among women with a history of chest radiation, 47.3% (95% CI; 41.6%-53.0%) of those younger than 40 years had never had a mammogram and only 52.6% (95% CI; 46.4%-58.8%) of women aged 40 through 50 years were being regularly screened (2 mammograms within 4 years). Screening rates were higher among women who reported a physician recommendation than those who did not (ages 25-39 years, 76.0% vs 17.6%; ages 40-50 years, 87.3% vs 58.3%). In multivariate models, the association was particularly strong for younger women (ages 25-39 years, prevalence ratio [PR], 3.0; 95% CI, 2.0-4.0; ages 40-50 years, PR, 1.3; 95% CI, 1.1-1.6).

*Conclusions.*—In this cohort of women who had childhood cancer treated with chest radiation, 63.5% of those aged 25 through 39 years and 23.5% of those aged 40 through 50 years had not had mammography screening for breast cancer within the previous 2 years despite a guideline recommendation that survivors of childhood cancer who were treated with chest radiation should undergo annual screening mammography.

▶ It is well understood that women who have had chest radiation for a pediatric malignancy have a significant increase in the risk of breast cancer at a relatively young age. This risk is so significant that estimates suggest a risk of breast cancer development of 12% to 20% by age 45. Because of this very substantial risk, these patients are to receive annual screening mammography. The fact that in this study of 625 such women 63.5% of these patients ages 25 to 39 and 23.5% of these patients ages 40 to 50 had not had a screening mammogram in the past 2 years is frightening. It is imperative that we as radiation oncologists get this message out to primary care doctors and this patient population. Simple screening mammograms can help diagnose these cancers early and help reduce the chances of another life-threatening cancer in patients who have already faced this crisis as a child.

**C. A. Lawton, MD**

**ACR appropriateness criteria® on postmastectomy radiotherapy: Expert Panel on Radiation Oncology—Breast**

Taylor ME, Haffty BG, Rabinovitch R, et al (Washington Univ, Saint Louis, MO; Univ of Medicine and Dentistry, New Brunswick, NJ; Univ of Colorado Cancer Ctr, Denver; et al)

*Int J Radiat Oncol Biol Phys* 73:997-1002, 2009

This summary focuses on the role of postoperative radiation therapy in patients treated with modified radical mastectomy for invasive breast cancer, particularly in patients receiving systemic therapy.

▶ Standards of practice are exceedingly helpful for all practicing radiation oncologists. However, working to develop such standards takes the dedication and perseverance of many. The appropriateness criteria on postmastectomy radiotherapy (ACR) has taken a leadership role in developing standards for many aspects of radiation therapy, and this article on postmastectomy radiotherapy is another example of that fine work. The authors of this article represent a group of dedicated experts in the field of breast radiation therapy who come from institutions that literally spread from one end of the United States to the other. The method that they use to address the topic was also very beneficial and enlightening. Starting with local, regional failure rates in nonirradiated patients was important so as to address the potential effects of chemotherapy and hormone therapy (tamoxifen) on the local regional control of breast cancer. The authors next focused on the clear but important benefit of local regional control of breast cancer (with postmastectomy radiation therapy) and its improvement on both disease free and overall survival. Finally, they outlined the treatment volumes, techniques, and doses that allow for the benefit of local regional control and yet limit the potential toxicities.

These standards of practice are not only important to note and follow, but also must be updated on a regular basis as new data emerges. This article represents such an update, as the original guideline was developed in 1996. We look forward to more of these in the future.

**C. A. Lawton, MD**

**High Prevalence of Vitamin D Deficiency Despite Supplementation in Premenopausal Women With Breast Cancer Undergoing Adjuvant Chemotherapy**

Crew KD, Shane E, Cremers S, et al (Columbia Univ, NY)

*J Clin Oncol* 27:2151-2156, 2009

*Purpose*.—Vitamin D deficiency is associated with increased breast cancer risk and decreased breast cancer survival. The purpose of this study was to determine the prevalence of vitamin D deficiency, as measured by serum 25-hydroxyvitamin D (25-OHD), in premenopausal women at initiation of adjuvant chemotherapy for breast cancer and after 1 year of vitamin D supplementation.

*Patients and Methods.*—The study included 103 premenopausal women from the northeastern United States with stages I to III breast cancer who received adjuvant chemotherapy and participated in a 1-year zoledronate intervention trial. All patients were prescribed vitamin $D_3$ (cholecalciferol) 400 IU and calcium carbonate 1,000 mg daily. At baseline and at 6 and 12 months, bone mineral density (BMD) measurements were obtained and blood was collected and analyzed in batches for serum 25-OHD. Vitamin D deficiency was defined as serum 25-OHD less than 20 ng/mL, insufficiency as 20 to 29 ng/mL, and sufficiency as 30 ng/mL or greater.

*Results.*—At baseline, 74% of women were vitamin D deficient (median, 17 ng/mL). Vitamin D deficiency was slightly less common in white women (66%) compared with black (80%) and Hispanic (84%) women. After vitamin D supplementation for 1 year, less than 15% of white and Hispanic women, and no black women, achieved sufficient 25-OHD levels. Vitamin D levels did not correlate with baseline BMD and were not altered by chemotherapy or bisphosphonate use.

*Conclusion.*—Vitamin D deficiency is highly prevalent in women with breast cancer. The current recommended dietary allowance of vitamin D is too low to increase serum 25-OHD greater than 30 ng/mL. Optimal dosing for bone health and, possibly, improved survival has yet to be determined.

▶ Deficiency of vitamin D, in addition to adverse effects on the integrity of the bones, has been associated with an increased risk for the development of breast cancer and an increased risk for recurrence and death in those who have had breast cancer. In patients who have had breast cancer, supplementation with 1200 mg of calcium and 400 units of vitamin D daily has been recommended. This study looked at patients with breast cancer to determine the frequency with which vitamin deficiency is observed and the adequacy of recommended supplementation.

The study included 103 premenopausal women with stages I to III breast cancer who received adjuvant chemotherapy and participated in a 1-year trial involving intervention with zoledronate. All patients received 400 units of vitamin D and 1000 mg of calcium carbonate daily, with baseline, 6-, and 12-month assessments of bone mineral density and vitamin D levels. At baseline, 74% of women were vitamin D deficient (66% of Caucasian and 80% of black women). After the 1 year of vitamin D supplementation, less than 15% of Caucasian women and none of the black women achieved sufficient vitamin D levels. These levels did not correlate with baseline vitamin D levels and were not altered by chemotherapy or bisphosphanate use.

The bottom line of the study is that vitamin D deficiency is highly prevalent and that current recommendations for supplementation is not adequate. Physicians need to monitor this closely in their patients with breast cancer and to take appropriate measures to achieve adequate vitamin D levels in their patients.

**J. T. Thigpen, MD**

---

**Comparison of Sentinel Lymph Node Biopsy Alone and Completion Axillary Lymph Node Dissection for Node-Positive Breast Cancer**

Bilimoria KY, Bentrem DJ, Hansen NM, et al (American College of Surgeons, Chicago, IL; Northwestern Univ, Chicago, IL; et al)

*J Clin Oncol* 27:2946-2953, 2009

---

*Purpose.*—For women with breast cancer, the role of completion axillary lymph node dissection (ALND) after identification of nodal metastases by sentinel lymph node biopsy (SLNB) has been questioned. Our objectives were to assess national nodal evaluation practice patterns and to examine differences in recurrence and survival for SLNB alone versus SLNB with completion ALND.

*Patients and Methods.*—From the National Cancer Data Base (1998 to 2005), women with clinically node-negative breast cancer who underwent SLNB and who had nodal metastases were identified. Practice patterns and outcomes were examined for patients who underwent SLNB alone versus SLNB with completion ALND (median follow-up, 63 months).

*Results.*—Of 97,314 patients, 20.8% underwent SLNB alone, and 79.2% underwent SLNB with completion ALND. In 2004 to 2005, patients were significantly more likely to undergo SLNB alone if they were older, had smaller tumors, or were treated at non-National Cancer Institute–designated cancer centers. In patients with macroscopic nodal metastases (n = 20,075 during 1998 to 2000), there was a nonsignificant trend toward better outcomes for completion ALND (*v* SLNB alone) after analysis was adjusted for differences between the two groups: axillary recurrence (hazard ratio [HR], 0.58; 95% CI, 0.32 to 1.06) and overall survival (HR, 0.89; 95% CI, 0.76 to 1.04). In patients with microscopic nodal metastases (n = 2,203 during 1998 to 2000), there were no significant differences in axillary recurrence or survival for patients who underwent SLNB alone versus completion ALND.

*Conclusion.*—Compared with SLNB alone, completion ALND does not appear to improve outcomes for breast cancer patients with microscopic nodal metastases; however, there was a nonsignificant trend toward better outcomes with completion ALND for those with macroscopic disease.

► The determination of whether axillary lymph nodes are involved at the time of breast cancer diagnosis provides the physician and patient with information on the single most important prognostic factor for outcome. Complete removal of axillary lymph nodes through axillary dissection, however, does not in and of itself appear to improve outcome. With the development of sentinel node biopsy as a means of assessing the likelihood of axillary lymph node involvement, the question then becomes whether there is any reason to perform a subsequent axillary lymph node dissection with its attendant morbidity. An attempt to address this question in a prospective randomized trial by American College of Surgeons Oncology Group ended in premature closure because of the lack of accrual, and the reason for low accrual was the unwillingness of physicians and patients potentially to forgo the standard-of-care node dissection as a part of randomization.

This article attempts to address this question through a retrospective look at patients in the National Cancer Data Base over the 8-year period from 1998-2005. A total of 97 314 patients with clinically node-negative breast carcinoma were included. Of these, 20.8% underwent sentinel node biopsy alone; the rest had a completion axillary node dissection after sentinel node biopsy. No statistically significant differences in axillary recurrence or ultimate outcome were observed. One subset of patients, those with macroscopic involvement of lymph nodes, demonstrated a trend toward decreased axillary recurrence and improved overall survival, but these differences were not statistically significant.

It therefore appears that only patients who have macroscopic nodal involvement have a potential to benefit from completion axillary node dissection. A randomized trial will be required to answer definitively the role of completion axillary dissection in this patient population.

**J. T. Thigpen, MD**

---

### Impact of Micrometastases in the Sentinel Node of Patients With Invasive Breast Cancer

Hansen NM, Grube B, Ye X, et al (John Wayne Cancer Inst at Saint John's Health Ctr, Santa Monica, CA)
*J Clin Oncol* 27:4679-4684, 2009

---

*Purpose.*—Lymph node metastases are the most significant prognostic indicator for patients with breast cancer. Sentinel node biopsy (SNB) has led to an increase in the detection of micrometastases in the sentinel node (SN). This prospective study was designed to determine the survival impact of micrometastases in SNs of patients with invasive breast cancer. This study is based on the new sixth edition of the American Joint Committee on Cancer (AJCC) staging criteria.

*Patients and Methods.*—Between January 1, 1992 and April 30, 1999, 790 patients entered this prospective study at the John Wayne Cancer Institute. The SN was examined first by hematoxylin and eosin (HE), and if the SN was negative with HE, then immunohistochemical staining was performed. The patients were then divided into four groups based on AJCC nodal staging: pN0(i−), no evidence of tumor (n = 486); pN0(i+), tumor deposit ≤ 0.2 mm (n = 84); pN1mi, tumor deposit more than 0.2 mm but ≤ 2 mm (n = 54), and pN1, tumor deposit more than 2 mm (n = 166). Disease-free survival (DFS) and overall survival (OS) were estimated using the Kaplan-Meier method. The log-rank test was used to determine differences in DFS and OS of patients from different groups.

*Results.*—At a median follow-up of 72.5 months, the size of SN metastases was a significant predictor of DFS and OS.

*Conclusion.*—Patients with micrometastatic tumor deposits, pN0(i+) or pN1mi, do not seem to have a worse 8-year DFS or OS compared with SN-negative patients. As expected, there was a significant decrease in 8-year DFS and OS in patients with pN1 disease in the SN.

▶ Involvement of lymph nodes with metastatic deposits has been shown to be a major prognostic factor in early breast cancer. This observation was based on evaluation of lymph nodes on hematoxylin and eosin (HE) specimens. More recently, more sophisticated techniques have made detection of microscopic metastases not detectable by HE and light microscopy possible. This has an important question: do these micrometastases account for much of the 20% to 30% of patients with negative nodes who have recurrence or do these micrometastases have essentially no impact on outcome?

This study looks retrospectively at 790 patients who underwent sentinel node biopsy between 1992 and 1999 to determine whether detection of micrometastases by immunohistochemical staining identifies a group of patients at greater risk of recurrence. There are 4 groups of patients identified: pN0(i–) with no evidence of disease (n = 486); pN0+ with tumor deposits ≤0.2 mm (n = 84); pN1mi with tumor deposits between 0.2 mm and 2.0 mm in size (n = 54); and pN1 with deposits > 2.0 mm (n = 166). The bottom line is that there were no detectable differences in outcome among the first 3 of these groups. This strongly suggests that these micrometastases have no adverse effect on prognosis and would also suggest that these patients should manage as though they were node negative.

**J. T. Thigpen, MD**

---

### Independent Review of E2100: A Phase III Trial of Bevacizumab Plus Paclitaxel Versus Paclitaxel in Women With Metastatic Breast Cancer

Gray R, Bhattacharya S, Bowden C, et al (Dana-Farber Cancer Inst, Boston, MA; Genentech, South San Francisco, CA; Indiana Univ Melvin and Bren Simon Cancer Ctr, Indianapolis; et al)

*J Clin Oncol* 27:4966-4972, 2009

---

*Purpose.*—E2100, an open-label, randomized, phase III trial conducted by the Eastern Cooperative Oncology Group (ECOG), demonstrated a significant improvement in progression-free survival (PFS) and overall response rate (ORR) with paclitaxel plus bevacizumab compared with paclitaxel alone as initial chemotherapy for patients with HER2-negative metastatic breast cancer.

*Methods.*—An independent, blinded review of radiologic and clinical data was performed, assessing progression and response according to Response Evaluation Criteria in Solid Tumors. In addition, ECOG's investigator assessments were reanalyzed using the same methods applied to the independent review. The primary end point was PFS as assessed by an independent review facility (IRF).

*Results.*—The addition of bevacizumab to paclitaxel resulted in a statistically significant improvement in PFS using both the IRF and investigator assessments. Hazard ratios for PFS (0.48, 95% CI, 0.385 to 0.607; $P < .0001$ for the IRF *v* 0.42, 95%CI, 0.34 to 0.52; $P < .0001$ for ECOG investigators) and the improvement in median PFS (11.3 *v* 5.8 months for the IRF *v* 11.4 *v* 5.8 months for ECOG investigators) were similar. Among patients with measurable disease at baseline, the IRF-assessed ORR was significantly higher in patients treated with paclitaxel and bevacizumab (48.9% *v* 22.2%; $P < .0001$).

*Conclusion.*—The risk of progression was reduced by more than half and the ORR more than doubled with the addition of bevacizumab to weekly paclitaxel in both analyses, confirming a substantial and robust bevacizumab treatment effect. The consistency between the IRF and ECOG analyses validates the original data previously reported by ECOG in this open-label trial.

▶ This article is a report of an independent analysis of Eastern Cooperative Oncology Group trial E2100, which randomized HER2-negative patients with metastatic breast cancer to paclitaxel with or without bevacizumab. A review of these data by the Oncology Drugs Advisory Committee of the Food and Drug Administration led to a vote not to approve bevacizumab for use in metastatic breast cancer; thus, it is important that each oncologist review these data to determine whether he or she feels that bevacizumab has a role to play in the management of metastatic breast cancer. The independent review essentially confirmed the original report.[1] Patients assigned to the paclitaxel/bevacizumab regimen, as opposed to paclitaxel alone, exhibited a superior response rate (48.9% vs 22.2%, $P < .0001$) and superior progression-free survival (PFS) (hazard ratio = 0.48, $P < .0001$; median 11.3 vs 5.8 months). This would seem to represent clear evidence that paclitaxel/bevacizumab was clearly superior and that bevacizumab should be a part of the therapy for these patients. The principal controversy seems to focus on the use of PFS instead of overall survival as a measure of clinical benefit. One must, however, consider that for responsive cancers such as breast cancer and ovarian cancer, overall survival suffers from the fact that investigators cannot control therapy received by the patient after progression. This introduces multiple variables that can blur any ability to detect survival improvement; hence PFS, assessed carefully and correctly, would seem to be the most appropriate end point for these trials. PFS is clearly improved with bevacizumab added to paclitaxel.

**J. T. Thigpen, MD**

*Reference*

1. Miller K, Wang M, Gralow J, et al. Paclitaxel plus bevacizumab versus paclitaxel alone for metastatic breast cancer. *N Engl J Med*. 2007;357:2666-2676.

## Trastuzumab for Patients With Axillary-Node–Positive Breast Cancer: Results of the FNCLCC-PACS 04 Trial

Spielmann M, Roché H, Delozier T, et al (Institut Gustave Roussy, Villejuif; Institut Claudius Régaud, Toulouse; Centre François Baclesse, Caen; et al)
*J Clin Oncol* 27:6129-6134, 2009

*Purpose.*—To evaluate the efficacy of trastuzumab in patients with node-positive breast cancer treated with surgery, adjuvant chemotherapy, radiotherapy, and hormone therapy if applicable.

*Patients and Methods.*—Three thousand ten patients with operable node-positive breast cancer were randomly assigned to receive adjuvant anthracycline-based chemotherapy with or without docetaxel. Patients who presented human epidermal growth factor receptor 2 (HER2) -overexpressing tumors were secondary randomly assigned to either a sequential regimen of trastuzumab (6 mg/kg every 3 weeks) for 1 year or observation. The primary end point was disease-free survival (DFS).

*Results.*—Overall 528 patients were randomly assigned between trastuzumab (n = 260) and observation (n = 268) arm. Of the 234 patients (90%) who received at least one administration of trastuzumab, 196 (84%) received at least 6 months of treatment, and 41 (18%) discontinued treatment due to cardiac events (any grade). At the date of analysis (October 2007), 129 DFS events were recorded. Random assignment to the trastuzumab arm was associated with a nonsignificant 14% reduction in the risk of relapse (hazard ratio, 0.86; 95% CI, 0.61 to 1.22; *P* = .41, log-rank stratified on pathologic node involvement). Three-year DFS rates were 78% (95% CI, 72.3 to 82.5) and 81% (95% CI, 75.3 to 85.4) in the observation and trastuzumab arms, respectively.

*Conclusion.*—After a 47-month median follow-up, 1 year of trastuzumab given sequentially after adjuvant chemotherapy was not associated with a statistically significant decrease in the risk of relapse.

▶ The administration of trastuzumab in addition to chemotherapy in the adjuvant setting to patients with human epidermal growth factor receptor 2 (HER2) + breast carcinoma is widely accepted as the standard of care at the current time. This is based on the results of 5 separate phase III trials. In each of those studies, trastuzumab was given concurrently with chemotherapy and was followed with maintenance trastuzumab alone for a period of 1 year. This study differed from these other 5 trials in that it is the only one to use trastuzumab only as a maintenance therapy after the completion of chemotherapy. Among 528 patients randomized to trastuzumab or no trastuzumab after completion of chemotherapy, there was no difference in disease-free survival (hazard ratio [HR] = 0.86, $P = .41$). There are several possible explanations for this result. First, as noted above, this is the only study to report the use of trastuzumab only as a single agent in the maintenance setting. Second, this result is supported by a report, presented but not yet published, from the North Central Cancer Treatment Group trial of no benefit associated with the use of trastuzumab only as a single agent maintenance after chemotherapy. Third, this is the smallest dataset among the various studies of trastuzumab and hence may simply be underpowered, although the HR is substantially smaller than that observed in the other trials. In short, it is not clear why this result does not support the use of trastuzumab as maintenance only.

From a practical standpoint, the weight of evidence supports the use of trastuzuamb both concurrently with and following adjuvant chemotherapy in patients overexpressing HER2/neu.

**J. T. Thigpen, MD**

**Meta-Analysis of Breast Cancer Outcomes in Adjuvant Trials of Aromatase Inhibitors Versus Tamoxifen**

Dowsett M, Cuzick J, Ingle J, et al (Royal Marsden Hosp, London; Queen Mary Univ of London; Royal Free and Univ College London Med School; et al)

*J Clin Oncol* 28:509-518, 2010

*Purpose.*—To conduct meta-analyses of randomized trials of aromatase inhibitors (AIs) compared with tamoxifen either as initial monotherapy (cohort 1) or after 2 to 3 years of tamoxifen (cohort 2).

*Materials and Methods.*—Data submitted to the Early Breast Cancer Trialists' Collaborative Group were used in separate meta-analyses of two cohorts. Primary analyses involve postmenopausal women with tumors reported to be estrogen receptor positive. Log-rank $P$ values are two-sided.

*Results.*—Cohort 1 comprised 9,856 patients with a mean of 5.8 years of follow-up. At 5 years, AI therapy was associated with an absolute 2.9% (SE = 0.7%) decrease in recurrence (9.6% for AI *v* 12.6% for tamoxifen; $2P < .00001$) and a nonsignificant absolute 1.1% (SE = 0.5%) decrease in breast cancer mortality (4.8% for AI *v* 5.9% for tamoxifen; $2P = .1$). Cohort 2 comprised 9,015 patients with a mean of 3.9 years of follow-up. At 3 years from treatment divergence (ie, approximately 5 years after starting hormonal treatment), AI therapy was associated with an absolute 3.1% (SE = 0.6%) decrease in recurrence (5.0% for AI *v* 8.1% for tamoxifen since divergence; $2P < .00001$) and an absolute 0.7% (SE = 0.3%) decrease in breast cancer mortality (1.7% for AI *v* 2.4% for tamoxifen since divergence; $2P = .02$). There was no convincing heterogeneity in the proportional recurrence reduction with respect to age, nodal status, tumor grade, or progesterone receptor status and no indication of an increase in nonbreast deaths with AIs in either cohort.

*Conclusion.*—AIs produce significantly lower recurrence rates compared with tamoxifen, either as initial monotherapy or after 2 to 3 years of tamoxifen. Additional follow-up will provide clearer information on long-term survival.

► For hormonal therapy in postmenopausal patients with breast cancer, tamoxifen was long considered to be the initial therapy of choice. With the development of better-tolerated inhibitors of aromatase, studies have been conducted to compare the effect of these agents with tamoxifen. This meta-analysis focuses on 2 such trials which compare 5 years of an aromatase inhibitor with 5 years of tamoxifen and 4 such trials which give all patients 2 to 3 years of tamoxifen and then randomize patients to either continued tamoxifen for 5 years or an aromatase inhibitor for 5 years. The pooled data include 18 871 patients. The use of an aromatase inhibitor produced an absolute 3% reduction in recurrence and an absolute 0.7% reduction in mortality. These data suggest that an aromatase inhibitor should be a part of the adjuvant hormonal therapy for postmenopausal patients with breast cancer. One should also keep in mind that the absolute gain is greater in those patients with a greater risk for recurrence.

**J. T. Thigpen, MD**

## Inflammatory Breast Cancer

Woodward WA, Cristofanilli M (The Univ of Texas M. D. Anderson Cancer Ctr, Houston)

*Semin Radiat Oncol* 19:256-265, 2009

Inflammatory breast cancer (IBC) represents the most virulent form of breast cancer, characterized by involvement of the skin and rapid progression of the disease. Management involves careful coordination of all multidisciplinary modalities, including imaging, systemic chemotherapy, surgery, and radiation therapy. The use of neoadjuvant chemotherapy has contributed significantly to improvement in overall survival since the first descriptions of this entity and has made the role of locoregional therapy, including surgery and radiation critical to continued improvements in this disease. In this article, we examine the unique epidemiology and pathology of IBC and review the various treatment modalities noting the significance of a multimodality approach and delineating each of the specific components. Moreover, we briefly describe the current research in IBC that will hopefully contribute further to improve systemic therapies.

► Breast cancer affects approximately 1 in 8 women in the United States, with inflammatory breast cancer being the most virulent. This form of breast cancer is associated with skin involvement and rapid progression of disease and often death.

Advances in chemotherapy have helped this previously almost uniformly fatal disease to become one that is systemically treatable and in some cases curable. These authors have written an excellent review of the history of this disease as well as the current treatments of choice. Their discussion of risk factors, clinical signs, and conventional biomarkers, in addition to the treatment aspects, serves as a fine overview of the state of the art of treatment for this terrible form of breast cancer.

Despite major advances in treatment for inflammatory breast cancer there remain some patients who do not respond well to neoadjuvant chemotherapy. Thus the author's discussion of ongoing research is helpful and necessary.

**C. A. Lawton, MD**

---

**Local Excision Alone Without Irradiation for Ductal Carcinoma In Situ of the Breast: A Trial of the Eastern Cooperative Oncology Group**

Hughes LL, Wang M, Page DL, et al (North Georgia Radiation Therapy/The Hope Ctr, Cartersville; Emory Univ, Atlanta, GA; Dana-Farber Cancer Inst, Boston, MA; et al)

*J Clin Oncol* 27:5319-5324, 2009

---

*Purpose.*—To determine the risk of ipsilateral breast events in patients with ductal carcinoma in situ (DCIS) treated with local excision without irradiation.

*Patients and Methods.*—Patients with either low- or intermediate-grade DCIS measuring 2.5 cm or smaller, or high-grade DCIS measuring 1 cm or smaller who had microscopic margin widths of 3 mm or wider and no residual calcifications on postoperative mammograms were eligible for a prospective trial conducted from 1997 to 2002 by the Eastern Cooperative Oncology Group and North Central Cancer Treatment Group. Patients entered in 2000 and later could take tamoxifen if they wished. Median age at last surgery for the entire population was 60 years (range, 28 to 88 years), and median tumor sizes in the two strata were 6 mm and 5 mm, respectively.

*Results.*—With a median follow-up of 6.2 years, the 5-year rate of ipsilateral breast events in the 565 eligible patients in the low/intermediate grade stratum was 6.1% (95% CI, 4.1% to 8.2%). With a median follow-up of 6.7 years, this incidence for the 105 eligible patients in the high-grade stratum was 15.3% (95% CI, 8.2% to 22.5%).

*Conclusion.*—Rigorously evaluated and selected patients with low- to intermediate-grade DCIS with margins 3 mm or wider had an acceptably low rate of ipsilateral breast events at 5 years after excision without irradiation. Patients with high-grade lesions had a much higher rate, suggesting that excision alone is inadequate treatment. Further follow-up is necessary to document long-term results.

▶ Prospective (randomized if possible) trials represent the type of data that oncologists wish they had for each medical decision they make. And while we do have many such trials, the majority of the decisions we make are based on lesser evidence.

Ductal carcinoma in situ (DCIS) is not invasive breast cancer. Thus, radical treatment, be it mastectomy or lumpectomy plus whole-breast irradiation, presents concerns for overtreatment in a disease that in many cases will never progress. This trial of the Eastern Cooperative Oncology Group (ECOG) presents an excellent resource for patients and oncologists alike in trying to decide next steps after lumpectomy in patients with the diagnosis of DCIS.

With a median follow-up of 6.2 years, which is short in breast cancer terms, this data certainly supports the need for postlumpectomy radiation therapy in patients with high-grade DCIS. For patients with low- and intermediate-grade DCIS, longer follow-up is needed to reinforce the low risk of recurrence seen to date with lumpectomy alone. We also await the results of RTOG 98-04, a phase III trial with case selection similar to this trial, but randomized to post-lumpectomy radiation versus observation.

**C. A. Lawton, MD**

---

**Effect of oral clodronate on bone mass, bone turnover and subsequent metastases in women with primary breast cancer**

McCloskey E, Paterson A, Kanis J, et al (Univ of Sheffield Med School, UK; Tom Baker Cancer Centre, Calgary, Alberta, Canada; et al)

*Eur J Cancer* 46:558-565, 2010

---

Breast cancer treatments have been associated with accelerated bone loss and increased osteoporosis risk. In a subgroup analysis of a randomised, double-blind, placebo-controlled study, we compared the changes in spine and total hip bone mineral density (BMD) and biochemical markers of bone turnover in women with primary breast cancer who had received standard therapy plus either oral clodronate 1600 mg/d ($n = 419$) or placebo ($n = 432$) for 2 years. After 2 years, spine BMD was 1.92% higher in patients who received clodronate instead of placebo ($P < 0.0001$) and total hip BMD was 1.29% higher ($P = 0.002$ versus placebo). Patients who received clodronate had a median 26% reduction in levels of serum N-terminal pro-peptide of type I procollagen (PINP) – a marker of bone turnover – after 2 years of therapy. This compares with a median 5% increase in patients who received placebo ($P < 0.0001$). Effects on BMD, but not biochemical markers, persisted for up to 3 years post-treatment. Early changes in PINP were associated with changes in BMD and the likelihood of developing bone metastases.

**This study shows the use of oral clodronate during primary breast cancer treatment is associated with reduced bone turnover and protection against bone metastases.**

▶ In this interesting article, McCloskey and colleagues describe the effects of oral clodronate administered to patients with primary breast cancer.

The objective of this subgroup analysis was to evaluate the effect of oral clodronate treatment on spine and total hip BMD during a 2-year treatment period and during the 3 years of posttreatment follow-up. In addition, in a group of participants who had serum and urine samples collected, McCloskey and colleagues evaluated the relationship between early changes in BMD and bone turnover biochemical markers and incident bone metastases.

The trial was designed as a double-blind, multicenter, randomized, placebo-controlled study. As mentioned above, McCloskey and colleagues evaluated the long-term effect of adjuvant oral clodronate 1600 mg/day for 2 years on the incidence of bone and other metastases and on long-term survival in women with primary operable breast cancer. Of the 1069 patients enrolled in the main study, 516 (48%) had BMD data available for review, and 566 (53%) had serum and urine samples collected for analysis.

After 2 years, spine BMD was 1.92% higher in patients who received clodronate compared to those who received a placebo, and total hip BMD was 1.29% higher. McCloskey and colleagues found that adding oral clodronate to standard adjuvant therapy for primary breast cancer prevented bone loss and reduced bone turnover in both pre and postmenopausal women.

McCloskey and colleagues also found that bone metabolism at the time of breast cancer diagnosis, as assessed by bone mass and turnover markers, is not significantly associated with the subsequent risk of bone metastasis. However, they noted that early changes in serum PINP were associated with changes in BMD and the likelihood of developing bone metastases. The relationship between PINP progression and the development of bone metastases persisted, with the incidence of bone disease in the progressive group being 17.6% compared with 5.2% in the other groups combined ($P = 0.015$). They concluded that serum PINP has the potential to be a marker of response to therapy and possibly provide early detection of skeletal metastases.

Since this was a subset analysis, the number of patients was small, with only 230 women with paired measurements at baseline and 1 year. Another prospective study will be needed to confirm these observations and place them in a clinical context.

It is important to understand how bone metabolism markers influence bone loss and bone metastases. There is evidence that bisphosphonates prevent bone loss,[1,2] but whether or not bisphosphonates are appropriate adjuvant therapy and have antitumor effects is a controversial issue. If a bone marker that influences bone loss and the development of bone metastases were found, we could effectively select patients for whom bisphosphonate therapy prevents bone loss and bone metastases and prolongs survival.

The results of this analysis add to the growing body of literature suggesting that there is a role for the adjuvant use of bisphosphonates. The proper selection of patients at risk of bone disease, avoidance of bisphosphonate-associated toxicities, and the best agent and means of administration are subjects of ongoing research. In this study, McCloskey and colleagues used clodronate, a bisphosphonate not available in the United States, so American clinicians unfortunately cannot apply this approach to their practice.

**N. Niikura, MD**

**R. L. Theriault, DO, MBA**

*References*

1. Eidtmann H, de Boer R, Bundred N, et al. Efficacy of zoledronic acid in postmenopausal women with early breast cancer receiving adjuvant letrozole: 36-month results of the ZO-FAST Study [published online ahead of print May 5, 2010]. *Ann Oncol.* doi:10.1093/annonc/mdq217.
2. Brufsky AM, Bosserman LD, Caradonna RR, et al. Zoledronic acid effectively prevents aromatase inhibitor-associated bone loss in postmenopausal women with early breast cancer receiving adjuvant letrozole: Z-FAST study at 36-month follow-up results. *Clin Breast Cancer.* 2009;9:77-85.

---

**Surgeon Recommendations and Receipt of Mastectomy for Treatment of Breast Cancer**

Morrow M, Jagsi R, Alderman AK, et al (Memorial Sloan-Kettering Cancer Ctr, NY; Univ of Michigan Health System, Ann Arbor; et al)

*JAMA* 302:1551-1556, 2009

---

*Context.*—There is concern that mastectomy is overused in the United States.

*Objectives.*—To evaluate the association of patient-reported initial recommendations by surgeons and those given when a second opinion was sought with receipt of initial mastectomy; and to assess the use of mastectomy after attempted breast-conserving surgery (BCS).

*Design, Setting, and Patients.*—A survey of women aged 20 to 79 years with intraductal or stage I and II breast cancer diagnosed between June 2005 and February 2007 and reported to the National Cancer Institute's Surveillance, Epidemiology, and End Results registries for the metropolitan areas of Los Angeles, California, and Detroit, Michigan. Patients were identified using rapid case ascertainment, and Latinas and blacks were oversampled. Of 3133 patients sent surveys, 2290 responded (73.1%). A mailed survey was completed by 96.5% of respondents and 3.5% completed a telephone survey. The final sample included 1984 female patients (502 Latinas, 529 blacks, and 953 non-Hispanic white or other).

*Main Outcome Measures.*—The rate of initial mastectomy and the perceived reason for its use (surgeon recommendation, patient driven, medical contraindication) and the rate of mastectomy after attempted BCS.

*Results.*—Of the 1984 patients, 1468 had BCS as an initial surgical therapy (75.4%) and 460 had initial mastectomy, including 13.4% following surgeon recommendation and 8.8% based on patient preference. Approximately 20% of patients (n = 378) sought a second opinion; this was more common for those patients advised by their initial surgeon to undergo mastectomy (33.4%) than for those advised to have BCS (15.6%) or for those not receiving a recommendation for one procedure over another (21.2%) ($P < .001$). Discordance in treatment recommendations between surgeons occurred in 12.1% (n = 43) of second opinions and did not differ on the basis of patient race/ethnicity, education, or geographic site. Among the 1459 women for whom BCS was attempted, additional surgery was required in 37.9% of patients, including 358 with reexcision (26.0%) and 167 with mastectomy (11.9%). Mastectomy was most common in patients with stage II cancer ($P < .001$).

*Conclusion.*—Breast-conserving surgery was recommended by surgeons and attempted in the majority of patients evaluated, with surgeon recommendation, patient decision, and failure of BCS all contributing to the mastectomy rate.

► This article by Morrow and colleagues presents a compelling landmark view of the decision-making process of patients undergoing breast cancer treatment. The authors utilized the National Cancer Institute's Surveillance, Epidemiology, and End Results (SEER) data set to find patients recently treated (within 9 months) then used a survey, for which the patients were reimbursed, to collect the corollary information regarding the patients' decisions about the primary treatment of their breast cancer. Critical to the study and cogent to the arguments about surgeon influence in the decision-making process is the fact that surgeons were very accurate and on task relative to their recommendations, with only 6.2% of patients receiving a recommendation for mastectomy when there was no compelling contraindication to lumpectomy. Furthermore, 11.9% of patients underwent conversion to mastectomy when lumpectomy was initially recommended, and conversely, 46.5% of patients for whom mastectomy was initially recommended ultimately required mastectomy when they chose against the recommendation and opted for lumpectomy. Aside from the decision-based observations, several benchmarks of treatment can be derived from these data and are consistent with the published literature. The overall lumpectomy reexcision rate was 26.0%, and of the patients who underwent lumpectomy reexcision, 30.7% had ductal carcinoma in situ, 23.7% had stage I disease, and 24.0% had stage II disease. A compelling finding was that 37.9% of all BCS patients required a second operation. Furthermore, of the patients who underwent BCS conversion to mastectomy, 18.0% had stage II disease, 12.0% had ductal carcinoma in situ, and 8.3% had stage I disease.

The discussion by Morrow and colleagues is thorough and complete. It points out some potential flaws of generalizing the data collected from large metropolitan areas and qualifies that patient recall of the presentation of the complex information in this decision-making process is subject to bias from

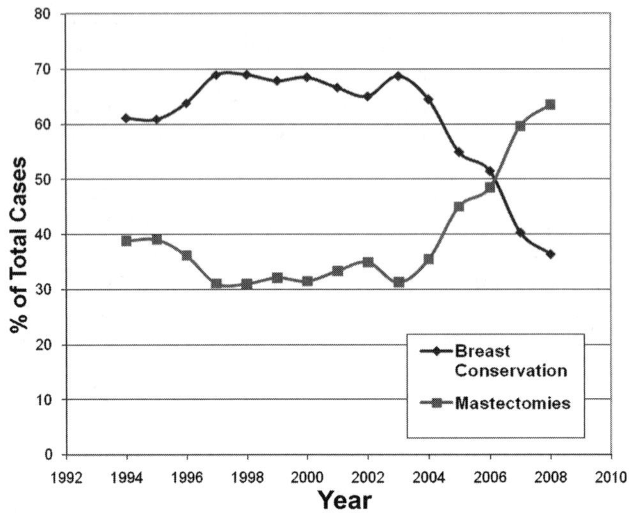


FIGURE 1.—

the patient and researcher alike. That aside, the information collected from the patients is extremely accurate and consistent with the literature and thus has extreme validity in our eyes. The data demonstrate that in these major metropolitan academic centers, the rate of lumpectomy remains 66%.

We are not sure that this study truly addresses the "overuse of mastectomy" as a community-based issue since the metropolitan academic medical center surgeon base of the SEER study group is keenly aware of lumpectomy and its use. Many influences in the community setting may not apply here. Economic credentialing of surgeons within insurance plans could influence recommendations. Surgeons performing mastectomies alone would represent a better bottom line to the insurer since they would not be adding a second procedure 38% of the time and would be utilizing costly irradiation infrequently, making them the preferred providers. As the authors pointed out, patient preferences can vary and social networks can have a profound influence on the patient decision-making process. Recent compilations from the Mayo Clinic[1] and the Moffitt Cancer Center[2] have demonstrated a dramatic shift in patient choice within the same time frame as this study (Fig). Clearly, practice patterns at large referral centers with large geographic draws may indeed have various socioeconomic and decision-making influences at play. Additional factors that have been cited as possible causes of this shift away from lumpectomy include younger age, higher education level, and earlier disease stage in patients with a family history of breast cancer. Furthermore, increased use of magnetic resonance imaging (MRI) for preoperative planning is a commonly referenced cause.[3] The Moffitt Cancer Center and Mayo Clinic studies, while assessing this as a contributory factor, could not attribute more than an 8% to 10% shift away from lumpectomy to MRI overinterpretation.[1,2]

Affluence, mobility, and the ability of patients to choose and travel to a "center of excellence," as well as access to social networks through the Internet, are causing huge changes in this decision-making process, in which the physician has little control and about which little research exists. Patients can now go online and seek opinions anonymously. The author-initiated group FACTors (Fighting Against Cancer Together), which was designed in the 1980s as the first peer-to-peer support group to allow lumpectomy patients to contact each other for treatment and outcome information, was instrumental in increasing the rate of lumpectomy at the Moffitt Cancer Center to nearly 70%,[2] compared with the Florida statewide rate of only 20% (Florida Cancer Data System 1987-1997). Other organizations, including Susan G. Komen for the Cure, Why me? and the American Cancer Society's Reach for Recovery program, as well as local social support groups, were also developed during the 1980s. These programs now pale in comparison to the anonymity, availability, and universality of Web-based blogs, Facebook, and Twitter. Rarely does a patient present without a sheaf of papers, questions, and commentary harvested from the Internet. Never have there been as many well-informed patients.

More than 60% of patients with breast cancer in the SEER database have undergone BCS over the past 20 years; therefore, many survivors have experienced BCS or mastectomy for recurrence after BCS, each of whom has passed through several decision-making steps over the course of their care. After BCS, the constant reminders of one's breast cancer diagnosis are punctuated by mammograms, biopsies, MRIs, recurrent calcifications, chest wall discomfort, and breast size or contour discrepancies associated with radiotherapy. In addition, the need for reconstructive surgery following mastectomy for recurrence after BCS and the many reconstructive options available (autologous reconstruction with latissimus dorsi, deep inferior epigastric perforator, transverse rectus abdominis musculocutaneous, or gluteal flaps, as well as implant-based reconstruction) add to these complexities. Furthermore, chemotherapy and its complications—alopecia, paresthesia, weight gain, hot flashes, and bone pain—as well as decisions regarding the use of hormone therapy, are just a few more issues faced by patients who have undergone BCS. These survivors, who are informed and willing to share, are the first to say they are alive as a result of their treatment, but they would likely trade their breast to avoid the "fear of recurrence" and all the mammograms, biopsies, and MRIs. Who is to say that they are not right?

Breast salvage is a tremendous advance in breast cancer care and has saved many lives and led to excellent outcomes in the majority of patients over the last 2 decades. However, the pendulum of social networking, whether based on knowledge or patient experience, is a significant driving force in the decision-making process and one that has yet to be investigated. Blogs have existed since 1994 and gained popularity in 2002 when they became the vehicle for former US Senator Trent Lott's resignation. By 2004, they had become mainstream; they were being used by news media to find news stories and were truly functioning as a social networking tool. These Web-based tools and other social networks that exist in communities, the workplace, churches, and even within families have an impact on the decision-making process. Fear is a powerful motivator for women, mothers, and wives, who when confronted with a diagnosis of BRCA genetic risk or cancer recurrence, often perceive their breasts as changing from a sexual asset to a life-or-death liability.

In the 1980s, BCS was tied to the Equal Rights Amendment and a woman's right to choose her fate.[4] Rose Kushner's legacy of patient and women's advocacy, born through Bernie Fischer's validation of lumpectomy as a treatment choice, thrives today.[5] Their vocal and strident efforts will remain their legacy for generations. Yet, the pendulum is swinging back in the other direction for all the reasons mentioned herein, a trend that has little to do with women's rights but perhaps much to do with the right to live unfettered by fear.[6,7]

**C. E. Cox, MD**
**M. Wilson, MD**
**M. M. Williams, MD**

*References*


1. Katipamula R, Degnim AC, Hoskin T, et al. Trends in mastectomy rates at the Mayo Clinic Rochester: effect of surgical year and preoperative magnetic resonance imaging. *J Clin Oncol.* 2009;27:4082-4088.
2. McGuire K, Santillan AA, Kaur P, et al. Are mastectomies on the rise? A 13-year trend analysis of the selection of mastectomy versus breast conservation therapy in 5865 patients. *Ann Surg Oncol.* 2009;16:2682-2690.
3. Lee MC, Rogers K, Griffith K, et al. Determinants of breast conservation rates: reasons for mastectomy at a comprehensive cancer center. *Breast J.* 2009;15: 34-40.
4. Wikipedia contributors. Rose Kushner. Wikipedia, The Free Encyclopedia, http://en.wikipedia.org/wiki/Rose_Kushner. Updated May 21, 2010. Accessed June 14, 2010.
5. Lerner BH. No shrinking violet: Rose Kushner and the rise of American breast cancer activism. *West J Med.* 2001;174:362-365.
6. Balch CM, Jacobs LK. Mastectomies on the rise for breast cancer: "the tide is changing". *Ann Surg Oncol.* 2009;16:2669-2672.
7. Balch C. Choosing Between a Mastectomy or Lumpectomy, http://mycanceradvisor.com/2010/01/22/choosing-between-a-mastectomy-or-lumpectomy/. Accessed January 22, 2010.


## Radiation Dose and Breast Cancer Risk in the Childhood Cancer Survivor Study

Inskip PD, Robison LL, Stovall M, et al (Natl Insts of Health, Bethesda, MD; St Jude Children's Res Hosp, Memphis, TN; Univ of Texas MD Anderson Cancer Ctr, Houston; et al)
*J Clin Oncol* 27:3901-3907, 2009

*Purpose.*—The purpose of this study was to quantify the risk of breast cancer in relation to radiation dose and chemotherapy among survivors of childhood cancer.

*Methods.*—We conducted a case-control study of breast cancer in a cohort of 6,647 women who were 5-year survivors of childhood cancer and who were treated during 1970 through 1986. One hundred twenty patients with histologically confirmed breast cancer were identified and were individually matched to four selected controls on age at initial cancer and time since initial cancer. Medical physicists estimated radiation dose to the breast tumor site and ovaries on the basis of medical records.

*Results.*—The odds ratio for breast cancer increased linearly with radiation dose, and it reached 11-fold for local breast doses of approximately 40 Gy relative to no radiation ($P$ for trend < .0001). Risk associated with breast irradiation was sharply reduced among women who received 5 Gy or more to the ovaries ($P$ =.002). The excess odds ratio per Gy was 0.36 for those who received ovarian doses less than 5 Gy and was 0.06 for those who received higher doses. Radiation-related risk did not vary significantly by age at exposure. Borderline significantly elevated risks were seen for doxorubicin, dactinomycin, dacarbazine, and carmustine.

*Conclusion.*—Results confirm the radiation sensitivity of the breast in girls age 10 to 20 years but do not demonstrate a strong effect of age at exposure within this range. Irradiation of the ovaries at doses greater than 5 Gy seems to lessen the carcinogenic effects of breast irradiation, most likely by reducing exposure of radiation-damaged breast cells to stimulating effects of ovarian hormones.

▶ This study by Inskip and colleagues addresses an important gap in knowledge regarding the risk of second breast cancers related to breast radiation dose received during breast development. This case-control study was conducted as part of the Childhood Cancer Survivor Study. The study included a large cohort of 6647 women who were 5-year survivors of childhood cancer. The study included patients who were treated for 1 of 8 types of first cancers: leukemia, craniospinal cancer, Hodgkin's lymphoma, non-Hodgkin's lymphoma, kidney cancer, soft tissue sarcoma, neuroblastoma, and bone sarcoma.

This study showed that individuals who developed second breast cancers were 2.7 times more likely to have been exposed to radiation. A significant finding of this study was that the data followed a linear dose-response model with a slope (excess odds ratio) of 0.27 per Gy. There was no downturn in the response for high doses, a finding that differs from many theoretical dose-response relationships that assume extensive cell killing at high doses. When data were adjusted for radiation dose and age at irradiation, differences by type of first cancer were not statistically significant. As such, the dose-response model applies for all types of first cancers.

When data were separated for women whose treatment for the initial cancer included a sterilizing dose to the ovaries (≥5 Gy), the data still followed a linear dose-response curve, but the slope decreased to 0.06 per Gy. This information translates into the tangible finding that women who received breast doses of 40 Gy had an overall 11-fold higher risk for developing second breast cancers as compared to nonirradiated patients. However, women whose treatment for the initial cancer included 5 Gy or more to the ovaries had a lower risk of developing a second breast cancer, showing only a 3.4-fold higher risk relative to nonirradiated patients. Chemotherapy for the initial cancer was not found to significantly affect breast cancer risk when analyses were adjusted for radiation dose to the breast and ovaries.

A notable strength of this study is that it has substantial information regarding the patients as well as their radiation and chemotherapy treatments. Data on surgical procedures and all chemotherapeutic agents, including cumulative doses and routes of administration, were obtained from the medical record of each study participant. Furthermore, the radiation therapy records were abstracted to identify the dates of therapy, beam energy, field size, field location, number of treatment fractions, and total dose to each field. This information was then used to reconstruct the dose distributions for each case-control set to the most specific breast tumor location possible. The dosimetric reconstructions also considered the stage of breast development by changing the size of the breast for dose calculations on the basis of stage of development. The dose reconstructions were also used to determine the dose to the ovaries for each case-control set. An additional strength of this study is that statistical power was maximized by using individually matched controls, with a control-to-case ratio of 4:1.

This study by Inskip and colleagues is by far one of the best studies to date that addresses second breast cancers. Its main strengths include the large number of patients in the study as well as patient-specific information, most notably the excellent patient-specific dosimetry. The overarching implications of this work are the demonstration of a linear dose-response model and the associated inference that every effort should be made to minimize the dose to healthy breast tissue during radiation therapy for patients under 20 years of age.

**R. M. Howell, PhD**

**S. F. Kry, PhD**

# 15 Central Nervous System

**American College of Radiology appropriateness criteria on multiple brain metastases**

Expert Panel on Radiation Oncology–Brain Metastases, Videtic GMM (Cleveland Clinic Foundation, OH; Univ of Colorado Penver. Aurora; Van Elslander Cancer ctr, Grosse Point, MI; et al)

*Int J Radiat Oncol Biol Phys* 75:961-965, 2009

As many as 170,000 cancer patients will develop brain metastases each year (1). Brain metastases represent the most common neurologic manifestation of cancer, occurring in 15% cancer patients, particularly those with lung and breast cancer diagnoses (2). Clinical (2), imaging (3), and autopsy (4) series have shown that approximately half of brain metastases will be solitary and half will be multiple. Among patients with multiple lesions, the majority of metastases (70%) are found supratentorially (2). The most common symptoms of brain metastases are headache, altered mental status, and focal weakness, occurring in up to half of patients. The next most common symptoms include seizures and gait ataxia, which are seen in approximately 10–20% of patients (2).

Whole-brain radiotherapy (WBRT) is the established standard of care for the vast majority of patients with multiple brain metastases, although there have been no randomized trials showing that WBRT offers a survival advantage over supportive care. Even a recent randomized pilot study that compared primary chemotherapy for newly diagnosed non–small-cell lung cancer brain metastases with up-front WBRT found no differences in survival or response rates (5). Nonetheless, attempts to improve outcomes in patients with multiple brain metastases are warranted given the modest outcomes and have included the use of different dose/fractionation schedules, radiation sensitizers, surgery, and stereotactic radiosurgery (SRS).

▶ Guidelines for the treatment of many cancers are helpful parameters for clinical radiation oncologists across the United States and beyond. With ever-changing technology within radiation oncology and other related fields such as surgical oncology and medical oncology, such appropriateness criteria can be a source of great comfort in reinforcing best care/state-of-the-art care for patients with cancer.

This article addresses the American College of Radiology (ACR) appropriateness criteria for patients with multiple brain metastases. Given that the number of patients who suffer from brain metastases each year exceeds 150 000 worldwide, this is an important topic to address.

The standard-of-care treatment for patients with multiple brain metastases has been whole brain radiation therapy. Because the survival of these patients usually ranges from 4 to 6 months, one has to wonder if this is the best option because it is well understood that this treatment has toxicity. Hair loss and neurocognitive decline are known side effects of whole brain radiation therapy. Therefore, its application to the patient with multiple brain metastases has to be considered with some caution. The benefit of the ACR approach to these appropriateness criteria is that it is done based on clinical cases (a sampling of which is in the article). It is definitely worth the reader's time to examine each of the clinical vignettes presented and the recommended approach for each by this panel of brain metastasis experts.

**C. A. Lawton, MD**

---

**Technological Advances in Radiation Oncology for Central Nervous System Tumors**

Noda S-E, Lautenschlaeger T, Siedow MR, et al (Massachusetts General Hosp, Boston; et al)

*Semin Radiat Oncol* 19:179-186, 2009

---

Advances in computer software technology have led to enormous progress that has enabled increasing levels of complexity to be incorporated into radiotherapy treatment planning systems. Because of these changes, the delivery of radiotherapy evolved from therapy designed primarily on plain 2-dimensional X-ray images and hand calculations to therapy based on 3-dimensional images incorporating increasingly complex computer algorithms in the planning process. In addition, challenges in treatment planning and radiation delivery, such as problems with setup error and organ movement, have begun to be systematically addressed, ushering in an era of so-called 4-dimensional radiotherapy. This review article discusses how these advances have changed the way in which many common neoplasms of the central nervous system are being treated at present.

▶ Multiple technological advances have occurred in the delivery of radiotherapy over the last 2 decades. These advances have allowed for a revolution in the identification of central nervous system tumors, and therefore, the ability to target and treat them with radiotherapy. These authors have reviewed the advances and have outlined the relative results of these technologies: intensity-modulated radiation therapy (IMRT) stereotactic radiosurgery, image-guided radiation therapy (IGRT), protons and other particle therapies such as carbon ions and boron neutron capture therapy, and brachytherapy.

What is clear is that each of these technologies has a particular role and should be used and understood accordingly. For example, IMRT clearly has resulted in less dose to critical organs such as the brain stem, optic chiasm, etc in the treatment of gliomas of the brain, yet major improvements in terms of survival with IMRT-treated glioma patients has not been seen. Additionally, the whole question of stereotactic treatment of brain metastasis in addition to whole brain radiotherapy has been studied extensively. It appears that there is a role for stereotactic radiosurgery in patients with a solitary brain metastasis, but not for patients with multiple metastasis. Finally, with regard to proton therapy, the value of this treatment for pediatric central nervous system tumors is unquestioned due to the increased conformality, yet there is no clear role that has been established for proton therapy of adult central nervous system tumors. As technologies for radiation therapy advance, we must scientifically evaluate their potential role and use that data to guide our appropriate use of these technologies.

**C. A. Lawton, MD**

# 16 Chemotherapy: Mechanisms and Side Effects

---

**Effective Strategies for Management of Hypertension After Vascular Endothelial Growth Factor Signaling Inhibition Therapy: Results From a Phase II Randomized, Factorial, Double-Blind Study of Cediranib in Patients With Advanced Solid Tumors**

Langenberg MHG, van Herpen CML, De Bono J, et al (Univ Med Ctr Utrecht, the Netherlands; Radboud Univ Nijmegen Med Centre, the Netherlands; The Netherlands Cancer Inst; et al)

*J Clin Oncol* 27:6152-6159, 2009

---

*Purpose.*—Hypertension is a commonly reported adverse effect after administration of vascular endothelial growth factor (VEGF) inhibitors. Cediranib is a highly potent and selective VEGF signaling inhibitor of all three VEGFRs. This study prospectively investigated hypertension management to help minimize dose interruptions/reductions to maximize cediranib dose intensity.

*Patients and Methods.*—Patients ($n = 126$) with advanced solid tumors were randomly assigned to one of four groups: cediranib 30 or 45 mg/d with or without antihypertensive prophylaxis. All patients developing hypertension on cediranib treatment were treated with a standardized, predefined hypertension management protocol.

*Results.*—Cediranib was generally well tolerated, and all groups achieved high-dose intensities in the first 12 weeks (> 74% in all groups). Antihypertensive prophylaxis did not result in fewer dose reductions or interruptions. Increases in blood pressure, including moderate and severe readings of hypertension, were seen early in treatment in all groups and successfully managed. Severe hypertension occurred in one patient receiving prophylaxis versus 18 in the nonprophylaxis groups. Overall, there were nine partial responses, and 38 patients experienced stable disease ≥ 8 weeks.

*Conclusion.*—To our knowledge, this is the first prospective investigation of hypertension management during administration of a VEGF signaling inhibitor. All four regimens were well tolerated with high-dose intensities and no strategy was clearly superior. The current cediranib hypertension management protocol appears to be effective in managing hypertension compared with previous cediranib studies where no plan was in place, and early recognition and treatment of hypertension is likely to reduce the number of severe hypertension events. This protocol is included in all ongoing cediranib clinical studies.

▶ Antiangiogenic therapy with a number of agents is associated with hypertension as a major adverse effect. One of these agents in particular, cediranib, exhibited a 16% frequency of grade 3 to 4 hypertension and a 4% frequency of hypertensive crisis. Many patients on the initial phase II study were unable to complete the assigned 8 weeks of therapy. Hypertension therefore posed a major problem.

This study sought to determine whether prophylaxis for hypertension and organized treatment of hypertension that developed would reduce the frequency with which the drug had to be discontinued. Patients were randomized to either 30 mg/d or 45 mg/d of cediranib and then rerandomized to either antihypertensive prophylaxis or no prophylaxis. Those assigned to prophylaxis with a baseline blood pressure between 110/70 and 150/100 were started on prophylactic low-dose calcium channel blocker (nifedipine) 3 to 7 days before the start of cediranib, while those with a baseline lower than 110/70 were started on prophylaxis on the same day that cediranib was started. If hypertension developed during treatment, patients were treated with a defined protocol outlined in the figure in the original article and dependent on the severity of the observed hypertension. In the trial, 19 patients developed elevated blood pressure meeting the criteria for severe hypertension, 1 on the prophylaxis regimen and 18 among those not receiving prophylaxis. These findings suggest that prophylaxis can decrease the frequency of severe hypertension and that management with a defined protocol results in fewer patients having to stop therapy early. This in turn can theoretically improve outcome with cediranib.

**J. T. Thigpen, MD**

# 17 Genitourinary

**Adjuvant Radiotherapy for Pathological T3N0M0 Prostate Cancer Significantly Reduces Risk of Metastases and Improves Survival: Long-Term Followup of a Randomized Clinical Trial**

Thompson IM, Tangen CM, Paradelo J, et al (Univ of Texas Health Science Ctr at San Antonio; The Fred Hutchinson Cancer Res Ctr, Seattle, WA; The Kansas City Community Clinical Oncology Program, MO; et al)

*J Urol* 181:956-962, 2009

*Purpose.*—Extraprostatic disease will be manifest in a third of men after radical prostatectomy. We present the long-term followup of a randomized clinical trial of radiotherapy to reduce the risk of subsequent metastatic disease and death.

*Materials and Methods.*—A total of 431 men with pT3N0M0 prostate cancer were randomized to 60 to 64 Gy adjuvant radiotherapy or observation. The primary study end point was metastasis-free survival.

*Results.*—Of 425 eligible men 211 were randomized to observation and 214 to adjuvant radiation. Of those men under observation 70 ultimately received radiotherapy. Metastasis-free survival was significantly greater with radiotherapy (93 of 214 events on the radiotherapy arm vs 114 of 211 events on observation; HR 0.71; 95% CI 0.54, 0.94; $p = 0.016$). Survival improved significantly with adjuvant radiation (88 deaths of 214 on the radiotherapy arm vs 110 deaths of 211 on observation; HR 0.72; 95% CI 0.55, 0.96; $p = 0.023$).

*Conclusions.*—Adjuvant radiotherapy after radical prostatectomy for a man with pT3N0M0 prostate cancer significantly reduces the risk of metastasis and increases survival.

► The question of if and when to initiate postoperative irradiation after surgery for patients with pathologic T3 adenocarcinoma of the prostate has been a source of controversy for decades. Proponents of postoperative radiation closer to the time of the prostatectomy cite smaller volume of disease and therefore more cures as their premise. Yet many urologists and radiation oncologists are concerned about the potential additional toxicity from the radiation for these patients given the fact that some may never relapse. Thus we have to commend the Southwestern Oncology Group (SWOG) for conducting this study of 431 patients with pathologic T3N0M0 prostate cancer and randomizing them to immediate postoperative irradiation versus observation. Their findings of a positive effect of immediate postoperative irradiation on both metastasis-free survival and overall survival leaves little question as to the benefit of immediate (within 18 weeks) postoperative irradiation for pathologic T3 patients. Given the positive outcome and quality of life results, postoperative irradiation needs to be offered to all patients with pathologic T3 disease who are able to receive radiation.

**C. A. Lawton, MD**

## Long-Term Outcomes in Younger Men Following Permanent Prostate Brachytherapy

Shapiro EY, Rais-Bahrami S, Morgenstern C, et al (North Shore-Long Island Jewish Health System, New Hyde Park, NY)
*J Urol* 181:1665-1671, 2009

*Purpose.*—We reviewed the long-term outcomes in men undergoing permanent prostate brachytherapy with a focus on those presenting before age 60 years.

*Materials and Methods.*—Between 1992 and 2005 a total of 2,119 patients with clinical stage T1–T2, N0, M0 prostate cancer treated with permanent prostate brachytherapy were included in this study. Treatment regimens consisted of permanent prostate brachytherapy with or without hormone therapy, permanent prostate brachytherapy with external beam radiotherapy, or all 3 modalities. Biochemical recurrence was defined using the Phoenix definition. Multivariate analysis was performed to determine if age and/or other clinicopathological features were associated with disease progression. The Kaplan-Meier method was used to calculate rates of freedom from progression with the log rank test to compare patients younger than 60 vs 60 years or older.

*Results.*—Median followup was 56.1 months. In the study population 237 patients were younger than 60 years at diagnosis (11%). The 5 and 10-year freedom from progression rates were 90.1% and 85.6%, respectively, for the entire population. Multivariate analysis demonstrated that prostate specific antigen ($p < 0.01$), biopsy Gleason score ($p < 0.0001$) and year of treatment ($p < 0.001$) were associated with freedom from progression while age ($p = 0.95$) and clinical stage ($p = 0.11$) were not. There was no significant difference in freedom from progression between men younger than 60, or 60 years or older (log rank $p = 0.46$). In the younger cohort the 10-year freedom from progression for patients presenting with low, intermediate and high risk disease was 91.3%, 80.0% and 70.2% compared to 91.8%, 83.4% and 72.1%, respectively, for men 60 years or older.

*Conclusions.*—Our long-term results confirm favorable outcomes after permanent prostate brachytherapy in men younger than 60 years. Outcomes are impacted by disease related risk factors but not by age or clinical stage. Definitive treatment options for younger men with clinically localized prostate cancer should include permanent prostate brachytherapy.

▶ Prostate brachytherapy has gained acceptance in the cancer community as an effective alternative to surgery or external beam irradiation, especially for patients who present with low-risk disease (ie, prostate specific antigen [PSA] < 10, Gleason score [GS] < 6, and T stage < clinical T2a). Yet as PSA screening has become more widespread, resulting in younger patients presenting with low-risk disease, the question as to the appropriateness of prostate brachytherapy in this population has been raised. The issues at hand relate to long-term control of the disease and potential toxicities. These authors have addressed these issues in a review of over 2100 prostate cancer patients treated with brachytherapy, of whom 237 were less than 60 years of age. Given a median follow-up of just under 5 years, and excellent freedom from progression rates for the entire cohort, age was not associated with worse outcome. Outcomes were affected by increasing PSA and increasing GS as expected. This data clearly sets the stage for the appropriate use of prostate brachytherapy in young patients with low-risk disease, but we await the 10- and 15-year results along with toxicity profiles to ensure that this option remains equivalent to surgery and external beam therapy for these patients.

**C. A. Lawton, MD**

---

**Screening and Prostate-Cancer Mortality in a Randomized European Study**

Schröder FH, for the ERSPC Investigators (Erasmus Med Ctr, Rotterdam, the Netherlands; et al)

*N Engl J Med* 360:1320-1328, 2009

---

*Background.*—The European Randomized Study of Screening for Prostate Cancer was initiated in the early 1990s to evaluate the effect of screening with prostate-specific–antigen (PSA) testing on death rates from prostate cancer.

*Methods.*—We identified 182,000 men between the ages of 50 and 74 years through registries in seven European countries for inclusion in our study. The men were randomly assigned to a group that was offered PSA screening at an average of once every 4 years or to a control group that did not receive such screening. The predefined core age group for this study included 162,243 men between the ages of 55 and 69 years. The primary outcome was the rate of death from prostate cancer. Mortality follow-up was identical for the two study groups and ended on December 31, 2006.

*Results.*—In the screening group, 82% of men accepted at least one offer of screening. During a median follow-up of 9 years, the cumulative incidence of prostate cancer was 8.2% in the screening group and 4.8% in the control group. The rate ratio for death from prostate cancer in the screening group, as compared with the control group, was 0.80 (95% confidence interval [CI], 0.65 to 0.98; adjusted P = 0.04). The absolute risk difference was 0.71 death per 1000 men. This means that 1410 men would need to be screened and 48 additional cases of prostate cancer would need to be treated to prevent one death from prostate cancer. The analysis of men who were actually screened during the first round (excluding subjects with noncompliance) provided a rate ratio for death from prostate cancer of 0.73 (95% CI, 0.56 to 0.90).

*Conclusions.*—PSA-based screening reduced the rate of death from prostate cancer by 20% but was associated with a high risk of overdiagnosis. (Current Controlled Trials number, ISRCTN49127736.)

▶ The controversy over screening with prostate-specific antigen (PSA) for prostate cancer has been continuing for years. The cost versus the benefit has caused many primary care doctors to wonder if PSA screening truly has merit. Overdiagnosis which results in overtreatment is the concern, yet in the United States approximately 29 000 men die of prostate cancer annually.

A good screening test such as the mammogram in breast cancer will result in a decrease in deaths from the disease. The results of this large study show that PSA screening does result in a decrease in prostate cancer deaths after a follow-up period of approximately 9 years. This decrease in death rate from prostate cancer corresponds to a 20% relative reduction in the death rate from prostate cancer for patients in the age range of 55 to 69 years. Indolent cancers were found as well and concern for overdiagnosis and overtreatment persists. Yet, the end point of decreased prostate cancer deaths was reached with PSA screening. Future work needs to focus on appropriate populations for screening (ie, those where the diagnosis of the disease will likely affect the patients longevity or quality of life). This is not different than appropriate use of screening mammography in the female population. Screening women with mammograms in their 80s is not likely to be beneficial unless an individual patient has extensive longevity in their family history and is healthy.

**C. A. Lawton, MD**

---

**Cardiovascular Mortality After Androgen Deprivation Therapy for Locally Advanced Prostate Cancer: RTOG 85-31**

Efstathiou JA, Bae K, Shipley WU, et al (Massachusetts General Hosp, Boston; Dept of Statistics; Fox Chase Cancer Ctr, Philadelphia, PA; et al)

*J Clin Oncol* 27:92-99, 2008

---

*Purpose.*—Gonadotropin-releasing hormone (GnRH) agonists are associated with greater risk of coronary heart disease and myocardial infarction in men with prostate cancer, but little is known about potential impact on cardiovascular mortality. We assessed the relationship between

GnRH agonists and cardiovascular mortality in a large randomized phase III trial of men treated with or without adjuvant goserelin after radiation therapy (RT) for locally advanced prostate cancer.

*Patients and Methods.*—Between 1987 and 1992, 945 men with locally advanced prostate cancer were randomly assigned to RT and adjuvant goserelin or RT alone. Fine and Gray's regression was used to evaluate treatment effect on cardiovascular mortality. Covariates included age, prevalent cardiovascular disease (CVD), hypertension, diabetes mellitus (DM), body mass index, race, Gleason score, stage, acid phosphatase level, prostatectomy history, and nodal involvement.

*Results.*—After a median follow-up of 8.1 years, there were 117 cardiovascular-related deaths but no treatment-related increase in cardiovascular mortality. At 9 years, cardiovascular mortality for men receiving adjuvant goserelin was 8.4% v 11.4% for men treated without adjuvant goserelin (Gray's $P = .17$). In multiple regression analyses, treatment arm was not significantly associated with increased risk of cardiovascular mortality (adjusted hazard ratio [HR] = 0.73; 95% CI, 0.47 to 1.15; $P = .16$; when censoring at time of salvage goserelin therapy, HR = 0.99; 95% CI, 0.58 to 1.69; $P = .97$). Traditional cardiac risk factors, including prevalent CVD and DM, were significantly associated with greater cardiovascular mortality.

*Conclusion.*—GnRH agonists do not seem to increase cardiovascular mortality in men with locally advanced prostate cancer. Further studies are warranted to evaluate adverse effects of GnRH agonists in men with lower cancer-specific mortality.

▶ The role of androgen deprivation in addition to radiation therapy is an accepted standard for patients with locally advanced and/or high-risk prostate cancer. Yet the toxicities of androgen deprivation in terms of hot flashes, sexual dysfunction, bone loss, muscle mass loss, etc cannot be overlooked. Given these toxicities and the weight gain often associated with androgen deprivation, some authors have concluded that androgen deprivation has an associated increase in cardiovascular mortality.

The above concepts taken together are very confusing. If androgen deprivation has proven to increase overall survival and disease-specific survival in multiple phase III trials as it clearly has, then how can it also increase cardiovascular mortality?

Radiation Therapy Oncology Group (RTOG) protocol 85-31 is an excellent trial to address the cardiovascular question. Patients on this trial were randomized to either no hormone therapy (ie, radiation alone) or indefinite hormone therapy along with radiation treatments. The trial has long follow-up and does not show an increase in cardiovascular mortality. This is important data, and it helps the treating physician to understand that the benefit of androgen suppression does not come with an increase in cardiovascular mortality. It is also important to realize and not minimize the real toxicities of hormone therapy and to be as vigilant as possible with efforts to decrease these toxicities.

**C. A. Lawton, MD**

---

**Duration of Androgen Suppression in the Treatment of Prostate Cancer**

Bolla M, for the EORTC Radiation Oncology Group and Genito-Urinary Tract Cancer Group (Centre Hospitalier Régional Universitaire de Grenoble, France; et al)

*N Engl J Med* 360:2516-2527, 2009

---

*Background.*—The combination of radiotherapy plus long-term medical suppression of androgens (≥2 years) improves overall survival in patients with locally advanced prostate cancer. We compared the use of radiotherapy plus short-term androgen suppression with the use of radiotherapy plus long-term androgen suppression in the treatment of locally advanced prostate cancer.

*Methods.*—We randomly assigned patients with locally advanced prostate cancer who had received external-beam radiotherapy plus 6 months of androgen suppression to two groups, one to receive no further treatment (short-term suppression) and the other to receive 2.5 years of further treatment with a luteinizing hormone–releasing hormone agonist (long-term suppression). An outcome of noninferiority of short-term androgen suppression as compared with long-term suppression required a hazard ratio of more than 1.35 for overall survival, with a one-sided alpha level of 0.05. An interim analysis showed futility, and the results are presented with an adjusted one-sided alpha level of 0.0429.

*Results.*—A total of 1113 men were registered, of whom 970 were randomly assigned, 483 to short-term suppression and 487 to long-term suppression. After a median follow-up of 6.4 years, 132 patients in the short-term group and 98 in the long-term group had died; the number of deaths due to prostate cancer was 47 in the short-term group and 29 in the long-term group. The 5-year overall mortality for short-term and longterm suppression was 19.0% and 15.2%, respectively; the observed hazard ratio was 1.42 (upper 95.71% confidence limit, 1.79; $P = 0.65$ for noninferiority). Adverse events in both groups included fatigue, diminished sexual function, and hot flushes.

*Conclusions.*—The combination of radiotherapy plus 6 months of androgen suppression provides inferior survival as compared with radiotherapy plus 3 years of androgen suppression in the treatment of locally advanced prostate cancer. (ClinicalTrials.gov number, NCT00003026.)

▶ It is clear from multiple clinical trials performed during the 1980s through the mid-1990s that the combination of hormone therapy and radiation produces superior results in terms of survival compared with radiation therapy alone in patients with locally advanced prostate cancer. The next question was just how long does one need the hormone therapy to get the survival advantage?

The Radiation Therapy Oncology Group (RTOG) performed trial 92-02 looking at 4 months of total androgen suppression (2 months neoadjuvantly and 2 months concurrent with radiation) versus the same treatment plus 2 years of luteinizing hormone-releasing hormone (LHRH) therapy adjuvantly. The results showed a survival advantage to the adjuvant 2 years of LHRH therapy arm. Yet as a treating radiation oncologist who understands the potential toxicities of longer term LHRH therapy, we want to know if perhaps something short of the 2 years of adjuvant therapy would still be effective? This question has been addressed at some level by the results of this European Organization for Research and Treatment of Cancer (EORTC) trial 22961. These researchers have shown that 6 months of total androgen suppression plus 2.5 years of adjuvant LHRH therapy and radiation therapy is superior to 6 months of total androgen suppression plus radiation in terms of overall survival via a phase III randomized trial of over 1000 patients. In addition, the long-term LHRH therapy did not result in a decrease in overall quality of life for these patients compared with the shorter 6-month course. So to date, for optimal treatment of locally advanced prostate cancer (based now on 2 prospective randomized phase III trials) one should use hormone therapy on a long term adjuvant basis with radiation (ie, 2-2.5 years).

**C. A. Lawton, MD**

---

**Overall Survival and Updated Results for Sunitinib Compared With Interferon Alfa in Patients With Metastatic Renal Cell Carcinoma**

Motzer RJ, Hutson TE, Tomczak P, et al (Memorial Sloan-Kettering Cancer Ctr, NY; Baylor Sammons Cancer Ctr-Texas Oncology, Dallas; Massachusetts General Hosp Cancer Ctr, Boston; et al)

*J Clin Oncol* 27:3584-3590, 2009

---

*Purpose.*—A randomized, phase III trial demonstrated superiority of sunitinib over interferon alfa (IFN-$\alpha$) in progression-free survival (primary end point) as first-line treatment for metastatic renal cell carcinoma (RCC). Final survival analyses and updated results are reported.

*Patients and Methods.*—Seven hundred fifty treatment-naïve patients with metastatic clear cell RCC were randomly assigned to sunitinib 50 mg orally once daily on a 4 weeks on, 2 weeks off dosing schedule or to IFN-$\alpha$ 9 MU subcutaneously thrice weekly. Overall survival was compared by two-sided log-rank and Wilcoxon tests. Progression-free survival, response, and safety end points were assessed with updated follow-up.

*Results.*—Median overall survival was greater in the sunitinib group than in the IFN-$\alpha$ group (26.4 *v* 21.8 months, respectively; hazard ratio [HR] = 0.821; 95% CI, 0.673 to 1.001; $P$ =.051) per the primary analysis of unstratified log-rank test ($P = .013$ per unstratified Wilcoxon test). By stratified log-rank test, the HR was 0.818 (95% CI, 0.669 to 0.999; $P = .049$). Within the IFN-$\alpha$ group, 33% of patients received sunitinib, and 32% received other vascular endothelial growth factor–signaling inhibitors after discontinuation from the trial. Median progression-free survival was 11 months for sunitinib compared with 5 months for IFN-$\alpha$ ($P < .001$). Objective response rate was 47% for sunitinib compared with 12% for IFN-$\alpha$ ($P < .001$). The most commonly reported sunitinib-related grade 3 adverse events included hypertension (12%), fatigue (11%), diarrhea (9%), and hand-foot syndrome (9%).

*Conclusion.*—Sunitinib demonstrates longer overall survival compared with IFN-$\alpha$ plus improvement in response and progression-free survival in the first-line treatment of patients with metastatic RCC. The overall survival highlights an improved prognosis in patients with RCC in the era of targeted therapy.

▶ The approval of sunitinib for metastatic renal cell carcinoma (RCC) was based on superior response rates and progression-free survival (PFS) because overall survival (OS) benefit had not yet been demonstrated. This report follows up on the outcomes of patients treated on the randomized phase III trial comparing sunitinib with interferon alpha. Reaffirming the improvement in response rate and PFS, the article presents the OS data, which demonstrate that despite a large number of the patients receiving either sunitinib or another vascular endothelial growth factor (VEGF)-targeted therapy at the time of progression, there was still a survival benefit though this was only borderline statistically significant. This trial highlights several critical issues: First, that salvage therapy with a tyrosine kinase inhibitor (TKI) or VEGF-directed therapy has the ability to improve OS significantly and second, that the improvement in PFS translated into longer OS compared with historical and this randomized control. One of the controversies in the treatment of RCC has been the issue of whether or not patients should undergo high-dose interleukin-2 (HD IL-2) before treatment with a TKI. I believe that this study reaffirms the fact that patients who receive a delayed or deferred TKI therapy may expect to receive similar OS advantage. Hence, I believe that for selective patients, the use of HD IL-2 as frontline therapy is warranted to ensure that the opportunity for cure is not lost. Subsequent VEGF-targeted therapy should be considered.

**M. S. Gordon, MD**

# 18 Gynecology

**The Role of Adjuvant Radiation in Endometrial Cancer**

Diavolitsis V, Boyle J, Singh DK, et al (Robert H. Lurie Comprehensive Cancer Ctr of Northwestern Univ, Chicago, IL)

*Oncology* 23:342-349, 2009

Endometrial cancer treatment ideally begins with a staging procedure including abdominopelvic washing, total abdominal hysterectomy, bilateral salpingo-oophorectomy, and lymph node evaluation. Recommendations for postoperative adjuvant radiotherapy are determined by recurrence risk. Patients who have undergone staging and have early stage I disease and an absence of high-risk features for recurrence generally are treated with surgery alone. Intermediate-risk patients—those with high-risk stage I disease and some stage II patients—may benefit from adjuvant radiation therapy. Several randomized trials show that radiation therapy improves locoregional control among intermediate-risk patients. The optimal type of radiation therapy; whether vaginal brachytherapy or whole-pelvic radiation therapy, remains undetermined, though treatment decision can be guided by risk factors not encompassed by the current staging system. Patients with high-risk stage II disease and stage III disease generally receive external-beam radiotherapy, often in combination with chemotherapy. Chemotherapy alone in advanced-stage patients is a consideration, given the results of the Gynecologic Oncology Group (GOG)-122 trial.

▶ Endometrial carcinoma is the most common gynecologic malignancy in women in the United States with over 40 000 cases diagnosed in 2008 and over 7000 deaths. Obesity and increasing age along with other factors predispose women to this disease. We know that the first appropriate step in treating this disease (assuming no evidence of metastatic disease) is surgery in the form of a total abdominal hysterectomy with salpingo-oophorectomy, abdominal pelvic washings, and lymph node assessment. When to add postoperative radiation and exactly how to apply it (ie, vaginal brachytherapy vs external beam to the pelvis vs extended field radiation vs some combination) can be confusing. The authors have done a service to the radiation oncology community in outlining the current data with regards to postoperative radiation. While the data are rather clear for very low-risk patients (ie, they don't need postoperative radiation), the data are much more confusing for patients with intermediate-risk features and even those with advanced disease (ie, stage III). These authors after outlining the current data make recommendations for vaginal brachytherapy for most intermediate-risk patients. They also advocate for radiation and chemotherapy for stage III patients. Given the data presented, these are reasonable conclusions. In addition, the 2 authors who reviewed the article, Dr Kathryn Greven and Dr Patricia Eifel, both suggest opportunities for further studies to elucidate the best treatment for these patients. We are a country that is getting older and more obese, which will increase the incidence of this disease. Trials to answer the questions posed should be done so as to provide the best care possible for this.

**C. A. Lawton, MD**

---

**Dose-dense paclitaxel once a week in combination with carboplatin every 3 weeks for advanced ovarian cancer: a phase 3 open-label randomised controlled trial**

Katsumata N, for the Japanese Gynecologic Oncology Group (Natl Cancer Ctr Hosp, Tokyo, Japan; et al)

*Lancet* 374:1331-1338, 2009

---

*Background.*—Paclitaxel and carboplatin given every 3 weeks is standard treatment for advanced ovarian carcinoma. Attempts to improve patient survival by including other drugs have yielded disappointing results. We compared a conventional regimen of paclitaxel and carboplatin with a dose-dense weekly regimen in women with advanced ovarian cancer.

*Methods.*—Patients with stage II to IV epithelial ovarian cancer, fallopian tube cancer, or primary peritoneal cancer were eligible for enrolment in this phase 3, open-label, randomised controlled trial at 85 centres in Japan. Patients were randomly assigned by computer-generated randomisation sequence to receive six cycles of either paclitaxel (180 mg/m$^2$; 3-h intravenous infusion) plus carboplatin (area under the curve [AUC] 6 mg/mL per min), given on day 1 of a 21-day cycle (conventional regimen; n=320), or dose-dense paclitaxel (80 mg/m$^2$; 1-h intravenous infusion) given on days 1, 8, and 15 plus carboplatin given on day 1 of a 21-day cycle (dose-dense regimen; n=317). The primary endpoint was progression-free survival. Analysis was by intention to treat (ITT). This trial is registered with ClinicalTrials.gov, number NCT00226915.

*Findings.*—631 of the 637 enrolled patients were eligible for treatment and were included in the ITT population (dose-dense regimen, n=312; conventional regimen, n=319). Median progression-free survival was longer in the dose-dense treatment group (28·0 months, 95% CI 22·3–35·4) than in the conventional treatment group (17·2 months, 15·7–21·1; hazard ratio [HR] 0·71; 95% CI 0·58–0·88; p=0·0015). Overall survival at 3 years was higher in the dose-dense regimen group (72·1%) than in the conventional treatment group (65·1%; HR 0·75, 0·57–0·98; p=0·03). 165 patients assigned to the dose-dense regimen and

117 assigned to the conventional regimen discontinued treatment early. Reasons for participant dropout were balanced between the groups, apart from withdrawal because of toxicity, which was higher in the dose-dense regimen group than in the conventional regimen group (n=113 *vs* n=69). The most common adverse event was neutropenia (dose-dense regimen, 286 [92%] of 312; conventional regimen, 276 [88%] of 314). The frequency of grade 3 and 4 anaemia was higher in the dose-dense treatment group (214 [69%]) than in the conventional treatment group (137 [44%]; $p<0{\cdot}0001$). The frequencies of other toxic effects were similar between groups.

*Interpretation.*—Dose-dense weekly paclitaxel plus carboplatin improved survival compared with the conventional regimen and represents a new treatment option in women with advanced epithelial ovarian cancer.

▶ The standard of care for advanced ovarian carcinoma is surgical cytoreduction followed by 6 cycles of paclitaxel/carboplatin. This standard has been in place since the Third Ovarian Cancer Consensus Conference in September 2004. Two significant phase III trials have challenged this standard; one of these 2 studies is reported in this article from the Japanese Gynecologic Oncology Group (GOG). The study is a large phase III trial that is well designed. One aspect of the design to take note of is the fact that there is no break during the 18 weeks of weekly paclitaxel in the experimental regimen. The results provide 3 surprises: (1) that there is an advantage for the weekly regimen in light of prior data, suggesting no advantage for weekly paclitaxel, (2) that the progression-free survival difference was as large as it was, and (3) that there was an overall survival advantage. This 1 study, however, does not establish weekly paclitaxel plus every 3-week carboplatin as the standard of care. First, the study results may only apply to the Japanese population in which it was run. Secondly, the toxicity of the regimen (myelosuppression and neurotoxicity) is substantial. Thirdly, a confirmatory trial is essential; and at least 3 cooperative groups have one under way. In addition, it would be wrong to conclude, as some apparently already have, that the use of weekly paclitaxel obviates the need to add bevacizumab to the front-line regimen, an addition that is under study at the current time. In short, this is an interesting study, which needs confirmation before it impacts the standard of care. This and other issues will be under debate at the upcoming Fourth Ovarian Cancer Consensus Conference in Vancouver, Canada, in June 2010.

**J. T. Thigpen, MD**

## Phase III Trial of Four Cisplatin-Containing Doublet Combinations in Stage IVB, Recurrent, or Persistent Cervical Carcinoma: A Gynecologic Oncology Group Study

Monk BJ, Sill MW, McMeekin DS, et al (Univ of California, Irvine; Choa Family Comprehensive Cancer Ctr, Orange, CA; Roswell Park Cancer Inst, Buffalo, NY; et al)

*J Clin Oncol* 27:4649-4655, 2009

*Purpose.*—Assess toxicity and efficacy of cisplatin (Cis) doublet combinations in advanced and recurrent cervical carcinoma.

*Patients and Methods.*—Patients were randomly assigned to paclitaxel 135 mg/m$^2$ over 24 hours plus Cis 50 mg/m$^2$ day 2 every 3 weeks (PC, reference arm); vinorelbine 30 mg/m$^2$ days 1 and 8 plus Cis 50 mg/m$^2$ day 1 every 3 weeks (VC); gemcitabine 1,000 mg/m$^2$ day 1 and 8 plus Cis 50 mg/m$^2$ day 1 every 3 weeks (GC); or topotecan 0.75 mg/m$^2$ days 1, 2, and 3 plus Cis 50 mg/m$^2$ day 1 every 3 weeks (TC). Survival was the primary end point with a 33% improvement relative to PC considered important (85% power, alpha = 5%). Quality-of-life data were prospectively collected.

*Results.*—A total of 513 patients were enrolled when a planned interim analysis recommended early closure for futility. The experimental-to-PC hazard ratios of death were 1.15 (95% CI, 0.79 to 1.67) for VC, 1.32 (95% CI, 0.91 to 1.92) for GC, and 1.26 (95% CI, 0.86 to 1.82) for TC. The hazard ratios for progression-free survival (PFS) were 1.36 (95% CI, 0.97 to 1.90) for VC, 1.39 (95% CI, 0.99 to 1.96) for GC, and 1.27 (95% CI, 0.90 to 1.78) for TC. Response rates (RRs) for PC, VC, GC, and TC were 29.1%, 25.9%, 22.3%, and 23.4%, respectively. The arms were comparable with respect to toxicity except for leucopenia, neutropenia, infection, and alopecia.

*Conclusion.*—VC, GC, and TC are not superior to PC in terms of overall survival (OS). However, the trend in RR, PFS, and OS favors PC. Differences in chemotherapy scheduling, pre-existing morbidity, and toxicity are important in individualizing therapy.

▶ The management of disseminated or recurrent carcinoma of the cervix is a major challenge because essentially all of the patients have had prior radiation. The current Food and Drug Administration approved standard of care for this group of patients was established with the results of prior Gynecologic Oncology Group (GOG) study (GOG 179), which showed that topotecan/cisplatin produced a superior response rate, progression-free survival (PFS), and overall survival as compared with cisplatin alone. The GOG had also shown a superior response rate and PFS but not overall survival in a study which compared the doublet of paclitaxel/cisplatin to cisplatin alone (GOG 169). In addition, the GOG had studied 2 additional doublets and shown significant activity for them (gemcitabine/cisplatin and vinorelbine/cisplatin). This study seeks to determine which of the 4 regimens might represent the best choice for these patients.

This study (GOG 204), which was started before the results of GOG 179 were known, randomizes patients with disseminated or recurrent carcinoma of the cervix to 1 of 4 doublets: paclitaxel/cisplatin (control), topotecan/cisplatin, vinorelbine/cisplatin, or gemcitabine/cisplatin. A total of 513 patients were randomized on study. The bottom line is that while no doublet demonstrated a statistically significant superiority, strong and clear trends favored paclitaxel/cisplatin with regard to PFS and overall survival. Patients with disseminated or recurrent carcinoma of the cervix should receive therapy with paclitaxel/cisplatin.

**J. T. Thigpen, MD**

### Impact of Human Papillomavirus (HPV)-6/11/16/18 Vaccine on All HPV-Associated Genital Diseases in Young Women

Muñoz N, Kjaer SK, Sigurdsson K, et al (Natl Inst of Cancer, Bogotá, Colombia; Univ of Copenhagen, Denmark; Natl Cancer Detection Clinic, Reykjavik, Iceland; et al)

*J Natl Cancer Inst* 102:325-339, 2010

*Background.*—The impact of the prophylactic vaccine against human papillomavirus (HPV) types 6, 11, 16, and 18 (HPV6/11/16/18) on all HPV-associated genital disease was investigated in a population that approximates sexually naive women in that they were "negative to 14 HPV types" and in a mixed population of HPV-exposed and-unexposed women (intention-to-treat group).

*Methods.*—This analysis studied 17 622 women aged 15–26 years who were enrolled in one of two randomized, placebo-controlled, efficacy trials for the HPV6/11/16/18 vaccine (first patient on December 28, 2001, and studies completed July 31, 2007). Vaccine or placebo was given at day 1, month 2, and month 6. All women underwent cervicovaginal sampling and Papanicolaou (Pap) testing at day 1 and every 6–12 months thereafter. Outcomes were any cervical intraepithelial neoplasia; any external anogenital and vaginal lesions; Pap test abnormalities; and procedures such as colposcopy and definitive therapy. Absolute rates are expressed as women with endpoint per 100 person-years at risk.

*Results.*—The average follow-up was 3.6 years (maximum of 4.9 years). In the population that was negative to 14 HPV types, vaccination was up to 100% effective in reducing the risk of HPV16/18-related high-grade cervical, vulvar, and vaginal lesions and of HPV6/11-related genital warts. In the intention-to-treat group, vaccination also statistically significantly reduced the risk of any high-grade cervical lesions (19.0% reduction; rate vaccine = 1.43, rate placebo = 1.76, difference = 0.33, 95% confidence interval [CI] = 0.13 to 0.54), vulvar and vaginal lesions (50.7% reduction; rate vaccine = 0.10, rate placebo = 0.20, difference = 0.10, 95% CI = 0.04 to 0.16), genital warts (62.0% reduction;

rate vaccine = 0.44, rate placebo = 1.17, difference = 0.72, 95% CI = 0.58 to 0.87), Pap abnormalities (11.3% reduction; rate vaccine = 10.36, rate placebo = 11.68, difference = 1.32, 95% CI = 0.74 to 1.90), and cervical definitive therapy (23.0% reduction; rate vaccine = 1.97, rate placebo = 2.56, difference = 0.59, 95% CI = 0.35 to 0.83), irrespective of causal HPV type.

*Conclusions.*—High-coverage HPV vaccination programs among adolescents and young women may result in a rapid reduction of genital warts, cervical cytological abnormalities, and diagnostic and therapeutic procedures. In the longer term, substantial reductions in the rates of cervical, vulvar, and vaginal cancers may follow.

▶ Cervical cancer remains a major killer of women worldwide, even though both incidence and mortality related to invasive procedures have declined dramatically in the United States over the last 6 decades since the introduction of the papaincolaou (Pap) smear in 1950. The recent development of 2 vaccines directed against human papilloma virus (HPV) (a bivalent vaccine directed primarily against types 16 and 18 and a quadrivalent vaccine directed against primarily types 6, 11, 16, and 18) has sparked hope of eradication of the disease as we know it today. Widespread vaccination, however, has become somewhat controversial in some areas and, because of cost, may be impractical in the underdeveloped world where it might have the greatest impact. It is in this context that this study looks at benefits other than impact on cervical epithelial neoplasia.

The study focuses on 17 622 women aged 15 to 26 years who participated in 1 of 2 randomized placebo-controlled efficacy trials. Investigators evaluated impact of vaccination and observed a number of benefits: reduction of high-grade cervical, vulvar, and vaginal lesions related to HPV, reduction in genital warts, and reduction of Pap smear abnormalities. In addition, there was a significant reduction in the frequency of diagnostic and therapeutic procedures required by the vaccinated population. Further follow-up will be required to document a reduction in the long-term risk for cervical, vulvar, and vaginal cancers.

This study thus documents a number of beneficial effects of HPV vaccination in addition to control of cancers of the cervix.

**J. T. Thigpen, MD**

**Absolute Risk of Endometrial Carcinoma During 20-Year Follow-Up Among Women With Endometrial Hyperplasia**

Lacey JV Jr, Sherman ME, Rush BB, et al (Natl Cancer Inst, Rockville, MD; Johns Hopkins Med Institutions, Baltimore, MD; Univ of Maryland Med Ctr, Baltimore; et al)

*J Clin Oncol* 28:788-792, 2010

*Purpose.*—The severity of endometrial hyperplasia (EH)—simple (SH), complex (CH), or atypical (AH)—influences clinical management, but valid estimates of absolute risk of clinical progression to carcinoma are lacking.

*Materials and Methods.*—We conducted a case-control study nested in a cohort of 7,947 women diagnosed with EH (1970-2002) at one prepaid health plan who remained at risk for at least 1 year. Patient cases (N = 138) were diagnosed with carcinoma, on average, 6 years later (range, 1 to 24 years). Patient controls (N = 241) were matched to patient cases on age at EH, date of EH, and duration of follow-up, and they were counter-matched to patient cases on EH severity. After we independently reviewed original slides and medical records of patient controls and patient cases, we combined progression relative risks (AH *v* SH, CH, or disordered proliferative endometrium [ie, equivocal EH]) from the case-control analysis with clinical censoring information (ie, hysterectomy, death, or left the health plan) on all cohort members to estimate interval-specific (ie, 1 to 4, 5 to 9, and 10 to 19 years) and cumulative (ie, through 4, 9, and 19 years) progression risks.

*Results.*—For nonatypical EH, cumulative progression risk increased from 1.2% (95% CI, 0.6% to 1.9%) through 4 years to 1.9% (95% CI, 1.2% to 2.6%) through 9 years to 4.6% (95% CI, 3.3% to 5.8%) through 19 years after EH diagnosis. For AH, cumulative risk increased from 8.2% (95% CI, 1.3% to 14.6%) through 4 years to 12.4% (95% CI, 3.0% to 20.8%) through 9 years to 27.5% (95% CI, 8.6% to 42.5%) through 19 years after AH.

*Conclusion.*—Cumulative 20-year progression risk among women who remain at risk for at least 1 year is less than 5% for nonatypical EH but is 28% for AH.

▶ Endometrial hyperplasia has long been recognized as a risk factor for endometrial carcinoma. The degree of atypia has been recognized as a factor in determining the level of risk, and prior estimates suggest that risk in patients with atypical endometrial hyperplasia is very high. This article quantitates this risk in a large population of almost 8000 cases of endometrial hyperplasia. Patients with atypical hyperplasia are shown to have risks as high as 28% for endometrial hyperplasia. The one caveat about this estimate is the recent study by the Gynecologic Oncology Group (GOG) that showed that distinguishing between endometrial carcinoma and atypical endometrial hyperplasia is difficult with substantial disagreement among experienced gynecologic pathologists as well as members of an expert review panel. Nevertheless, while the precise risk for the subsequent development of endometrial carcinoma may remain in question, it is clear that the risk is high. Patients with atypical endometrial hyperplasia should undergo measures to eliminate the problem with the definitive treatment remaining: hysterectomy.

**J. T. Thigpen, MD**

---

**The potential benefit of 6 vs. 3 cycles of chemotherapy in subsets of women with early-stage high-risk epithelial ovarian cancer: An exploratory analysis of a Gynecologic Oncology Group study**

Chan JK, Tian C, Fleming GF, et al (Univ of California, San Francisco; Roswell Park Cancer Inst, Buffalo, NY; Univ of Chicago, IL; et al)

*Gynecol Oncol* 116:301-306, 2010

---

*Objectives.*—A prior clinical trial on early-stage high risk ovarian cancer showed a lower recurrence rate in those treated with six vs. three cycles of chemotherapy. We proposed to identify subsets of patients who may benefit from more cycles of chemotherapy.

*Methods.*—Outcomes of patients who underwent six vs. three cycles of chemotherapy were analyzed based on clinico-pathologic factors. Kaplan–Meier estimates and Cox Regression Model were used for analyses.

*Results.*—Of 427 patients (median age: 55 years), 69% had stage I disease, 30% had clear cell, 25% endometrioid, 23% serous, 7% mucinous, and 15% had other cell types. The risk of recurrence in those who had six vs. three cycles of chemotherapy was not different based on age, performance status, stage, grade of disease, presence of ascites, tumor rupture, or positive cytology. However, those with serous tumors had a significantly lower risk of recurrence after six vs. three cycles of chemotherapy (HR = 0.33, CI = 0.14–0.77; $p = 0.04$) in contrast to non-serous tumors (HR = 0.94, CI = 0.60–1.49). Nevertheless, a test of homogeneity did not show a difference in treatment effects across cell types ($p = 0.285$). Of those with serous tumors, the 5-year recurrence-free survival was 83% and 60% in those who received six vs. three cycles of chemotherapy, respectively ($p = 0.007$).

*Conclusions.*—In this exploratory analysis of early-stage high risk ovarian cancer, our data suggest that six rather than three cycles of chemotherapy may decrease the recurrence of patients with serous tumors. Further studies are needed to confirm these findings.

▶ The current standard of care for patients with high-risk stage I ovarian carcinoma in the United States is surgical resection followed by adjuvant chemotherapy. Although phase III data to support a particular treatment are lacking, the vast majority of patients receive paclitaxel/carboplatin. In an attempt to define precisely how much adjuvant therapy was necessary, the Gynecologic Oncology Group (GOG) conducted GOG 157, which randomized patients with stage I to II ovarian carcinoma exhibiting high-risk features (grade-3 disease, positive peritoneal cytology, the presence of ascites, disease on the surface of the ovaries, or disease outside the ovaries) to receive paclitaxel/carboplatin for either 3 or 6 cycles. The study demonstrated an advantage for 6 cycles with a hazard ratio (HR) of 0.69, but this difference was not statistically significant because the study was powered to detect a HR of 0.5. Since the completion of the study, there has been much controversy about whether the HR of 0.69 was real and thus a reason to give 6 cycles. The report of Chan and colleagues is an exploratory analysis of various tumor features to determine if there is a subset of patients who clearly benefit from the additional chemotherapy.

A total of 427 patients are included in the analysis. The analysis revealed that serous histology was associated with a large and clear decrease in the risk of recurrence with 6 cycles as compared with 3 (HR = 0.33, $P = .04$), which translated into 83% recurrence-free survival at 5 years with 6 cycles as compared with 60% recurrence-free survival with 3 cycles. No other histology benefited from the additional cycles. The authors conclude that serous tumors may well benefit from the additional treatment. Should this then become the standard of care? Further study would be required to draw that conclusion, but strong consideration to 6 cycles should be given in patients with serous histology until further data are available.

**J. T. Thigpen, MD**

**Smoking behavior in women with locally advanced cervical carcinoma: a Gynecologic Oncology Group study**

Waggoner SE, Darcy KM, Tian C, et al (Univ Hosps of Cleveland, OH; Roswell Park Cancer Inst, Buffalo, NY; et al)

*Am J Obstet Gynecol* 202:283.e1-283.e7, 2010

*Objective.*—The purpose of this study was to assess cigarette use and environmental smoke exposure in women with cervical cancer.

*Study Design.*—Smoking behavior was recorded prospectively in a clinical trial of women with locally advanced cervical carcinoma.

*Results.*—Of 315 participants, 133 women (42%) were current smokers; 72 women (23%) were former smokers, and 110 women (35%) were never smokers. Current smokers began smoking earlier (16 vs 18 years; $P = .009$), for more years (29 vs 24 years; $P = .005$), and in greater amounts (20 vs 11 cigarettes/d; $P < .001$) than former smokers. Active smokers lived more often with another smoker (63.3%), compared with former smokers (35.0%; $P < .001$) or never-smokers (28.7%; $P < .001$). Agreement between self-report and urine cotinine level was high (kappa = 0.872; $P < .001$). A significant decrease in cotinine level during treatment occurred in 5.2% of current smokers.

*Conclusion.*—Prevalence of smoking and tobacco consumption was twice that of the North American female population. Few smokers quit or decreased consumption during treatment.

▶ Cigarette smoking is a recognized risk factor for the development of a number of cancers; one among them is squamous cell carcinoma of the uterine cervix. Not only do a high proportion of patients with cervix carcinoma smoke, but continued smoking during treatment is a predictor of both disease progression and death. The Gynecologic Oncology Group, in a study of concurrent chemoradiation, evaluated the smoking behavior of the participants. Of the 328 participants, 42% were current smokers at the time of treatment on study. Although there was no standard intervention under study in the trial, patients were counseled about the risks of more frequent progression and death associated with smoking. Despite this, very few quit smoking. This study emphasizes the magnitude of smoking problems in patients with cervix carcinoma and the difficulty of cessation despite patients being warned about those risks. Although the study itself does not provide an answer to the problem of tobacco use during treatment for cervix carcinoma, it does underline the need for an aggressive effort to change patient behavior with regard to tobacco use and the need for further improvements in those approaches.

**J. T. Thigpen, MD**

**Quality of care in advanced ovarian cancer: The importance of provider specialty**

Mercado C, Zingmond D, Karlan BY, et al (David Geffen School of Medicine at UCLA, Los Angeles, CA; Women's Cancer Res Inst, Los Angeles, CA; et al)
*Gynecol Oncol* 117:18-22, 2010

*Background.*—One of the cornerstones of ovarian cancer therapy is cytoreductive surgery, which can be performed by surgeons with different specialty training. We examined whether surgeon specialty impacts quality of life (as proxied by presence of ostomy) and overall survival for women with advanced ovarian cancer.

*Methods.*—Stage IIIC/IV ovarian cancer patients were identified using 4 state cancer registries: California, Washington, New York, and Florida and linked records to the corresponding inpatient-hospital discharge file, AMA Masterfile, and 2000 U.S. Census SF4 File. Predictors of receipt of care by a general surgeon and creation of fecal ostomy were analyzed. Multivariate modeling was performed to assess the association of hospital volume (low volume (LV) [0–4 cases], middle volume (MV) [5–9], high volume (HV) [10–19], and very high volume (VHV) [20+]) and surgeon specialty training (gynecologic oncologists/gynecologists, general surgeons, and other specialty) on survival.

*Results.*—We identified 31,897 Stage IIIC/IV patients; mean age was 64 years. Treatment of patients by a general surgeon was predicted by LV, rural patient residence, poverty, and high level of comorbidity. Patients had lower hazard of death when treated in higher volume hospitals as compared to LV [VHV hazard ratio (HR) = 0.79, $P < .0001$; HV HR = 0.89, $P < 0.001$]. Patients treated by a general surgeon had higher likelihood of an ostomy (OR = 4.46, $P < .0001$) and hazard of death (HR = 1.63, $P < .0001$) compared to gynecologic oncologist/gynecologist.

*Conclusions.*—Advanced stage ovarian cancer patients have better survival when treated by gynecologic oncology/gynecology trained surgeons. Data suggest that referral to these specialists may optimize surgical debulking and minimize the creation of a fecal ostomy.

▶ The standard of care for patients with newly diagnosed advanced ovarian carcinoma has been defined by an international consortium of cooperative groups conducting trials in ovarian carcinoma as an aggressive attempt at cytoreductive surgery followed by 6 cycles of paclitaxel plus carboplatin. It is important to note that this consensus considered management to begin with aggressive bulk-reductive surgery, which, if successful, results in improved survival and improved response to chemotherapy. This study seeks to determine the best circumstances for the patient in terms of the likelihood of achieving adequate bulk reduction (preferably no gross residual disease remaining at the conclusion of surgery).

The study identified from 4 state cancer registries 31 897 stage IIIC/IV patients and examined patient outcomes by hospital and by surgical specialty of the provider of the initial surgery. Hospitals seeing a higher volume of ovarian cancer patients exhibited better outcome (hazard ratio [HR] for mortality = 0.79, $P < .0001$ favoring higher volume hospitals) and a lower likelihood of the patient having an ostomy (HR = 4.46, $P = < .0001$). Similarly, outcome was better if the surgeon was a gynecologic oncologist as opposed to a general surgeon.

These results underline the importance of having a gynecologic oncologist perform the bulk-reductive surgery. Patients should be referred to a gynecologic oncologist even if this requires significant travel for the patient.

**J. T. Thigpen, MD**

# 19 Hematologic Malignancies

---

**Treating Childhood Acute Lymphoblastic Leukemia without Cranial Irradiation**

Pui C-H, Campana D, Pei D, et al (St Jude Children's Res Hosp, Memphis, TN; et al)

*N Engl J Med* 360:2730-2741, 2009

---

*Background.*—Prophylactic cranial irradiation has been a standard treatment in children with acute lymphoblastic leukemia (ALL) who are at high risk for central nervous system (CNS) relapse.

*Methods.*—We conducted a clinical trial to test whether prophylactic cranial irradiation could be omitted from treatment in all children with newly diagnosed ALL. A total of 498 patients who could be evaluated were enrolled. Treatment intensity was based on presenting features and the level of minimal residual disease after remission-induction treatment. The duration of continuous complete remission in the 71 patients who previously would have received prophylactic cranial irradiation was compared with that of 56 historical controls who received it.

*Results.*—The 5-year event-free and overall survival probabilities for all 498 patients were 85.6% (95% confidence interval [CI], 79.9 to 91.3) and 93.5% (95% CI, 89.8 to 97.2), respectively. The 5-year cumulative risk of isolated CNS relapse was 2.7% (95% CI, 1.1 to 4.3), and that of any CNS relapse (including isolated relapse and combined relapse) was 3.9% (95% CI, 1.9 to 5.9). The 71 patients had significantly longer continuous complete remission than the 56 historical controls ($P = 0.04$). All 11 patients with isolated CNS relapse remained in second remission for 0.4 to 5.5 years. CNS leukemia (CNS-3 status) or a traumatic lumbar puncture with blast cells at diagnosis and a high level of minimal residual disease (≥1%) after 6 weeks of remission induction were significantly associated with poorer event-free survival. Risk factors for CNS relapse included the genetic abnormality t(1;19)(*TCF3-PBX1*), any CNS involvement at diagnosis, and T-cell immunophenotype. Common adverse effects included allergic reactions to asparaginase, osteonecrosis, thrombosis, and disseminated fungal infection.

*Conclusions.*—With effective risk-adjusted chemotherapy, prophylactic cranial irradiation can be safely omitted from the treatment of childhood ALL. (ClinicalTrials.gov number, NCT00137111.)

▶ The improved outcome of children with acute lymphoblastic leukemia (ALL) has been one of the more gratifying stories in oncology. Many lessons have been learned in the process, including the novel use of conventional agents, the timing of intensification regimens, and the prophylaxis of leukemia sanctuary sites such as the central nervous system (CNS). Traditionally, intrathecal chemotherapy and cranial radiation have been used and proven to be effective at reducing, although not eradicating, CNS relapses. One of the most unfortunate adverse sequelae of CNS radiation is the neurocognitive deficits that result especially in young children and, in particular, females. Thus, over the past 20 years, the use of cranial radiation has become increasingly restricted and reserved for those patients with higher risk of CNS relapse. Pui et al report the superb overall outcome results of children with ALL in St Jude total trials but also push the envelope by completely omitting prophylactic cranial radiation for all patients. The frequency of CNS relapse is low and in line with other studies, including in the group of patients who would have historically met criteria for receiving prophylactic CNS irradiation (~1.4%—1 of 71). Out of a total of 33 relapses, 11 showed isolated CNS relapse, 4 had combined CNS and hematologic relapse, and 17 had only hematologic relapse. Outcome for the 11 patients with isolated CNS relapse was an 85.6% 5-year event-free survival. It should be kept in mind that this study used only a historic group of patients for comparison, which could be problematic in terms of potential bias. In addition, the number of patients is quite small on which to base secure and definitive conclusions. Nevertheless, this is an important step in the right direction. Even if those patients who have isolated CNS relapse ultimately receive cranial irradiation, the approach reported here shows that the vast majority of children with ALL do not require this type of treatment. It is of note that more than 25 years ago, the work of Simone and colleagues at St Jude's also contributed to the profound increase in cure rate by using CNS prophylaxis, ironically with cranial radiation.

**R. J. Arceci, MD, PhD**

---

**New Developments in Tyrosine Kinase Inhibitor Therapy for Newly Diagnosed Chronic Myeloid Leukemia**

le Coutre P, Schwarz M, Kim TD (Charité Universitätsmedizin, Berlin, Germany)

*Clin Cancer Res* 16:1771-1780, 2010

---

The biology of chronic myeloid leukemia (CML) has enabled pioneering studies with targeted therapies. BCR-ABL inhibition with imatinib results in high levels of efficacy in patients with newly diagnosed CML in chronic phase (CP), but an estimated 35% of patients could benefit from more effective treatment. Several novel treatment strategies are being investigated in newly diagnosed CML-CP. These strategies include upfront treatment with next-generation tyrosine kinase inhibitors, such as dasatinib, nilotinib, or bosutinib, which also target BCR-ABL but with increased *in vitro* potency compared with imatinib, and possibly a reduced potential for resistance. Recent *in vitro* studies have shown that short-term exposure to dasatinib or continuous exposure to imatinib result in equivalent levels of apoptosis, indicating that potent intermittent inhibition is a successful strategy for improving dasatinib tolerability. Modified imatinib regimens are also being investigated in newly diagnosed CML-CP, including higher doses and combination with alternative classes of agents, such as interferon. Existing data suggest that both newer agents and combination approaches can improve treatment responses compared with standard imatinib treatment, although further data are needed, particularly from ongoing phase 3 trials, before the standard of care is revised.

▶ This article provides an excellent summary of the evolving strategies in the treatment and management of chronic myeloid leukemia (CML) with regard to the evolution of orally administered tyrosine kinase inhibitor (TKI) therapies. As new agents have been developed and are being tested in newly diagnosed, TKI-resistant or TKI-intolerant, and accelerating/blast crisis phases, it is clear that the management of CML requires a deeper understanding of the mechanism of action for these agents and an appreciation of the data to determine proper sequencing of these agents. This review does an excellent job of highlighting the various options for therapy.

**M. S. Gordon, MD**

# 20 Melanoma

**Interferon Alpha Adjuvant Therapy in Patients With High-Risk Melanoma: A Systematic Review and Meta-analysis**

Mocellin S, Pasquali S, Rossi CR, et al (Univ of Padova, Italy)

*J Natl Cancer Inst* 102:493-501, 2010

*Background.*—Based on previous meta-analyses of randomized controlled trials (RCTs), the use of interferon alpha (IFN-α) in the adjuvant setting improves disease-free survival (DFS) in patients with high-risk cutaneous melanoma. However, RCTs have yielded conflicting data on the effect of IFN-α on overall survival (OS).

*Methods.*—We conducted a systematic review and meta-analysis to examine the effect of IFN-α on DFS and OS in patients with high-risk cutaneous melanoma. The systematic review was performed by searching MEDLINE, EMBASE, Cancerlit, Cochrane, ISI Web of Science, and ASCO databases. The meta-analysis was performed using time-to-event data from which hazard ratios (HRs) and 95% confidence intervals (CIs) of DFS and OS were estimated. Subgroup and meta-regression analyses to investigate the effect of dose and treatment duration were also performed. Statistical tests were two-sided.

*Results.*—The meta-analysis included 14 RCTs, published between 1990 and 2008, and involved 8122 patients, of which 4362 patients were allocated to the IFN-α arm. IFN-α alone was compared with observation in 12 of the 14 trials, and 17 comparisons (IFN-α vs comparator) were generated in total. IFN-α treatment was associated with a statistically significant improvement in DFS in 10 of the 17 comparisons (HR for disease recurrence = 0.82, 95% CI = 0.77 to 0.87; $P <$ 001) and improved OS in four of the 14 comparisons (HR for death = 0.89, 95% CI = 0.83 to 0.96; $P =$ 002). No between-study heterogeneity in either DFS or OS was observed. No optimal IFN-α dose and/or treatment duration or a subset of patients more responsive to adjuvant therapy was identified using subgroup analysis and meta-regression.

*Conclusion.*—In patients with high-risk cutaneous melanoma, IFN-α adjuvant treatment showed statistically significant improvement in both DFS and OS.

▶ The use of high-dose interferon alpha in patients with high-risk melanoma is controversial. Initial trials performed by the Eastern Cooperative Oncology Group demonstrated an improvement in both disease-free survival (DFS) and overall survival (OS). Subsequent trials, while continuing to show a DFS advantage, failed to demonstrate an OS improvement. The authors took advantage of the large number of randomized trials using high-dose interferon as either the comparator or experimental arm and performed a meta-analysis on 14 large randomized controlled trials in the published literature. The result, not surprisingly, confirmed the improvement in DFS because this has been seen in 10 of the 17 conducted trials. Of importance, however, is the improvement in OS, which reached statistically significant levels. This meta-analysis of more than 8000 subjects receiving interferon confirms that at the present time, this therapy is the only one to promote improved DFS and OS in high-risk melanoma. The major problem at the present time is represented by the change in the definition of high-risk disease and the fact that so many patients are being diagnosed with node-positive disease on the basis of microscopically involved sentinel lymph nodes (SLNs). It is clear that the survival of patients with a microscopically positive SLN is different than that of a patient with relapsed macroscopic disease. Hence, while interferon is clearly the adjuvant therapy of choice, the determination of which patients should receive this therapy in 2010 is evolving. In addition, interferon regimens of shorter duration are being explored in this setting.

**M. S. Gordon, MD**

---

**Indoor Tanning and Risk of Melanoma: A Case-Control Study in a Highly Exposed Population**

Lazovich D, Vogel RI, Berwick M, et al (Univ of Minnesota, Minneapolis; Univ of New Mexico Cancer Ctr, Albuquerque; et al)

*Cancer Epidemiol Biomarkers Prev* 19:1557-1568, 2010

---

*Background.*—Indoor tanning has been only weakly associated with melanoma risk; most reports were unable to adjust for sun exposure, confirm a dose-response, or examine specific tanning devices. A population-based case-control study was conducted to address these limitations.

*Methods.*—Cases of invasive cutaneous melanoma, diagnosed in Minnesota between 2004 and 2007 at ages 25 to 59, were ascertained from a statewide cancer registry; age-matched and gender-matched controls were randomly selected from state driver's license lists. Self-administered questionnaires and telephone interviews included information on ever use of indoor tanning, types of device used, initiation age, period of use, dose, duration, and indoor tanning–related burns. Odds ratios (OR) and 95% confidence intervals (CI) were adjusted for known melanoma risk factors.

*Results.*—Among 1,167 cases and 1,101 controls, 62.9% of cases and 51.1% of controls had tanned indoors (adjusted OR 1.74; 95% CI, 1.42-2.14). Melanoma risk was pronounced among users of UVB-enhanced (adjusted OR, 2.86; 95% CI, 2.03-4.03) and primarily UVA-emitting devices (adjusted OR, 4.44; 95% CI, 2.45-8.02). Risk increased with use: years ($P < 0.006$), hours ($P < 0.0001$), or sessions ($P = 0.0002$). ORs were elevated within each initiation age category; among indoor tanners, years used was more relevant for melanoma development.

*Conclusions.*—In a highly exposed population, frequent indoor tanning increased melanoma risk, regardless of age when indoor tanning began. Elevated risks were observed across devices.

*Impact.*—This study overcomes some of the limitations of earlier reports and provides strong support for the recent declaration by the IARC that tanning devices are carcinogenic in humans.

▶ For years, it has been debated as to whether artificial sunlight in tanning booths can increase the risk of melanoma. Previous studies have demonstrated an increased risk but have been criticized for being too small or too biased. In this trial, the authors performed a case control study to try and address the question. All cases of melanoma diagnosed in Minnesota between 2004 and 2007 were matched to comparators from the Minnesota driver's license bank. Questionnaires and telephone interviews included questions about exposure to sun and tanning salon booths. As one of the largest studies exploring the question of this relationship, it gets away from one of the major flaws of previous studies, which is size. The trial clearly identified that the use of tanning booths was associated with a greater risk of developing melanoma. Risk factors included the age at which subjects first started tanning, and consequently, there was a greater risk as the number of tanning sessions increased. Subjects who had experienced 100 sessions of tanning or had tanned in booths for more than 10 years had the highest risk, though this same increase in the odds ratio was seen at 5 years and earlier. The risk was the same regardless of whether the booths were ultraviolet A or ultraviolet B booths. Hence, this study confirms that artificial tanning in booths is associated with an increased risk of developing melanoma and that the risk increases the longer and more frequently that subjects are exposed.

**M. S. Gordon, MD**

# 21 Supportive Care

**Patterns of Use and Risks Associated With Erythropoiesis-Stimulating Agents Among Medicare Patients With Cancer**

Hershman DL, Buono DL, Malin J, et al (Columbia Univ and New York Presbyterian Hosp)

*J Natl Cancer Inst* 101:1633-1641, 2009

*Background.*—Erythropoiesis-stimulating agents (erythropoietin and darbepoietin) have been approved to reduce the number of blood transfusions required during chemotherapy; however, concerns about the risks of venous thromboembolism and mortality exist.

*Methods.*—We identified patients who were aged 65 years or older in the Surveillance, Epidemiology, and End Results–Medicare database; who were diagnosed with colon, non–small cell lung, or breast cancer or with diffuse large B-cell lymphoma from January 1, 1991, through December 31, 2002; and who received chemotherapy. The main outcome measures were claims for use of an erythropoiesis-stimulating agent, blood transfusion, venous thromboembolism (ie, deep vein thrombosis or pulmonary embolism), and overall survival. We used multivariable logistic regression models to analyze the association of erythropoiesis-stimulating agent use with clinical and demographic variables. We used time-dependent Cox proportional hazards models to analyze the association of time to receipt of first erythropoiesis-stimulating agent with venous thromboembolism and overall survival. All statistical tests were two-sided.

*Results.*—Among 56210 patients treated with chemotherapy from 1991 through 2002, 15 346 (27%) received an erythropoiesis-stimulating agent. The proportion of patients receiving erythropoiesis-stimulating agents increased from 4.8% in 1991 to 45.9% in 2002 ($P < .001$). Use was associated with more recent diagnosis, younger age, urban residence, comorbidities, receipt of radiation therapy, female sex, and metastatic or recurrent cancer. The rate of blood transfusion per year during 1991–2002 remained constant at 22%. Venous thromboembolism developed in 1796 (14.3%) of the 12 522 patients who received erythropoiesis-stimulating agent and 3400 (9.8%) of the 34820 patients who did not (hazard ratio = 1.93, 95% confidence interval = 1.79 to 2.07). Overall survival was similar in both groups.

*Conclusion.*—Use of erythropoiesis-stimulating agent increased rapidly after its approval in 1991, but the blood transfusion rate did not change.

## Use of erythropoiesis-stimulating agents was associated with an increased risk of venous thromboembolism but not of mortality.

▶ This article studies the patterns of use and risks associated with erythropoiesis-stimulating agents (ESAs) and reviews the data on which the current Food and Drug Administration's (FDA) position on ESAs was presumably based. The investigators used the Surveillance, Epidemiology, and End Results (SEER)-Medicare database and selected patients who were diagnosed with colon, non-small cell lung, and breast cancer and also those with diffuse large B-cell lymphoma. Among the 56 210 individuals included, 27% received an ESA. This number represents an increased frequency of use from 4.8% in 1991 to 45.9% in 2002. The investigators present several noteworthy findings. First, it seems clear that there is an increased risk of venous thromboembolism associated with the use of ESAs. Second, the authors found no evidence of increased mortality associated with the use of ESAs in patients receiving chemotherapy. Third, they could find no evidence of a decrease in transfusions with the use of ESAs; but they do note that others have identified a decrease in the use of transfusions.[1] Finally, this article does not take into account any of the data on the improvement of quality of life published in the 1990s.

The FDA currently permits the use of ESAs in patients receiving chemotherapy, the group identified as having no increase in mortality in this study. It also requires, however, that patients sign a form, indicating that ESAs increase mortality in several cancers including carcinoma of the cervix. The basis for this last contention is a trend only in 1 study of carcinoma of the cervix by the Gynecologic Oncology Group. The study actually showed no difference in survival in a study closed early solely because of the increased observation of venous thromboembolism.

**J. T. Thigpen, MD**

*Reference*

1. Bohlius J, Wilson J, Seidenfeld J, et al. Erythropoietin or darbepoetin for patients with cancer. *Cochrane Database Syst Rev.* 2006;3:CD003407.

# 22 Thoracic Cancer

**Compliance with Fleischner Society Guidelines for Management of Small Lung Nodules: A Survey of 834 Radiologists**

Eisenberg RL, Bankier AA, Boiselle PM (Beth Israel Deaconess Med Ctr, Boston, MA)

*Radiology* 255:218-224, 2010

*Purpose.*—To determine the familiarity of radiologists with the Fleischner Society guidelines for management of small lung nodules and to assess whether their decisions for nodule management are consistent with these recommendations.

*Materials and Methods.*—Institutional review board exemption was granted for this electronic survey, which was sent to a sample of 7000 radiologists randomly selected from the Radiological Society of North America (RSNA) directory. Three clinical scenarios for nodule management were presented. Information about policies and guidelines for nodule management, awareness of published guidelines, and respondent demographics was obtained. Associations between these parameters and management recommendations were assessed by using a $\chi^2$ test. Respondents were also asked about tube current settings for routine chest computed tomographic examinations and those performed solely for nodule follow-up.

*Results.*—Of 834 respondents (response rate, 11.9%), 649 (77.8%) were aware of the Fleischner Society guidelines and 490 (58.8%) worked in practices that employed them or similar guidelines. Management selections were consistent with the Fleischner guidelines in 34.7%–60.8% of responses for the three scenarios. A significantly higher rate of concordance was associated with awareness of the Fleischner guidelines, presence of written policies based on them, a teaching practice setting, practice in a group with at least one member having chest radiology fellowship training, and fewer than 5 years of experience practicing radiology ($P < .05$ for all associations). The spectrum of tube current settings used was similar between the subgroups of respondents who were aware and those who were unaware of the Fleischner guidelines.

*Conclusion.*—Among survey respondents, there was high awareness and adoption of the Fleischner guidelines, but radiologists showed varying degrees of conformance with these recommendations. Future efforts are necessary to bridge the gap between awareness and implementation of these evidence-based guidelines.

▶ The authors surveyed 7000 randomly selected radiologists from the Radiological Society of North America (RSNA) directory. The purpose of the study was to identify familiarity and compliance with the Fleischner Society guidelines for managing pulmonary nodules. The increased utilization of CT scans has created an ever-expanding issue of managing unplanned findings. The individuals frequently ordering CT scans of the chest are not the same individuals who would be necessarily familiar with guidelines for managing pulmonary nodules and are thus reliant on radiologic recommendations. Only 824 (11.9%) of those surveyed responded, possibly creating a selection bias toward radiologists most familiar with the Fleischner Society guidelines. Having stated that, the compliance to following guidelines and understanding them was 35% to 61% for 3 different scenarios. This selection bias may be overestimating knowledge of the guidelines across all radiologists in RSNA.

The study reminds not only radiologists but also other physicians as to the existence of these guidelines and their recommendations. Failure to follow these will result in unnecessary surgeries or extra CT scans and thus radiation exposure. These occurrences typically occur for fear of missing cancer or of legal recourse. These guidelines provide a solid basis for following pulmonary nodules and should be thoroughly understood by any physician dealing with CT scans of the chest and pulmonary nodules.

**T. L. Bauer II, MD**

---

**Details and Difficulties Regarding the New Lung Cancer Staging System**

Detterbeck FC, Boffa DJ, Tanoue LT, et al (Yale Univ School of Medicine, New Haven, CT)

*Chest* 137:1172-1180, 2010

---

The new lung cancer stage classification system is the culmination of 10 years of work and an unprecedented analysis and validation process. This article reviews details of the rules governing how to implement the system and discusses areas in which ambiguities and difficulties exist.

▶ The authors review the entire new edition for the staging of lung cancer by the International Association for the Study of Lung Cancer. They review each of the changes in the staging system and discuss several concerns in detail at each level of tumor, nodal, and metastasis. They elucidate several concerns about the management of multiple pulmonary nodules and ground glass opacities and provide sound advice regarding the interpretation of the staging system in these areas. The article, as well as the staging system, is a must read for those dealing with the management of lung cancer.

**T. L. Bauer II, MD**

# 23 Miscellaneous

**Issues in Using Progression-Free Survival When Evaluating Oncology Products**

Fleming TR, Rothmann MD, Lu HL (Univ of Washington, Seattle; US Food and Drug Administration, Silver Spring, MD)

*J Clin Oncol* 27:2874-2880, 2009

Several challenging and often controversial issues arise in oncology trials with the use of the end point progression-free survival (PFS), defined to be the time to detection of progressive disease or death. While this end point does not directly measure how a patient feels, functions, or survives, it does provide insights about whether an intervention affects the tumor burden process, the intended mechanism through which it is hoped that most anticancer agents will provide benefit. However, simply achieving statistically significant effects on PFS is insufficient to obtaining reliable evidence of important clinical benefit, and even is insufficient to justifying the conclusion that the experimental intervention is "reasonably likely to provide clinical benefit." The magnitude of the effect on PFS in addition to the statistical strength of evidence is of great importance in interpreting the reliability of the evidence regarding clinical efficacy. PFS has several important properties, including being a direct measure of the effect of treatment on the tumor burden process, being sensitive to cytostatic as well as cytotoxic mechanisms of interventions, and incorporating the clinically relevant event of death, increasing its sensitivity to influential harmful mechanisms and avoiding substantial bias that arises when deaths are censored. To obtain reliable evidence about the effect of an intervention on PFS and patient survival, randomized trials should be conducted where all patients are followed to progression and death, and where patients in a control arm do not cross-in at progression unless the experimental regimen has already been established to be effective rescue treatment.

▶ Establishing an appropriate end point for a clinical trial is critical to the trial's success. The gold standard of end points has always been considered to be overall survival. As the number of therapeutic options has increased and efficacy has improved, however, the reliability and appropriateness of overall survival have been brought into question. Essentially no studies attempt to control all therapy from entry into a trial to the death of the patient because of numerous factors, not the least of which is the availability of multiple options after progression of disease. Because these options are not uniformly applied, subsequent therapy can blur differences in survival that otherwise might have been seen.

This problem is particularly true of ovarian carcinoma. This disease is very responsive to initial chemotherapy with clinical complete responses observed in at least half of the patients with bulky advanced disease. In those who do develop complete responses and relapse more than 6 months later, high response rates and complete response rates are reported with retreatment with a platinum-based doublet. In patients who have exhibited clinical resistance to platinum-based regimens, at least 20 different agents have shown definite activity. Most patients receive multiple lines of therapy after clinical resistance has developed. If one insists on overall survival as the only valid end point for clinical trials, it will be very difficult to achieve approval of a new agent because of this impact of postprogression therapy. The most rational end point for such trials would appear to be progression-free survival (PFS) as it assesses the impact of the particular regimen on an end point that assesses treatment impact on disease burden.

The authors of this article, however, contend that PFS is not a measure of clinical benefit. This, of course, depends on how one defines clinical benefit. PFS, measured carefully to avoid falsely prolonging this end point (identical assessments and timing of assessment for all patients and either blinding or careful review of dates of progression), correlates clinically with better quality of life and freedom from disease effects and thus is a measure of clinical benefit. In the case of ovarian carcinoma, PFS has also been shown to be a surrogate for survival in presentations by Mark Brady and Mark Buyse at the FDA Endpoints Conference in April 2006. At least in ovarian carcinoma, PFS is the only end point that makes sense because of the confounding impact of subsequent therapy on overall survival. It is to be hoped that an accommodation between investigators in the field of ovarian carcinoma and the FDA on the use of PFS as a primary end point can be reached so that progress in ovarian carcinoma does not come to a screeching halt.

**J. T. Thigpen, MD**

## Stereotactic body radiotherapy is effective salvage therapy for patients with prior radiation of spinal metastasis

Sahgal A, Ames C, Chou D, et al (Univ of California San Francisco; et al)
*Int J Radiat Oncol Biol Phys* 74:723-731, 2009

*Purpose.*—To provide actuarial outcomes and dosimetric data for spinal/paraspinal metastases, with and without prior radiation, treated with stereotactic body radiotherapy (SBRT).

*Methods and Materials.*—A total of 39 consecutive patients (60 metastases) were treated with SBRT between April 2003 and August 2006 and retrospectively reviewed. In all, 23 of 60 tumors had no previous radiation (unirradiated) and 37/60 tumors had previous irradiation (reirradiated).

Of 37 reirradiated tumors, 31 were treated for "salvage" given image-based tumor progression. Local failure was defined as progression by imaging and/or clinically.

*Results.*—At last follow-up, 19 patients were deceased. Median patient survival time measured was 21 months (95% CI = 8–27 months), and the 2-year survival probability was 45%. The median total dose prescribed was 24 Gy in three fractions prescribed to the 67% and 60% isodose for the unirradiated and reirradiated cohorts, respectively. The median tumor follow-up for the unirradiated and reirradiated group was 9 months (range, 1–26) and 7 months (range, 1-48) respectively. Eight of 60 tumors have progressed, and the 1- and 2-year progression-free probability (PFP) was 85% and 69%, respectively. For the salvage group the 1 year PFP was 96%. There was no significant difference in overall survival or PFP between the salvage reirradiated vs. all other tumors treated ($p = 0.08$ and $p = 0.31$, respectively). In six of eight failures the minimum distance from the tumor to the thecal sac was≤1 mm. Of 60 tumors treated, 39 have ≥6 months follow-up and no radiation-induced myelopathy or radiculopathy has occurred.

*Conclusion.*—Spine SBRT has shown preliminary efficacy and safety in patients with image-based progression of previously irradiated metastases.

▶ When cancer patients with metastatic disease to the spine present with pain and/or cord compression symptoms, radiation is the next logical step. Radiation therapy for such patients can effectively reduce painful symptoms and often reduce or prevent progression of neurologic sequelae. Typical treatments to the spine of 30 Gy in 10 fractions are effective, but leave little room for further radiation in case of progression of disease in the same region. Given the increasing effectiveness of systemic therapies, the likelihood of a need to readdress spinal metastasis after one course of radiation is also increasing. Many institutions have considered re-irradiation but have used limited fields and doses because of the concern regarding spinal cord toxicity. With the advent of image-guided radiotherapy (IGRT) and intensity-modulated radiotherapy (IMRT), a potential role for stereotactic body radiation therapy (SBRT) to retreat such patients seems warranted. These authors have evaluated such patients treated with SBRT (23/60 had no previous radiation and 37/60 had previous radiation). Although the data are preliminary, this work certainly suggests a potential role for SBRT in these patients and should help to augment interest in the RTOG protocol 06-31 evaluating SBRT for such patients.

**C. A. Lawton, MD**

**PART FOUR**

# KIDNEY, WATER, AND ELECTROLYTES

RENEE GARRICK, MD

# Introduction

Selections this year demonstrate that prevalence of renal insufficiency among the elderly is continuing to rise. Population studies suggest that most patients with stage 3 chronic kidney disease (CKD) will die, typically from cardiovascular complications, before they reach dialysis. This finding has prompted studies designed to define risk factors that might be used to predict renal cardiovascular outcomes. The presence of microalbuminuria has been previously shown to be a risk factor for renal and cardiovascular disease in hypertensive patients and diabetics. Studies this year extend that observation to the normal population. Large database analyses demonstrate that even within normal individuals, microalbuminuria is an independent risk factor for cardiovascular and renal morbidity and mortality. It is not yet definitively known whether treatment of early stage microalbuminuria will alter patient outcome.

Other risk factors for renal disease progression have also been identified. Some factors such as fructose, phosphate, and B vitamins (at least in patients with diabetes) may worsen renal disease. Others such as vitamin D, bicarbonate, and citrate may slow disease progression.

Also included are selections that focus on our knowledge, or lack thereof, regarding the use of erythropoietin-stimulating agents in predialysis and dialysis patients. Despite 20 years of postmarketing experience and numerous treatment and dosing guidelines, there still appear to be gaps in our knowledge of the most appropriate way to use these agents. The articles included here highlight that fact and the need for careful risk-benefit assessment and modified dosing guidelines.

The ASTRAL trial, which evaluated the role of stent placement in patients with atherosclerotic renal artery stenosis, concluded that in the population studied, medical management had the same outcomes as intervention and posed fewer risks. This important trial is another example of the need to perform well-designed appropriately powered trials before therapeutic modalities are deemed beneficial and widely implemented.

Attention continues to focus on communication and safety issues that surround the care of patients with renal disease. Several selections highlight the fact that therapeutic regimens that are appropriate for one population cannot be safely generalized to those with kidney disease or dialysis patients. In addition, the studies reviewed here indicate that medication errors are all too common among this population of patients, and the data suggest that the presence, or significance, of renal disease is not always appreciated. Effective communication and handoff tools, likely via an electronic record, will need to be developed to mitigate these risks.

Additional studies have focused on the continuum of care in the elderly, and the study included here evaluated the utility of dialysis care in elderly nursing home residents. These data should help patients and families set reasonable expectations and assist both patients and physicians as they work together to formulate care plans.

Overall, basic science and clinical nephrology research continues to focus on ways to identify risk factors, slow the progression of renal disease, and improve patient safety throughout the continuum of care.

*Topical Summaries*

METABOLIC FACTORS AND RENAL DISEASE PROGRESSION

Utilizing the KEEP, NHANES, and Medicare cohorts, Stevens and colleagues evaluated the prevalence of CKD and comorbid conditions in elderly patients. Their findings demonstrate that CKD is common in the elderly population and is associated with a high frequency of comorbid conditions. Current incident and prevalence data suggest that most patients with stage 3 CKD will succumb to cardiovascular and cerebrovascular injury before dialysis is reached. This has led to the suggestion that, for many patients, the reduction in glomerular filtration rate (GFR) that defines stage 3 CKD may be as much a marker for underlying cardiovascular illness as for the presence of renal disease.

Along these lines, the first series of studies included here focus on albuminuria and provide evidence that microalbuminuria is a predictor of both chronic renal insufficiency and of cardiovascular outcomes and mortality. For example, the MAGIC study tracked approximately 900 nondiabetic hypertensive patients for almost 12 years. The findings suggest that in this nondiabetic population, microalbuminuria is an independent risk factor for renal and cardiovascular complications. The study by Rifkin and colleagues focused specifically on patients over the age of 65 and evaluated the association between GFR (defined by cystatin C) and microalbuminuria on cardiovascular outcomes and mortality. The results demonstrated that either preclinical renal disease or microalbuminuria was associated with a 50% increase in mortality risk, and the presence of both kidney disease and microalbuminuria conferred a 4-fold increased risk of mortality.

Together, the studies of Coresh and van der Velde demonstrated that in the general population, microalbuminuria, and microalbuminuria and eGFR can predict mortality, and it can identify individuals at risk for the development of renal disease, respectively.

These results open the question as to whether screening for (and possibly treating) microalbuminuria in asymptomatic normotensive patients is appropriate. The screening for microalbuminuria is relatively inexpensive, but the jury is out as to whether therapeutic intervention is either safe or appropriate in asymptomatic normotensive patients. This will certainly be an area of future study.

Turing to the diabetic population, the ADVANCE collaborative group examined the independent predictive power of albuminuria and GFR on cardiovascular and renal outcomes in individuals with type 2 diabetes. The data are quite impressive. A urinary albumin-to-creatinine ratio of greater than 300 mg/g and an eGFR of less than 60 yields about a 3-fold higher risk for cardiovascular events and a 22-fold higher risk for renal events.

Unlike the general population of asymptomatic patients with microalbuminuria, there is of course a large body of literature on the treatment of proteinuria and the diabetic population. The study of Mehdi and colleagues showed us that despite similar blood pressure control, the addition of spironolactone, but not losartan, to a regimen of maximal angiotensin-converting enzyme inhibition provided increased renal protection. This small, well-designed trial will likely open the way for a larger multicenter study. The SMART investigators studied the effect of super maximal doses of candesartan in proteinuric diabetics and nondiabetics. The candesartan dose was escalated to 128 mg daily for 30 weeks, and it resulted in a 33% greater reduction in proteinuria than that achieved with the 16 mg daily dose. Blood pressure was not different among the groups, but serum potassium levels required extra monitoring.

As increased attention is focused on the significance and treatment of microalbuminuria, it is important to know how to measure albumin excretion. A very interesting and relevant study by Heerspink, and colleagues rigorously evaluated the various methodologies for the determination of urinary protein and albumin excretion. They demonstrated that the first morning void albumin-to-creatinine ratio is superior to a 24-hour collection, and is the most appropriate method for predicting renal disease progression in patients with type 2 diabetes and nephropathy.

The next series of studies focuses on other metabolic factors that may alter the risk or rate of progression of renal disease. Included is a study that evaluated the soluble vascular endothelial growth factor receptor sFlt1 as a marker of endothelial dysfunction, which may predict cardiovascular disease in CKD. Also included is a basic science study demonstrating that fructose leads to an increase in intracellular uric acid in human proximal tubular cells, and this study provides insight into the possible link between fructose and renal dysfunction.

The last selections focus on slowing the progression of renal disease, and they end on a bright note. Brito-Ashurst demonstrated that bicarbonate supplementation (aiming for a serum bicarbonate of greater than 23 mol/L) is safe, well-tolerated, and may slow the progression of renal disease. Phisitkul, utilizing sodium citrate (a "bicarbonate equivalent"), demonstrated some mechanistic insight into the mode of action by showing that citrate therapy reduced markers of kidney tubular interstitial injury.

The fact that such simple therapies may reduce the progression of kidney disease is indeed appealing.

## Diabetic Nephropathy and Chronic Kidney Disease

The articles in this section were selected because they provide important new clinical information regarding diabetic nephropathy. The articles by Perkins and Waden focus on type 1 Diabetes. Virtually every textbook of medicine suggests that microalbuminuria is the primary predictive marker for type 1 diabetic renal disease. A progressive increase in urinary protein excretion from microalbuminuria to macroalbuminuria, to nephrotic range proteinuria has been the standard model used to define the onset and progression of type 1 diabetic renal injury, and it has typically been taught that proteinuria preceded renal injury. The longitudinal study by Perkins utilized a cohort of type 1 diabetics with new onset microalbuminuria. Patients were studied for 12 years. Contrary to classical teaching, about a third of the patients with type 1 diabetes had advanced kidney disease develop very soon after the onset of microalbuminuria, and in the majority of patients, proteinuria was not an antecedent event but rather occurred concomitant with the development of CKD. The findings suggest that proteinuria is not a perfect surrogate marker of renal injury, and studies that focus on the mechanisms of the progression of proteinuria in type 1 diabetes may ultimately not be as meaningful as studies that focus on other mechanisms of renal injury.

The study by Waden was included because it provides new information regarding the utility of hemoglobin $A_1C$ variability as a marker of incident cardiovascular disease. The data suggest that glycemic excursions and their effects on oxidative stress in individuals with type 2 diabetes may be linked to cardiovascular events. This sheds new light on the clinical usefulness of monitoring hemoglobin $A_1C$ variability.

The routine measurement of homocysteine led to widespread therapy with B vitamins ($B_6$, $B_{12}$, and folic acid). Unfortunately, once again observational data could not withstand the scrutiny of a randomized controlled trial, A particularly bothersome finding was that supplementation with B vitamins could actually hasten the progression of renal disease in diabetics. The findings again certainly indicate the critical importance of carefully designed randomized studies.

### Calcium, Phosphate, Vitamin D, and Renal Injury

The last decade saw an enormous explosion of research related to the role of the renin-angiotensin system in progressive renal insufficiency. Currently, attention has turned to the potential role of the calcium, phosphate, and vitamin D axis in renal and vascular systems. It has become clear that hyperphosphatemia, itself, can influence the outcomes in patients with renal failure. Recent studies have demonstrated that in patients with moderate renal insufficiency (eGFR less than 16 mL/min per 1.73 $m^2$), serum phosphorus levels at the high end of normal are associated with increased vascular calcification.[1] The elegant basic science study of Ohnishi and Razzaque utilized Klotho knockout mice to evaluate the effects of phosphorus and dietary phosphate manipulation on the cellular mechanisms associated with accelerated aging and calcification. The results of their genetic and dietary manipulations provided an in vivo demonstration that phosphate toxicity can accelerate aging and promote vascular and soft tissue calcification.

Against this background, studies by Melamed and colleagues suggest that low levels of 25-hydroxyvitamin D may increase the risk of progressive renal insufficiency especially in African Americans. It is not yet known what, if any, effect vitamin D supplementation may have on clinical renal disease progression. However, vitamin D therapy can increase serum phosphate, and the findings Ohnishi certainly suggest that phosphate levels should be monitored when vitamin D supplementation is prescribed.

Secondary hyperparathyroidism is a common complication in patients with progressive renal insufficiency who are not yet on dialysis. The studies by Chonchol demonstrate that cinacalcet can be used to control PTH levels in the predialysis population. However, unlike patients on dialysis, in predialysis patients, cinacalcet increases the serum phosphate. This raises the risk/benefit questions that must be addressed before cinacalcet is widely used in these patients. The final selection draws attention to the renal and systemic roles of Klotho, which are quite fascinating, and is clearly an area of intense cardiorenal research.

### Chronic Renal Failure and Transplantation

With the implementation of medical homes and accountable care organizations, it is extremely likely that non-nephrologists will become increasingly involved in the care of patients with CKD. Therefore, it will be important for these practitioners to be aware of the diverse metabolic and laboratory abnormalities that develop as kidney disease progresses. Moranne and colleagues sought to evaluate the timeline for the occurrence of these various complications over the continuum of renal disease. Their findings should help non-nephrologists be better able to anticipate the metabolic perturbations of CKD.

The next series of articles investigated the management of common complications of kidney disease. Kalra and colleagues evaluated over 10 million patients age 66 and older over a 13-year period and noted that at the time-dependent variable, atherosclerotic renovascular disease was associated with an excess mortality. The much-anticipated ASTRAL trial evaluated medical management versus revascularization for the treatment of renal artery stenosis. The results suggested that medical management is superior. Autosomal dominant polycystic kidney disease is the most common inherited renal disorder, and Pei and colleagues have developed a scheme for radiographic screening that is inexpensive, sensitive, and specific. The study by Karami-Djurabi focuses on a diagnosis of pulmonary embolism, which is a common complication in patients with renal insufficiency. They demonstrated that a normal D-dimer coupled with a low clinical likelihood of risk can obviate the need for contrast imaging, and thereby reduce the risk of contrast induced nephropathy. Erythropoietin stimulating agents (ESAs) have been available for more than 20 years and, surprisingly enough, appropriate dosing targets in the pre-ESRD population are only now being carefully assessed. The carefully controlled TREAT trial evaluated the use of darbepoetin alpha (Aranesp), in nondialysis patients with CKD and type 2 diabetes. The use of ESAs to maintain a hemoglobin of 13 g/dL did not reduce the risk of either death or of a cardiovascular or renal event but was associated with an increased risk of stroke. This study has caused practitioners to rethink the risk-benefit ratio of these agents, and has led the US Food and Drug Administration to impose new warnings and dosing guidelines to govern the use of these agents.

The next series of articles evaluated the occurrence of adverse events in patients with CKD. The studies demonstrate that these potentially preventable events are shockingly common, and they occur across the entire spectrum of care settings. Failure to recognize the presence, or significance, of kidney disease frequently contributes to medication errors. Most of these mistakes could be avoided by improved handoffs, communication tools, and checklists.

### Dialysis Dependent Kidney Disease

The first series of papers in this section call attention to the fact that even common medications, many of which were initially believed to be innocuous (such as gadolinium), must be approached with caution in dialysis patients. Clinicians must recognize that therapeutic parameters established in one population cannot be generalized to dialysis patients. The results of Brookhart's study regarding the use of ESAs in dialysis patients are quite interesting, especially when considered in the context of the results of the TREAT trial. Although the mechanisms are not clear, the data do suggest an increased risk of mortality with the use of higher doses of ESA growth factor and iron in patients higher (33% to 35.9%) hematocrits. Unfortunately, when ESAs were first introduced, it was presumed they would be beneficial and placebo-controlled trials were not performed. If nothing else, this prescribing experience should teach us that non–placebo-controlled trials can never be used to assess a risk-benefit relationship.

The data regarding the continued use of statins in the dialysis population, despite the negative results of the 4D trial, are quite interesting. As the review mentions, there are numerous possible explanations for this; regardless of the reasons, the findings provide an interesting window into the psychodynamics of the physician-patient relationship. The last selection demonstrates that dialysis may be of limited benefit in elderly patients residing in skilled nursing facilities. Data such as these may help patients and families form realistic expectations regarding the risks and benefits of dialysis in this population.

**Renee Garrick, MD**

*Reference*

1. Adeney KL, Siscovick DS, Ix JH, et al. Association of serum phosphate with vascular and valvular calcification in moderate CKD. *J Am Soc Nephrol.* 2009; 20:381-387.

# 24 Metabolic Factors and Renal Disease Progression

---

**Prevalence of CKD and Comorbid Illness in Elderly Patients in the United States: Results From the Kidney Early Evaluation Program (KEEP)**

Stevens LA, Li S, Wang C, et al (Tufts Med Ctr, Boston, MA; Minneapolis Med Res Foundation, MN; et al)

*Am J Kidney Dis* 55:S23-S33, 2010

---

*Background.*—Elderly individuals with chronic kidney disease (CKD) have high rates of comorbid conditions, including cardiovascular disease and its risk factors, and CKD-related complications. In individuals aged ≥ 65 years, we sought to describe the prevalence of CKD determined from laboratory test results in the Kidney Early Evaluation Program (KEEP; n = 27,017) and National Health and Nutrition Examination Survey (NHANES) 1999-2006 (n = 5,538) and the prevalence of diagnosed CKD determined from billing codes in the Medicare 5% sample (n = 1,236,946). In all 3 data sources, we also explored comorbid conditions and CKD-related complications.

*Methods.*—CKD was identified as decreased estimated glomerular filtration rate (<60 mL/min/1.73 m$^2$) or increased albumin-creatinine ratio in KEEP and NHANES; CKD was identified using *International Classification of Diseases, Ninth Revision, Clinical Modification* codes in Medicare. Investigated comorbid conditions included diabetes, hypertension, high cholesterol level, coronary artery disease, congestive heart failure, cerebrovascular disease, peripheral vascular disease, and cancer, and CKD-related complications included anemia, hypocalcemia, hyperphosphatemia, and hyperparathyroidism.

*Results.*—The prevalence of CKD was ~44% in both KEEP and NHANES participants, and the prevalence of diagnosed CKD was 7% in Medicare beneficiaries. In all 3 data sets, the prevalence of CKD or diagnosed CKD was higher in participants aged ≥ 80 years and those with comorbid conditions. For KEEP and NHANES participants, the prevalence of most comorbid conditions and CKD complications increased with decreasing estimated glomerular filtration rate. For participants with CKD stages 3-5, a total of 29.2% (95% CI, 27.8-30.6) in KEEP and 19.9% (95% CI, 17.0-23.1) in NHANES had anemia, 0.7% (95% CI, 0.4-0.9) and 0.6% (95% CI, 0.3-1.3) had hypocalcemia, 5.4% (95% CI, 4.7-6.1) and 6.4% (95% CI, 5.1-8.0) had hyperphosphatemia, and 52.0% (95% CI, 50.4-53.6) and 30.0% (95% CI, 25.9-34.3) had hyperparathyroidism, respectively.

*Conclusions.*—CKD is common in the elderly population and is associated with high frequencies of concomitant comorbid conditions and biochemical abnormalities. Because CKD is not commonly diagnosed, greater emphasis on physician education may be beneficial (Table 3).

▶ Currently, the fastest growing group of incident dialysis patients is comprised of those who are older than 75 years.[1] From a public health perspective, it is important that we understand the road ahead of us in terms of both manpower analysis and access to care. Using 3 large cohorts drawn from the Kidney Early Evaluation Program (KEEP), the National Health and Nutrition Examination Survey (NHANES-1999-2006), and the Medicare 5% sample (n = 1,236,946), the prevalence of chronic kidney disease (CKD) and the associated comorbid conditions were evaluated. Terminology and diagnostic criteria were standardized, and where available, the laboratory data were verified. For the Medicare 5% sample, CKD was defined as at least 1 inpatient claim or 2 outpatient claims or physician or supplier claims with the appropriate International Classification of Diseases, Ninth Edition, Clinical Modification codes. In both the KEEP and the NHANES population, approximately 44% of patients older than 65 years were determined to have CKD. Among the KEEP participants, 77% had stage 3 and 5% had stage 4 to 5 CKD. The comparative

**TABLE 3.—Prevalence of Comorbid Conditions in Patients With and Without CKD**

| | KEEP | | | NHANES 1999-2006 | | | Medicare 2006 | | |
|---|---|---|---|---|---|---|---|---|---|
| Comorbid Conditions[a] | CKD | No CKD | *P* | CKD | No CKD | *P* | CKD | No CKD | *P* |
| Diabetes | 45.1 | 37.4 | <0.001 | 21.4 | 12.1 | <0.001 | 46.2 | 19.5 | <0.001 |
| Hypertension | 94.5 | 84.9 | <0.001 | 91.6 | 69.0 | <0.001 | 89.8 | 54.6 | <0.001 |
| High cholesterol | 38.8 | 42.1 | <0.001 | 50.5 | 56.0 | 0.01 | NA | NA | NA |
| Coronary artery disease | 21.0 | 14.6 | <0.001 | 26.7 | 16.8 | <0.001 | 48.0 | 18.5 | <0.001 |
| Congestive heart failure | 7.5 | 4.2 | <0.001 | 13.5 | 4.2 | <0.001 | 37.9 | 7.8 | <0.001 |
| Peripheral vascular disease | 1.3 | 1.0 | 0.09 | 8.5 | 4.0 | 0.002 | 32.3 | 9.7 | <0.001 |
| Cerebrovascular disease | 11.1 | 7.8 | <0.001 | 12.4 | 5.7 | <0.001 | 20.6 | 7.5 | <0.001 |
| Cancer | 20.3 | 18.6 | <0.001 | 13.2 | 4.0 | 0.03 | 19.2 | 9.4 | <0.001 |
| Frequency[b] (no. of conditions) | | | | | | | | | |
| 0 | 1.6 | 5.4 | <0.001 | 2.1[c] | 6.2 | <0.001 | 2.3 | 32.6 | <0.001 |
| 1 | 25.2 | 30.0 | <0.001 | 16.8 | 31.8 | <0.001 | 14.6 | 30.8 | <0.001 |
| 2 | 40.1 | 39.3 | 0.2 | 40.1 | 38.0 | 0.4 | 24.3 | 21.0 | <0.001 |
| 3 | 22.6 | 18.3 | <0.001 | 26.1 | 17.0 | <0.001 | 24.0 | 9.9 | <0.001 |
| >3 | 10.5 | 7.0 | <0.001 | 15.0 | 7.1 | <0.001 | 34.8 | 5.6 | <0.001 |

Abbreviations: CKD, chronic kidney disease; KEEP, Kidney Early Evaluation Program; NA, not available; NHANES, National Health and Nutrition Examination Survey.

[a]In KEEP, diabetes is defined as self-reported or fasting glucose level ≥ 126 mg/dL or nonfasting glucose level ≥ 200 mg/dL (7.1 or 11.1 mmol/L); hypertension is defined as self-reported or blood pressure ≥ 130/80 mm Hg for patients with diabetes or CKD and ≥ 140/90 otherwise; other conditions are defined as in Table 1. In NHANES, comorbid conditions are defined as in Table 1.

[b]Because of data limitations, frequency results are for NHANES 1999-2004 only.

[c]Estimate is not reliable.

percentages in NHANES were approximately 70% and 4.8%, respectively. In the Medicare data set, 7% of the beneficiary claims included a diagnosis of CKD. As indicated in Table 3, patients with CKD have a very high prevalence of comorbid conditions. This was true of all 3 data sets.

Current incidence and prevalence data have suggested that many patients with stage 3 CKD will succumb to cardiovascular and cerebrovascular injury before dialysis is reached. The large number of patients with stage 3 disease as compared with those with stage 4 and 5 disease is in keeping with this observation. These data are compelling for several reasons. First, the large number of elderly patients with stage 3 CKD identified in these cohorts is similar to that detected by other analyses.[2-5] This finding again demonstrates the need for caregivers to always be aware of kidney function before prescribing drugs or interventions in this at-risk population. There is an ongoing discussion in the renal community as to whether, for many patients, the reduction in glomerular filtration rate in stage 3 CKD represents actual primary kidney disease or is a marker for underlying cardiovascular illnesses. These data do not answer this question but do highlight that from a prevention and intervention standpoint, practitioners must appreciate that comorbid conditions are plentiful and that to be useful, prevention will most likely need to both occur early and be multifaceted.

**R. Garrick, MD**

*References*

1. US Renal Data System. *USRDS 2005 Annual Data Report*. Bethesda, MD: National Institutes of Health, National Institute of Diabetes and Digestive and Kidney Diseases; 2005.
2. Coresh J, Selvin E, Stevens LA, et al. Prevalence of chronic kidney disease in the United States. *JAMA*. 2007;298:2038-2047.
3. Stevens LA, Coresh J, Levey AS. CKD in the elderly—old questions and new challenges: World Kidney Day 2008. *Am J Kidney Dis*. 2008;51:353-357.
4. Levey AS, Stevens LA, Schmid CH, et al. A new equation to estimate glomerular filtration rate. *Ann Intern Med*. 2009;150:604-612.
5. Manjunath G, Tighiouart H, Coresh J, et al. Level of kidney function as a risk factor for cardiovascular outcomes in the elderly. *Kidney Int*. 2003;63:1121-1129.

## Microalbuminuria Is a Predictor of Chronic Renal Insufficiency in Patients without Diabetes and with Hypertension: The MAGIC Study

Viazzi F, Leoncini G, Conti N, et al (Univ of Genoa, Italy; et al)
*Clin J Am Soc Nephrol* 5:1099-1106, 2010

*Background and Objectives.*—Increased urinary albumin excretion is a known risk factor for cardiovascular events and clinical nephropathy in patients with diabetes. Whether microalbuminuria predicts long-term development of chronic renal insufficiency (CRI) in patients without diabetes and with primary hypertension remains to be documented.

*Design, Setting, Participants, & Measurements.*—We conducted an 11.8-year follow-up of 917 patients who did not have diabetes and had hypertension and were enrolled in the Microalbuminuria: A Genoa Investigation on Complications (MAGIC) cohort between 1993 and 1997. Urinary albumin-to-creatinine ratio (ACR) was assessed at baseline in untreated patients in a core laboratory. Microalbuminuria was defined as ACR ≥22 mg/g in men and ACR ≥31 mg/g in women.

*Results.*—A total of 10,268 person-years of follow-up revealed that baseline microalbuminuria was associated with an increased risk for developing CRI (relative risk [RR] 7.61; 95% confidence interval [CI] 3.19 to 8.16; $P < 0.0001$), cardiovascular events (composite of fatal and nonfatal cardiac and cerebrovascular events; RR 2.11; 95% CI 1.08 to 4.13; $P < 0.028$), and cardiorenal events (composite of former end points; RR 3.21; 95% CI 1.86 to 5.53; $P < 0.0001$). Microalbuminuria remained significantly related to CRI (RR 12.75; 95% CI 3.62 to 44.92; $P < 0.0001$) and cardiorenal events (RR 2.58; 95% CI 1.32 to 5.05; $P = 0.0056$) even after adjustment for several baseline covariates.

*Conclusions.*—Microalbuminuria is an independent predictor of renal and cardiovascular complications in patients without diabetes and with primary hypertension.

▶ To investigate the significance of microalbuminuria as a predictor of renal disease in nondiabetic patients with hypertension, Pontremoli and colleagues performed long-term follow-up on a cohort of patients who were enrolled in the Microalbuminuria: A Genoa Investigation on Complications (MAGIC) trial. This trial enrolled 1230 patients between 1993 and 1997. Pontremoli and colleagues performed 11.8 years of follow-up on 917 of these patients who had a diagnosis of hypertension without diabetes. Hypertension was defined as a blood pressure exceeding 140/90 mmHg on at least 3 occasions; chronic renal insufficiency was defined as a hospitalization with an ICD-9 code for chronic kidney disease; and microalbuminuria was defined by the urinary albumin-to-creatinine ratio (ACR) (ACR > 22 mg/g in men and ACR > 31 mg/g in women). Patients with known congestive heart failure, ischemic cardiomyopathy, or advanced pulmonary disease were excluded. Patients with microalbuminuria at the start of the study were 7.6 times as likely to develop chronic kidney disease and 2.1 times as likely to develop fatal and nonfatal cardiovascular and cerebrovascular events. Overall, after multiple statistical adjustments for a number of baseline differences and comorbid conditions, such as gender, body mass index, cholesterol, and smoking, patients with microalbuminuria were still 2.6 times more likely to develop combined kidney and cardiovascular problems as compared with people who have normal protein excretion.

Several trials have evaluated the cardiovascular significance of microalbuminuria. For example, the randomized HOPE trial[1] evaluated patients at high risk for cardiovascular diseases and demonstrated that the presence of microalbuminuria was associated with an increased risk of cardiovascular death, myocardial infarction, and stroke. The population data from the PREVEND study[2] evaluated albumin excretion rates in a general population of 40 548 from the Netherlands. After 2.6 years of follow-up, those investigators reported that a 2-fold increase in urinary albumin excretion rate was associated with a 1.29-fold increased relative risk of cardiovascular mortality. Similarly, the Framingham heart trial[3] evaluated very low levels of albumin excretion rate (urinary ACRs of less than 30 mg/g) and demonstrated an increased risk of cardiovascular mortality in nonhypertensive patients with microalbuminuria.

The current observation from the MAGIC trial extends our understanding of the long-term renal risks of microalbuminuria. A strength this study has is that the demographics of the patients were well defined. A limitation of the study is that the washout period before the baseline determinations was 4 weeks, which may not be long enough to completely clear the antiproteinuric effect of all agents. And there are no data available to evaluate the possible relationship between renal and cardiovascular risks and the type of antihypertensive therapy used. However, the finding of a 7-fold higher risk of chronic renal insufficiency among hypertensive nondiabetic patients with microalbuminuria certainly suggests the need for additional research aimed at determining whether specific therapies aimed at reducing microalbuminuria will have an effect on long-term renal outcomes in the nondiabetic population. Pending definitive long-term data, the results of the present trial do suggest that prudent medical management would include periodic determination of the urinary microalbumin-to-creatinine ratio and that elevated steps be taken to minimize the cardiovascular and renal risks. In the absence of definitive data, such steps may currently include therapy directed at the activity of the renin-angiotensin system, cholesterol and weight reduction, and an evaluation for the presence of underlying proinflammatory conditions, such as periodontal or gastric disease.

**M. Brogan, MD**

*References*

1. Gerstein HC, Mann JF, Yi Q, et al. Albuminuria and risk of cardiovascular events, death, and heart failure in diabetic and nondiabetic individuals. *JAMA*. 2001;286: 421-426.
2. Hillege HL, Fidler V, Diercks GF, et al. Urinary albumin excretion predicts cardiovascular and noncardiovascular mortality in general population. *Circulation*. 2002;106:1777-1782.
3. Arnlöv J, Evans JC, Meigs JB, et al. Low-grade albuminuria and incidence of cardiovascular disease events in nonhypertensive and nondiabetic individuals: the Framingham Heart Study. *Circulation*. 2005;112:969-975.

## Albuminuria, impaired kidney function and cardiovascular outcomes or mortality in the elderly

Rifkin DE, Katz R, Chonchol M, et al (Tufts Med Ctr and Tufts Univ School of Medicine, Boston, MA; Univ of Washington, Seattle; Univ of Colorado Health Sciences Centre; et al)

*Nephrol Dial Transplant* 25:1560-1567, 2010

*Background.*—Kidney disease is a risk factor for mortality and cardiovascular disease in older adults, but the separate and combined effects of albuminuria and cystatin C, a novel marker of glomerular filtration, are not known.

*Methods.*—We examined associations of these markers with mortality and cardiovascular outcomes during a median follow-up of 8.3 years in 3291 older adults in the Cardiovascular Health Study. Kidney disease was assessed using urinary albumin/creatinine ratio (ACR), cystatin C and Modification of Diet in Renal Disease estimated glomerular filtration rate (eGFR). We defined subgroups based on presence of microalbuminuria (MA, ACR > 30 mg/g) and categories of normal kidney function (cystatin C < 1.0 mg/L and eGFR > 60 mL/min/1.73 m$^2$); preclinical kidney disease (cystatin C level > 1.0 mg/l but eGFR > 60 mL/min/1.73 m$^2$); and chronic kidney disease (CKD) (eGFR < 60 mL/min/1.73 m$^2$). Cox proportional hazards models were used to examine associations between these six subgroups and all-cause or cardiovascular mortality, myocardial infarction and heart failure.

*Results.*—One thousand one hundred fifty (34.9%) had normal kidney function (12.2% with MA), 1518 (46.1%) had preclinical kidney disease (17.9% with MA) and 622 (18.9%) had CKD (47% with MA). After adjustment, the presence of either preclinical kidney disease or MA was associated with an over 50% increase in mortality risk; the presence of both was associated with a 2.4-fold mortality risk. Those with CKD and MA were at highest risk, with a nearly 4-fold mortality risk.

*Conclusion.*—Elevated cystatin C and albuminuria are common, identify different subsets of the older population, and are independent, graded risk factors for cardiovascular disease and mortality.

► Participants in the Cardiovascular Health Study represent a cohort of adults aged 65 years and older who are Medicare eligible and live within 4 communities (North Carolina, California, Maryland, and Pittsburgh). The present study evaluated the utility of the combined markers of cystatin C and albuminuria as risk factors for mortality and cardiovascular disease. Subgroups were defined based on the presence of microalbuminuria (albumin/creatinine ratio more than 30 mg/gm), and kidney function was classified as normal (cystatin C < 1 mg/L and estimated glomerular filtration rate [eGFR] > 60 mL/min/1.73 m$^2$), preclinical renal disease (cystatin C > 1 mg/L and eGFR > 60 mL/min/1.73 m$^2$), and chronic kidney disease (eGFR < 60 mL/min/1.73 m$^2$). The relationship between the subgroups and all-cause or cardiovascular mortality, myocardial infarction, and heart failure was evaluated. Approximately, 35% of the patients had normal renal function with microalbuminuria, 46% of the patients had preclinical renal disease, and 19% of the patients had an eGFR less than 60 mL/min/1.73 m$^2$. The presence of microalbuminuria was variably distributed across these groups.

Interestingly, and similar to the results of the ADVANCE trial, both microalbuminuria and impaired GFR (as measured by elevated cystatin C) were independently associated with more than 50% increase in mortality risk. Patients with both microalbuminuria and preclinical renal disease had a 2.4-fold increase in mortality risk. Not surprisingly, patients with the most significant

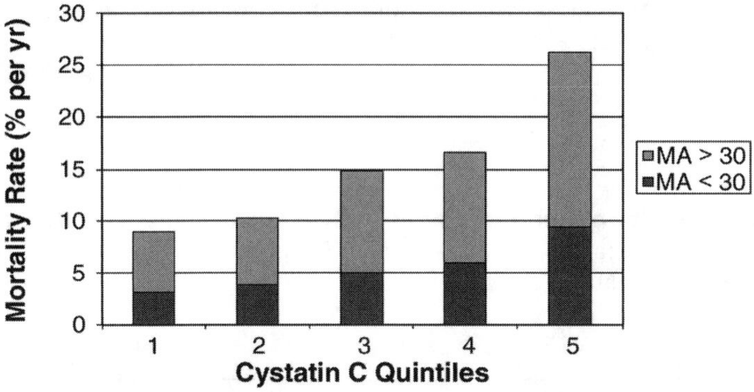


**FIGURE 1.**—Mortality rates by quintiles of kidney function and microalbuminuria cystatin C quintiles: (1) <0.91 mg/L; (2) 0.92–1.02 mg/L; (3) 1.03–1.13 mg/L; (4) 1.14–1.32 mg/L; (5) >1.32 mg/L. (Courtesy of Rifkin DE, Katz R, Chonchol M, et al. Albuminuria, impaired kidney function and cardiovascular outcomes or mortality in the elderly. *Nephrol Dial Transplant.* 2010;25:1560-1567.)

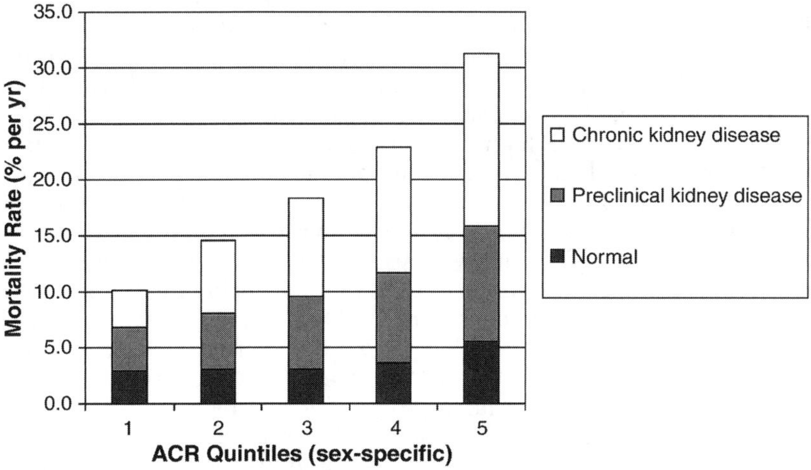


**FIGURE 2.**—Mortality rates by ACR quintile and category of kidney disease. (Courtesy of Rifkin DE, Katz R, Chonchol M, et al. Albuminuria, impaired kidney function and cardiovascular outcomes or mortality in the elderly. *Nephrol Dial Transplant.* 2010;25:1560-1567.)

renal disease had the highest mortality risk. Also of interest was the finding that as shown in Figs 1 and 2, a pattern of increasing mortality rates was observed with both increased microalbuminuria and higher cystatin C levels. Both cystatin C and microalbuminuria conferred increased, independent risk to all-cause and cardiovascular mortality in this elderly population. The observational nature of this study cannot explain the physiologic mechanism responsible for the results. However, the results are quite interesting as they do demonstrate that the measurement of cystatin C coupled with microalbuminuria suggests that a large population of patients (approximately 70% of the cohort studies) appear to be at increased risk of cardiovascular events. Further studies will be required to better define the independent prognostic role of these markers in defining cardiovascular disease and mortality risk.

**R. Garrick, MD**

**Screening for Albuminuria Identifies Individuals at Increased Renal Risk**

van der Velde M, Halbesma N, de Charro FT, et al (Univ Med Ctr Groningen, Netherlands; RENINE, Registry for Renal Replacement Therapy, Rotterdam, Netherlands)

*J Am Soc Nephrol* 20:852-862, 2009

It is unknown whether screening for albuminuria in the general population identifies individuals at increased risk for renal replacement therapy (RRT) or accelerated loss of renal function. Here, in a general population-based cohort of 40,854 individuals aged 28 to 75 yr, we collected a first morning void for measurement of urinary albumin. In a subset of 6879 individuals, we measured 24-h urinary albumin excretion and estimated GFR at baseline and during 6 yr of follow-up. Linkage with the national RRT registry identified 45 individuals who started RRT during 9 yr of follow-up. The quantity of albuminuria was associated with increased renal risk: the higher the level of albuminuria, the higher the risk of need for renal replacement therapy and the more rapid renal function decline. A urinary albumin concentration of ≥20 mg/L identified individuals who started RRT during follow-up with 58% sensitivity and 92% specificity. Of the identified individuals, 39% were previously unknown to have impaired renal function, and 50% were not being medically treated. Restricting screening to high-risk groups (*e.g.*, known hypertension, diabetes, cardiovascular disease [CVD], older age) reduced the sensitivity of the test only marginally but failed to identify 45% of individuals with micro- and macroalbuminuria. In conclusion, individuals with elevated levels of urinary albumin are at increased risk for RRT and accelerated loss of renal function. Screening for albuminuria identifies patients at increased risk for progressive renal disease, 40 to 50% of whom were previously undiagnosed or untreated.

▶ The Prevention of Renal and Vascular Endstage Disease (PREVEND) study is a prospective cohort study designed to evaluate whether the presence of albuminuria predicts the development of cardiovascular and renal disease in the general population. Prior elements of the PREVEND study have been previously reviewed. Conducted in the Netherlands, The PREVEND trial included 40 845 individuals. In the present subset study of 6879 individuals, 24-hour urinary albumin excretion and estimated glomerular filtration rate were measured at baseline and during a 6-year follow-up. Renal replacement therapy was begun in 45 individuals during a 9-year follow-up period. Urinary albumin concentration of 20 mg per liter or greater identified individuals who required

**TABLE 4.**—Screening Test Characteristics for Various Cutoff Points of UAC in a Single First Morning Void Urine to Identify Individuals Who Started RRT During Follow-Up[a]

| | | Test Characteristics UAC | | | | |
|---|---|---|---|---|---|---|
| UAC (mg/L) | Sensitivity (%) | Specificity (%) | PPV (%) | NPV (%) | LR+ | LR− |
| General population | | | | | | |
| >10 | 67 | 76 | 0.3 | 99.9 | 2.74 | 0.44 |
| >20 | 58 | 92 | 0.8 | 99.9 | 7.43 | 0.46 |
| >100 | 49 | 99 | 4.2 | 99.9 | 39.51 | 0.52 |
| >200 | 36 | 99 | 5.7 | 99.9 | 54.55 | 0.65 |
| CVD history | | | | | | |
| >10 | 16 | 99 | 1.5 | 99.9 | 13.5 | 0.85 |
| >20 | 16 | 99 | 2.8 | 99.9 | 26.1 | 0.85 |
| >100 | 11 | 99 | 6.7 | 99.9 | 64.8 | 0.89 |
| >200 | 7 | 99 | 7.1 | 99.8 | 69.8 | 0.93 |
| With known hypertension/diabetes | | | | | | |
| >10 | 49 | 96 | 1.4 | 99.9 | 12.7 | 0.53 |
| >20 | 44 | 98 | 2.6 | 99.9 | 24.3 | 0.57 |
| >100 | 38 | 99 | 8.4 | 99.9 | 82.9 | 0.63 |
| >200 | 31 | 99 | 11.6 | 99.9 | 118.7 | 0.69 |
| Age >55 yr | | | | | | |
| >10 | 47 | 92 | 0.6 | 99.9 | 5.5 | 0.58 |
| >20 | 44 | 96 | 1.3 | 99.9 | 12.1 | 0.58 |
| >100 | 36 | 99 | 5.2 | 99.9 | 46.7 | 0.65 |
| >200 | 27 | 99 | 7.1 | 99.9 | 68.9 | 0.74 |
| At least one of above risk factors | | | | | | |
| >10 | 58 | 90 | 0.7 | 99.9 | 6.0 | 0.47 |
| >20 | 53 | 96 | 1.4 | 99.9 | 12.8 | 0.49 |
| >100 | 44 | 99 | 5.7 | 99.9 | 54.5 | 0.56 |
| >200 | 33 | 99 | 7.6 | 99.9 | 74.7 | 0.67 |

[a]LR+, likelihood ratio of a positive test; LR−, likelihood ratio of a negative test; NPV, negative predictive value; PPV, positive predictive value.

renal replacement therapy, and approximately half the patients who required renal placement therapy had microalbuminuria. Surprisingly, almost 40% of the individuals identified were previously unknown to have impaired renal function. Screening confined to patients in high-risk groups (hypertension, diabetes, and cardiovascular disease; older than 55 years) identified 55% of patients with microalbuminuria and 87% of the individuals who progressed to renal placement therapy.

The authors calculated the screening test characteristics of a single morning urine sample for both the general population and high-risk groups (Table 4). Fig 2 in the original article demonstrates that the rate of renal function decline increases continuously with increasing levels of albuminuria. Together the results demonstrate that microalbuminuria (especially a urinary albumin excretion of more than 150 mg/24 hours) is a risk factor for renal events in both the general population and in patients with known underlying risk factors. One possible drawback of this study is that the relative renal risk of albuminuria may be underestimated because patients with renal disease often die from cardiovascular complications before dialysis is reached. In addition, the number of renal events was small and longer follow-up will likely improve the power of this study. Whether or not the results of the study should be used to change care guidelines such that microalbuminuria becomes a routine screening tool for the general population will require cost-benefit analyses. The results from the previous PREVEND Intervention Trial[1] study demonstrated a marginally beneficial effect of fosinopril and pravastatin on renal and cardiovascular outcomes in a small number of patients with low-grade albuminuria. However, these results were not robust enough to support the routine screening for microalbuminuria in the general population. Thus, although measuring microalbuminuria is relatively inexpensive, whether therapeutic intervention in asymptomatic normotensive patients with microalbuminuria of the degree noted here will be clinically safe and appropriate will require further study.

**M. Brogan, MD**

*Reference*

1. Atthobari J, Asselbergs FW, Boersma C, et al. PREVEND IT Study Group. Cost-effectiveness of screening for albuminuria with subsequent fosinopril treatment to prevent cardiovascular events: a pharmacoeconomic analysis linked to the prevention of renal and vascular endstage disease (PREVEND) study and the prevention of renal and vascular endstage disease intervention trial (PREVEND IT). *Clin Ther.* 2006;28:432-444.

---

**Association of estimated glomerular filtration rate and albuminuria with all-cause and cardiovascular mortality in general population cohorts: a collaborative meta-analysis**

Chronic Kidney Disease Prognosis Consortium (Johns Hopkins Bloomberg School of Public Health, Baltimore, MD; Univ of Groningen, Netherlands; et al)

*Lancet* 375:2073-2081, 2010

---

*Background.*—Substantial controversy surrounds the use of estimated glomerular filtration rate (eGFR) and albuminuria to define chronic kidney disease and assign its stages. We undertook a meta-analysis to assess the independent and combined associations of eGFR and albuminuria with mortality.

*Methods.*—In this collaborative meta-analysis of general population cohorts, we pooled standardised data for all-cause and cardiovascular mortality from studies containing at least 1000 participants and baseline information about eGFR and urine albumin concentrations. Cox proportional hazards models were used to estimate hazard ratios (HRs) for all-cause and cardiovascular mortality associated with eGFR and albuminuria, adjusted for potential confounders.

*Findings.*—The analysis included 105 872 participants (730 577 person-years) from 14 studies with urine albumin-to-creatinine ratio (ACR) measurements and 1 128 310 participants (4 732 110 person-years) from seven studies with urine protein dipstick measurements. In studies with ACR measurements, risk of mortality was unrelated to eGFR between 75 mL/min/1·73 m$^2$ and 105 mL/min/1·73 m$^2$ and increased at lower

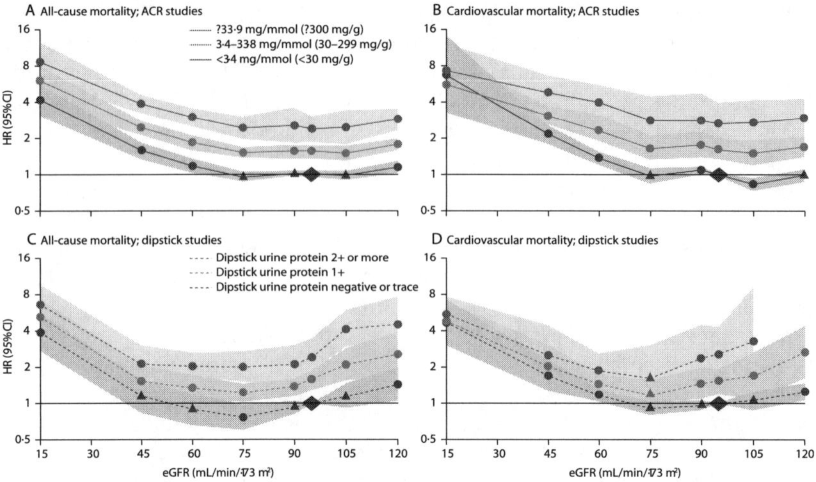


**FIGURE 3.**—Hazard ratios and 95% CIs for all-cause and cardiovascular mortality according to spline estimated glomerular filtration rate (eGFR) and categorical albuminuria. Shaded areas represent 95% CIs. Models included spline eGFR, categorical albuminuria, and their interaction terms as well as adjustment for age, sex, ethnic origin, history of cardiovascular disease, systolic blood pressure, diabetes, smoking, and total cholesterol. The reference (diamond) was eGFR 95 mL/min/1·73 $m^2$ plus ACR less than 3·4 mg/mmol (30 mg/g) or dipstick test result negative or trace. Circles represent statistically significant and triangles represent not significant. The estimated HR and 95% CI at eGFR 120 mL/min/1·73 $m^2$ with dipstick 2+ or more for cardiovascular mortality were omitted, since only two studies contributed to reliable estimation. To convert ACR in mg/g to mg/mmol multiply by 0·113. (Reprinted from Chronic Kidney Disease Prognosis Consortium. Association of estimated glomerular filtration rate and albuminuria with all-cause and cardiovascular mortality in general population cohorts: a collaborative meta-analysis. *Lancet* 2010;375:2073-2081, with permission from Elsevier.)

eGFRs. Compared with eGFR 95 mL/min/1·73 $m^2$, adjusted HRs for all-cause mortality were 1·18 (95% CI 1·05–1·32) for eGFR 60 mL/min/1·73 $m^2$, 1·57 (1·39–1·78) for 45 mL/min/1·73 $m^2$, and 3·14 (2·39–4·13) for 15 mL/min/1·73 $m^2$. ACR was associated with risk of mortality linearly on the log-log scale without threshold effects. Compared with ACR 0·6 mg/mmol, adjusted HRs for all-cause mortality were 1·20 (1·15–1·26) for ACR 1·1 mg/mmol, 1·63 (1·50–1·77) for 3·4 mg/mmol, and 2·22 (1·97–2·51) for 33·9 mg/mmol. eGFR and ACR were multiplicatively associated with risk of mortality without evidence of interaction. Similar findings were recorded for cardiovascular mortality and in studies with dipstick measurements.

*Interpretation.*—eGFR less than 60 mL/min/1·73 $m^2$ and ACR 1·1 mg/mmol (10 mg/g) or more are independent predictors of mortality risk in the general population. This study provides quantitative data for use of both kidney measures for risk assessment and definition and staging of chronic kidney disease.

► Physicians tend to be cautious in the interpretation of observational data derived from meta-analyses. However, the sheer size and the findings of this meta-analysis are worthy of comment. The meta-analysis pooled data from the general population on cardiovascular and all-cause mortality from studies that enrolled at least 1000 patients and contain data on urine protein/albumin excretion and estimated glomerular filtration rate (eGFR). Data regarding urine albumin-to-creatinine ratio were available in 105 872 participants (730 577 person-years) and urine protein (measured by dipstick) were available in 1 128 310 participants (4 732 110 person-years).

The data are compelling. Fig 3 demonstrates the hazard ratios for all-cause and cardiovascular mortality according to eGFR and albuminuria. In its totality, this enormous database demonstrates that eGFR of less than 60 and albumin-to-creatinine ratio of greater than 10 mg/g are independent predictors of cardiovascular and all-cause mortality in the general population.

These data are very reminiscent of those of the PREVEND trial[1] and demonstrate that even small amounts of albumin in the urine are abnormal and can predict cardiovascular and all-cause mortality. Whether measurement of microalbuminuria will become the standard of care for the general population will require further cost-benefit analysis. However, the findings of this meta-analysis certainly support the measurement of eGFR and urine albumin-to-creatinine ratio in members of the general population who may be at increased risk but are without current evidence of cardiovascular or renal disease. Such individuals might include those with a family history of diabetes or cardiovascular disease and hypertension.

**R. Garrick, MD**

*Reference*

1. van der Velde M, Halbesma N, de Charro FT, et al. Screening for albuminuria identifies individuals at increased renal risk. *J Am Soc Nephrol.* 2009;20:852-862.

---

**Addition of Angiotensin Receptor Blockade or Mineralocorticoid Antagonism to Maximal Angiotensin-Converting Enzyme Inhibition in Diabetic Nephropathy**

Mehdi UF, Adams-Huet B, Raskin P, et al (The Univ of Texas Southwestern Med Ctr, Dallas)

*J Am Soc Nephrol* 20:2641-2650, 2009

---

Aldosterone promotes glomerular and tubular sclerosis independent of angiotensin II in animal models of diabetic nephropathy. Most human studies testing the renoprotective benefit of adding an angiotensin receptor blocker or a mineralocorticoid receptor antagonist to a regimen based on inhibition of angiotensin-converting enzyme (ACE) used relatively low doses of ACE inhibitors. Furthermore, these studies did not determine whether antiproteinuric effects were independent of BP lowering. We conducted a double-blind, placebo-controlled trial in 81 patients with diabetes, hypertension, and albuminuria (urine albumin-to-creatinine ratio ≥300 mg/g) who all received lisinopril (80 mg once daily). We randomly assigned the patients to placebo, losartan (100 mg daily), or spironolactone (25 mg daily) for 48 wk. We obtained blood and urine albumin, urea, creatinine, electrolytes, A1c, and ambulatory BP at baseline, 24, and 48 wk. Compared with placebo, the urine albumin-to-creatinine ratio decreased by 34.0% (95% CI, −51.0%, −11.2%, $P = 0.007$) in the group assigned to spironolactone and by 16.8% (95% CI, −37.3%, +10.5%, $P = 0.20$) in the group assigned to losartan. Clinic and ambulatory BP, creatinine clearance, sodium and protein intake, and glycemic control did not differ between groups. Serum potassium level was significantly higher with the addition of either spironolactone or losartan. In conclusion, the addition of spironolactone, but not losartan, to a regimen including maximal ACE inhibition affords greater renoprotection in diabetic nephropathy despite a similar effect on BP. These results support the need to conduct a long-term, large-scale, renal failure outcomes trial.

▶ This is a very interesting study. Prior animal studies[1,2] and small trials in humans with diabetes[3,4] suggested that in patients with diabetic nephropathy adding an angiotensin receptor antagonist or a mineralocorticoid receptor antagonist to an angiotensin-converting enzyme inhibitor (ACEi)-based regimen may further reduce proteinuria and slow the progression of renal disease. However, it remains unclear whether the beneficial effects were related to the specific actions of the antagonist or to the effects of blood pressure lowering. In addition, the ACEi dosage used in these studies was often submaximal. This well-designed and well-conducted study demonstrates that the addition of spironolactone (25 mg/d) but not losartan (100 mg/d) to a regimen, including maximum ACE inhibition (lisinopril 80 mg/d), affords greater renal protection in diabetic nephropathy.

These are very welcome data. The recall of the results of the COOPERATE trial[5] and the incidence of acute renal injury (likely related to episode of hypotension in a high-risk population) that occurred in the ONTARGET trial[6] have left clinicians a bit uncertain as to the correct management of the at-risk diabetics with proteinuria. One caveat is that the dropout rate in the study was a bit higher than anticipated, but the baseline characteristics of the patients who dropped out were similar to those of the patients who finished the trial. Additionally, there was a higher incidence of hyperkalemia in the spironolactone group. Lower doses of spironolactone (12.5 mg/d) were not studied, so it is unknown as to whether lower dose therapy would carry the same efficacy with less risk. Nonetheless, these are new observations drawn from a carefully conducted, albeit small, clinical trial. The findings open the way for a larger multicenter trial and do offer evidence that will allow clinicians appropriately extend the therapeutic regimen in this at-risk population.

**R. Garrick, MD**

*References*

1. Juknevicius I, Segal Y, Kren S, Lee R, Hostetter TH. Effect of aldosterone on renal transforming growth factor-β. *Am J Physiol Renal Physiol.* 2004;286: F1059-F1062.

2. Ponda MP, Hostetter TH. Aldosterone antagonism in chronic kidney disease. *Clin J Am Soc Nephrol.* 2006;1:668-677.
3. Rossing K, Schjoedt KJ, Smidt UM, Boomsma F, Parving HH. Beneficial effects of adding spironolactone to recommended antihypertensive treatment in diabetic nephropathy: a randomized, doublemasked, cross-over study. *Diabetes Care.* 2005;28:2106-2112.
4. Sato A, Hayashi K, Naruse M, Saruta T. Effectiveness of aldosterone blockade in patients with diabetic nephropathy. *Hypertension.* 2003;41:64-68.
5. Retraction–Combination treatment of angiotensin-II receptor blocker and angiotensin-converting-enzyme inhibitor in non-diabetic renal disease (COOPERATE): a randomised controlled trial. *Lancet.* 2009;374:1226.
6. Mann JF, Schmieder RE, McQueen M, et al. Renal outcomes with telmisartan, ramipril, or both, in people at high vascular risk (the ONTARGET study): a multicenter, randomized, double-blind, controlled trial. *Lancet.* 2008;372:547-553.

## Supramaximal Dose of Candesartan in Proteinuric Renal Disease

Burgess E, the SMART (Supra Maximal Atacand Renal Trial) Investigators (Univ of Calgary, Alberta, Canada; et al)
*J Am Soc Nephrol* 20:893-900, 2009

High levels of proteinuria predict renal deterioration, suggesting that interventions to reduce proteinuria may postpone the development of severe renal impairment. This multicenter Canadian trial evaluated whether supramaximal dosages of candesartan would reduce proteinuria to a greater extent than the maximum approved antihypertensive dosage. The authors randomly assigned 269 patients who had persistent proteinuria (≥1 g/d) despite 7 wk of treatment with the highest approved dosage of candesartan (16 mg/d) to 16, 64, or 128 mg/d candesartan for 30 wk. The median serum creatinine level was 130.0 μmol/L (1.47 mg/dl), and the median urinary protein excretion was 2.66 g/d; most (53.9%) patients had diabetic nephropathy. The mean difference of the percentage change in proteinuria for patients receiving 128 mg/d candesartan compared with those receiving 16 mg/d candesartan was −33.05% (95% confidence interval −45.70 to −17.44; $P < 0.0001$). Reductions in BP were not different across the three treatment groups. Elevated serum potassium levels ($K^+ > 5.5$ mEq/L) led to the early withdrawal of 11 patients, but there were no dosage-related increases in adverse events. In conclusion, proteinuria that persists despite treatment with the maximum recommended dosage of candesartan can be reduced by increasing the dosage of candesartan further, but serum potassium levels should be monitored during treatment (Table 2).

▶ Proteinuria has been used as a surrogate marker of renal disease outcome and predictive marker for all-cause and cardiovascular mortality. Several trials in a variety of disease states have suggested that the use of angiotensin-converting enzyme inhibitors (ACEIs) and angiotensin type 1 receptor blockers (ARBs) leads to a reduction in proteinuria and a preservation of renal function

**TABLE 2.**—Proteinuria Results in g/d and Percentage Change at Various Dosages of Candesartan[a]

| Urinary Protein Values[b] | 16 mg | 64 mg | 128 mg |
|---|---|---|---|
| Randomization (SEM) | 2.80 ± 0.07 | 2.83 ± 0.06 | 2.85 ± 0.07 |
| Completion | 2.59 ± 0.08 | 2.20 ± 0.08 | 1.79 ± 0.11 |
| Δ Randomization (%) | −7.49 ± 5.69 | −22.23 ± 6.17 | −36.95 ± 7.05 |
| Δ *versus* 16 mg | NA | −16.91 | −33.05 |

[a]Analysis of covariance model with center and proteinuria at baseline as covariates.
[b]Geometric means were used to calculate the urinary protein values, because these values are presented as a percentage change.

that is better than what would be achieved by blood pressure control alone.[1,2] Blockade of the renin-angiotensin system is believed to have beneficial effects on inflammation and fibrosis that are independent from blood pressure control. Some, but not all, studies have demonstrated a discordant affect between proteinuria and blood pressure control with ACEI and ARB use such that super maximal doses of the agents result in a reduction in proteinuria without causing hypotension.[3,4] To better understand the potential risks and benefits of using high-dose therapy, the Supra Maximal Atacand Renal Trial was initiated in patients with proteinuria of more than 1 g/d with primary glomerular disease, diabetes, or hypertensive glomerulosclerosis. After the run-in period, during which time all patients received the usual maximum dose of 16 mg/d of candesartan, 269 patients continued to have persistent proteinuria (more than 1 g/d) and were assigned to the high-dose candesartan groups. The maximum dose of candesartan was 128 mg/d for 30 weeks. As shown in Table 2, high-dose candesartan was associated with a substantial reduction in proteinuria without an adverse affect on blood pressure. Adverse effects included hyperkalemia (no difference between the groups); hypotension (1 patient in the 16-mg/d group); and an elevated serum creatinine (1 patient receiving 16 mg/d and 2 receiving 128 mg/d).

The results are thought provoking because the higher dosage clearly has an improved antiproteinuric effect and does not seem to be associated with a substantial increase in adverse events. However, whether or not these doses are truly renal protective or cardioprotective is unclear because surrogate markers are being used. Clearly, as pointed out by de Zeeuw and Lambers-Heerspink,[5] appropriate efficacy and safety studies are needed to better address this question. In the meantime, if clinicians chose to exceed the maximum recommended therapeutic dose and use supramaximal doses, it would seem wise to advise patients of the current state of our knowledge and carefully monitor their clinical status.

**R. Garrick, MD**

*References*

1. Eijkelkamp WBA, Zhang Z, Remuzzi G, et al. Albuminuria is a target for renoprotective therapy independent from blood pressure in patients with type 2 diabetic nephropathy: post hoc analysis from the Reduction of Endpoints in NIDDM

with Angiotensin II Antagonist Losartan (RENAAL) trial. *J Am Soc Nephrol.* 2007;18:1540-1546.
2. de Zeeuw D, Remuzzi G, Parving HH, et al. Proteinuria, a target for renoprotection in patients with type 2 diabetic nephropathy: lessons from RENAAL. *Kidney Int.* 2004;65:2309-2320.
3. Rossing K, Schjoedt KJ, Jensen BR, Boomsma F, Parving HH. Enhanced renoprotective effects of ultrahigh doses of irbesartan in patients with type 2 diabetes and microalbuminuria. *Kidney Int.* 2005;68:1190-1198.
4. Hollenberg NK, Parving HH, Viberti G, et al. Albuminuria response to very high-dose valsartan in type 2 diabetes mellitus. *J Hypertens.* 2007;25:1921-1926.
5. de Zeeuw D, Lambers-Heerspink H. Drug dosing for renoprotection: maybe it's time for drug efficacy-safety score? *J Am Soc Nephrol.* 2009;20:681-691.

## Comparison of Different Measures of Urinary Protein Excretion for Prediction of Renal Events

Lambers Heerspink HJ, Gansevoort RT, Brenner BM, et al (Univ of Groningen, The Netherlands; Brigham and Women's Hosp and Harvard School of Medicine, Boston, MA; et al)
*J Am Soc Nephrol* 21:1355-1360, 2010

There are many methods to screen for abnormal amounts of proteinuria to identify patients at risk for progression of renal disease, but which method best predicts renal risk is unknown. Here, we analyzed a subset of 701 patients with type 2 diabetes and nephropathy participating in the Reduction of Endpoints in Non Insulin Dependent Diabetes Mellitus with the Angiotensin II Antagonist Losartan (RENAAL) trial to compare the ability of urinary protein excretion (UPE) and urinary albumin excretion (UAE) from a 24-hour urine collection and urinary albumin concentration (UAC) and the albumin:creatinine ratio (ACR) from a first-morning void in predicting renal events. The primary outcome measure was the time to a doubling of serum creatinine or end-stage renal disease. During follow-up, 202 events occurred. The hazard ratios for the risk of a renal outcome (95% CIs) associated with 1-SD increment in the log-transformed measures were 3.16 (2.60 to 3.86) for UAE, 3.02 (2.53 to 3.62) for UPE, 3.23 (2.67 to 3.91) for UAC, and 4.36 (3.50 to 5.45) for ACR. The area under the ROC curve was significantly higher for ACR compared with the other measures. In conclusion, measurement of the albumin:creatinine ratio in a first-morning void is the superior method to predict renal events in patients with type 2 diabetes and nephropathy.

▶ Proteinuria and microalbuminuria are recognized as risk factors for renal disease progression and cardiovascular events. During the last decade, several different methods have been used to quantify urine protein and albumin excretion. Initially, the 24-hour urine collection was the mainstay for these determinations. However, these collections are cumbersome and often hampered by errors in collection. Several different methodologies have been used to estimate

**TABLE 2.**—Area Under the ROC Curve and 95% CIs for the Prediction of the Composite of Doubling of Serum Creatinine or End-Stage Renal Disease Based on Baseline Proteinuria Measures

| | | Doubling of Serum Creatinine or End-Stage Renal Disease | | | |
|---|---|---|---|---|---|
| | | 24-Hour Urine | | First-Morning Void | |
| | Subjects/Events | UAE (mg/24 h) | UPE (mg/24 h) | UAC (mg/L) | ACR (mg/g) |
| Overall | 701/202 | 0.78 [0.74, 0.82] | 0.78 [0.75, 0.82] | 0.79 [0.75 to 0.83] | 0.82 [0.79, 0.86][a,b,c] |
| Subgroups | | | | | |
| Gender | | | | | |
| Men | 436/107 | 0.76 [0.71, 0.81] | 0.76 [0.70, 0.81] | 0.77 [0.72, 0.82] | 0.79 [0.73, 0.84] |
| Women | 265/95 | 0.81 [0.76, 0.87] | 0.83 [0.77, 0.88] | 0.82 [0.77, 0.87] | 0.86 [0.82, 0.91][a,c] |
| Age | | | | | |
| ≤61.0 years | 351/120 | 0.78 [0.72, 0.83] | 0.79 [0.74, 0.84] | 0.80 [0.75, 0.85] | 0.84 [0.79, 0.88][a,b,c] |
| >61.0 years | 350/82 | 0.77 [0.71, 0.83] | 0.76 [0.70, 0.83] | 0.77 [0.71, 0.83] | 0.80 [0.75, 0.86] |
| Race | | | | | |
| Caucasian | 323/75 | 0.76 [0.70, 0.82] | 0.77 [0.71, 0.83] | 0.79 [0.73, 0.85] | 0.79 [0.74, 0.85] |
| African American | 144/33 | 0.75 [0.64, 0.86] | 0.76 [0.65, 0.86] | 0.77 [0.68, 0.87] | 0.83 [0.74, 0.91] |
| Hispanic | 192/78 | 0.78 [0.71, 0.85] | 0.78 [0.71, 0.85] | 0.78 [0.71, 0.85] | 0.82 [0.75, 0.88][a,b] |
| Gender, age, and race adjusted | 701/202 | 0.79 [0.75, 0.83] | 0.79 [0.75, 0.83] | 0.80 [0.76 to 0.83] | 0.82 [0.79, 0.86][a,b,c] |

Bonferroni correction was applied in AUC comparison to adjust for multiple testing. ACR, first-morning void albumin:creatinine ratio; AUC, area under the ROC curve; UAE, 24-hour urinary albumin excretion; UPE, 24-hour urinary protein excretion.

[a]$P < 0.01$ *versus* UAE.

[b]$P < 0.01$ *versus* UPE.

[c]$P < 0.01$ *versus* UAC.

protein and albumin excretion. The 24-hour urine protein excretion, and urine albumin excretion, and the urinary albumin concentration and albumin-to-creatinine ratio on single-voided samples have all been used to predict renal events. The present study is drawn from the well-described database of patients with type 2 diabetes who participated in the Reduction of Endpoints in Non Insulin Dependent Diabetes Mellitus with the Angiotensin II Antagonist Losartan study[1] and methodically compares these various methods for the detection of the proteinuria. The primary outcome measure was the time to doubling the serum creatinine or end-stage renal disease. The baseline proteinuria measurements have a positive and continuous relationship with the risk for the occurrence of the primary end points. As shown in Table 2, for prediction of the primary end points, the area under the curve of the first-morning void albumin-to-creatinine ratio was significantly better than the 3 other proteinuria measurements. Interestingly, the authors also demonstrated that the predictive value for a primary outcome event was improved by using the first-morning void albumin-to-creatinine ratio as compared with the 24-hour urine albumin excretion rate. In fact, increase in the albumin-to-creatinine ratio by one standard deviation approximately quadrupled the likelihood of an adverse renal event.

This study represents the first rigorous evaluation of the various methodologies for the determination of urinary protein and albumin excretion. Moreover, the result is linked to a primary outcome end point in a very well-defined population. This is an important study because it demonstrates that the determination of the first-morning void albumin-to-creatinine ratio, which is currently the favored clinical practice, is the most appropriate method for predicting renal disease progression in patients with type 2 diabetes and nephropathy.

**R. Garrick, MD**

*Reference*

1. de Zeeuw D, Remuzzi G, Parving HH, et al. Proteinuria, a target for renoprotection in patients with type 2 diabetic nephropathy: lessons from RENAAL. *Kidney Int.* 2004;65:2309-2320.

## The Soluble VEGF Receptor sFlt1 Contributes to Endothelial Dysfunction in CKD

Di Marco GS, Reuter S, Hillebrand U, et al (Univ Clinics Münster, Germany; et al)

*J Am Soc Nephrol* 20:2235-2245, 2009

Endothelial dysfunction contributes to the increased cardiovascular risk that accompanies CKD. We hypothesized that the soluble VEGF receptor 1 (sFlt-1), a VEGF antagonist, plays a role in endothelial dysfunction and decreased angiogenesis in CKD. We enrolled 130 patients with CKD stages

3 to 5 and 56 age- and gender-matched control patients. Plasma sFlt-1 levels were higher in patients with CKD and, after multivariate regression analyses, exclusively associated with renal function and levels of vWF, a marker of endothelial dysfunction. Compared with serum from control patients, both recombinant sFlt-1 and serum from patients with CKD had antiangiogenic activity in the chick chorioallantoic membrane (CAM) assay, induced endothelial cell apoptosis *in vitro*, and decreased nitric oxide generation in two different endothelial cell lines. Pretreating the sera with an antibody against sFlt-1 abrogated all of these effects. Furthermore, we observed increased sFlt1 levels in 5/6-nephrectomized rats compared with sham-operated animals. Finally, using real-time PCR and ELISA, we identified monocytes as a possible source of increased sFlt-1 in patients with CKD. Our findings show that excess sFlt-1 associates with endothelial dysfunction in CKD and suggest that increased sFlt-1 may predict cardiovascular risk in CKD.

▶ It is well described that there is an increased risk of cardiovascular morbidity in patients with chronic kidney disease.[1] It has also been demonstrated that endothelial dysfunction is independently associated with impaired renal function.[2] These risks have usually been attributed to the presence of hypertension with increased shear stress,[3] inflammation,[4] advanced glycated end products (in diabetics),[5] uremic calcification due to secondary hyperparathyroidism and hyperphosphatemia,[6] or other uremic toxins.

sFlt1, a soluble vascular endothelial growth factor (VEGF) receptor, is known to antagonize VEGF both by sequestering VEGF and by occupying the tissue receptors. This leads to decreased angiogenesis and endothelial dysfunction. By these mechanisms, sFlt1 has been implicated in the pathogenesis of preeclampsia with its associated proteinuria, hypertension, and renal dysfunction.

This study by Di Marco et al elegantly demonstrated that the plasma concentration of sFlt1 is negatively correlated with estimated glomerular filtration rate. The investigators demonstrated that monocytes isolated from uremic patients expressed more sFlt1 than controls. The sFlt1 level seemed to be positively correlated with markers of endothelial dysfunction, Framingham risk scores, and more relevantly, clinical outcomes, such as myocardial infarction and stroke. When tested in vivo, patients' sera rich in sFlt1, had sera that was proapoptotic and had decreased nitric oxide availability. Recombinant sFlt1 had the same effects, while sFlt1 neutralization had the opposite effect.

These data strongly suggest that sFlt1, probably expressed by monocytes, accumulates in uremic plasma and may be a critical factor in the vascular pathology, which results in excess cardiovascular morbidity. Surprisingly, statin use increased the levels of sFlt1, a finding that will no doubt spark further investigation. The findings of this study will certainly lead to additional studies directed at better understanding and modifying the influence of sFlt1 on vascular health in chronic kidney disease.

**M. Klein, MD, JD**

*References*

1. Sarnak MJ, Levey AS, Schoolwerth AC, et al. Kidney disease as a risk factor for development of cardiovascular disease: a statement from the American Heart Association Councils on Kidney in Cardiovascular Disease, High Blood Pressure Research, Clinical Cardiology, and Epidemiology and Prevention. *Hypertension.* 2003;42:1050-1065.
2. Thambyrajah J, Landray MJ, McGlynn FJ, Jones HJ, Wheeler DC, Townend JN. Abnormalities of endothelial function in patients with predialysis renal failure. *Heart.* 2000;83:205-209.
3. Ballermann BJ, Dardik A, Eng E, Liu A. Shear stress and the endothelium. *Kidney Int Suppl.* 1998;54:S100-S108.
4. Kaysen GA. The microinflammatory state in Uremia: causes and potential consequences. *J Am Soc Nephrol.* 2001;12:1549-1557.
5. Linden E, Cai W, He JC, et al. Endothelial dysfunction in patients with chronic kidney disease results from advanced glycation end products (AGE)-mediated inhibition of endothelial nitric oxide synthase through RAGE activation. *Clin J Am Soc Nephrol.* 2008;3:691-698.
6. De Boer IH, Gorodetskaya I, Young B, Hsu CY, Chertow GM. The severity of secondary hyperparathyroidism in chronic renal insufficiency is GFR-Dependent, race-dependent, and associated with cardiovascular disease. *J Am Soc Nephrol.* 2002;13:2762-2769.

## Ketohexokinase-Dependent Metabolism of Fructose Induces Proinflammatory Mediators in Proximal Tubular Cells

Cirillo P, Gersch MS, Mu W, et al (Univ of Florida, Gainesville; et al)
*J Am Soc Nephrol* 20:545-553, 2009

Increased consumption of fructose may play an important role in the epidemic of metabolic syndrome and may presage the development of diabetes, cardiovascular disease, and chronic kidney disease. Once in the cell, fructose is phosphorylated by ketohexokinase (KHK), leading to consumption of ATP, formation of AMP, and generation of uric acid through xanthine oxidoreductase (XOR). This study aimed to examine the direct effects of fructose in human kidney proximal tubular cells (HK-2) and whether they are mediated by the fructose metabolism *via* KHK. At a similar concentration to that observed in peripheral blood after a meal, fructose induced production of monocyte chemotactic protein 1 (MCP-1) and reactive oxygen species in HK-2 cells. Knockdown of KHK by stable transfection with small hairpin RNA demonstrated that these processes were KHK dependent. Several antioxidants, including specific inhibitors of NADPH oxidase and XOR, prevented MCP-1 secretion. We detected XOR mRNA in HK-2 cells and confirmed its activity by identifying uric acid by mass spectrometry. Fructose increased intracellular uric acid, and uric acid induced production of MCP-1 as well. In summary,

**postprandial concentrations of fructose stimulate redox- and urate-dependent inflammatory mediators in proximal tubular cells.**

▶ Worldwide obesity is reaching alarming proportions.[1,2] The most recent National Health and Nutrition Examination Survey data set suggests that the prevalence of obesity (body mass index greater than 30) ranges between 33% and 35% for men and women. Metabolic syndrome and the associated risk of renal disease has been a matter of intense investigation. Several studies[3-5] have suggested that fructose ingestion (as high-fructose corn syrup) may be a key intermediary in the pathogenesis of obesity, the metabolic syndrome, and renal injury. Several lines of investigation have suggested that fructose-induced changes in uric acid metabolism may be associated with endothelial dysfunction, the production of proinflammatory mediators, oxidative stress, and alterations in the nitric oxide pathway with related changes in renal hemodynamics. The studies on human cultured proximal tubular cells demonstrate that typical postprandial concentrations of fructose generate urate-dependent inflammatory mediators in proximal tubular cells. Moreover, they demonstrated that ketohexokinase, the first enzyme of the main pathway of fructose metabolism, is required for this proinflammatory effect. These findings provide direct insight into a possible link between fructose and renal dysfunction. This exciting translational research provides significant new insight into what has become a worrisome and an ever-expanding clinical problem.

**R. Garrick, MD**

*References*


1. World Health Organization Western Pacific Region. *International Association for the Study of Obesity, International Obesity Task Force. The Asia-Pacific Perspective: Redefining Obesity and its Treatment.* Sydney: Health Communications Australia Pty Limited; 2000.
2. Chang CJ, Wu CH, Chang CS, et al. Low body mass index but high percent body fat in Taiwanese subjects: implications of obesity cutoffs. *Int J Obes Relat Metab Disord.* 2003;27:253-259.
3. Neilson EG. The fructose nation. *J Am Soc Nephrol.* 2007;18:2619-2621.
4. Sanchez-Lozada LG, Tapia E, Jiménez A, et al. Fructose-induced metabolic syndrome is associated with glomerular hypertension and renal microvascular damage in rats. *Am J Physiol Renal Physiol.* 2007;292:F423-F429.
5. Nakagawa T, Hu H, Zharikov S, et al. A causal role for uric acid in fructose-induced metabolic syndrome. *Am J Physiol Renal Physiol.* 2006;290:F625-F631.

**Bicarbonate Supplementation Slows Progression of CKD and Improves Nutritional Status**

de Brito-Ashurst I, Varagunam M, Raftery MJ, et al (William Harvey Res Inst and Barts and the London NHS Trust, UK)

*J Am Soc Nephrol* 20:2075-2084, 2009

Bicarbonate supplementation preserves renal function in experimental chronic kidney disease (CKD), but whether the same benefit occurs in humans is unknown. Here, we randomly assigned 134 adult patients with CKD (creatinine clearance [CrCl] 15 to 30 ml/min per 1.73 $m^2$) and serum bicarbonate 16 to 20 mmol/L to either supplementation with oral sodium bicarbonate or standard care for 2 yr. The primary end points were rate of CrCl decline, the proportion of patients with rapid decline of CrCl (>3 ml/min per 1.73 $m^2$/yr), and ESRD (CrCl <10 ml/min). Secondary end points were dietary protein intake, normalized protein nitrogen appearance, serum albumin, and mid-arm muscle circumference. Compared with the control group, decline in CrCl was slower with bicarbonate supplementation (5.93 *versus* 1.88 ml/min 1.73 $m^2$; $P < 0.0001$). Patients supplemented with bicarbonate were significantly less likely to experience rapid progression (9 *versus* 45%; relative risk 0.15; 95% confidence interval 0.06 to 0.40; $P < 0.0001$). Similarly, fewer patients supplemented with bicarbonate developed ESRD (6.5 *versus* 33%; relative risk 0.13; 95% confidence interval 0.04 to 0.40; $P < 0.001$). Nutritional parameters improved significantly with bicarbonate supplementation, which was well tolerated. This study demonstrates that bicarbonate supplementation slows the rate of progression of renal failure to ESRD and improves nutritional status among patients with CKD.

▶ As the authors note, metabolic acidosis is a common complication of chronic renal disease and is typically noted when glomerular filtration rate falls below 30 ml/min.[1] Several animal studies[2] as well as small studies in patients on dialysis[3] and with chronic renal insufficiency[4] have suggested that control of the acid-base status may slow disease progression and reduce protein breakdown. The results of this randomized controlled trial by de Brito-Ashurst and colleagues are very important. The results demonstrate that daily supplementation with oral sodium bicarbonate (600 mg twice daily increased as necessary to achieve and maintain the bicarbonate level ≥23 mmol/L) can reduce the rate of progression of renal disease and improve nutritional parameters. The primary end point, the rate of decline in creatinine clearance, was proximally 6 versus 1.88 ml/min/1.73 $m^2$ in the control versus treated group. At the end of year one, 14 patients in the control group, but none in the bicarbonate group, began dialysis. At the end of year two, 22 patients in the control group as compared with 4 in the treatment group progressed to dialysis. The positive renal effects of sodium bicarbonate supplementation were not associated with any untoward effects on blood pressure control or proteinuria. This is especially important because both of these parameters are believed to be relevant risk factors for the progression of chronic renal disease. This well-designed randomized controlled trial is the first to demonstrate that oral bicarbonate supplementation is associated with a positive effect on clinically relevant end points in patients with chronic renal insufficiency. The therapy is safe, inexpensive, easily tolerated, and readily available. One caveat: sodium bicarbonate is marketed in many dosage strengths and both powder and pill formulations. Clinicians should specify the dose desired and avoid substituting powdered sodium bicarbonate for sodium bicarbonate tablets as patients are often confused by the dosage conversions of the powdered formulations.

**R. Garrick, MD**

*References*

1. Kraut JA, Kurtz I. Metabolic acidosis of CKD: diagnosis, clinical characteristics, and treatment. *Am J Kidney Dis*. 2005;45:978-993.
2. Bailey JL, Wang X, England BK, Price SR, Ding X, Mitch WE. The acidosis of chronic renal failure activates muscle proteolysis in rats by augmenting transcription of genes encoding proteins of the ATP-dependent ubiquitin-proteasome pathway. *J Clin Invest*. 1996;97:1447-1453.
3. Graham KA, Reaich D, Channon SM, Downie S, Goodship TH. Correction of acidosis in hemodialysis decreases whole-body protein degradation. *J Am Soc Nephrol*. 1997;8:632-637.
4. Rustom R, Grime JS, Costigan M, et al. Oral sodium bicarbonate reduces proximal renal tubular peptide catabolism, ammoniogenesis, and tubular damage in renal patients. *Ren Fail*. 1998;20:371-382.

---

## Amelioration of metabolic acidosis in patients with low GFR reduced kidney endothelin production and kidney injury, and better preserved GFR

Phisitkul S, Khanna A, Simoni J, et al (Texas Tech Univ Health Sciences Ctr, Lubbock; et al)
*Kidney Int* 77:617-623, 2010

---

Metabolic acidosis often accompanies low glomerular filtration rate and induces secretion of endothelin, which in turn might mediate kidney injury. Here we tested whether treatment of metabolic acidosis in patients with low glomerular filtration rate reduced the progression of kidney disease. Fifty-nine patients with hypertensive nephropathy and metabolic acidosis had their blood pressure reduced with regimens that included angiotensin-converting enzyme inhibition. Thirty patients were then prescribed sodium citrate, and the remaining 29, unable or unwilling to take sodium citrate, served as controls. All were followed for 24 months with maintenance of their blood pressure reduction. Urine endothelin-1 excretion, a surrogate of kidney endothelin production, and *N*-acetyl-β-D-glucosaminidase, a marker of kidney tubulointerstitial injury, were each significantly lower, while the rate of estimated glomerular filtration rate decline was significantly slower. The estimated glomerular filtration rate was statistically higher after 24 months of sodium citrate treatment compared to the control group. Hence it appears that sodium citrate is an effective kidney-protective adjunct to blood pressure reduction and angiotensin-converting enzyme inhibition.

▶ This study by Phisitkul and colleagues extends the observations of de Brito-Ashurst.[1] Patients with hypertensive nephropathy in stage 3 chronic kidney disease (mean estimated glomerular filtration rate [eGFR], 33 ml/min/ 1.73 $m^2$) were enrolled in a 2-year trial. Thirty patients were prescribed sodium citrate at 1 meq bicarbonate/kg body weight per day in 3 divided doses to maintain a serum $CO_2$ of approximately 23 mmol/L. Renal function measured as eGFR and cystatin C, and urine albumin excretion, and markers of endothelin production and tubular interstitial injury were monitored. Blood pressure control and the use of diuretics and angiotensin-converting enzyme inhibitor therapy were similar in both groups. Sodium citrate therapy was associated with reduction in urine albumin excretion, an improvement in the rate of decline of GFR as measured by plasma cystatin C, an increase in serum bicarbonate level, and improvement in levels of endothelin-1 and *N*-acetyl-β-D-glucosaminidase, a marker of tubular-interstitial injury.

This study offers some insight into the possible pathophysiological mode of action of bicarbonate therapy and opens the way for further larger randomized controlled trials. This study and the study of de Brito-Ashurst certainly suggest that simple and readily available therapy with bicarbonate or the bicarbonate equivalent, citrate, has a place in the armamentaria of agents aimed at slowing the progression of renal disease. In fact, if the data hold up, the effect of bicarbonate may be significantly greater than that of much more expensive therapies.

**R. Garrick, MD**

*Reference*

1. de Brito-Ashurst I, Varagunum M, Raftery MJ, Yaqoob MM. Bicarbonate supplementation slows progression of CKD and improves nutritional status. *J Am Soc Nephrol.* 2009;20:2075-2084.

---

**Effect of B-Vitamin Therapy on Progression of Diabetic Nephropathy: A Randomized Controlled Trial**

House AA, Eliasziw M, Cattran DC, et al (Univ of Western Ontario, London, Canada; Univ of Calgary, Alberta, Canada; Univ of Toronto, Ontario, Canada; et al)

*JAMA* 303:1603-1609, 2010

---

*Context.*—Hyperhomocysteinemia is frequently observed in patients with diabetic nephropathy. B-vitamin therapy (folic acid, vitamin $B_6$, and vitamin $B_{12}$) has been shown to lower the plasma concentration of homocysteine.

*Objective.*—To determine whether B-vitamin therapy can slow progression of diabetic nephropathy and prevent vascular complications.

*Design, Setting, and Participants.*—A multicenter, randomized, double-blind, placebo-controlled trial (Diabetic Intervention with Vitamins to Improve Nephropathy [DIVINe]) at 5 university medical centers in Canada conducted between May 2001 and July 2007 of 238 participants who had type 1 or 2 diabetes and a clinical diagnosis of diabetic nephropathy.

*Intervention.*—Single tablet of B vitamins containing folic acid (2.5 mg/d), vitamin $B_6$ (25 mg/d), and vitamin $B_{12}$ (1 mg/d), or matching placebo.

*Main Outcome Measures.*—Change in radionuclide glomerular filtration rate (GFR) between baseline and 36 months. Secondary outcomes were dialysis and a composite of myocardial infarction, stroke, revascularization, and all-cause mortality. Plasma total homocysteine was also measured.

*Results.*—The mean (SD) follow-up during the trial was 31.9 (14.4) months. At 36 months, radionuclide GFR decreased by a mean (SE) of 16.5 (1.7) mL/min/1.73 $m^2$ in the B-vitamin group compared with 10.7 (1.7) mL/min/1.73 $m^2$ in the placebo group (mean difference, −5.8; 95% confidence interval [CI], −10.6 to −1.1; $P = .02$). There was no difference in requirement of dialysis (hazard ratio [HR], 1.1; 95% CI, 0.4-2.6; $P = .88$). The composite outcome occurred more often in the B-vitamin group (HR, 2.0; 95% CI, 1.0-4.0; $P = .04$). Plasma total homocysteine decreased by a mean (SE) of 2.2 (0.4) μmol/L at 36 months in the B-vitamin group compared with a mean (SE) increase of 2.6 (0.4) μmol/L in the placebo group (mean difference, −4.8; 95% CI, −6.1 to −3.7; $P < .001$, in favor of B vitamins).

*Conclusion.*—Among patients with diabetic nephropathy, high doses of B vitamins compared with placebo resulted in a greater decrease in GFR and an increase in vascular events.

*Trial Registration.*—isrctn.org Identifier: ISRCTN41332305.

▶ The authors point out that there are approximately 21 million diabetics in the United States and approximately 40% of these individuals are at risk for developing renal disease.[1] Several observational studies[2-4] suggested that supplementation with vitamin B6, vitamin B12, and folic acid could reduce homocysteine levels and improve endothelial function in this at-risk population. The authors designed a randomized double-blind placebo-controlled trial in type 1 and type 2 diabetics with diabetic nephropathy to test whether therapy with B vitamins would slow the progression of nephropathy and prevent vascular events. The participants had stage 4 or 5 chronic kidney disease (CKD) (glomerular filtration rate [GFR] less than 30 mL/min as defined by Modification of Diet in Renal Disease [MDRD] equation)[5] and received folic acid (2.5 mg/d), vitamin B6 (25 mg/d) and vitamin B12 (1 mg/d), or placebo. Previous studies such as Heart Outcomes Prevention Evaluation (HOPE)-2[6] that used slightly higher doses of vitamin B6 in patients with vascular disease or diabetes suggested that the supplements did not reduce the risk of major cardiovascular event. The NORVIT trial[7] that included patients with a recent acute myocardial infarction and used lower doses of B supplements suggested that such therapy was associated with a slight worsening of cardiovascular event rate. The results of the current trial are striking. After a median follow-up of 31.4 months, the group that received B vitamins had lower homocysteine levels, a greater decrease in GFR, and an increase in vascular events as compared with the placebo group. As the authors note, there are several metabolic possibilities that may explain these results. For example, folic acid and vitamin B12 might increase the production of the nitric oxide synthase inhibitor asymmetric dimethyl arginine and/or folic acid may act to promote cell proliferation. While the exact explanation for these findings remains to be elucidated the results are extremely worrisome. Vitamin supplements and diabetes are both ubiquitous. Moreover, these supplements are routinely available in dosages that far exceed those used in this trial. B vitamin supplements are recommended by nutraceutical advocates for a variety of conditions ranging from carpal tunnel syndrome and fibromyalgia to memory loss. It is extremely important that practitioners be aware of these results and caution patients with diabetes to avoid excessive use of these supplements.

**R. Garrick, MD**

*References*


1. Palmer AJ, Valentine WJ, Chen R, et al. A health economic analysis of screening and optimal treatment of nephropathy in patients with type 2 diabetes and hypertension in the USA. *Nephrol Dial Transplant.* 2008;23:1216-1223.
2. Becker A, Smulders YM, van Guldener C, Stehouwer CD. Epidemiology of homocysteine as a risk factor in diabetes. *Metab Syndr Relat Disord.* 2003;1:105-120.
3. Looker HC, Fagot-Campagna A, Gunter EW, et al. Homocysteine as a risk factor for nephropathy and retinopathy in type 2 diabetes. *Diabetologia.* 2003;6:766-772.
4. Refsum H, Nurk E, Smith AD, et al. The Hordaland homocysteine study: a community-based study of homocysteine, its determinants, and associations with disease. *J Nutr.* 2006;136:1731S-1740S.
5. Levey AS, Bosch JP, Lewis JB, Greene T, Rogers N, Roth D. Modification of Diet in Renal Disease Study Group. A more accurate method to estimate glomerular filtration rate from serum creatinine: a new prediction equation. *Ann Intern Med.* 1999;130:461-470.
6. Lonn E, Yusuf S, Arnold MJ, et al. Heart Outcomes Prevention Evaluation (HOPE) 2 Investigators. Homocysteine lowering with folic acid and B vitamins In vascular disease. *N Engl J Med.* 2006;354:1567-1577.
7. Bønaa KH, Njolstad I, Ueland PM, et al. NORVIT Trial Investigators. Homocysteine lowering and cardiovascular events after acute myocardial infarction. *N Engl J Med.* 2006;354:1578-1588.


## 25-Hydroxyvitamin D Levels, Race, and the Progression of Kidney Disease

Melamed ML, Astor B, Michos ED, et al (Albert Einstein College of Medicine, Bronx, NY; Johns Hopkins Bloomberg School of Public Health, Baltimore, MD; Johns Hopkins Univ School of Medicine, Baltimore, MD; et al)

*J Am Soc Nephrol* 20:2631-2639, 2009

Black individuals have lower 25-hydroxyvitamin D [25(OH)D] levels and experience a disproportionate burden of ESRD compared with white individuals. Animal studies suggest that vitamin D has renoprotective effects. We evaluated the contribution of low 25(OH)D levels on incidence of ESRD using data from the Third National Health and Nutrition Examination Survey–linked Medicare claims files ($n = 13{,}328$). We included baseline (1988 through 1994) measurements of 25(OH)D and assessed the incidence of ESRD through July 31, 2001. Overall, 34% of non-Hispanic black individuals had 25(OH)D levels <15 ng/ml compared with 5% of non-Hispanic white individuals ($P < 0.001$). During a median of 9.1 yr, 65 participants developed ESRD. After adjustment for demographic, socioeconomic, and clinical and laboratory factors (including diabetes, hypertension, estimated GFR, and albuminuria), participants with 25(OH)D levels <15 ng/ml had a 2.6-fold greater incidence of ESRD than those with levels ≥15 ng/ml (incidence rate ratio 2.64; 95% confidence interval [CI] 1.00 to 7.05; $P = 0.05$). After adjustment for clinical covariates but not 25(OH)D levels, non-Hispanic black individuals had a 2.83-fold (95% CI 1.03 to 7.77) higher risk for developing ESRD compared with non-Hispanic white individuals. Additional adjustment for 25(OH)D levels reduced the risk by 58% (incidence rate ratio 1.77; 95% CI 0.38 to 8.21). In summary, low 25(OH)D levels associate with development of ESRD even after adjustment for multiple risk factors. Low 25(OH)D levels may account for a substantial proportion of the increased risk for ESRD experienced by black individuals.

▶ Low levels of 25-hydroxyvitamin $D_3$ have been associated with cardiovascular disease and increased mortality.[1,2] In animal studies, alterations in the level of the active form of vitamin D, 1,25-dihydroxyvitamin $D_3$, had been demonstrated to reduce proteinuria and preserve the structure of the glomerular podocyte.[3,4] Previous reports in humans have suggested that vitamin D may potentially slow the progression of renal disease.

In this study, the authors used data from the Third National Health and Nutrition Examination Survey to evaluate the effect of 25-hydroxyvitamin D levels and race on the progression of kidney disease. Data were adjusted for multiple cofounders, including age, gender, hypertension, diabetes, body mass index, cholesterol, estimated glomerular filtration rate, baseline proteinuria, and baseline markers of inflammation such as C-reactive protein.

Multivariate analysis demonstrated that individuals with 25-hydroxyvitamin $D_3$ levels of less than 15 ng/mL were 2.6 times more likely to progress to end-stage renal disease (ESRD) than were individuals with higher levels of 25-hydroxyvitamin $D_3$. Non-Hispanic blacks had a 2.83-fold higher risk for developing ESRD compared with non-Hispanic white individuals. After adjustment for 25-hydroxyvitamin $D_3$ levels, this risk was reduced by 58% to 1.77 (95% confidence interval 0.38-8.21).

As the authors note, these data must be cautiously interpreted, and it would be premature to generalize this small observational sample to the population at large. Nonetheless, the data are interesting. Given its important role in cellular function, it is not surprising that alterations in the vitamin D level may be associated with a variety of physiological alterations and clinical disease states.

These data will generate interesting testable hypotheses regarding a possible renoprotective role for vitamin D. At present, given the risks of excess vitamin D (hypercalcemia and hyperphosphatemia), practitioners should be cautious regarding overzealous use of these agents. At present, it seems reasonable to ensure that patients are receiving adequate intake to maintain serum levels within the normal range (30-90 ng/mL) and to periodically monitor the serum chemistries and renal function during exogenous supplementation.

**R. Garrick, MD**

*References*


1. Wang TJ, Pencina MJ, Booth SL, et al. Vitamin D deficiency and risk of cardiovascular disease. *Circulation*. 2008;117:503-511.
2. Giovannucci E, Liu Y, Hollis BW, Rimm EB. 25-hydroxyvitamin D and risk of myocardial infarction in men: a prospective study. *Arch Intern Med*. 2008;168: 1174-1180.
3. Li YC, Qiao G, Uskokovic M, Xiang W, Zheng W, Kong J. Vitamin D: a negative endocrine regulator of the renin-angiotensin system and blood pressure. *J Steroid Biochem Mol Biol*. 2004;89-90:387-392.
4. Migliori M, Giovannini L, Panichi V, et al. Treatment with 1,25-dihydroxyvitamin D3 preserves glomerular slit diaphragm-associated protein expression in experimental glomerulonephritis. *Int J Immunopathol Pharmacol*. 2005;18:779-790.

# 25 Diabetes

**In patients with type 1 diabetes and new-onset microalbuminuria the development of advanced chronic kidney disease may not require progression to proteinuria**

Perkins BA, Ficociello LH, Roshan B, et al (Univ of Toronto, Ontario, Canada; Joslin Diabetes Ctr, Boston, MA; Beth Israel-Deaconess Med Ctr and Joslin Diabetes Ctr, Boston, MA)

*Kidney Int* 77:57-64, 2010

We sought to study new-onset microalbuminuria, its progression, and the decline of renal function in patients with type 1 diabetes. Using a cohort of 109 patients who developed new-onset microalbuminuria in the first 4 years following enrollment in the 1st Joslin Kidney Study, we simultaneously tracked the change in their renal function and urinary albumin excretion. Of these, 79 patients were followed for an average of 12 years after microalbuminuria onset, wherein their glomerular filtration rate was estimated by the Modification of Diet in Renal Disease Study formula and compared with their microalbuminuria and proteinuria. The concordance between these outcomes was weak. Only 12 of the 23 patients who progressed to advanced (stage 3–5) chronic kidney disease developed proteinuria, which, in general, did not precede but accompanied the progression to advanced chronic kidney disease. The remaining 11 patients who developed advanced disease had persistent microalbuminuria or returned to normal albuminuria. Thus, we found that one-third of patients with type 1 diabetes developed advanced chronic kidney disease relatively soon after the onset of microalbuminuria and this was not conditional on the presence of proteinuria. Contrary to the existing concept of early nephropathy in type 1 diabetes, less emphasis should be placed on the mechanisms of progression to proteinuria and more placed on mechanisms initiating and promoting the early decline of renal function that eventually progresses to advanced chronic kidney disease.

▶ Several publications have been drawn from the First Joslin Kidney Study (also known as the Joslin Kidney Study). The Joslin Study enrolled 1602 patients between January 1991 and April 1992. A previous publication by the same authors[1] focused on patients who developed microalbuminuria within the first 4 years of follow-up (109 patients), along with the 312 prevalent cases of microalbuminuria. The results from that study demonstrated that the "risk for early renal function decline depended on whether microalbuminuria regressed, remained stable, or progressed, rising from 16 to 32 and 68%, respectively

TABLE 2.—Estimated Glomerular Filtration Rate and Urinary Albumin Excretion at Baseline and in the Final 2-Year Evaluation Interval[a]

| Characteristic | Controls (*N*=56) GFR > 60 ml/ min per 1.73 m$^2$ 'CKD Stages 1–2' (*N*=56) | Cases (*N*=23) GFR ≤ 60 ml/ min per 1.73 m$^2$ 'CKD Stages 3–4' (*N*=17) | ESRD 'CKD Stage 5' (*N*=6) | *P*[b] |
|---|---|---|---|---|
| $GFR_{MDRD}$ (ml/min/1.73 m$^2$) | | | | |
| *Mean (min, max)* | | | | |
| Baseline | 107 (60, 164) | 98 (73, 156) | 101 (69, 134) | 0.77 |
| Final interval[a] | 84 (61, 126) | 50 (22, 59) | 27 (4, 58) | — |
| Urinary albumin excretion rate (in µg/min) | | | | |
| *Median (interquartile range)* | | | | |
| Baseline | 49 (34, 68) | 40 (34, 45) | 46 (33, 69) | 0.33 |
| Final interval[a] | 35 (16, 71) | 52 (18, 241) | 1285 (856, 2805) | 0.06 |
| *Albumin excretion changes during 12 years of follow up* | | | | |
| Remission to normo-albuminuria | 28 (50%) | 3 (18%) | 0 (0%) | |
| Persistent microalbuminuria | 19 (34%) | 8 (47%) | 0 (0%) | 0.001[c] |
| Progression to proteinuria | 9 (16%) | 6 (35%) | 6 (100%) | |
| Total | 56 (100%) | 17 (100%) | 6 (100%) | |
| *Treatment with reno-protective drugs during the final interval*[a] | | | | |
| ACE-inhibitor and ARB[d] | 41 (73%) | 11 (65%) | 5 (83%) | 0.45 |

CKD, chronic kidney disease; ESRD, end-stage renal disease; GFR, glomerular filtration rate.

[a]The final interval represents the 2-year interval at the end of observation for controls and cases with CKD stage 3–4, but the preceding interval for cases with CKD stage 5.

[b]Comparison of cases and controls. As $GFR_{MDRD}$ in the final interval was involved in defining cases and controls, this variable was not tested. *P*-values for comparison of proportions of cases in each albumin excretion rate class were calculated according to the $\chi^2$-statistic using the contingency table method.

[c]In the 2 × 3 table of case–control status versus course of urinary albumin excretion, $\chi^2 = 13.7$, $P = 0.001$.

[d]Angiotensin receptor blocker (ARB) use was uncommon and present in five subjects, all of whom received valsartan. All exposure to valsartan was beyond 8 years after microalbuminuria onset and was used in combination with angiotensin-converting enzyme (ACE) inhibitors in three of the five patients.

($P < 0.001$)." The authors concluded that "progressive renal function decline in type 1 diabetes is an early event that occurs in a large proportion of patients with microalbuminuria."[1]

The present study focuses on the follow-up of only the incident cohort of 109 patients from the same Joslin Kidney Study. Data were available on 79 of the 109 patients. Of these, 56 patients maintained a normal glomerular filtration rate (GFR) (measured by estimated GFR using the Modification of Diet in Renal Disease equation),[2] and 23 patients progressed to stage 3-5 kidney disease. Patients who maintained a normal GFR were used as the control group. The average follow-up was 12 years. As shown in the accompanying table (Table 2), 17 patients progressed to stage 3-4 chronic kidney disease (CKD) and 6 patients progressed to end-stage renal disease requiring dialysis. Therefore, approximately one-third of the patients with type I diabetes developed stage 3 or 4 without the microalbuminuria advancing to a higher grade of proteinuria. Of interest is the finding that all of the patients who did progress to stage 5 CKD had either persistent microalbuminuria or had progressed to macroproteinuria (defined as 300 µg/min or greater).

Together these findings indicate that the absence of macroalbuminuria does not protect type I diabetics from disease progression. These long-term clinical observations do extend our thinking regarding the classic concept that in type I diabetes, proteinuria worsens before renal disease progression occurs. Rather, the data shown suggest that macroproteinuria portends a bad prognosis and that for a significant number of patients, the same is true for microalbuminuria. One caveat is that the patient number is small. In addition, although there was no difference between the groups with regard to the use of angiotensin-converting enzyme inhibitor/angiotensin receptor blocker therapy, only 65% of the patients with microalbuminuria received therapy with these agents. This may represent a confounding variable as these agents may have multiple effects on renal function that are independent from their antiproteinuric effects. Overall, the study is important as it highlights that proteinuria is not a perfect surrogate marker for kidney injury and that attention needs to be focused on other factors, such as blood pressure, cholesterol, obesity, and glycemic control, which might also influence disease progression.

**R. Garrick, MD**

*References*

1. Perkins BA, Ficociello LH, Ostrander BE, et al. Microalbuminuria and the risk for early progressive renal function decline in type 1 diabetes. *J Am Soc Nephrol.* 2007;18:1353-1361.
2. National Kidney Foundation. K/DOQI clinical practice guidelines for chronic kidney disease: evaluation, classification, and stratification. *Am J Kid Dis.* 2002; 39:S1-S266.

**A1C Variability Predicts Incident Cardiovascular Events, Microalbuminuria, and Overt Diabetic Nephropathy in Patients With Type 1 Diabetes**

Wadén J, on behalf of the Finnish Diabetic Nephropathy Study Group (Folkhälsan Inst of Genetics, Helsinki, Finland)
*Diabetes* 58:2649-2655, 2009

*Objective.*—Recent data from the Diabetes Control and Complications Trial (DCCT) indicated that A1C variability is associated with the risk of diabetes microvascular complications. However, these results might have been influenced by the interventional study design. Therefore, we investigated the longitudinal associations between A1C variability and diabetes complications in patients with type 1 diabetes in the observational Finnish Diabetic Nephropathy (FinnDiane) Study.

*Research Design and Methods.*—A total of 2,107 patients in the FinnDiane Study had complete data on renal status and serial measurements of A1C from baseline to follow-up (median 5.7 years), and 1,845 patients had similar data on cardiovascular disease (CVD) events. Intrapersonal SD of serially measured A1C was considered a measure of variability.

*Results.*—During follow-up, 10.2% progressed to a higher albuminuria level or to end-stage renal disease, whereas 8.6% had a CVD event. The

SD of serial A1C was 1.01 versus 0.75 ($P < 0.001$) for renal status and 0.87 versus 0.79 ($P = 0.023$) for CVD in progressors versus nonprogressors, respectively. In a Cox regression model, SD of serial A1C was independently associated with progression of renal disease (hazard ratio 1.92 [95% CI 1.49–2.47]) and of a CVD event (1.98 [1.39–2.82]) even when adjusting for mean A1C and traditional risk factors. Interestingly for CVD, mean serial A1C itself was not predictive even though SD of A1C was.

*Conclusions.*—In patients with type 1 diabetes, A1C variability was not only predictive of incident microalbuminuria and progression of renal disease but also of incident CVD events.

▶ Hemoglobin A1C (HbA1c) has long been considered the ideal marker of extended-term glycemic control in patients with diabetes mellitus.[1] This was confirmed in the Diabetes Control and Complications Trial (DCCT) that demonstrated a delay in the development of overt nephropathy with intensive lowering of HbA1c.[2]

Wadén et al, using data from the Finnish Diabetic Nephropathy Study, viewed the HbA1c in a novel fashion, which may give more insight into the effect of HbA1c on nephropathy and also on cardiovascular outcomes. From this study it appears that the absolute value of HbA1c, though important as noted in DCCT, may be further interpreted by looking at relative changes of HbA1c over time. Patients who have both high variability in HbA1c readings and high absolute HbA1c readings had the worst renal outcomes over time. Conversely, those with the lowest variability and lowest absolute values for HbA1c had the best. Renal outcomes were intermediate between these extremes where either the variability of HbA1c or the absolute value of HbA1c was high but not both.

They also found that the intrapatient variability of HbA1c was predictive of cardiovascular outcomes even if HbA1c was not significantly different between the groups of those with cardiovascular events and those without.

The authors point out that these findings are consistent with studies of glycemic excursions and their effects on oxidative stress, at least in patients with type 2 diabetes.[3] It also supports prior findings that glycemic variation is detrimental to in vitro cellular effects.[4]

From this study we can see that single measure of HbA1c may not tell a complete story. Serial follow-up and monitoring of HbA1c variability may give clinicians clues that may indicate cardiovascular and renal risks.

**M. Klein, MD, JD**

*References*

1. Koenig RJ, Peterson CM, Jones RL, Saudek C, Lehrman M, Cerami A. Correlation of glucose regulation and hemoglobin AIc in diabetes mellitus. *N Engl J Med.* 1976;295:417-420.
2. The effect of intensive treatment of diabetes on the development and progression of long-term complications in insulin-dependent diabetes mellitus. The Diabetes Control and Complications Trial Research Group. *N Engl J Med.* 1993;329: 977-986.

3. Monnier L, Mas E, Ginet C, et al. Activation of oxidative stress by acute glucose fluctuations compared with sustained chronic hyperglycemia in patients with type 2 diabetes. *JAMA*. 2006;295:1681-1687.
4. Risso A, Mercuri F, Quagliaro L, Damante G, Ceriello A. Intermittent high glucose enhances apoptosis in human umbilical vein endothelial cells in culture. *Am J Physiol Endocrinol Metab*. 2001;281:E924-E930.


### Albuminuria and Kidney Function Independently Predict Cardiovascular and Renal Outcomes in Diabetes

Ninomiya T, on behalf of the ADVANCE Collaborative Group (Univ of Sydney, Australia; et al)

*J Am Soc Nephrol* 20:1813-1821, 2009

There are limited data regarding whether albuminuria and reduced estimated GFR (eGFR) are separate and independent risk factors for cardiovascular and renal events among individuals with type 2 diabetes. The Action in Diabetes and Vascular disease: preterAx and diamicroN-MR Controlled Evaluation (ADVANCE) study examined the effects of routine BP lowering on adverse outcomes in type 2 diabetes. We investigated the effects of urinary albumin-to-creatinine ratio (UACR) and eGFR on the risk for cardiovascular and renal events in 10,640 patients with available data. During an average 4.3-yr follow-up, 938 (8.8%) patients experienced a cardiovascular event and 107 (1.0%) experienced a renal event. The multivariable-adjusted hazard ratio for cardiovascular events was 2.48 (95% confidence interval 1.74 to 3.52) for every 10-fold increase in baseline UACR and 2.20 (95% confidence interval 1.09 to 4.43) for every halving of baseline eGFR, after adjustment for regression dilution. There was no evidence of interaction between the effects of higher UACR and lower eGFR. Patients with both UACR >300 mg/g and eGFR <60 ml/min per 1.73 $m^2$ at baseline had a 3.2-fold higher risk for cardiovascular events and a 22.2-fold higher risk for renal events, compared with patients with neither of these risk factors. In conclusion, high albuminuria and low eGFR are independent risk factors for cardiovascular and renal events among patients with type 2 diabetes.

▶ The Action in Diabetes and Vascular disease: preterAx and diamicroN-MR Controlled Evaluation (ADVANCE) trial is a factorial, randomized, controlled trial evaluating the effects of blood pressure lowering and intensive blood glucose control in vascular outcomes in patients with type 2 diabetes. Previous data from the advanced trial evaluated the role of tight glucose control with gliclazide[1] and blood pressure control with perindopril and indapamide.[2] This study reports the observational analyses of the association between albuminuria and glomerular filtration rate (GFR) at baseline and during follow-up and the risk for renal and cardiovascular events in 10 640 patients with available data during an average 4.3-year follow-up. Approximately 9% of patients experienced a cardiovascular event (cardiovascular death, nonfatal myocardial infarction, or nonfatal stroke), and 1% of patients experienced renal events (death as a result of kidney disease, initiation of dialysis or transplantation, or doubling the serum creatinine greater than 2.27 mg%). As shown in Fig 2 in the original article, the hazard ratio for cardiovascular events was approximately 2.5 for every 10-fold increase in the baseline urinary albumin-to-creatinine ratio and approximately 2.2 for every halving of the baseline estimated GFR (eGFR). Patients with both macroalbuminuria and eGFR of less than 60 mL/min/1.73 $m^2$ at baseline had a 3.2-fold greater risk for cardiovascular events and a 22.2-fold higher risk for renal events. There was no evidence of an interaction between effects of a higher urinary albumin-to-creatinine ratio and eGFR. These data suggest that albuminuria and eGFR are independent risk factors for cardiovascular and renal events in patients with type 2 diabetes.

The strengths of the study include the large sample size and follow-up period. The study does use an eGFR drawn from the Modification of Diet in Renal Disease equation,[3] and limitations of this estimate across the wide range of clearances present in this study may result in some misclassification of renal function; however, it is unlikely that that misclassification would affect the conclusions. I included this study because despite what some might have anticipated, the data suggest that in type 2 diabetes, albuminuria and eGFR are independent, and continuous, risk factors for adverse cardiovascular and kidney outcomes. Thus, from an experimental and therapeutic standpoint, it is important for payors, practitioners, and patients to be cognizant of the fact that specific therapeutic modalities directed at either cardiovascular or renal outcomes may not necessarily have beneficial effects on the other. As the science of comparative effectiveness research and outcome analysis continues to be applied to health care resource management, it is important for all stakeholders to realize that only continued scientific investigation will provide accurate insight into the complex array of interrelated, but independent, factors that ultimately result in a single patient outcome.

**R. Garrick, MD**

*References*


1. ADVANCE Collaborative Group, Patel A, MacMahon S, Chalmers J, et al. Intensive blood glucose control and vascular outcomes in patients with type 2 diabetes. *N Engl J Med.* 2008;358:2560-2572.
2. ADVANCE Collaborative Group, Patel A, MacMahon S, Chalmers J, et al. Effects of a fixed combination of perindopril and indapamide on macrovascular and microvascular outcomes in patients with type 2 diabetes mellitus (the ADVANCE trial): a randomised controlled trial. *Lancet.* 2007;370:829-840.
3. National Kidney Foundation. K/DOQI clinical practice guidelines for chronic kidney disease: evaluation, classification, and stratification. *Am J Kidney Dis.* 2002;39:S1-S266.

# 26 Calcium, Phosphorus, and Bone

---

**Dietary and genetic evidence for phosphate toxicity accelerating mammalian aging**

Ohnishi M, Razzaque MS (Harvard School of Dental Medicine, Boston, MA)

*FASEB J* 24:3562-3571, 2010.

---

Identifying factors that accelerate the aging process can provide important therapeutic targets for slowing down this process. Misregulation of phosphate homeostasis has been noted in various skeletal, cardiac, and renal diseases, but the exact role of phosphate toxicity in mammalian aging is not clearly defined. Phosphate is widely distributed in the body and is involved in cell signaling, energy metabolism, nucleic acid synthesis, and the maintenance of acid-base balance by urinary buffering. In this study, we used an *in vivo* genetic approach to determine the role of phosphate toxicity in mammalian aging. Klotho-knockout mice (*klotho*$^{-/-}$) have a short life span and show numerous physical, biochemical, and morphological features consistent with premature aging, including kyphosis, uncoordinated movement, hypogonadism, infertility, severe skeletal muscle wasting, emphysema, and osteopenia, as well as generalized atrophy of the skin, intestine, thymus, and spleen. Molecular and biochemical analyses suggest that increased renal activity of sodium-phosphate cotransporters (NaPi2a) leads to severe hyperphosphatemia in *klotho*$^{-/-}$ mice. Genetically reducing serum phosphate levels in *klotho*$^{-/-}$ mice by generating a *NaPi2a* and *klotho* double-knockout (*NaPi2a*$^{-/-}$/*klotho*$^{-/-}$) strain resulted in amelioration of premature aging-like features. The *NaPi2a*$^{-/-}$/*klotho*$^{-/-}$ double-knockout mice regained reproductive ability, recovered their body weight, reduced their organ atrophy, and suppressed ectopic calcifications, with the resulting effect being prolonged survival. More important, when hyperphosphatemia was induced in *NaPi2a*$^{-/-}$/*klotho*$^{-/-}$ mice by feeding with a high-phosphate diet, premature aging-like features reappeared, clearly suggesting that phosphate toxicity is the main cause of premature aging in *klotho*$^{-/-}$ mice. The results of our dietary and genetic manipulation studies provide *in vivo* evidence for phosphate toxicity accelerating the aging process and suggest a novel role for phosphate in mammalian aging.

▶ Hyperphosphatemia and secondary hyperparathyroidism are common complications of progressive kidney failure. In the last decade, it has become apparent that hyperphosphatemia, itself, can directly influence outcomes in patients with renal failure.[1] It has been suggested that elevated serum phosphate levels directly contribute to the increased cardiovascular mortality seen in these patients. Several lines of investigation have suggested that this increased cardiovascular risk may be related to the effects of elevated phosphate on vascular calcification. Of great interest is the finding that serum phosphorus levels in the high-normal range in healthy young adults appear to be associated with increased cardiovascular disease.[2,3]

In this study, the effects of phosphorus on the cellular mechanisms associated with accelerated aging and calcification were evaluated. Prior studies have suggested that in klotho$^{-/-}$ mice, increased renal activity of the sodium phosphate cotransporter (NaPi2a) leads to hyperphosphatemia. Using a variety of biochemical and genetic manipulations, this study demonstrated that mice that were double knockout (NaPi2a$^{-/-}$ and klotho$^{-/-}$) had reduced serum phosphate levels and improved signs of premature aging, which included a reduction in the presence of ectopic calcification. Moreover, when hyperphosphatemia was induced in this model, via a high-phosphate diet, these protective effects were lost, and signs of premature aging again occurred.

These elegant studies suggest that phosphate toxicity can accelerate the aging process and promote vascular and soft tissue calcification. With new research highlighting the possible increased cardiovascular mortality in patients with high-normal phosphate levels, this study has possible bioepidemiological implications. While further studies are required to understand the molecular basis of the so-called phosphate toxicity, it would seem prudent to take steps now to closely control phosphate in at-risk populations.

**S. Raayasa, MD**

*References*

1. Young EW, Albert JM, Satayathum S, et al. Predictors and consequences of altered mineral metabolism: the Dialysis Outcomes and Practice Patterns study (DOPPS). *Kidney Int.* 2005;67:1179-1187.
2. Dhingra R, Sullivan LM, Fox CS, et al. Relations of serum phosphorus and calcium levels to the incidence of cardiovascular disease in the community. *Arch Intern Med.* 2007;167:879-885.
3. Foley RN, Collins AJ, Herzog CA, Ishani A, Kalra PA. Serum phosphorus associate with coronary atherosclerosis in young adults. *J Am Soc Nephrol.* 2009;20:397-404.

## Klotho Prevents Renal Calcium Loss

Alexander RT, Woudenberg-Vrenken TE, Buurman J, et al (Nijmegen Centre for Molecular Life Sciences, The Netherlands; et al)
*J Am Soc Nephrol* 20:2371-2379, 2009

Disturbed calcium ($Ca^{2+}$) homeostasis, which is implicit to the aging phenotype of klotho-deficient mice, has been attributed to altered vitamin D metabolism, but alternative possibilities exist. We hypothesized that failed tubular $Ca^{2+}$ absorption is primary, which causes increased urinary $Ca^{2+}$ excretion, leading to elevated 1,25-dihydroxyvitamin $D_3$ [$1,25(OH)_2D_3$] and its sequelae. Here, we assessed intestinal $Ca^{2+}$ absorption, bone densitometry, renal $Ca^{2+}$ excretion, and renal morphology via energy-dispersive x-ray microanalysis in wild-type and klotho$^{-/-}$ mice. We observed elevated serum $Ca^{2+}$ and fractional excretion of $Ca^{2+}$ ($FE_{Ca}$) in klotho$^{-/-}$ mice. Klotho$^{-/-}$ mice also showed intestinal $Ca^{2+}$ hyperabsorption, osteopenia, and renal precipitation of calcium-phosphate. Duodenal mRNA levels of transient receptor potential vanilloid 6 (TRPV6) and calbindin-$D_{9K}$ increased. In the kidney, klotho$^{-/-}$ mice exhibited increased expression of TRPV5 and decreased expression of the sodium/calcium exchanger (NCX1) and calbindin-$D_{28K}$, implying a failure to absorb $Ca^{2+}$ through the distal convoluted tubule/connecting tubule (DCT/CNT) via TRPV5. Gene and protein expression of the vitamin D receptor (VDR), 25-hydroxyvitamin D-1-$\alpha$-hydroxylase (1$\alpha$OHase), and calbindin-$D_{9K}$ excluded renal vitamin D resistance. By modulating the diet, we showed that the renal $Ca^{2+}$ wasting was not secondary to hypercalcemia and/or hypervitaminosis D. In summary, these findings illustrate a primary defect in tubular $Ca^{2+}$ handling that contributes to the precipitation of calcium-phosphate in DCT/CNT. This highlights the importance of klotho to the prevention of renal $Ca^{2+}$ loss, secondary hypervitaminosis D, osteopenia, and nephrocalcinosis.

▶ Disturbances in phosphorus and calcium metabolism have been linked to many renal complications, including cardiovascular disease, peripheral arterial disease, and bone disease. In addition, abnormalities of these cellular mediators may contribute to premature cellular aging. The klotho gene is located on chromosome 13q12 and encodes proteins belonging to the β-glycosidase family.

Klotho has a variety of renal effects. Through its role as a fibroblast growth factor 23 coreceptor, klotho inhibits the production of 1,25-dihydroxyvitamin $D_3$, and it affects the expression and function of the epithelial Ca channel transient receptor potential vanilloid 5 (TRPV5) in the distal nephron. TRPV5, located on the apical surface of the distal convoluted tubule, is essential for the renal handling of calcium.

Klotho knockout mice have hypercalcemia and hypercalciuria, along with calcium phosphate precipitation in the distal nephron.

This study suggests that the hypercalciuria observed is a primary renal defect because the renal calcium leak persisted even after the serum calcium and active vitamin D were normalized. TRPV5 expression was paradoxically elevated, but the receptors were presumably not located in the apical membrane and, therefore, not active, allowing for hypercalciuria and nephrocalcinosis. The net result in the klotho-deficient mice was a primary renal calcium leak, hypercalciuria, increased active vitamin D synthesis, increased calcium absorption from intestines and bone (with concomitant osteopenia), and ultimately hypercalcemia and nephrocalcinosis.

We included this article because research into the mechanisms of action of klotho is helping to unravel cellular processes that underlie aging. The renal effects of klotho will likely be pivotal, and certainly more data regarding klotho's effects on the kidney, bone, and cardiovascular system will be forthcoming.

**J. Michaud, DO**

# 27 Chronic Renal Failure and Transplantation

**Timing of Onset of CKD-Related Metabolic Complications**

Moranne O, the NephroTest Study Group (Université Paris-Sud, France; et al)

*J Am Soc Nephrol* 20:164-171, 2009

Chronic kidney disease (CKD) guidelines recommend evaluating patients with GFR <60 ml/min per 1.73 $m^2$ for complications, but little evidence supports the use of a single GFR threshold for all metabolic disorders. We used data from the NephroTest cohort, including 1038 adult patients who had stages 2 through 5 CKD and were not on dialysis, to study the occurrence of metabolic complications. GFR was measured using renal clearance of $^{51}$Cr-EDTA (mGFR) and estimated using two equations derived from the Modification of Diet in Renal Disease study. As mGFR decreased from 60 to 90 to <20 ml/min per 1.73 $m^2$, the prevalence of hyperparathyroidism increased from 17 to 85%, anemia from 8 to 41%, hyperphosphatemia from 1 to 30%, metabolic acidosis from 2 to 39%, and hyperkalemia from 2 to 42%. Factors most strongly associated with metabolic complications, independent of mGFR, were younger age for acidosis and hyperphosphatemia, presence of diabetes for acidosis, diabetic kidney disease for anemia, and both male gender and the use of inhibitors of the renin-angiotensin system for hyperkalemia. mGFR thresholds for detecting complications with 90% sensitivity were 50, 44, 40, 39, and 37 ml/min per 1.73 $m^2$ for hyperparathyroidism, anemia, acidosis, hyperkalemia, and hyperphosphatemia, respectively. Analysis using estimated GFR produced similar results. In summary, this study describes the onset of CKD-related complications at different levels of GFR; anemia and hyperparathyroidism occur earlier than acidosis, hyperkalemia, and hyperphosphatemia.

▶ Utilizing the NephroTest cohort that included 1038 adult patients with stage 2 to 5 chronic kidney disease (CKD), the authors sought to correlate the timing of the onset of various metabolic perturbations with the stage of kidney disease. If possible, this would be clinically useful because it might allow practitioners to implement laboratory testing and therapeutic intervention within a framework that is evidence based and potentially cost effective. A strength of the study is that it used both estimated glomerular filtration rate (eGFR) (derived from the Modification of Diet in Renal Disease equation) and measured GFR using $^{51}$Cr-EDTA. Not surprisingly, as shown in Fig 1 in the original article, the investigators demonstrated that the incidence of each of the major metabolic abnormalities associated with progressive kidney disease (hyperparathyroidism, metabolic acidosis, anemia, and hyperparathyroidism) increases as renal function declines. In keeping with the previous observation of Levin and colleagues,[1] almost 20% of the patients with stage 2 CKD have hyperparathyroidism. Independent of the GFR level and of other patient characteristics, the risk of hyperphosphatemia was more pronounced among those who were younger than 65 years. Hyperkalemia was most prevalent among men who were receiving concomitant angiotensin-converting enzyme inhibitor or angiotensin receptor blocker treatment. Overall, this large population-based study should help to alert nonnephrologists as to the timing of the occurrence and the prevalence of the metabolic complications that are commonly associated with progressive renal disease. Each of these metabolic disorders can be associated with their own adverse outcomes. Practitioners should be aware of the general timing of these metabolic alterations so that appropriate diagnosis, therapeutic intervention, and when necessary specialty referral can occur.

**R. Garrick, MD**

*Reference*

1. Levin A, Bakris GL, Molitich M, et al. Prevalence of abnormal serum vitamin D, PTH, calcium and phosphorus in patients with chronic kidney disease: results of the study to evaluate early kidney disease. *Kidney Int.* 2007;71:31-38.

---

**Atherosclerotic renovascular disease in the United States**

Kalra PA, Guo H, Gilbertson DT, et al (Salford Royal Hosp, UK; United States Renal Data System Coordinating Ctr, Minneapolis, MN)

*Kidney Int* 77:37-43, 2010

---

Atherosclerotic renovascular disease (ARVD) is an increasingly recognized clinical condition that is diagnosed predominantly in older patients. Here we used annual United States Medicare 5% Denominator Files and studied 16,036,904 patients, 66 years of age and older, to quantify trends in diagnostic rates, associations, treatment, and outcomes of ARVD over a 13-year period. Overall, there was an ARVD rate of 3.09 per 1000 patient-years, which rose progressively with an adjusted hazard ratio of 3.35, comparing data from 1992 to 2004. Within 6 months of disease diagnosis, 13.4% of patients had undergone revascularization. A biphasic pattern of revascularization was found where the adjusted hazard ratios significantly increased in a progressive manner until 1999, following which there was a decline through 2004, which was not significant. The method of revascularization changed markedly over time with endovascular intervention steadily replacing direct surgical revascularization. As a time-dependent variable, ARVD was associated with excess mortality in each calendar year, albeit with declining hazard ratio estimates in more recent years. Among patients with this disease, revascularization was associated with mortality adjusted hazard ratios <1 in each year. Our study shows the diagnosis of ARVD has substantially risen in the United States but the survival implications were not fully explained by other comorbid vascular diseases.

▶ Kalra et al reviewed 16 million Medicare files in order to quantify trends in diagnostic rates, associations, treatment, and outcomes of atherosclerotic renal vascular disease over a 13-year period. They found that the hazard ratios for diagnosis rose steadily during the period, while revascularization rates increased to a peak in 1999 and then steadily declined. The authors note that this early upward trend may well have been driven by early studies supporting stenting for ostial stenoses,[1] whereas the subsequent downward trend may have been the result of later negative studies, such as those published at the turn of the millennium.[2] It was also noted that the preferred revascularization modality progressively shifted from surgical to percutaneous methods during the survey period. It does seem likely from the data that the increase in the diagnosis of atherosclerotic renovascular disease between 1992 and 2002 was least in part related to improvements in noninvasive diagnostic imaging techniques. Thus, it became easier to make the diagnosis of renal artery disease, but the correct therapeutic approach remained quite controversial. These observations highlight the confusion and the need for further guidance regarding the treatment of this common condition. The need to establish the most appropriate therapeutic approach is even more critical in view of recent concerns regarding gadolinium-related nephrogenic systemic fibrosis. Thus, if intervention for atherosclerotic renovascular disease is rarely indicated, then practitioners should be less likely to expose patients to potentially harmful studies of diagnostic but not therapeutic use.

**M. Klein, MD, JD**

*References*

1. Blum U, Krumme B, Flügel P, et al. Treatment of ostial renal-artery stenoses with vascular endoprostheses after unsuccessful balloon angioplasty. *N Engl J Med.* 1997;336:459-465.
2. van Jaarsveld BC, Krijnen P, Pieterman H, et al. The effect of balloon angioplasty on hypertension in atherosclerotic renal-artery stenosis. Dutch Renal Artery Stenosis Intervention Cooperative Study Group. *N Engl J Med.* 2000;342:1007-1014.

---

**Revascularization versus Medical Therapy for Renal-Artery Stenosis**

The ASTRAL Investigators (Univ of Birmingham, UK; et al)

*N Engl J Med* 361:1953-1962, 2009

---

*Background.*—Percutaneous revascularization of the renal arteries improves patency in atherosclerotic renovascular disease, yet evidence of a clinical benefit is limited.

*Methods.*—In a randomized, unblinded trial, we assigned 806 patients with atherosclerotic renovascular disease either to undergo revascularization in addition to receiving medical therapy or to receive medical therapy alone. The primary outcome was renal function, as measured by the reciprocal of the serum creatinine level (a measure that has a linear relationship with creatinine clearance). Secondary outcomes were blood pressure, the time to renal and major cardiovascular events, and mortality. The median follow-up was 34 months.

*Results.*—During a 5-year period, the rate of progression of renal impairment (as shown by the slope of the reciprocal of the serum creatinine level) was $-0.07\times10^{-3}$ liters per micromole per year in the revascularization group, as compared with $-0.13\times10^{-3}$ liters per micromole per year in the medical-therapy group, a difference favoring revascularization of $0.06\times10^{-3}$ liters per micromole per year (95% confidence interval [CI], −0.002 to 0.13; P = 0.06). Over the same time, the mean serum creatinine level was 1.6 μmol per liter (95% CI, −8.4 to 5.2 [0.02 mg per deciliter; 95% CI, −0.10 to 0.06]) lower in the revascularization group than in the medical-therapy group. There was no significant between-group difference in systolic blood pressure; the decrease in diastolic blood pressure was smaller in the revascularization group than in the medical-therapy group. The two study groups had similar rates of renal events (hazard ratio in the revascularization group, 0.97; 95% CI, 0.67 to 1.40; P = 0.88), major cardiovascular events (hazard ratio, 0.94; 95% CI, 0.75 to 1.19; P = 0.61), and death (hazard ratio, 0.90; 95% CI, 0.69 to 1.18; P = 0.46). Serious complications associated with revascularization occurred in 23 patients, including 2 deaths and 3 amputations of toes or limbs.

*Conclusions.*—We found substantial risks but no evidence of a worthwhile clinical benefit from revascularization in patients with atherosclerotic renovascular disease. (Current Controlled Trials number, ISRCTN59586944.)

▶ The earlier study by Kalra et al[1] demonstrated that the incidence of the diagnosis of atherosclerotic renal vascular disease has increased steadily over the last decades, but the indications and beneficial effects of revascularization have remained uncertain. The Angioplasty and Stenting for Renal Artery Lesions (ASTRAL) trial was a multicenter, nonblinded, prospective, randomized controlled trial with more than 800 patients, which was designed to help determine whether the benefits of revascularization outweigh the risks. The decision to submit a patient to the risk of invasive angiography and potential stenting has always given careful clinicians pause because this procedure has inherent dangers, including atheroembolism, vascular injury, bleeding, and infection. But faced with the specter of worsening renal function and severe hypertension, many physicians have been inclined to recommend intervention. Previous small underpowered trials failed to demonstrate the benefit of revascularization over medical therapy alone.

This ASTRAL trial compared medical therapy, including statins, antiplatelet agents, and multiagent blood pressure control, with revascularization that included angioplasty and, in 95% of patients, stenting. There was a 6% rate of crossover from medical therapy alone to the intervention group. The investigators found that glomerular filtration rates decline and that average systolic blood pressures, cardiovascular event rates, and overall survival rates were not different in the 2 groups. Furthermore, the medical therapy group actually had slightly lower diastolic pressures. The complication rates were significant, with 23 events, including 2 deaths and 3 amputations.

The important conclusion drawn is that invasive intervention in atherosclerotic renal disease offers substantial risks, without substantial evidence of clinical benefit. It is important to note that this study did not address fibromuscular dysplasia which responds very well to revascularization with a low rate of vascular morbidity.[2] An additional caveat is that future subgroup analyses of the ASTRAL datasets may yet uncover specific subsets of patients who would benefit from intervention.

**M. Klein, MD, JD**

*References*

1. Kalra PA, Guo H, Gilbertson DT, et al. Atherosclerotic renovascular disease in the United States. *Kidney Int.* 2010;77:37-43.
2. Klow NE, Paulsen D, Vatne K, Rokstad B, Lien B, Fauchald P. Percutaneous transluminal renal artery angioplasty using the coaxial technique. Ten years of experience from 591 procedures in 419 patients. *Acta Radiol.* 1998;39:594-603.

### Unified Criteria for Ultrasonographic Diagnosis of ADPKD

Pei Y, Obaji J, Dupuis A, et al (Univ of Toronto, Ontario, Canada; Hosp for Sick Children, Toronto, Ontario, Canada; et al)
*J Am Soc Nephrol* 20:205-212, 2009

Individuals who are at risk for autosomal dominant polycystic kidney disease are often screened by ultrasound using diagnostic criteria derived from individuals with mutations in *PKD1*. Families with mutations in *PKD2* typically have less severe disease, suggesting a potential need for different diagnostic criteria. In this study, 577 and 371 at-risk individuals from 58 *PKD1* and 39 *PKD2* families, respectively, were assessed by renal ultrasound and molecular genotyping. Using sensitivity data derived from genetically affected individuals and specificity data derived from genetically unaffected individuals, various diagnostic criteria were compared. In addition, data sets were created to simulate the *PKD1* and *PKD2* case mix expected in practice to evaluate the performance of diagnostic criteria for families of unknown genotype. The diagnostic criteria currently in use performed suboptimally for individuals with mutations in *PKD2* as a result of reduced test sensitivity. In families of unknown genotype, the presence of three or more (unilateral or bilateral) renal cysts is sufficient for establishing the diagnosis in individuals aged 15 to 39 y, two or more cysts in each kidney is sufficient for individuals aged 40 to 59 y, and four or more cysts in each kidney is required for individuals ≥60 yr. Conversely, fewer than two renal cysts in at-risk individuals aged ≥40 yr is sufficient to exclude the disease. These unified diagnostic criteria will be useful for testing individuals who are at risk for autosomal

**dominant polycystic kidney disease in the usual clinical setting in which molecular genotyping is seldom performed.**

▶ The most common hereditary kidney disease is autosomal dominant polycystic kidney disease (ADPKD). Although the pathology of this disease is not yet fully understood, the genetics have become quite clear over the past few years. Mutations of *PKD1* and *PKD2* genes account for more than 85% of all PKD cases in the population.[1] Because these mutations manifest different severities of the condition, genetic testing for each mutation is still the gold standard for the diagnosis and the prognosis, especially for genetic counseling and kidney donation planning. A sensitive and specific test for these genotypes, that would be less expensive than genotyping, would be very useful. Standardized ultrasound criteria for patients with PKD1 are currently in use. The diagnosis depends on a minimum number of cysts appearing after certain defined ages. The disease can be excluded by a radiographic paucity of cysts after a certain age in an at-risk individual.

Pei et al used the current radiographic diagnostic criteria and compared them with available genotypes in 948 subjects. Because of PKD2 being a milder and later appearing syndrome than PKD1, the diagnostic sensitivity of imaging in patients with PKD2 was 71.9%, which was far inferior to the greater than 98% sensitivity found in patients with PKD1. In both cohorts the specificity was nearly 100%. The investigators concluded that diagnostic criteria in use for PKD1 did not perform well when applied to PKD2 because of the higher risk of false negatives (lower sensitivity). They noted, however, that this deficiency was mostly in the patients aged 30 to 39 years. In older at-risk patients with greater than 4 cysts per kidney, the sensitivity and specificity were nearly 100% for both syndromes.

This study demonstrated a scheme for radiographic screening that is inexpensive, sensitive, and specific. Their conclusion is that for individuals at risk for ADPKD, a diagnosis is confirmed by the presence of at least 3 renal cysts (unilateral or bilateral) in individuals aged 15 to 39 years. This minimizes the small risk of false positives in this age bracket. Two or more cysts in each kidney in patients aged 40 to 59 years or 4 cysts or greater in each kidney if patients are older than 60 years of age confirms diagnosis. The absence of any cysts after the age of 40 years in individuals at risk, is a virtual exclusion of PKD and may be helpful in making decisions regarding kidney donation to family members with ADPKD.

**M. Klein, MD, JD**

*Reference*

1. Igarashi P, Somlo S. Genetics and pathogenesis of polycystic kidney disease. *Am Soc Nephrol.* 2002;13:2384-2398.

**D-dimer Testing in Patients with Suspected Pulmonary Embolism and Impaired Renal Function**

Karami-Djurabi R, Klok FA, Kooiman J, et al (Leiden Univ Med Ctr, the Netherlands)

*Am J Med* 122:1050-1053, 2009

*Background.*—Determination of pretest probability and D-dimer tests are the first diagnostic steps in patients with suspected pulmonary embolism, which can be ruled out when clinical probability is unlikely and D-dimer level is normal. We evaluated the utility of D-dimer testing in patients with impaired renal function.

*Methods.*—D-dimer tests were performed in consecutive patients with suspected pulmonary embolism and an unlikely clinical probability. Creatinine levels were assessed as clinical routine. Glomerular filtration rate was calculated using the Modification of Diet in Renal Disease formula. Correlation between D-dimer level and renal function and proportions of patients with normal D-dimer in different categories of estimated glomerular filtration rate (eGFR) were assessed. Different categories of decreasing eGFR were defined as: normal renal function (eGFR >89 mL/min), mild decrease in eGFR (eGFR 60-89 mL/min), and moderate decrease in eGFR (eGFR 30-59 mL/min).

*Results.*—Creatinine levels were assessed in 351 of 385 patients (91%). D-dimer levels significantly increased in 3 categories of decreasing eGFR ($P=.027$ and $P=.021$ for moderate renal impairment compared with mild renal impairment and normal renal function, respectively). Normal D-dimer levels were found in 58% of patients with eGFR >89 mL/min, in 54% with eGFR 60-89 mL/min, and in 28% with eGFR 30-59 mL/min.

*Conclusions.*—The specificity of D-dimer testing in patients with suspected pulmonary embolism and decreased GFR is significantly decreased. Nonetheless, performing D-dimer tests is still useful because computed tomography scanning can be withheld in a significant proportion of these patients.

▶ The study is important because pulmonary embolism is a common clinical problem in patients with renal insufficiency and dialysis-dependent renal failure, and contrast tomography is often relatively contraindicated in this group. The clinical diagnosis of pulmonary embolism typically begins with the evaluation of the pretest clinical probability coupled with a D-dimer assay. If the D-dimer is normal and the clinical probability is low, further radiologic imaging and anticoagulation are not required. If either the D-dimer is abnormal or clinical probability is high, the diagnosis is typically established by either contrast-enhanced computer tomography or, if available, a ventilation-perfusion lung scan. The presence of chronic renal insufficiency complicates the diagnosis schema because the D-dimer levels are often abnormally elevated in the presence of renal disease. This study evaluates the use of the D-dimer assay for the diagnosis of pulmonary embolism in patients with chronic renal disease. The data demonstrate that the D-dimer levels vary with renal disease. Approximately 60% of patients with an eGFR of over 89 mL/min have normal D-dimer levels, whereas only about 30% of patients with an eGFR between 30 and 59 mL/min have normal D-dimer levels. Thus, although the specificity of the D-dimer test is reduced in patients with renal insufficiency, it is still worth obtaining because a normal D-dimer coupled with a low clinical likelihood can obviate the need for a contrast CT. One limitation of the study is that it did not include patients with creatinine clearance of < 30 mL/min, and the results may not be generalized to this population. The authors point out that in such patients lower extremity Doppler can be useful because if abnormal, anticoagulation can be initiated and a contrast study avoided.[1]

**R. Garrick, MD**

*Reference*

1. Righini M, Le Gal G, Aujesky D, et al. Diagnosis of pulmonary embolism by multidetector CT alone or combined with venous ultrasonography of the leg: a randomised non-inferiority trial. *Lancet*. 2008;371:1343-1352.

---

**A Trial of Darbepoetin Alfa in Type 2 Diabetes and Chronic Kidney Disease**

Pfeffer MA, for the TREAT Investigators (Brigham and Women's Hosp, Boston, MA; et al)

*N Engl J Med* 361:2019-2032, 2009

---

*Background.*—Anemia is associated with an increased risk of cardiovascular and renal events among patients with type 2 diabetes and chronic kidney disease. Although darbepoetin alfa can effectively increase hemoglobin levels, its effect on clinical outcomes in these patients has not been adequately tested.

*Methods.*—In this study involving 4038 patients with diabetes, chronic kidney disease, and anemia, we randomly assigned 2012 patients to darbepoetin alfa to achieve a hemoglobin level of approximately 13 g per deciliter and 2026 patients to placebo, with rescue darbepoetin alfa when the hemoglobin level was less than 9.0 g per deciliter. The primary end points were the composite outcomes of death or a cardiovascular event (nonfatal myocardial infarction, congestive heart failure, stroke, or hospitalization for myocardial ischemia) and of death or end-stage renal disease.

*Results.*—Death or a cardiovascular event occurred in 632 patients assigned to darbepoetin alfa and 602 patients assigned to placebo (hazard ratio for darbepoetin alfa vs. placebo, 1.05; 95% confidence interval [CI], 0.94 to 1.17; $P = 0.41$). Death or end-stage renal disease occurred in 652 patients assigned to darbepoetin alfa and 618 patients assigned to placebo (hazard ratio, 1.06; 95% CI, 0.95 to 1.19; $P = 0.29$). Fatal or nonfatal stroke occurred in 101 patients assigned to darbepoetin alfa and 53 patients assigned to placebo (hazard ratio, 1.92; 95% CI, 1.38 to 2.68; $P<0.001$). Red-cell transfusions were administered to 297 patients assigned to darbepoetin alfa and 496 patients assigned to placebo

(P<0.001). There was only a modest improvement in patient-reported fatigue in the darbepoetin alfa group as compared with the placebo group.

*Conclusions.*—The use of darbepoetin alfa in patients with diabetes, chronic kidney disease, and moderate anemia who were not undergoing dialysis did not reduce the risk of either of the two primary composite outcomes (either death or a cardiovascular event or death or a renal event) and was associated with an increased risk of stroke. For many persons involved in clinical decision making, this risk will outweigh the potential benefits. (ClinicalTrials.gov number, NCT00093015.)

▶ Many practitioners, in addition to nephrologists, participate in the treatment of anemia in patients with chronic kidney disease (CKD) who are not yet on dialysis. Therefore, it is important that every practitioner considering the use of erythropoietin agents in patients with renal insufficiency be familiar with the results of the Trial to Reduce Cardiovascular Events with Aranesp Therapy (TREAT) trial. After its introduction in the late 1980s, it was generally believed that correction of anemia with erythropoietin improved patient's quality of life, stabilized or improved ventricular function, and limited the need for red blood cell transfusions and their attendant risks. In 1998, The Normal Hematocrit study was conducted by Besarab and colleagues.[1] The study was designed to evaluate cardiovascular outcomes in patients with underlying ischemic heart disease who were undergoing dialysis. The target hematocrits were 30% ± 3% and 42% ± 3%. The study was terminated early because the high-hematocrit group had an increased risk of death and nonfatal cardiac infarction as compared with the low-hematocrit cohort. The Correction of Hemoglobin and Outcomes in Renal Insufficiency (CHOIR) study published in 2006 was conducted on patients not yet on dialysis, and a history of cardiac disease was not required for entrance into the study.[2] The CHOIR trial was also terminated early when it was determined that the patients in the target hemoglobin group of 13.5 g/dL as compared with those in the target group of 11.3 g/dL appeared to have a greater incidence of death and hospitalization from congestive heart failure.

The current TREAT trial was designed to evaluate whether treatment with the erythropoesis-stimulating agents (ESA) would reduce the risk of death and major cardiovascular events in patients with type 2 diabetes and CKD (estimated glomerular filtration rate of 20-60 mL/min/1.73 $m^2$) as calculated by the 4-variable Modification of Diet in Renal Disease equation. The hemoglobin targets were 13 g/dL in the treatment group, and rescue darbepoetin alpha was given to the comparison group when the hemoglobin was less than 9 g/dL. A complex dosing regimen agreed to by the Food and Drug Administration and the investigators was used to avoid overshooting the hemoglobin target. The use of the darbepoetin did not reduce the risk of either of the 2 primary composite outcomes; however, there was an increased risk of stroke in patients in the high-hemoglobin group. There was only a modest improvement in patient-reported well-being in the treatment group as compared with the control group.

Taken together, these studies suggest that in patients with CKD and end-stage renal disease, administration of erythropoietin to achieve the hemoglobin concentrations defined by these studies (13-14 g/dL), can be harmful. Whether this is related to the absolute amount of erythropoietin given[3] or to the rate of the rise of hemoglobin level is uncertain. These data are disheartening. Prior to ESA therapy, dialysis patients often had hemoglobin levels of 6 g/dL and received dangerous testosterone derivatives and blood products to keep the hemoglobin in this range. It is unfortunate that despite years of use, the most appropriate target hemoglobin for this high-risk population has not been carefully and definitively established. Practitioners should follow this literature closely, as new guidelines regarding ESA therapy, based on expert assessment of the data available, will surely be forthcoming.

**R. Garrick, MD**

*References*


1. Besarab A, Bolton WK, Browne JK, et al. The effect of normal as compared with low hematocrit values in patients with cardiac disease who are receiving hemodialysis and epoetin. *N Engl J Med.* 1998;339:584-590.
2. Singh AK, Szczech L, Tang KL, et al. Correction of anemia with epoetin alfa in chronic kidney disease. *N Engl J Med.* 2006;355:2085-2098.
3. Bookhart MA, Schneeweiss S, Avorn J, Bradbury BD, Liu J, Winkelmayer WC. Comparative mortality risks of anemia management practices and incident hemodialysis patients. *JAMA.* 2010;303:857-864.


## Adverse Safety Events in Chronic Kidney Disease: The Frequency of "Multiple Hits"

Chapin E, Zhan M, Hsu VD, et al (Univ of Maryland School of Medicine, Baltimore; Univ of Maryland School of Pharmacy, Baltimore)
*Clin J Am Soc Nephrol* 5:95-101, 2010

*Background and Objectives.*—Chronic kidney disease (CKD) lacks standardized patient safety indicators (PSIs); however, undetected safety events are likely to contribute to adverse outcomes in this disease. This study sought to determine the proportion of CKD patients who experience multiple potentially hazardous events from varied causes and to identify risk factors for the occurrence of "multiple hits."

*Design, Setting, Participants, & Measurements.*—A sample of patients with CKD ($n = 70{,}154$) in the Veterans Health Administration (VHA) were retrospectively examined for the occurrence of one or more safety events from a set of indicators defined *a priori*, including Agency for Healthcare Research and Quality (AHRQ) PSIs, hypoglycemia, hyperkalemia, and dosing for selected medications not accounting for CKD.

*Results.*—Approximately half of the cohort participants experienced one or two adverse safety events, whereas 7% had three or four (multiple) distinct events. Individuals with three or four of the predesignated safety events were more likely to be diabetic, non-Caucasian, have an estimated GFR (eGFR) < 30 ml/min/1.73 m$^2$, and be ≤65 yr of age. A "Safety Risk

Index" was developed using these characteristics, and those subjects that had all four traits were 25 times as likely to have three or four adverse safety events *versus* those with none of the characteristics.

*Conclusions.*—Patients with CKD are at a high risk for safety events pertinent to this disease and a substantial number are subject to multiple events from a diverse set of safety indicators, which could have important consequences in disease outcomes.

▶ Using safety events as defined by the Agency for Healthcare Research and Quality (AHRQ), which included hypoglycemia, hyperkalemia, errors in certain prescription drugs, or the occurrence of 1 or more AHRQ patient safety indicators (such as postoperative DVT, postoperative hemorrhage, or sepsis), patients with chronic kidney disease (classified by estimated glomerular filtration rate [eGFR]) were observed for the occurrence of adverse safety events.

The objective of this study was to determine the incidence and risk factors of patient safety events in this at-risk population. A Safety Risk Index was created using the factors that predicted the likelihood of multiple safety events. The Safety Risk Index range from a score of 0 to 4 predicated on the basis of a number of unweighted factors in any individual, including the presence of baseline diabetes, the index eGFR ($\leq$30 mL/min/1.73 $m^2$), non-Caucasian race, and age $\leq$65 years.

The results are very troubling. Approximately half of the 70 154 patients retrospectively studied had 1 or more adverse safety events, and a substantial number of patients (7%) had multiple distinct events. Individuals with a high Safety Risk Index were at greatest risk, and those patients who had all 4 traits of the Safety Risk Index were 25 times more likely to have a high number (3-4) of adverse safety events.

The data clearly indicate that patients with pre-end-stage renal disease are at high risk for a multitude of adverse safety events. The importance of the study is heightened by the fact that the adverse events studied were particularly pertinent to this disease population. Heightened attention to safety indicators, the use of checklists, and the use of computerized warning flags to advise prescribers, pharmacies, and other care givers of the presence of impaired kidney function may help improve these troubling statistics.

**R. Garrick, MD**

---

**Occurrence of adverse, often preventable, events in community hospitals involving nephrotoxic drugs or those excreted by the kidney**

Hug BL, Witkowski DJ, Sox CM, et al (Brigham and Women's Hosp, Boston, MA; Women's Healthcare Associates, P.C., Melrose, MA; Harvard Med School, Boston, MA)

*Kidney Int* 76:1192-1198, 2009

---

Medication errors in patients with reduced creatinine clearance are harmful and costly; however, most studies have been conducted in large academic hospitals. As there are few studies regarding this issue in smaller community hospitals, we conducted a multicenter, retrospective cohort study in six community hospitals (100 to 300 beds) to assess the incidence and severity of adverse drug events (ADEs) in patients with reduced creatinine clearance. A chart review was performed on adult patients hospitalized during a 20-month study period with serum creatinine over 1.5 mg/dl who were exposed to drugs that are nephrotoxic or cleared by the kidney. Among 109,641 patients, 17,614 had reduced creatinine clearance, and in a random sample of 900 of these patients, there were 498 potential ADEs and 90 ADEs. Among these ADEs, 91% were preventable, 51% were serious, 44% were significant, and 4.5% were life threatening. Of the potential ADEs, 54% were serious, 44% were significant, 1.6% were life threatening, and 96.6% were not intercepted. All 82 preventable events could have been intercepted by renal dose checking. Our study shows that ADEs were common in patients with impaired kidney function in community hospitals, and many appear potentially preventable with renal dose checking.

▶ This article is very important. Many health care providers believe that adverse patient safety events occur most often in teaching institutions where the complexity of disease is the greatest, and communication among multiple caregivers who are at various levels of training is the most challenging. The current well-defined, multicenter, retrospective cohort study involved 6 community hospitals and demonstrated that adverse drug reactions and their potential for patient harm is also a serious threat at the community hospital level. This study focused specifically on the prescription of potentially nephrotoxic drugs to patients with renal insufficiency.

The data are startling. Among a random sample of 900 patients with reduced renal function, there were almost 500 potential adverse drug events and 90 adverse drug events. This means that almost 1 in 10 patients with baseline renal insufficiency suffered an adverse drug event. Ninety-one percent of these actual adverse events were preventable, and all the preventable errors could have been intercepted if a system had been in place for renal dose verification. The actual cost of these types of adverse drug events to patients and to the health care system is almost incalculable.

Correct drug dosing, especially drug dosing in high-risk populations, such as those with renal insufficiency, is a long-standing safety goal. These errors are system issues and can only be corrected by appropriate allocation of resources so that hospitals of all size can implement a standardized approach to patient safety. Information technology that has been legitimately tested by the health care community before implementation will be an important part of any high-reliability system. Overzealous implementation of poorly planned and tested health care technology systems, with the idea that "we will get them all installed and see how they work," will likely increase the risk of adverse events. Practitioners and hospitals must be firmly committed to the goal of patient safety and must insist that resources be devoted to develop and implement high-reliability systems.

**R. Garrick, MD**

**A Randomized, Double-Blind, Placebo-Controlled Study to Assess the Efficacy and Safety of Cinacalcet HCl in Participants With CKD Not Receiving Dialysis**

Chonchol M, Locatelli F, Abboud HE, et al (Univ of Colorado Health Science Ctr, Denver; Azienda Ospedaliera di Lecco, Italy; Univ of Texas Health Science Ctr, San Antonio; et al)

*Am J Kidney Dis* 53:197-207, 2009

*Background.*—Secondary hyperparathyroidism is observed in patients with early chronic kidney disease (CKD). This study investigated the safety and efficacy of cinacalcet for secondary hyperparathyroidism in participants with CKD not receiving dialysis.

*Study Design.*—Double-blind, randomized, 32-week, phase 3 study.

*Setting & Participants.*—404 participants with stage 3 or 4 CKD from 73 centers in 9 countries.

*Interventions.*—Cinacalcet:placebo (3:1 ratio).

*Outcomes & Measurements.*—Proportion of participants with a mean decrease of 30% or greater in intact parathyroid hormone (iPTH) level, proportion with iPTH level of 70 or less or 110 or less pg/mL (stage 3 and 4 CKD, respectively), and mean percentage of iPTH change from baseline, all during the efficacy-assessment phase.

*Results.*—A greater proportion of cinacalcet than placebo participants achieved a 30% or greater decrease in iPTH level (74% versus 28%; $P < 0.001$), corresponding to a 43.1% decrease in iPTH level from baseline (cinacalcet) compared with a 1.1% increase (placebo). At week 32, serum calcium levels were 8.9 ± 0.8 mg/dL (+8.9%; cinacalcet) and 9.9 ± 0.6 mg/dL (+0.8%; placebo), phosphorus levels were 4.5 ± 1.0 mg/dL (+21.4%) and 4.0 ± 0.7 mg/dL (+6.8%), and calcium-phosphorus product values were 40.1 ± 8.3 $mg^2/dL^2$ (+18.9%) and 38.9 ± 6.9 $mg^2/dL^2$ (+17.1%), respectively. During the study course, 62% (cinacalcet) and 1% (placebo) of participants experienced 2 consecutive serum calcium concentrations less than 8.4 mg/dL. They generally were asymptomatic and without significant clinical consequences. Treatment generally was well tolerated, and most adverse events were mild to moderate in severity.

*Limitations.*—The study was not designed to assess the effects of cinacalcet on vascular calcification, bone histomorphometric parameters, or other clinical outcomes. It is not known whether the observed differences in changes in iPTH levels are clinically more important than observed differences in changes in serum calcium or phosphorus levels or dosages of vitamin D sterols and phosphate binders.

*Conclusions.*—These data show that cinacalcet treatment in patients with CKD not receiving dialysis can decrease plasma iPTH levels, but with frequent (albeit generally asymptomatic) serum calcium levels less than 8.4 mg/dL and increases in serum phosphorus levels (Figs 2-4).

▶ One of the mechanisms of action of cinacalcet is to increase the sensitivity of the calcium sensing receptor to serum calcium. This change allows the calcium

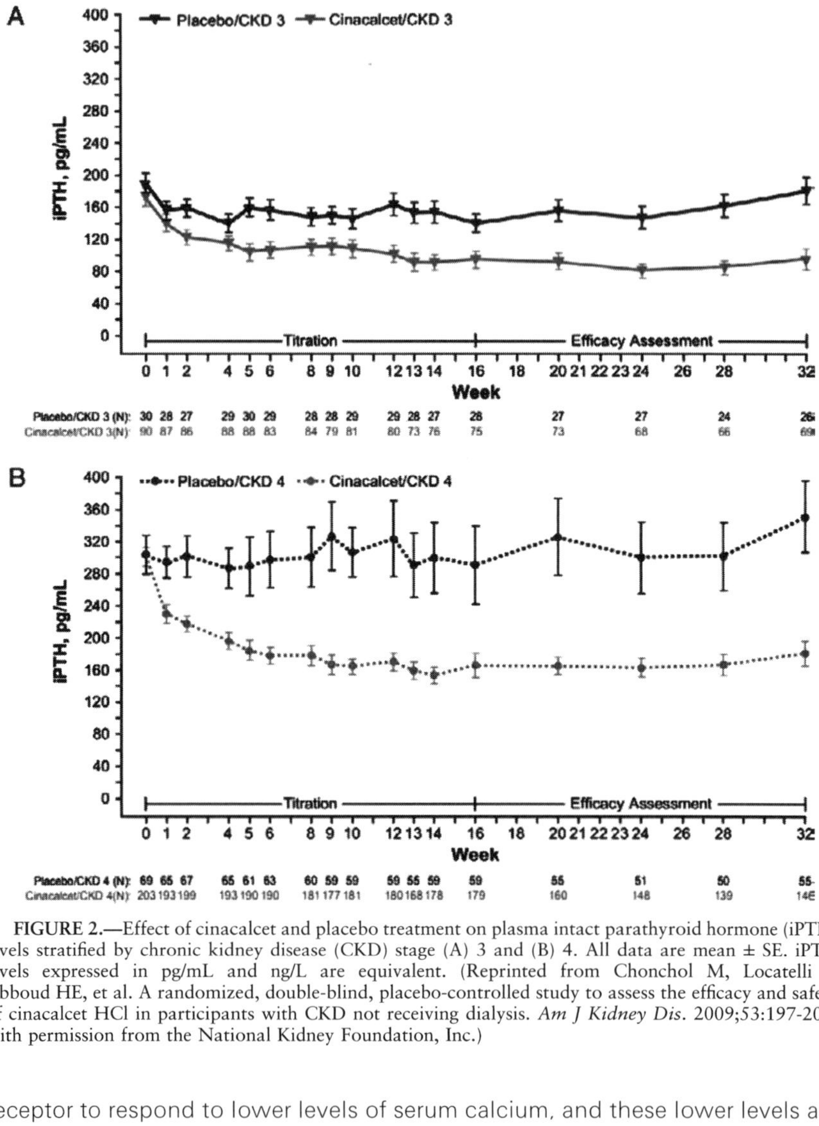


FIGURE 2.—Effect of cinacalcet and placebo treatment on plasma intact parathyroid hormone (iPTH) levels stratified by chronic kidney disease (CKD) stage (A) 3 and (B) 4. All data are mean ± SE. iPTH levels expressed in pg/mL and ng/L are equivalent. (Reprinted from Chonchol M, Locatelli F, Abboud HE, et al. A randomized, double-blind, placebo-controlled study to assess the efficacy and safety of cinacalcet HCl in participants with CKD not receiving dialysis. *Am J Kidney Dis*. 2009;53:197-207, with permission from the National Kidney Foundation, Inc.)

receptor to respond to lower levels of serum calcium, and these lower levels are able to effectively suppress calcium-sensing receptor-dependent parathyroid hormone (PTH) secretion.[1,2] In patients with chronic renal disease on dialysis, cinacalcet lowers serum phosphorus, calcium, alkaline phosphatase, and PTH levels. This constellation of changes makes it an ideal drug for the control of dialysis-related secondary hyperparathyroidism.

In patients not yet on dialysis, the overall effects of cinacalcet are slightly different. In the pre-end-stage renal disease (ESRD) population, the serum phosphate levels can increase in response to cinacalcet therapy.[3] The exact mechanism responsible for the rise in phosphate has not yet been fully

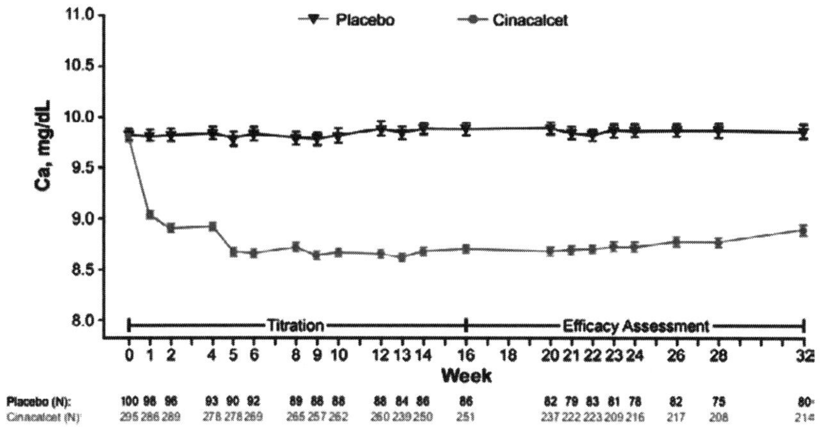


FIGURE 3.—Mean serum calcium (Ca) levels in participants receiving cinacalcet or placebo. All data are mean ± SE. To convert serum calcium in mg/dL to mmol/L, multiply by 0.2495. (Reprinted from Chonchol M, Locatelli F, Abboud HE, et al. A randomized, double-blind, placebo-controlled study to assess the efficacy and safety of cinacalcet HCl in participants with CKD not receiving dialysis. *Am J Kidney Dis*. 2009;53:197-207, with permission from the National Kidney Foundation, Inc.)

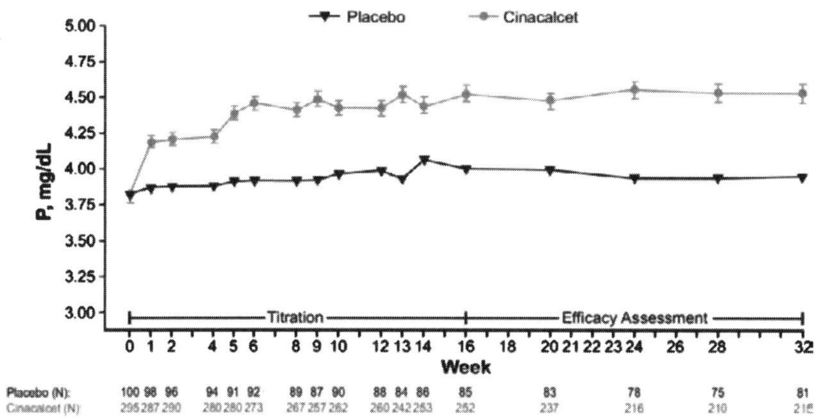


FIGURE 4.—Mean serum phosphorus (P) levels in participants receiving cinacalcet or placebo. All data are mean ± SE. To convert serum phosphorus in mg/dL to mmol/L, multiply by 0.3229. (Reprinted from Chonchol M, Locatelli F, Abboud HE, et al. A randomized, double-blind, placebo-controlled study to assess the efficacy and safety of cinacalcet HCl in participants with CKD not receiving dialysis. *Am J Kidney Dis*. 2009;53:197-207, with permission from the National Kidney Foundation, Inc.)

determined. It may be because of the reduced fibroblast growth factor 23 levels, with a resultant reduction in urine phosphate excretion and a rise in serum phosphate.[4]

The current 32-week phase 3 trial evaluated the use of cinacalcet in 404 individuals with stage 3 and 4 chronic kidney disease (estimated glomerular filtration rate less than 30 mL/min), measured by Modification of Diet in Renal Disease formula.[5] Cinacalcet lowered PTH levels in patients with both stage 3 and 4 disease and lowered the serum calcium level. However, as with other pre-ESRD studies,[3] the serum phosphorus levels increased (Figs 2-4).

And herein lays the conundrum. Do the potential risks of an elevated serum phosphate level offset the potential benefit of a lower PTH level in the pre-ESRD population? This question is very difficult to answer with any degree of certainty. Numerous studies have suggested that elevated serum phosphorus level, itself, is associated with an increase in mortality. Other studies I've previously reviewed have demonstrated that a serum phosphorus level that is at the high end of the normal range can be associated with an increased risk of cardiovascular events.[6-8] The fact that the appropriate PTH target in the pre-ESRD population remains uncertain further confounds the question.

On a bright note, unlike our prior experience with erythropoietin-stimulating agents, these investigators are attempting to determine the efficacy, appropriateness, risks, and benefits of cinacalcet, prior to its gaining widespread use for the treatment of secondary hyperparathyroidism in the pre-ESRD population. Until further long-term trials have been conducted cinacalcet should be used extremely judiciously in the pre-ESRD population and if used, the serum phosphorous (and calcium) level should be closely monitored.

**R. Garrick, MD**

*References*

1. Block GA, Martin KJ, de Francisco AL, et al. Cinacalcet for secondary hyperparathyroidism in patients receiving hemodialysis. *N Engl J Med.* 2004;350:1516-1525.
2. Lindberg JS, Culleton B, Wong G, et al. Cinacalcet HCl, an oral calcimimetic agent for the treatment of secondary hyperparathyroidism in hemodialysis and peritoneal dialysis: a randomized, double-blind, multicenter study. *J Am Soc Nephrol.* 2005;16:800-807.
3. Charytan C, Coburn JW, Chonchol M, et al. Cinacalcet hydrochloride is an effective treatment for secondary hyperparathyroidism in patients with CKD not receiving dialysis. *Am J Kidney Dis.* 2005;46:58-67.
4. Serra AL, Wuhrmann C, Wüthrich RP. Phosphatemic effect of cinacalcet in kidney transplant recipients with persistent hyperparathyroidism. *Am J Kidney Dis.* 2008;53:1151-1157.
5. Levey AS, Bosch JP, Lewis JB, Greene T, Rogers N, Roth D. A more accurate method to estimate glomerular filtration rate from serum creatinine: a new prediction equation. Modification of Diet in Renal Disease Study Group. *Ann Intern Med.* 1999;130:461-470.
6. Dhingra R, Sullivan LM, Fox CS, et al. Relations of serum phosphorus and calcium levels to the incidence of cardiovascular disease in the community. *Arch Intern Med.* 2007;167:879-885.
7. Kestenbaum B, Sampson JN, Rudser KD, et al. Serum phosphate levels and mortality risk among people with chronic kidney disease. *JAm Soc Nephrol.* 2005;16:520-528.
8. Gutiérrez OM, l Mannstadt M, Isakova T, et al. Fibroblast growth factor 23 and mortality among patients undergoing hemodialysis. *N Engl J Med.* 2008;359:584-592.

**Comparative Mortality Risk of Anemia Management Practices in Incident Hemodialysis Patients**

Brookhart MA, Schneeweiss S, Avorn J, et al (Univ of North Carolina, Chapel Hill; Brigham and Women's Hosp, Boston, MA; et al)

*JAMA* 303:857-864, 2010

*Context.*—Controversy exists about optimal management of anemia in end-stage renal disease.

*Objective.*—To compare the mortality risk of different dialysis center–level patterns of anemia management.

*Design, Setting, and Patients.*—Using data from Medicare's end-stage renal disease program (1999-2007), we characterized each US dialysis center's annual anemia management practice by estimating its typical use of erythropoiesis-stimulating agents (ESAs) and intravenous iron in hemodialysis patients within 4 hematocrit categories. We used Cox proportional hazards regression to correlate center-level patterns of ESA and iron use with 1-year mortality risk in 269 717 incident hemodialysis patients.

*Main Outcome Measure.*—One-year all-cause mortality.

*Results.*—Monthly mortality rates were highest in patients with hematocrit less than 30% (mortality, 2.1%) and lowest for those with hematocrit of 36%or higher (mortality, 0.7%). After adjustment for baseline case-mix differences, dialysis centers that used larger ESA doses in patients with hematocrit less than 30% had lower mortality rates than centers that used smaller doses (highest vs lowest dose group: hazard ratio [HR], 0.94; 95% confidence interval [CI], 0.90-0.97). Centers that administered iron more frequently to patients with hematocrit less than 33% also had lower mortality rates (highest vs lowest quintile, HR, 0.95; 95% CI, 0.91-0.98). However, centers that used larger ESA doses in patients with hematocrit between 33% and 35.9% had higher mortality rates (highest vs lowest quintile, HR, 1.07; 95% CI, 1.03-1.12). More intensive use of both ESAs and iron was associated with increased mortality risk in patients with hematocrit of 36% or higher. These findings persisted across a range of secondary analyses.

*Conclusions.*—Greater ESA and iron use were associated with decreased mortality risk at lower hematocrit levels, in which mortality rates are the highest. Although the overall mortality rate was lower at higher hematocrit levels, elevated mortality risk was associated with greater use of ESAs and iron in these patients.

▶ The outcome of the Trial to Reduce Cardiovascular Events with Aranesp Therapy (TREAT) trial demonstrated that the administration of darbepoetin alpha to patients with diabetes and chronic kidney disease (CKD) (estimated glomerular filtration rate [GFR] 20-60 ml/min) was associated with an increased risk of fatal and nonfatal stroke.[1] This study evaluated mortality and anemia management practices in incident dialysis patients. Using a novel study design based on the United States Renal Data System (USRDS), the authors were able to evaluate the anemia management profile for every US dialysis center. These data resulted in a set of predicted erythropoiesis-stimulating agent (ESA) and iron treatments received by patients with varying degrees of anemia. These data were then correlated with the 1-year mortality risk among patients initiating dialysis at each center. Based on this unique approach, the authors demonstrated that centers that used larger ESA doses in patients with levels less than 30% had lower mortality rates than centers that used smaller doses. Greater ESA and iron use were associated with decreased mortality risks among those with lower hemoglobin levels (where in the general mortality rates are the highest). However, patients with hematocrit levels between 33% and 35.9%, who received the highest ESA doses had higher mortality rates. The intensive use of both ESA and iron was associated with increased mortality risk in patients with hematocrits of 36% or higher. The data are thought provoking. The use of high-dose erythropoietin may, in and of itself, be problematic. Erythropoietin is a growth factor and is known to have a variety of extra-erythropoietic effects, including effects on platelets, blood pressure, and cellular proliferation. The authors point out that other existing trials were designed to compare the outcome effects of varying hematocrit concentrations. This study suggests that the ultimate dose of ESA/iron used relative to the hematocrit target may alter mortality outcomes. It is possible that the use of high-dose ESA to maintain a given target hemoglobin level (33%-36%) is contributing to the observed mortality. For example, certain patients may be relatively ESA resistant and require high doses to maintain a given hemoglobin level. This ESA resistance, and subsequent ESA dose, may contribute to an adverse outcome in the high-target hematocrit groups. This observational study has several limitations. For example, independent effects of iron therapy cannot be evaluated, it was confined to incident dialysis patients, and the exact ESA and iron management protocols were not available. Additional well-designed dosing studies will be required to better explore the possibilities raised by these observations. Certainly, the well-designed TREAT trial has demonstrated that despite its widespread use, much about ESA therapy remains unanswered.

**R. Garrick, MD**

*Reference*

1. Pfeffer MA, Burdman EA, Chen C-Y, et al. A trial of darbepoetin alpha in type 2 diabetes and chronic kidney disease. *N Engl J Med.* 2009;361:2019-2032.

---

**Contraindicated Medication Use in Dialysis Patients Undergoing Percutaneous Coronary Intervention**

Tsai TT, for the National Cardiovascular Data Registry (Denver VA Med Ctr, CO; et al)

*JAMA* 302:2458-2464, 2009

---

*Context.*—The US Food and Drug Administration guides clinicians through drug labeling of medications that are contraindicated or not recommended for use in specific patient groups. Little is known about the use of such medications and their effects on outcomes in clinical practice.

*Objective.*—To investigate the use of the contraindicated/not-recommended agents enoxaparin and eptifibatide among dialysis patients undergoing percutaneous coronary intervention (PCI) and their association with outcomes.

*Design, Setting, and Participants.*—Data from 829 US hospitals on 22 778 dialysis patients who underwent PCI between January 1, 2004, and August 31, 2008.

*Main Outcome Measures.*—In-hospital bleeding and death.

*Results.*—Five thousand eighty-four patients (22.3%) received a contraindicated antithrombotic; of these patients, 2375 (46.7%) received enoxaparin, 3261 (64.1%) received eptifibatide, and 552 (10.9%) received both. Compared with patients who did not receive a contraindicated antithrombotic, patients who did had higher rates of in-hospital bleeding (5.6% vs 2.9%; odds ratio [OR], 1.93; 95% confidence interval [CI], 1.66-2.23) and death (6.5% vs 3.9%; OR, 1.68; 95% CI, 1.46-1.95). After multivariable adjustment, patients receiving contraindicated antithrombotics had significantly higher risks of in-hospital bleeding (OR, 1.66; 95% CI, 1.43-1.92) and death (OR, 1.24; 95% CI, 1.04-1.48). In 10 158 patients matched by propensity scores, receipt of contraindicated antithrombotics remained significantly associated with in-hospital bleeding (OR, 1.63; 95% CI, 1.35-1.98) but not in-hospital death (OR, 1.15; 95% CI, 0.97-1.36).

*Conclusions.*—In a sample of dialysis patients undergoing PCI, 22.3% received a contraindicated antithrombotic medication. In propensity-matched analysis, receipt of these medications was significantly associated with an increased risk of in-hospital major bleeding.

▶ Tsai and colleagues draw attention to an important patient care and safety issue. In the current health care delivery system, many individuals participate in the care of patients with chronic kidney disease. These patients have varying degrees of renal function ranging from mild renal impairment to end-stage renal disease on dialysis. This study evaluated cardiac catheterization data obtained from 22 770 dialysis patients who underwent percutaneous coronary intervention during a 4-year period from January 2001 through August 2008. Using data from the National Cardiovascular Data Registry, the investigators demonstrated that 22.3% of these dialysis patients received eptifibatide (platelet glycoprotein IIb/IIIa inhibitor), enoxaparin (low-molecular weight heparin), or both. These drugs are both cleared by renal excretion, and their use is not recommended in dialysis patients because of the risk of bleeding complications. Patients who received these agents had a higher risk of in-hospital bleeding as compared with patients who did not receive these contraindicated antithrombotic agents. The study does have limitations in as much long-term follow-up is not available and the CathPCI registry does not capture all the elements of drug delivery (timing and exact dose). However, it is unlikely that specific drug errors would have been limited to one group versus another. It is noteworthy that a large number of patients received these agents, despite drug labeling that clearly states that they are contraindicated in patients on dialysis and despite the availability of other antithrombotic agents, such as abciximab and unfractionated heparin that are safer in the dialysis population. The investigators also found that the use of contraindicated medications was more common in centers with lower procedural volumes as compared with urban centers with training programs and higher procedural volumes.

The findings do appear to justify the current Food and Drug Administration's warnings regarding the use of these agents in dialysis patients. The prevalent dialysis population is continuing to grow and to age, and many practitioners besides nephrologists must be knowledgeable regarding drug utilization in this complex population. The results of this study highlight the clear need for ongoing aggressive education and the need to develop and implement treatment algorithms that take into account the underlying comorbidities of the population.[1]

**R. Garrick, MD**

*Reference*

1. Mehta SK, Frutkin AD, Lindsey JB, et al. Bleeding in patients undergoing percutaneous coronary intervention: the development of a clinical risk algorithm from the National Cardiovascular Data Registry. *Circ Cardiovasc Interv.* 2009;2: 222-229.

---

## Prevalence of nephrogenic systemic fibrosis in renal insufficiency patients: Results of the FINEST study

Janus N, Launay-Vacher V, Karie S, et al (Pitié-Salpêtrière Hosp, Paris, France; et al)

*Eur J Radiol* 73:357-359, 2010

---

*Purpose.*—Nephrogenic systemic fibrosis (NSF) is characterized by widespread tissue fibrosis, mainly affecting the skin. Gadolinium chelates have been implicated in the onset of NSF in patients with renal impairment (RI). The FINEST study (FIbrose Néphrogénique SysTémique) was designed to determine the prevalence of NSF after magnetic resonance imaging (MRI) in French RI patients.

*Materials and Methods.*—We studied all patients with RI who had at least one MRI examination during a one-year period, with or without gadolinium chelate administration. Data were collected retrospectively from 9 Nephrology Departments in France, and included sex, age, renal function, type of gadolinium administered, and subsequent cutaneous disorders. If a patient presented a cutaneous disorder, a skin biopsy was performed to confirm the diagnostic.

*Results.*—The 308 eligible patients had a mean age of 59.9 years, 59% were men, and 54% had stage 5 RI. 75% of those 308 patients received a Gadolinium chelate. Among those patients who received a gadolinium chelate, 76% received gadoterate, 20% gadopentetate, 3% gadodiamide and 1% gadobenate. No cutaneous disorders were recorded after MRI.

**TABLE 1.**—Renal Function of FINEST Study Patients According to the K/DOQI–KDIGO Classification (n = 308)

| GFR (mL/min/1.73 $m^2$) | Number of Patients | Percent of Patients |
|---|---|---|
| 60–90 | 22 | 7.1% |
| 30–60 | 56 | 18.2% |
| 15–30 | 62 | 20.1% |
| <15 | 165 | 53.6% |
| No data available | 3 | 1% |

K/DOQI: kidney disease outcomes quality initiative. KDIGO: kidney disease improving global outcomes. GFR: glomerular filtration rate.

*Conclusion.*—These results confirm that NSF is a rare disease. Based on a reported frequency, ~3.5% in patients with glomerular filtration rate <30 ml/min/1.73 $m^2$), some cases should have been observed in our study which included 308 patients. Most patients received gadoterate, a macrocyclic gadolinium chelate for which no case of NSF has been observed worldwide. This suggests that more stable macrocyclic agents may be less likely to induce NSF (Table 1).

▶ Nephrogenic systemic fibrosis (NSF) was first described in the early 2000s. Over the ensuing decade, it has become more widely recognized as an untreatable complication of gadolinium administration in patients with underlying kidney disease. Since then, several investigators have focused on the potential risk factors for NSF. Identified risk factors include the use of multiple doses and administration to patients with an estimated glomerular filtration rate (eGFR) of less than 30 mL/min. This study gathered data on approximately 300 patients with chronic kidney disease who were undergoing gadolinium imaging. Patients were stratified according to their kidney function[1] and were followed for 4 months after the MRI examination. Most patients (Table 1) had an estimated GFR of less than 15 mL/min. The most common gadolinium chelate administered was gadoterate, which is a macrocyclic gadolinium chelate. Only 2% of the patients received gadodiamide, which is a linear chelate and is the chelate most often linked to NSF in patients with underlying renal disease.[2]

It has been suggested that the formulation of gadolinium influences its stability, and this in turn influences the rate of transmetalation. No episodes of NSF occurred in patients who received gadoterate, despite the presence of significant renal impairment. The study does have limitations. The dose of gadolinium administered was not monitored, the follow-up period was limited to 4 months, and the lifetime history of gadolinium exposure was not always available.

These results should not be taken as an endorsement for the routine use of gadolinium in patients with advanced renal failure. Rather, they do suggest that if gadolinium-enhanced MRI imaging is clinically mandatory then a macrocyclic chelate should be used.

**R. Garrick, MD**

*References*

1. Levey AS, Eckardt KU, Tsukamoto Y, et al. Definition and classification of chronic kidney disease: a position statement from kidney disease: improving global outcomes (KDIGO). *Kidney Int.* 2005;67:2089-2100.
2. Kanal E, Broome DR, Martin DR, Thomsen HS. Responses to the FDA's May 23, 2007 nephrogenic systemic fibrosis update. *Radiology.* 2008;246:11-14.

## Results of a randomized controlled trial on statin use in dialysis patients had no influence on statin prescription

Lam NN, Jain AK, Hackam DG, et al (Univ of Western Ontario, London, Canada; et al)
*Kidney Int* 76:1172-1179, 2009

Randomized trials provide high-quality evidence for patient care. The Der Deutsche Diabetes Dialyse Studie (4D), a randomized study which demonstrated no benefit of statins among diabetic patients receiving hemodialysis, was published in July 2005. To determine effects of this study we conducted a retrospective, population-based, time series analysis with change-point regression to see if the rate of statin prescription to dialysis patients had been modified. We linked health administrative data for all diabetic hemodialysis patients living in Ontario, Canada, with similar characteristics to the 4D patient cohort. During the nearly 11-year period prior to study publication, the rate of statin use increased almost 14-fold, from 43 to 597 per 1000 patients. For 2.5 years after study publication, rather than diminish, statin use continued to rise to an absolute rate of 676 per 1000 patients. These temporal patterns in statin use closely mimicked trends in the diabetic population not receiving dialysis. The 4D trial had no impact on statin use when we restricted the analysis to incident statin prescriptions or expanded the characteristics of the dialysis patients considered for study. Thus, we found that publication of a large, expensive, randomized controlled trial in patients receiving hemodialysis had no immediate impact on clinical practice. The use of a common cardiovascular medication in this patient population appears to be influenced by other factors.

► The medical literature suffers from a paucity of high-quality randomized controlled trials involving patients with renal disease. Nephrologists often make clinical decisions based on the results of observational, cross-sectional, or retrospective studies or meta-analyses. Alternatively, nephrologists may generalize the results from other studies to their patients with renal disease. Therapies initiated based on these types of data may later be found to be ineffective or even harmful. The only randomized controlled trial studying the efficacy of statins on cardiovascular outcomes in patients with diabetic dialysis, Der Deutsche Diabetes Dialyse Studie (4D) trial published in 2005,[1] demonstrated a lack of benefit, and maybe even a trend toward an increased risk of stroke, in patients with diabetic dialysis who were treated with atorvastatin.

Noting that the use of statins had increased 13.9-fold between 1994 and the publication of 4D, Lam and colleagues tracked nephrologists' prescribing patterns in the years following the 4D trial. Surprisingly, they found that following the publication of 4D, nephrologists use of statin in dialysis patients did not decrease. Rather, the investigators found that the slope of the increase in statin use both before and after publication of 4D, were virtually identical. This was true even after accounting for incident prescriptions only, thereby precluding the suggested explanation that nephrologists were simply cautious about changing therapy in the face of a negative study.

There are many reasons why nephrologists, who care for this extremely morbid population, have been reluctant to incorporate the findings of 4D into their practice. It may be due to inertia, doubts about the validity or generalizability of the study, or the existence of highly persuasive data supporting statin use in other populations.

In any case, this study does throw doubt on the ability of even well-designed, expensive, and clinically important studies to influence the clinical behavior of nephrologists.

**M. Klein, MD, JD**

*Reference*

1. Wanner C, Krane V, März W, et al. Atorvastatin in patients with type 2 diabetes mellitus undergoing hemodialysis. *N Engl J Med.* 2005;353:238-248.

# 28 Dialysis

**Digoxin Associates with Mortality in ESRD**

Chan KE, Lazarus JM, Hakim RM (Fresenius Med Care NA, Waltham, MA)

*J Am Soc Nephrol* 21:1550-1559, 2010

The safety of prescribing digoxin in ESRD is unknown. Hypokalemia, which frequently occurs among dialysis patients, may enhance the toxicity of digoxin. Here, we analyzed the association between digoxin prescription and survival in a retrospective cohort using covariate- and propensity score–adjusted Cox models to minimize the potential for confounding by indication. Among 120,864 incident hemodialysis patients, digoxin use associated with a 28% increased risk for death (hazard ratio [HR] 1.28; 95% confidence interval 1.25 to 1.31). Increasing serum digoxin level was also significantly associated with mortality (HR 1.19 per ng/ml increase; 95% confidence interval 1.05 to 1.35). This increased mortality risk with level was most pronounced in patients with lower predialysis serum potassium (K) levels (HR 2.53 [$P = 0.01$] for K <4.3 mEq/L *versus* HR 0.86 [$P = 0.35$] for K >4.6 mEq/L). In conclusion, digoxin use among patients who are on hemodialysis associates with increased mortality, especially among those with low predialysis K concentrations.

▶ Digoxin therapy is often recommended for the treatment of atrial fibrillation, and occasionally the treatment of heart failure, in patients undergoing chronic renal replacement therapy. Electrolyte abnormalities and fluctuations in serum potassium levels are common in this population. This study used a database of almost 121 000 incident hemodialysis patients. Surprisingly, digoxin use was associated with a 28% increased risk of death. An increased risk of mortality was most significant in patients in whom the predialysis serum potassium was less than 4.3 mEq per liter. This potassium level is typical for many patients predialysis depending on their dietary compliance and concomitant medication use. There were no appreciable differences in the prescribed dialysis potassium or calcium among the groups. When data were adjusted for clinical comorbidities, increased risk for death remains in subanalyses, which compared the patients receiving digoxin with those with comparable indications but not on digoxin. As shown in Fig 1 in the original article, the crude survival rate decreased as the digoxin level increased. This observational study cannot be interpreted as showing causality. However, this is the first large database study to specifically evaluate this question. The data certainly suggest that the indication for digoxin use in this population be carefully evaluated and clinically warranted. In addition, the serum potassium and digoxin levels should be closely monitored.

**R. Garrick, MD**

---

**Functional Status of Elderly Adults before and after Initiation of Dialysis**

Tamura MK, Covinsky KE, Chertow GM, et al (Stanford Univ School of Medicine, Palo Alto, CA; Univ of California San Francisco)

*N Engl J Med* 361:1539-1547, 2009

---

*Background.*—It is unclear whether functional status before dialysis is maintained after the initiation of this therapy in elderly patients with end-stage renal disease (ESRD).

*Methods.*—Using a national registry of patients undergoing dialysis, which was linked to a national registry of nursing home residents, we identified all 3702 nursing home residents in the United States who were starting treatment with dialysis between June 1998 and October 2000 and for whom at least one measurement of functional status was available before the initiation of dialysis. Functional status was measured by assessing the degree of dependence in seven activities of daily living (on the Minimum Data Set–Activities of Daily Living [MDS–ADL] scale of 0 to 28 points, with higher scores indicating greater functional difficulty).

*Results.*—The median MDS–ADL score increased from 12 during the 3 months before the initiation of dialysis to 16 during the 3 months after the initiation of dialysis. Three months after the initiation of dialysis, functional status had been maintained in 39% of nursing home residents, but by 12 months after the initiation of dialysis, 58% had died and predialysis functional status had been maintained in only 13%. In a random-effects model, the initiation of dialysis was associated with a sharp decline in functional status, indicated by an increase of 2.8 points in the MDS–ADL score (95% confidence interval [CI], 2.5 to 3.0); this decline was independent of age, sex, race, and functional-status trajectory before the initiation of dialysis. The decline in functional status associated with the initiation of dialysis remained substantial (1.7 points; 95% CI, 1.4 to 2.1), even after adjustment for the presence or absence of an accelerated functional decline during the 3-month period before the initiation of dialysis.

*Conclusions.*—Among nursing home residents with ESRD, the initiation of dialysis is associated with a substantial and sustained decline in functional status.

▶ According to the United States renal data system,[1] the median age of new patients beginning end-stage renal disease therapy in 2008 was 64.4 years. The same database showed that the adjusted incident rate for those aged 75 years and older grew 11% since the year 2000 to 1744, and since 1996

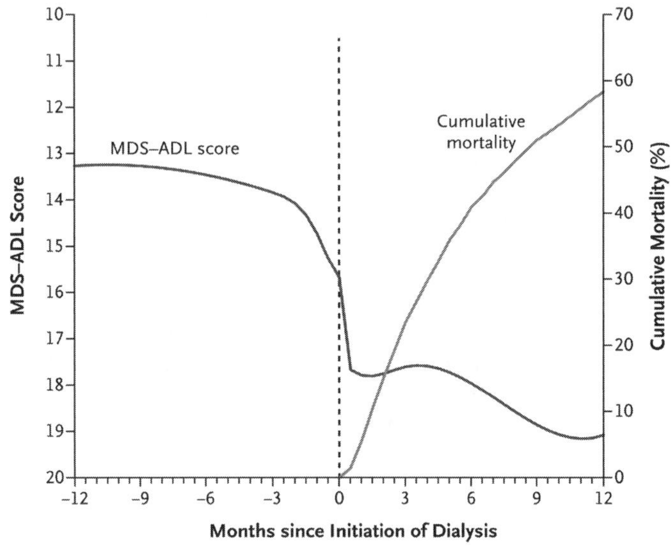


FIGURE 3.—Smoothed Trajectory of Functional Status before and after the Initiation of Dialysis and Cumulative Mortality Rate. The dashed vertical line indicates the initiation of dialysis in a hypothetical 75-year-old nursing home resident. MDS–ADL denotes Minimum Data Set–Activities of Daily Living. The numbers on the MDS–ADL axis run from highest to lowest. (Reprinted from Tamura MK, Covinsky KE, Chertow GM, et al. Functional status of elderly adults before and after initiation of dialysis. *N Engl J Med.* 2009;361:1539-1547. Copyright 2009 Massachusetts Medical Society. All rights reserved.)

the total prevalent number of patients aged 75 years and older has more than doubled. Taken within this context, the study by Tamura and colleagues is especially meaningful. By cross-linking a national registry of patients undergoing dialysis to a national registry of nursing home patients, the investigators were able to identify all 3702 individuals who initiated dialysis while residing in nursing homes between the years 1998 and 2000. The mean age of the resident was 73.4 ± 10 years. The investigators studied both the functional status and the mortality of nursing home patients following the initiation of dialysis. Their data demonstrate that the outcome of dialysis in the nursing home setting is quite bleak. Predialysis functional status (assessed by the ability to perform each of the 7 activities of daily living) was influenced by a number of factors, including older age, vascular disease, dementia, and low serum albumin (less than 3.5 g/dL). After the initiation of dialysis, functional status declined, and the trajectory of the decline was independent of age, sex, race, and the presence or absence of coexisting conditions. At the end of 3 months, only 39% of the patients had the same functional status as predialysis. The cumulative mortality rates were 24% at 3 months and 58% twelve months after the initiation of dialysis (Fig 3).

In 2006, Lambie and colleagues[4] used the data from the Dialysis Outcomes and Practice Pattern Study to evaluate the influence that patient characteristics have on nephrologist's opinions and practice patterns. They demonstrated that medical directors from different countries have varying opinions regarding the initiation of dialysis in patients with advanced renal dysfunction and multiple comorbidities. For example, medical directors from both France and the United Kingdom were less likely to routinely initiate dialysis for patients residing in nursing homes, for the very elderly, or for patients with major comorbidities than were medical directors from the United States.

This study does not allow us to assess whether or not the change in the patient's functional status was because of the initiation of dialysis or rather reflects the inexorable progress of disease.

Nonetheless, all practitioners who care for the elderly should be aware of these data when offering guidance about therapeutic options to patients and families. These data may help temper unrealistic expectations regarding the benefits of dialysis as patients move along the continuum of chronic disease. In addition, as the authors note, these data should heighten the practitioner's attention to other therapeutic modalities, such as rehabilitative interventions and dietary modifications[2,3] that may actually help improve the quality of life for the chronically ill nursing home patient with advanced renal disease.

**R. Garrick, MD**

*References*


1. US Renal Data System. *USRDS 2008 Annual Data Report: Atlas of Chronic Kidney Disease and End-Stage Renal Disease in the United States.* Bethesda, MD: National Institutes of Health, National Institute of Diabetes and Digestive and Kidney Diseases; 2008.
2. Fouque D, Aparicio M. Eleven reasons to control the protein intake of patients with chronic kidney disease. *Nat Clin Pract Nephrol.* 2007;3:383-392.
3. Brunori G, Viola BF, Parrinello G, et al. Efficacy and safety of a very-low-protein diet when postponing dialysis in the elderly: a prospective randomized multicenter controlled study. *Am J Kidney Dis.* 2007;49:569-580.
4. Lambie M, Rayner HC, Bragg-Gresham J. Starting and withdrawing haemodialysis—association between nephrologists' opinions, patient characteristics and practice patterns (data from the Dialysis Outcomes and Practice Patterns Study). *Nephrol Dial Transplant.* 2006;10:2814-2820.

**PART FIVE**

# PULMONARY DISEASE

JAMES A. BARKER, MD

# 29 Critical Care Medicine

---

**Decreased Mortality Associated With Prompt Gram Staining of Blood Cultures**

Barenfanger J, Graham DR, Kolluri L, et al (Memorial Med Ctr, Springfield, IL; Springfield Clinic, IL; Southern Illinois Univ School of Medicine, Springfield, IL; et al)

*Am J Clin Pathol* 130:870-876, 2008

---

Gram stains of positive blood cultures are the most important factor influencing appropriate therapy. The sooner appropriate therapy is initiated, the better. Therefore, it is reasonable to expect that the sooner Gram stains are performed, the better. To determine the value of timely Gram stains and whether improvement in Gram stain turnaround time (TAT) is feasible, we compared data for matched pairs of patients with cultures processed promptly (<1 hour TAT) with data for patients with cultures not processed promptly (≥1 hour TAT) and then monitored TAT by control charting.

In 99 matched pairs, average difference in time to detection of positive blood cultures within a pair of patients was less than 0.1 hour. For the less than 1 hour TAT group, the average TAT and crude mortality were 0.1 hour and 10.1%, respectively; for the 1 hour or longer TAT group, they were 3.3 hours and 19.2%, respectively ($P < .0001$ and $P = .0389$, respectively). After multifaceted efforts, we achieved significant improvement in the TAT for Gram stains.

▶ As there is incredible push for appropriate therapy for each patient as fast as possible, other processes logically have to follow suit. These researchers demonstrate the very nice relationship between quality improvement, scientific inquiry, and real patient outcomes. They even randomized their study to prove that rapid Gram stain and reporting as soon as blood culture broth is positive can be associated with an improved outcome. This is quality improvement research at its best.

Given the wide range of different positive organisms seen in this study (and in real life, I think) adjustment of antibiotics to the most optimal is clearly the best we can do. Hopefully, most microbiology labs in the United States will adopt this rapid detection and reporting sequence shown in this study.

**J. A. Barker, MD**

---

**Clinical predictors of mechanical ventilation in Fisher/Guillain–Barré overlap syndrome**

Funakoshi K, Kuwabara S, Odaka M, et al (Dokkyo Med Univ, Tochigi, Japan; Chiba Univ School of Medicine, Japan)

*J Neurol Neurosurg Psychiatry* 80:60-65, 2009

---

*Background.*—Some patients with Fisher syndrome (FS) developed subsequent descending tetraparesis (Fisher/Guillain–Barré overlapping syndrome: FS/GBS). The assumption is that such descending progression may frequently lead to respiratory failure.

*Objective.*—To investigate whether patients with FS/GBS more often require artificial ventilation than those with typical GBS and which clinical and serological findings are useful predictors.

*Methods.*—Medical records were reviewed of patients who had acute ophthalmoplegia, ataxia and areflexia, as well as subsequent tetraparesis with monophasic course. Forty-five patients fulfilled the FS/GBS criteria. Clinical and serological features were analysed, and clinical predictors of mechanical ventilation were investigated.

*Results.*—FS/GBS patients more frequently required mechanical ventilation than did GBS patients (24% vs 10%, $p = 0.04$). The former also needed artificial ventilation earlier than the latter ($p = 0.03$), but none of the FS patients required it. As the initial symptom, ventilated FS/GBS patients more frequently showed titubation than non-ventilated patients (55% vs 18%, $p = 0.04$). During the course of the illness, descending tetraparesis was more common in 11 ventilated FS/GBS patients than in the other 34 non-ventilated patients (64% vs 21%, $p = 0.02$). The need for artificial ventilation was not associated with anti-GQ1b IgG antibodies, monospecific anti-GT1a IgG antibodies or IgG antibodies to various ganglioside complexes.

*Conclusions.*—FS/GBS patients significantly needed mechanical ventilation more often. Such patients showing titubation and descending tetraparesis need to be carefully monitored as the illness progresses because those clinical features are helpful predictors of respiratory failure.

▶ Here in the United States we usually think of the Miller-Fisher (MF) variant of Guillain-Barré (GB) syndrome as being an atypical presentation, which begins with early facial involvement. And with that comes a connotation that MF variant more frequently and more rapidly proceeds to respiratory failure.

These Japanese investigators point out that there is a different syndromal approach (at least in their country). The Fisher syndrome is not always part of GB. This study focuses on those patients with Fisher syndrome who also have GB and whether they indeed have a worse prognosis than patients with typical GB.

Indeed these authors found that the vast majority of patients with Fisher syndrome do not progress to GB. As a non-neurologist, this is an important epiphany. Secondly, the patients with FGB syndrome do indeed have a much increased incidence of progression to respiratory failure, and a shorter timeline to respiratory failure when compared with patients with typical GB. The monitoring implications of this are significant. These patients obviously need to be in an ICU or step down ICU.

In addition, there is an excellent discussion here of serologic markers associated with both syndromes.

**J. A. Barker, MD**

---

**Outcome and prognostic factors of lung cancer patients admitted to the medical intensive care unit**

Adam AK, Soubani AO (Division of Pulmonary, Allergy, Critical Care and Sleep Medicine, Detroit, MI; Wayne State Univ School of Medicine and Karmanos Cancer Ctr, Detroit, MI)

*Eur Respir J* 31:47-53, 2008

---

The aim of the present study was to assess the outcome of lung cancer patients who were admitted to a medical intensive care unit (MICU) and to identify the measurable predictors of their MICU outcome.

The retrospective study took place at the MICUs of a university-affiliated medical centre and involved adult lung cancer patients admitted to the MICU between January 1998 and October 2005.

A total of 139 lung cancer patients were included during the study period. The mean age ± SD at MICU admission was 64.2 ± 10.2 yrs (48% males, 52% females). In total, 96 (69%) patients had nonsmall cell lung cancer, 18 (13%) patients had small cell lung cancer, and one patient had mesothelioma. The MICU mortality was 22% (31 patients), while the in-hospital mortality was 40% (56 patients). Sixty-eight (49%) patients required mechanical ventilation (MV), with MICU mortality of 38% and in-hospital mortality of 53%. The independent predictors of poor MICU outcome were: the need for MV; Acute Physiology And Chronic Health Evaluation III and Simplified Acute Physiology Score III scores; the use of vasopressors; positive blood cultures; high serum lactate; two or more organ system failures; and the need for adult cardiac life support. On multivariate analysis, only the need for vasopressors and the presence of two or more organ system failures predicted poor MICU outcome.

The present study shows that the medical intensive care unit outcome of lung cancer patients is better than previously reported. Intensive care and mechanical ventilation should not be considered futile care in this patient population. While there were no absolute predictors of mortality, the need for vasopressors and the presence of two or more organ system failures predicted poor medical intensive care unit care.

▶ Lung cancer is extremely common. The aggressive therapy of lung cancer is also common—both by oncologists and by ourselves (interventional pulmonary). Thus a significant number of patients with lung cancer are now commonly in our ICUs. As is often the case in patients with terminal illnesses or possibly terminal illnesses, we often seek guidance from the literature for meaningful predictive models as we work with families and patients. This nice article does give useful information for this population: the ICU mortality is not much higher than the general population. Even the 1-year mortality is not bad in comparison with certain other groups such as those with very advanced age or with advanced pulmonary fibrosis.

The correlates of poor outcome are likewise useful: positive blood cultures, need for pressors, need for mechanical ventilation, and multiorgan failure are all easily measurable end points.

**J. A. Barker, MD**

**Comparison of the Glidescope® and Airtraq® optical laryngoscopes in patients undergoing direct microlaryngoscopy**

Lange M, Frommer M, Redel A, et al (Univ of Würzburg, Germany; et al)
*Anaesthesia* 64:323-328, 2009

Optical laryngoscopes have been developed to facilitate difficult airway management. The Airtraq® is a single-use device and the GlideScope® is reusable. In this study, the Airtraq and the Glidescope were compared in 60 ASA I-III patients with tumours of the upper airway undergoing direct endoscopic microlaryngoscopy. Patients were randomly assigned to the Airtraq or the Glidescope group and the Cormack and Lehane grade was assessed by Macintosh laryngoscopy prior to tracheal intubation. There were no differences in tracheal intubation success rates or duration of intubation attempts between both devices. The Cormack and Lehane grade was improved in 77% and 82% of cases in the Airtraq and Glidescope group, respectively. Blood traces on the device and traumatic pharyngeal lesions were found more frequently in the Airtraq group. The Airtraq and Glidescope laryngoscopes are valuable tools for the management of patients with potentially difficult airways with the Glidescope appearing to be less traumatic (Figs 1 and 2).

▶ We began using a Glidescope 2 years ago. Looking back, I can't imagine how I practiced critical care without it for the past 20 years! In particular, it is a fantastic tool for both teaching and enhancing patient safety. No longer

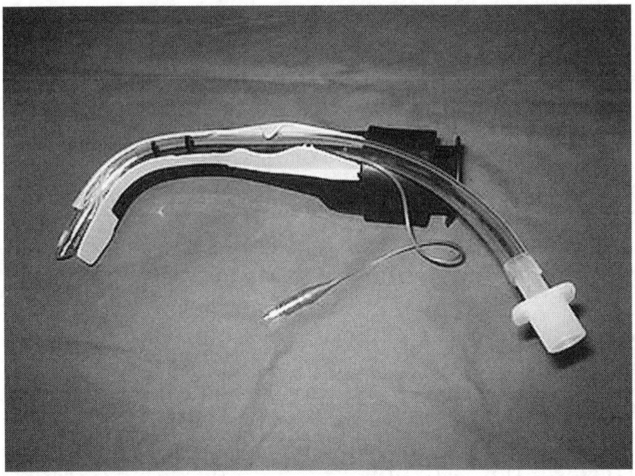

**FIGURE 1.**—The Airtraq optical laryngoscope with tracheal tube inserted in the adjacent channel. (Reprinted from Lange M, Frommer M, Redel A, et al. Comparison of the Glidescope® and Airtraq® optical laryngoscopes in patients undergoing direct microlaryngoscopy. *Anaesthesia.* 2009;64:323-328, with permission from John Wiley & Sons, Inc.)

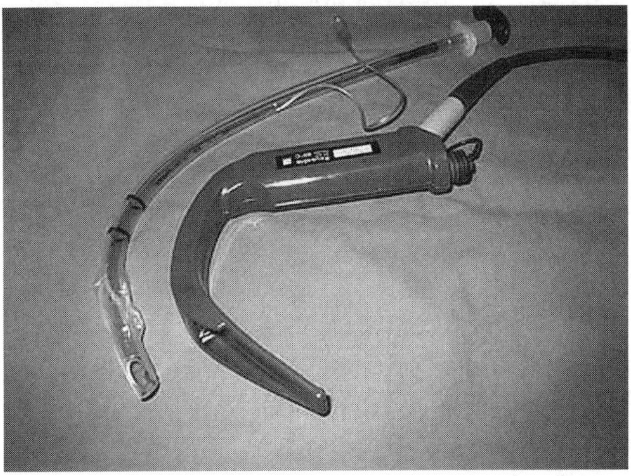

**FIGURE 2.**—The Glidescope video laryngoscope with tracheal tube and rigid stylet. (Reprinted from Lange M, Frommer M, Redel A, et al. Comparison of the Glidescope® and Airtraq® optical laryngoscopes in patients undergoing direct microlaryngoscopy. *Anaesthesia.* 2009;64:323-328, with permission from John Wiley & Sons, Inc.)

does one have to watch a trainee struggle, all the while feeling your own pulse rise as the Oxygen Saturation plummets. With this instrument, we can see the airway and larynx, and give directions to the trainee all in real time and with a real view. In addition, the Miller and Mac blade features are combined to give the best of all possibilities.

These authors demonstrate the efficacy of both devices in the most difficult of patients: those with upper airway tumors. The Glidescope intubation rate was 100%—enough said!

**J. A. Barker, MD**

---

**Efficacy of an expanded ventilator bundle for the reduction of ventilator-associated pneumonia in the medical intensive care unit**

Blamoun J, Alfakir M, Rella ME, et al (Seton Hall Univ, South Orange, NJ; Mt Sinai School of Medicine, NY; St Joseph's Regional Med Ctr, Paterson NJ)
*Am J Infect Control* 37:172-175, 2009

---

The ventilator bundle (VB) includes a group of clinical maneuvers (head-of-bed elevation, "sedation vacation," deep vein thrombosis prophylaxis, and peptic ulcer disease prophylaxis) to improve outcomes in patients undergoing mechanical ventilation. We modified the standard VB in our medical intensive care unit to include a group of respiratory therapist–driven protocols and, postimplementation, observed a statistically significant ($P = .0006$) reduction in ventilator-associated pneumonia (VAP), from a median of 14.1 cases/$10^3$ ventilator-days (interquartile range [IQR] = 12.1 to 20.6) to 0 cases/$10^3$ ventilator-days (IQR = 0 to 1.1) (Figs 1 and 2).

▶ Ventilator-associated pneumonia (VAP) is a big problem among our very ill, high acuity ICU patients of today. Previous approaches were really quite

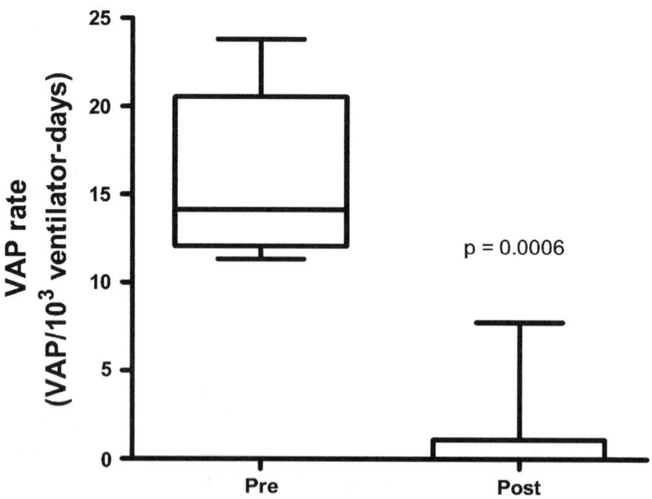


FIGURE 1.—Box-and-whisker plot of VAP rates preintervention and postintervention. (Reprinted from Blamoun J, Alfakir M, Rella ME, et al. Efficacy of an expanded ventilator bundle for the reduction of ventilator-associated pneumonia in the medical intensive care unit. *Am J Infect Control*. 2009;37:172-175.)

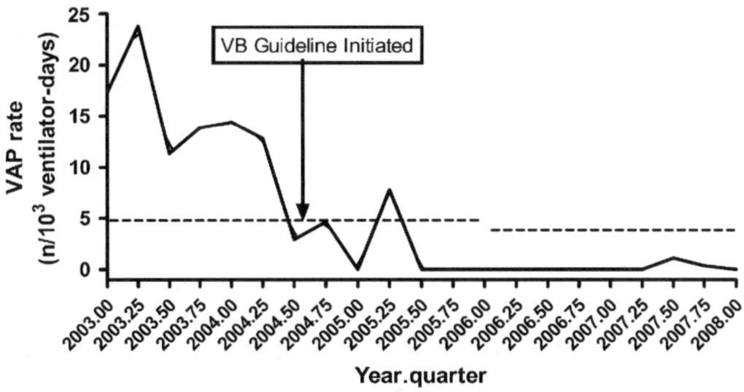


FIGURE 2.—Change in VAP rates after implementation of VB guidelines. Dotted lines indicate the national average of VAP for the indicated periods (2003 to 2006: 4.97 VAP/103 ventilator-days; 2006 to present: 3.6 VAP/103 ventilator-days). (Reprinted from Blamoun J, Alfakir M, Rella ME, et al. Efficacy of an expanded ventilator bundle for the reduction of ventilator-associated pneumonia in the medical intensive care unit. *Am J Infect Control.* 2009;37:172-175.)

nihilistic. This article, as have many others, demonstrates just how good the results can be with following a detailed plan to eradicate all possible risk. I very much like how they have displayed their data in Figs 1 and 2. The box and whisker plot in Fig 1 not only shows the significant data change, but the large distance between the 2 sets of data makes the magnitude of change very obvious. This is great work!

One quibble with the title: I don't know that this is truly an expanded VAP bundle so much as an optimized one. The authors have a central line bundle, nosocomial infection prevention plan, and an enforced, aggressive VAP bundle. Semantics aside, the results speak for themselves.

**J. A. Barker, MD**

---

**The Removal of Chest Tubes Despite an Air Leak or a Pneumothorax**

Cerfolio RJ, Minnich DJ, Bryant AS (Univ of Alabama at Birmingham)

*Ann Thorac Surg* 87:1690-1696, 2009

---

*Background.*—The presence of an air leak is currently a contraindication for removal of a chest tube. The objective of this series was to evaluate the safety of chest tube removal in patients with an air leak.

*Methods.*—This study was a retrospective cohort study of a prospective database. Patients who underwent elective pulmonary resection and were discharged home with a chest tube were eligible.

*Results.*—Between July 2000 and July 2007, 6,038 patients underwent elective pulmonary resection by one general thoracic surgeon. One hundred and ninety-nine patients (3.8%) with a persistent air leak had their chest tubes placed to a suctionless portable drainage device and were discharged home. One hundred ninety-four patients (97%) returned to our clinic (median, postdischarge day 16). One hundred thirty-seven patients had no air leak, and 57 patients still had an air leak. All 137 patients (including 26 with a nonexpanding pneumothorax) had their chest tubes removed. In addition, all 57 patients (including 19 who had pneumothorax as well) had their chest tubes removed without sequela (9 after provocative clamping). At 3 months' follow-up, all patients were asymptomatic without evidence of pleural space problems, except 3 (all in the persistent air leak group) in whom an empyema developed.

*Conclusions.*—Patients with air leaks can be safely discharged home with their chest tubes. These tubes can be safely removed even if the patients have a pneumothorax, if the following criteria are met: the patients have been asymptomatic, have no subcutaneous emphysema after 14 days on a portable device at home, and the pleural space deficit has not increased in size.

▶ This is an important and thought-provoking article. I encourage everyone to read it.

The problem of a persistent postoperative pneumothorax is a common one, yet there is little good data to support our common practices. These authors give us some very practical guidelines for dealing with these patients. We commonly send these same patients home with Heimlich valves or bulb syringe. These guidelines will make us comfortable with removing the tubes after an appropriate time out of the hospital. These authors pull them even with leak—but with no pneumothorax and after several days of suction.

**J. A. Barker, MD**

---

**Early physical and occupational therapy in mechanically ventilated, critically ill patients: a randomised controlled trial**

Schweickert WD, Pohlman MC, Pohlman AS, et al (Univ of Pennsylvania, Philadelphia; Univ of Chicago, IL; et al)

*Lancet* 373:1874-1882, 2009

---

*Background.*—Long-term complications of critical illness include intensive care unit (ICU)-acquired weakness and neuropsychiatric disease. Immobilisation secondary to sedation might potentiate these problems. We assessed the efficacy of combining daily interruption of sedation with physical and occupational therapy on functional outcomes in patients receiving mechanical ventilation in intensive care.

*Methods.*—Sedated adults (≥18 years of age) in the ICU who had been on mechanical ventilation for less than 72 h, were expected to continue for at least 24 h, and who met criteria for baseline functional independence were eligible for enrolment in this randomised controlled trial at two university hospitals. We randomly assigned 104 patients by computer-generated, permuted block randomisation to early exercise and mobilisation (physical and occupational therapy) during periods of daily interruption of sedation (intervention; n = 49) or to daily interruption of sedation with therapy as ordered by the primary care team (control; n = 55). The primary endpoint—the number of patients returning to independent functional status at hospital discharge—was defined as the ability to perform six activities of daily living and the ability to walk independently. Therapists who undertook patient assessments were blinded to treatment assignment. Secondary endpoints included duration of delirium and ventilator-free days during the first 28 days of hospital stay. Analysis was by intention to treat. This trial is registered with ClinicalTrials.gov, number NCT00322010.

*Findings.*—All 104 patients were included in the analysis. Return to independent functional status at hospital discharge occurred in 29 (59%) patients in the intervention group compared with 19 (35%) patients in the control group (p = 0·02; odds ratio 2·7 [95% CI 1·2–6·1]). Patients in the intervention group had shorter duration of delirium (median 2·0 days, IQR 0·0–6·0 vs 4·0 days, 2·0–8·0; p = 0·02), and more ventilator-free days (23·5 days, 7·4–25·6 *vs* 21·1 days, 0·0–23·8; p = 0·05) during the 28-day follow-up period than did controls. There was one serious adverse event in 498 therapy sessions (desaturation less than 80%). Discontinuation of therapy as a result of patient instability occurred in 19 (4%) of all sessions, most commonly for perceived patient-ventilator asynchrony.

*Interpretation.*—A strategy for whole-body rehabilitation—consisting of interruption of sedation and physical and occupational therapy in the earliest days of critical illness—was safe and well tolerated, and resulted in better functional outcomes at hospital discharge, a shorter duration of delirium, and more ventilator-free days compared with standard care.

► I applaud the investigators for this important study. A randomized controlled trial of standardized OT (occupational therapy) and PT (physical therapy) coupled with sedation interruption has to be inherently difficult (and obviously was because only 10% of those screened were entered into the study). The improvement in delirium severity and length is particularly important. I would guess that the expense of intense OT/PT therapy in ill, ventilated patients is probably less than the expense for medications and sitters for those with persistent delirium in ICU or even after discharge from ICU. Table 3 in the original article outlines all of the other significant outcomes. The marked difference in functional status at the time of discharge is impressive as well.

We have had a similar process in place for a couple of years. This study gives credence to the approach and some practical framework for others to follow.

**J. A. Barker, MD**

**Critical care checklists, the Keystone Project, and the Office for Human Research Protections: A case for streamlining the approval process in quality-improvement research**

Savel RH, Goldstein EB, Gropper MA (Montefiore Med Ctr, Bronx, NY; Maimonides Med Ctr, Brooklyn, NY; Univ of California San Francisco School of Medicine (UCSF))

*Crit Care Med* 37:725-728, 2009

Checklists have been recently promulgated as a method to enhance patient safety and improve outcomes for critically ill patients. Specifically, recent work performed by researchers from the Johns Hopkins Medical Institutions has demonstrated that the addition of checklists to usual care in the intensive care unit is associated with a decrease in the incidence of catheter-related bloodstream infections. Initially evaluated at the institutional level, this effort has been successfully expanded to the state level as part of the Michigan Keystone Project. Although this work has recently received significant positive attention in the lay press, the Office for Human Research Protections—as they felt that this was a research project requiring Institutional Review Board approval and informed consent—put the data collection on hold for lack of approval by the Institutional Review Board at the participating hospitals in Michigan as well as for not having obtained informed consent from each patient and clinician involved in the project. This article documents the recent events surrounding the Keystone Project and the response to the actions taken by the Office for Human Research Protections in the lay press and the new media (Internet and blogs), articulates how a determination can be made if a project is quality-improvement, human-subjects research, or both, and proposes some solutions to create a structured approach to this kind of research in the future.

► Our institution, Palmetto Richland Hospital, adopted the Pronovost ICU checklist in 2004 (which he and IHI distribute free of charge on the IHI Web site). Several immediate, tangible benefits were realized: infection rates markedly dropped, nurses showed improved job satisfaction and retention, respiratory therapy and nursing became teammates and traveler respiratory therapists (RTs) were no longer needed, and most importantly, patient mortality dropped.

The spread of the central line bundle and checklist in Michigan (Keystone project) is one of the most important critical care public health projects ever published. No one can argue that reducing ICU central line infections in an entire state from following a simple algorithm as outlined in the project is not fantastic and noteworthy. The sticky issues of what is research and what is quality improvement are important ones. Clearly, we must follow the tenets of patient confidentiality. Does every single patient need to give consent when quality improvement produces good results and needs to be shared in the scientific world? I don't think so.

The authors herein review these issues in detail. It is well worth reading.

**J. A. Barker, MD**

# 30 Lung Cancer

**Counseling and Interventions to Prevent Tobacco Use and Tobacco-Caused Disease in Adults and Pregnant Women: U.S. Preventive Services Task Force Reaffirmation Recommendation Statement**

U.S. Preventive Services Task Force

*Ann Intern Med* 150:551-555, 2009

*Description.*—Reaffirmation of the 2003 U.S. Preventive Services Task Force (USPSTF) recommendation on counseling to prevent tobacco use.

*Methods.*—The USPSTF reviewed new evidence in the U.S. Public Health Service's 2008 clinical practice guideline and determined that the net benefits of tobacco cessation interventions in adults and pregnant women remain well established.

*Recommendations.*—Ask all adults about tobacco use and provide tobacco cessation interventions for those who use tobacco products. (Grade A recommendation).

Ask all pregnant women about tobacco use and provide augmented, pregnancy-tailored counseling for those who smoke. (Grade A recommendation).

▶ This clinical guideline from the United States Preventive Services Task Force reiterates the need for clinicians to query all adult patients, particularly pregnant women, about tobacco use and to provide and facilitate smoking cessation interventions. It is clear that physicians are a powerful influence on patients' smoking behaviors, and even a few minutes of focused counseling make a difference. Use of pharmacotherapy is often beneficial and necessary to facilitate abstinence from nicotine, with the pharmacologic armamentarium now including 3 therapeutic options: nicotine replacement, bupropion, and varenicline. Assessment of an individual patient's ability to successfully quit should include an examination of social networks. Smoking behaviors are clustered; smoking cessation by a spouse has been reported to decrease an individual's chances of smoking by 67%, and it seems intuitive that smoking persistence by a spouse will adversely affect an individual's chances of successful abstinence.[1] Similarly, the smoking status of other social contacts will influence continuation or cessation and will need to be given consideration in counseling.

In 1964, at the time of the first Surgeon General's report on Smoking and Health, over 70% of American adult men were smoking.[2] At present, approximately 21% of all American adult men and women still smoke despite widespread appreciation of its morbidity.[3] That percentage has been relatively flat over the last few years; decreasing the numbers of smokers will require even more intense effort, in which physicians will play a key role.

**L. T. Tanoue, MD**

*References*

1. Christakis NA, Fowler JH. The collective dynamics of smoking in a large social network. *N Engl J Med.* 2008;358:2249-2258.
2. US Public Health Service. *Smoking and Health. Report of the Advisory committee to the Surgeon General of the Public Health Service, Publication No.1103.* Washington, DC: US Department of Health, Education, and Welfare, Public Health Service; 1964.
3. Maurice E, Trosclair A, Merritt R, et al. Cigarette smoking among adults—United States, 2004. *MMWR Morb Mortal Wkly Rep.* 2005;54:1121-1124.

## Data from The Society of Thoracic Surgeons General Thoracic Surgery database: The surgical management of primary lung tumors

Boffa DJ, Allen MS, Grab JD, et al (Cleveland Clinic, OH; Mayo Clinic School of Medicine, Rochester, MN; Duke Univ, Durham, NC; et al)
*J Thorac Cardiovasc Surg* 135:247-254, 2008

*Objective.*—Our objective was to investigate the surgical management of primary lung cancer by board-certified thoracic surgeons participating in the general thoracic surgery portion of The Society of Thoracic Surgeons database.

*Methods.*—We identified all pulmonary resections recorded in the general thoracic surgery prospective database from 1999 to 2006. Among the 49,029 recorded operations, 9033 pulmonary resections for primary lung cancer were analyzed.

*Results.*—There were 4539 men and 4494 women with a median age of 67 years (range 20–94 years). Comorbidity affected 79% of patients and included hypertension in 66%, coronary artery disease in 26%, body mass index of 30 kg/m$^2$ or more in 25.7%, and diabetes mellitus in 13%. The type of resection was a wedge resection in 1649 (18.1%), segmentectomy in 394 (4.4%), lobectomy in 6042 (67%), bilobectomy in 357 (4.0%), and pneumonectomy in 591 (6.5%). Mediastinal lymph nodes were evaluated in 5879 (65%) patients; via mediastinoscopy in 1928 (21%), nodal dissection 3722 (41%), nodal sampling in 1124 (12.4%), and nodal biopsy in 729 (8%). Median length of stay was 5 days (range 0–277 days). Operative mortality was 2.5% (179 patients). One or more postoperative events occurred in 2911 (32%) patients.

*Conclusion.*—The patients in the general thoracic surgery database are elderly, gender balanced, and afflicted by multiple comorbid conditions. Mediastinal lymph node evaluation is common and the pneumonectomy

TABLE 7.—All Databases Compared

| | STS Data (Current Study) | CCACS Survey (Little et al[2]) | NIS Dataset (Mequid et al[18]) | SEER–Medicare Database and NIS (Bach et al[1]) | NSQIP (Harpole et al[17]) | NHDS (Memtsoudis et al[15]) |
|---|---|---|---|---|---|---|
| Years | 1999–2006 | 2001 | 1998–2003 | 1985–1996 | 1991–1995 | 1988–2002 |
| Mortality defined | Hospital or 30-d | 30-d | Hospital mortality | 30-d | 30-d | Hospital mortality |
| Total resections | 9033 | 11,668 | 50,867 | 2118 | 3,516 | 512,758 |
| All resections | 2.5% (7859) | 5.2% (11,668) | 3.8% | 4% | NA | 4.8% |
| Lobectomy | 2% (5234) | 4.5% (7,869) | 3.3% | NA | 4.0% (2949) | NA |
| Bilobectomy | 4% (322) | NA | NA | NA | NA | NA |
| Pneumonectomy | 6.2% (512) | 8.5% (1,507) | 9.4% | NA | 11.5% (567) | NA |
| Segmentectomy | 2.9% (347) | NA | 3.3% | NA | NA | NA |
| Wedge resection | 2.7% (1,425) | 4.9% (1,737) | NA | NA | NA | NA |
| Median LOS (d) | 5 | | | 9 | | 10.8 (1–358) |

*STS*, The Society of Thoracic Surgeons; *CCACS*, Commission on Cancer of the American College of Surgeons; *NIS*, Nationwide Inpatient Sample; *SEER*, Surveillance Epidemiology and End Results; *NSQIP*, National Veterans Affairs Quality Improvement Program; *NHDS*, National Hospital Discharge Survey; *NA*, not available; *LOS*, length of stay.

rate is low. The length of stay is short and operative mortality is low, despite frequent postoperative events (Table 7).

▶ The Society of Thoracic Surgeons (STS) maintains a prospective database of patients undergoing cardiothoracic surgery. Submission to the database is voluntary; 97% of the 225 surgeons contributing data are board-certified thoracic surgeons. This report examines the 9033 pulmonary resections in the database performed for lung cancer from 1999 through 2006; 66% were lobectomies and 6.5% were pneumonectomies. The database confirmed previous observations that, as a group, patients undergoing lung cancer surgery have a high prevalence of other medical problems. Seventy-nine percent of patients had at least one comorbid medical condition, the most common of which were hypertension (66%), coronary artery disease (26%), and diabetes (13%). Thirty-two percent of patients experienced at least 1 postoperative complication, the most frequent of which were atrial arrhythmia requiring intervention (10.7%), prolonged air leak > 7 days (8%), pneumonia (3.9%), atelectasis requiring bronchoscopy (3.6%), and reintubation (3.4%). Video-assisted thoracoscopic surgery (VATS) was performed in 20% of patients undergoing lobectomy. Despite the preexisting comorbidities and frequent postoperative complications, mortality was remarkably low. Hospital and 30-day mortality for lobectomy and pneuomonectomy were 2% and 6.2%, respectively, lower than all other large surveys for lung cancer surgeries performed in a similar time period (Table 7). Further, median length of stay was only 5 days, compared to 9 days reported in comparable large studies.[1,2]

These impressive findings from the STS database merit consideration as to the reasons that such favorable results can be obtained in a population of medically complicated patients with lung cancer. Factors contributing to improved outcomes for lung cancer surgery commonly cited in other reports include larger hospital volume, and specialty training and experience of the surgeon.[1,3,4] This report reinforces the conclusion that, whenever feasible, lung cancer surgery should be performed by thoracic specialty-trained surgeons at high volume centers.

**L. T. Tanoue, MD**

*References*

1. Bach PB, Cramer LD, Schrag D, Downey RJ, Gelfand SE, Begg CB. The influence of hospital volume on survival after resection for lung cancer. *N Engl J Med.* 2001; 345:181-188.
2. Memtsoudis SG, Besculides MC, Zellos L, Patil N, Rogers SO. Trends in lung surgery: United States 1988 to 2002. *Chest.* 2006;130:1462-1470.
3. Silvestri GA, Handy J, Lackland D, Corley E, Reed CE. Specialists achieve better outcomes than generalists for lung cancer surgery. *Chest.* 1998;114:675-680.
4. Birkmeyer JD, Stukel TA, Siewers AE, Goodney PP, Wennberg DE, Lucas FL. Surgeon volume and operative mortality in the United States. *N Engl J Med.* 2003;349:2117-2127.

**Survival after Surgery in Stage IA and IB Non–Small Cell Lung Cancer**

Ost D, Goldberg J, Rolnitzky L, et al (New York Univ School of Medicine)

*Am J Respir Crit Care Med* 177:516-523, 2008

*Rationale.*—Whether histologic subtype of non–small cell lung cancer (NSCLC) has an important effect on prognosis after surgery is unknown.

*Objectives.*—We hypothesized that we could predict mortality more effectively by integrating precise tumor size and histology rather than relying on conventional staging.

*Methods.*—We used the SEER (Surveillance, Epidemiology, and End Results) registry. Inclusion criteria were as follows: (*1*) primary squamous cell or adenocarcinoma; (*2*) potentially curative surgery, defined as a lobectomy or bilobectomy; (*3*) lymph node dissection performed; and (*4*) pathologic stage IA or IB.

*Measurements and Main Results.*—From 1988 to 2000, 7,965 patients were included. For both all-cause and lung cancer–associated mortality, tumor size demonstrated the strongest association (log-rank $P < 0.0001$ for each). When tumors were small ($\leq 2$ cm), lung cancer–associated mortality was similar for adenocarcinoma when compared with squamous cell carcinoma. When tumors were 3 cm or larger in size, lung cancer–associated mortality was higher for adenocarcinoma. The increased risk of lung cancer–associated mortality with adenocarcinoma was more pronounced in those younger than 65 years. Survival prediction using precise size and histology had much better discriminatory power than conventional TNM (tumor-node-metastasis) staging ($P = 0.005$).

*Conclusions.*—Staging that takes into account size, histology, late recurrence risk, and patient age is more accurate than the current TNM system and is clinically relevant because improved prediction can facilitate better decisions on the use of adjuvant chemotherapy (Fig 1).

► This study by Ost and colleagues examined the effect of histology (adenocarcinoma vs squamous cell carcinoma), age, and tumor size on survival after curative resection for stage IA and IB nonsmall cell lung cancer (NSCLC). The study population included patients in the Surveillance, Epidemiology, and End Results (SEER) database between 1998 to 2000 with stage IA and IB NSCLC. Fig 1 demonstrates the major findings. Fig 1A demonstrates that tumor size, divided into 6 categories varying from <1 cm to >5 cm, affects outcome, with larger size associated with worse survival. This observation mirrors the large study performed by the International Association for the Study of Lung Cancer (IASLC) for the revision of the T descriptor in the new edition of the tumor-node metastasis (TNM) staging system.[1] Survival according to tumor size and histology are demonstrated in Fig 1C (squamous cell carcinoma) and 1D (adenocarcinoma). There was a significant difference in survival according to histology in patients with larger tumors; adenocarcinomas were associated with significantly higher mortality for tumors >3 cm and <4 cm (log-rank $P = .017$) and >4 cm (log-rank $P = .016$). This difference was particularly evident after 24 months and was felt to be related to late

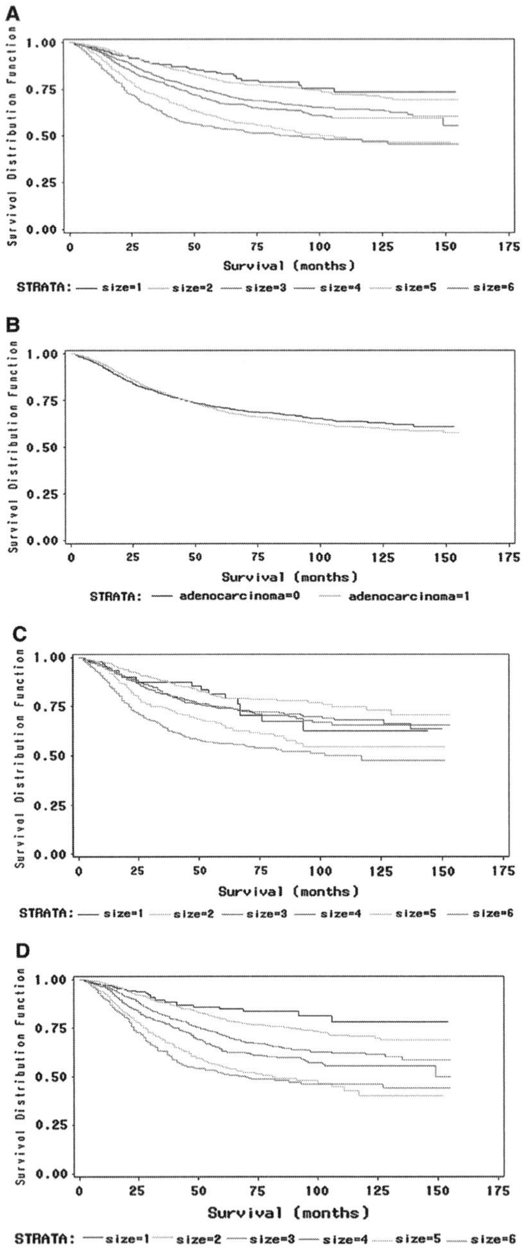


FIGURE 1.—Kaplan-Meier curves for mortality due to lung cancer in patients postlobectomy (*A*) according to size (log-rank $p < 0.0001$) and (*B*) according to histology, either adenocarcinoma (*red*) or squamous cell carcinoma (*black*). (*C*) Classified according to size for squamous cell carcinoma (log-rank $P < 0.0001$). (*D*) Classified according to size for adenocarcinomas (log-rank $P < 0.0001$). For interpretation of the references to color in this figure legend, the reader is referred to web version of this article. (Reprinted from Ost D, Goldberg J, Rolnitzky L, et al. Survival after surgery in stage IA and IB non–small cell lung cancer. *Am J Respir Crit Care Med.* 2008;177:516-523, with permission from the American Thoracic Society.)

recurrences. The authors concluded that, for this specific subset of patients with surgically treated Stage IA and IB NSCLC, staging according to tumor size and histology was more accurate in predicting survival than the standard TNM system.

The findings of this study are interesting as histology is becoming a major discriminator in the treatment of many patients with NSCLC. Tumor type is not included in the TNM staging system, which even in its new edition continues to be based on anatomic descriptors.[2] Other methods of evaluation, including molecular biomarkers, are needed to improve our ability to distinguish subgroups of patients within the same NSCLC stage who are destined to have different outcomes.[3] With particular reference to the population examined in this study, the ability to identify those patients with Stage I and II NSCLC at high risk of lung cancer relapse after surgical resection would have enormous clinical relevance, as that would provide an opportunity to intervene with adjuvant treatment to prevent late recurrence.

**L. T. Tanoue, MD**

*References*

1. Rami-Porta R, Ball D, Crowley J, et al. The IASLC Lung Cancer Staging Project: proposals for the revision of the T descriptors in the forthcoming (seventh) edition of the TNM classification for lung cancer. *J Thorac Oncol.* 2007;2:593-602.
2. Detterbeck FC, Boffa DJ, Tanoue LT. The new lung cancer staging system. *Chest.* 2009;136:260-271.
3. Herbst RS, Lippman SM. Molecular signatures of lung cancer–toward personalized therapy. *N Engl J Med.* 2007;356:76-78.

## Validation of a Model to Predict Perioperative Mortality from Lung Cancer Resection in the Elderly

Kates M, Perez X, Gribetz J, et al (Mount Sinai School of Medicine, NY; et al)
*Am J Respir Crit Care Med* 179:390-395, 2009

*Rationale.*—Surgical resection is the mainstay therapy for localized non–smallcell lung cancer (NSCLC), yet elderly patients are less likely to be treated due to concerns about morbidity and mortality related to surgery.

*Objectives.*—To validate and refine a clinical model to predict 30-day perioperative mortality (POM) in elderly patients undergoing curative resection for lung cancer.

*Methods.*—We identified 14,297 patients aged 65 years and older with stage I, II, or IIIA NCSLC from the Surveillance, Epidemiology, and End-Results Registry linked to Medicare claims. We used logistic regression analysis to identify independent risk factors for POM and to validate and refine a previously derived prediction model.

*Measurements and Main Results.*—Overall, POM was 4.6% (95% confidence interval, 4.2–4.9%). Multiple regression analysis revealed that greater age, male sex, resections of multiple lobes, advanced stage, greater tumor size, and certain comorbidities were associated with increased risk for POM. These risk factors were similar to those observed in the prior model. When patients were stratified according to their predicted risk of POM, the observed mortality increased from 1.2 to more than 10%.

*Conclusions.*—Among elderly patients with lung cancer, a prediction rule can identify those patients at higher risk for fatal complications from surgery. Further studies should evaluate whether use of the model can lead to improvements in treatment decision making.

▶ Surgical resection is the treatment of choice for patients with stage Ia non-small cell lung cancer (NSCLC), and it remains an integral part of first line treatment for all early-stage patients (stages I and II). Perioperative mortality related to resection is an important concern in all patients, but it is particularly important in the elderly. Lung cancer is largely a disease of older persons; the median age at diagnosis of 69 years is likely to rise as the population ages.[1] It is therefore reasonable that concerns related to performing major chest surgery in older individuals often arise. It is important to recognize the importance of surgery in the treatment of early-stage NSCLC, and decisions to operate or not should be guided whenever possible by evidence. This report by Kates and colleagues builds on a previous model predicting perioperative mortality in an older population undergoing lung cancer resection.[2] The authors developed a multivariable logistic regression model using the Surveillance, Epidemiology, and End Results (SEER)-Medicare database, examining 30-day perioperative mortality (POM) in patients over the age of 65 who are undergoing surgical resection for early-stage lung cancer. Factors associated with worse outcomes included increasing age, male sex, multilobe resection (bilobectomy or pneumonectomy), tumor size > 5 cm, higher stage, and higher comorbidity score. Overall, 30-day POM in the entire population was 4.6%. When stratified by the predictive model, patients in the lowest and highest quintiles of risk demonstrated 30-day POMs of 1.2% and over 10%, respectively.

This model is an important contribution to our ability to more accurately predict perioperative risk. It complements other evaluations performed in patients for whom lung resection is being considered – typically algorithms used to anticipate postoperative pulmonary function.[3,4] The identification of low risk should provide support for pursuing potentially curative surgery in an older patient. Conversely, identification of high risk may be useful in specific planning for the care of older patients pre- and post-operatively, or in counseling high-risk older patients about alternatives to surgical treatment. The model is limited in that it does not provide information about quality of life after surgical resection for lung cancer, an important parameter for which prediction is poorly defined. Further work enhancing our ability to stratify risk for perioperative mortality and to predict postoperative quality of life is necessary to improve our care of lung cancer patients.

**L. T. Tanoue, MD**

*References*

1. Wingo PA, Cardinez CJ, Landis SH, et al. Long-term trends in cancer mortality in the United States, 1930–1998. *Cancer.* 2003;97:3133-3275.
2. Strand TE, Rostad H, Møller B, Norstein J. Survival after resection for primary lung cancer: a population based study of 3211 resected patients. *Thorax.* 2006; 61:710-715.
3. Colice GL, Shafazand S, Griffin JP, et al. American College of Chest Physicians. Physiologic evaluation of the patient with lung cancer being considered for resectional surgery: ACCP evidenced-based clinical practice guidelines (2nd edition). *Chest.* 2007;132:161S-177S.
4. Wyser C, Stulz P, Solèr M, et al. Prospective evaluation of an algorithm for the functional assessment of lung resection candidates. *Am J Respir Crit Care Med.* 1999;159:1450-1456.

## Trends in End-of Life ICU Use Among Older Adults With Advanced Lung Cancer

Sharma G, Freeman J, Zhang D, et al (Univ of Texas Med Branch, Galveston)
*Chest* 133:72-78, 2008

*Background.*—There is increasing concern about the appropriateness of intensive medical care near the end of life in ICUs throughout the United States. As a result of hospice expansion in the 1990s, we hypothesized that ICU use decreased over time in older adults with advanced lung cancer.

*Methods.*—Retrospective analysis using the linked Surveillance, Epidemiology and End Results Medicare database. There were 45,627 Medicare beneficiaries ≥ 66 years of age with confirmed stage IIIB or IV lung cancer between January 1, 1992, and December 31, 2002, who died within a year of their cancer diagnosis from 1993 through 2002.

*Results.*—ICU use in the last 6 months of life increased from 17.5% in 1993 to 24.7% in 2002 ($p < 0.001$). After adjusting for patient characteristics, there was a 6.6% annual increase in ICU use from 1993 to 2002. During the same period, hospice use had risen from 28.8 to 49.9% ($p < 0.001$). A total of 6.2% of patients received both end-of-life ICU care and hospice care, a percentage that increased over time. The total health-care cost for Medicare fee-for-service patients during last 6 months was $40,929 for ICU users and $27,160 for non-ICU users ($p < 0.001$).

*Conclusion.*—Despite increasing hospice use, ICU utilization among older adults dying with advanced lung cancer continued to rise in the United States during the 1990s.

▶ Rising health care costs create an imperative for examination of medical services that appear to disproportionately consume dollars. End-of-life intensive care unit (ICU) care in the Medicare population is an area that has clearly been identified as such. This retrospective study by Sharma and colleagues examines end-of-life ICU care in the Medicare population with advanced lung cancer (stage IIIb or IV), utilizing the linked Surveillance, Epidemiology, and End Results (SEER)-Medicare database. In the Medicare population during the period 1992-2002, ICU use in the last 6 months of life increased from 17.5% to 24.7%. Hospice use rose from 28.8% to 49.9%, with a median duration of hospice care of 15 days. Chemotherapy use increased from 26.8% to 33.3%, with ICU use in the chemotherapy group also increasing from 20.7% to 24.2%. In the context of the time period of the study, these observations likely reflect a number of factors, including the development of platinum-based chemotherapy as standard first-line therapy, a wider appreciation that survival can be improved with chemotherapy even in advanced-stage disease, and a growing acceptance of hospice services across the country, within the context that our ability to accurately predict outcomes in a seriously ill population is still poor.

The commensurate increase in end-of-life ICU care and hospice use was contrary to the authors' original hypothesis that the growth of the hospice movement would decrease ICU utilization over time. Perhaps this seeming contradiction actually makes sense. The clinical trajectory of the study population (Fig 2 in the original article) demonstrates that more than half (58.7%) of ICU hospitalized patients with advanced lung cancer were discharged alive, and of these, more than half were discharged home. Their median survival after discharge was 50 days, during which nearly half (48.7%) were enrolled in Hospice care. A number of factors could be postulated to contribute to these findings. First, treatment for advanced lung cancer has improved. Longer expected cancer survival may contribute to a more aggressive approach with medical interventions overall, including critical care. Second, older patients with lung cancer are likely to have comorbid medical conditions that may be more likely to decompensate in the setting of cancer treatment, but are also likely to improve with intensive care. In fact, in this study, 38.1% of ICU users as well as 26.2% of non-ICU users had 3 or more hospitalizations in the last 6 months of life, implying that most of these hospitalizations had reversible causes. Third, the critical care setting often precipitates end-of-life discussions that may not previously have occurred. The paradox of the ICU physician advocating limitation of ICU care, including changing the goals of care to comfort in a hospice model, is actually a rational one.

The issue of the cost of health care in the last 6 months of life is real and pressing. Clearly, it is not limited to patients with advanced lung cancer. As treatments for lung cancer continue to evolve and improve this issue is likely to become even more complicated. Addressing this challenging area will require more study focused on improving our ability to predict both cancer and ICU outcomes more accurately, educating health care providers and patients in the benefits and limitations of cancer and ICU care, and examining quality of life during terminal illness.

**L. T. Tanoue, MD**

**Cannabis use and risk of lung cancer: a case–control study**

Aldington S, on behalf of the Cannabis and Respiratory Disease Research Group (Med Res Inst of New Zealand, Wellington; et al)

*Eur Respir J* 31:280-286, 2008

The aim of the present study was to determine the risk of lung cancer associated with cannabis smoking.

A case–control study of lung cancer in adults ≤55 yrs of age was conducted in eight district health boards in New Zealand. Cases were identified from the New Zealand Cancer Registry and hospital databases. Controls were randomly selected from the electoral roll, with frequency matching to cases in 5-yr age groups and district health boards. Interviewer-administered questionnaires were used to assess possible risk factors, including cannabis use. The relative risk of lung cancer associated with cannabis smoking was estimated by logistic regression.

In total, 79 cases of lung cancer and 324 controls were included in the study. The risk of lung cancer increased 8% (95% confidence interval (CI) 2–15) for each joint-yr of cannabis smoking, after adjustment for confounding variables including cigarette smoking, and 7% (95% CI 5–9) for each pack-yr of cigarette smoking, after adjustment for confounding variables including cannabis smoking. The highest tertile of cannabis use was associated with an increased risk of lung cancer (relative risk 5.7 (95% CI 1.5–21.6)), after adjustment for confounding variables including cigarette smoking.

In conclusion, the results of the present study indicate that long-term cannabis use increases the risk of lung cancer in young adults (Table 3).

▶ Cannabis (marijuana) smoke has been demonstrated to induce oncogenic changes in cell lines, and like cigarette smoke is known to contain carcinogenic polyaromatic hydrocarbons.[1] Cannabis tends to be smoked more intensely, with deeper inhalation and longer breathhold, than usual tobacco cigarettes. This behavior results in greater absorption of carbon monoxide from a cannabis joint than a tobacco cigarette, and plausibly may increase exposure of the respiratory tract to carcinogens present in cannabis smoke.[2] In this case-control

TABLE 3.—Cannabis Use and Tobacco Use, as Continuous Variables, and Risk of Lung Cancer

| Characteristic | RR of Lung Cancer | 95% CI |
|---|---|---|
| Pack-yr of cigarette smoking# | 1.07 | 1.05–1.09 |
| Joint-yr of cannabis smoking¶ | 1.08 | 1.02–1.15 |
| Joint-yrs to 5 yrs prior to diagnosis+ | 1.10 | 1.02–1.18 |

RR: relative risk; CI: confidence interval.

#: adjusted for age, sex, ethnicity, family history of lung cancer and joint-yrs of cannabis use.

¶: adjusted for age, sex, ethnicity, family history of lung cancer and pack-yrs.

+: adjusted for age, sex, ethnicity, family history of lung cancer, pack-yrs and age of onset of cannabis use.

study by Aldington and colleagues, cannabis smoking was defined as >20 joints in a lifetime, and a "joint-year" as 1 joint per day for 1 year. Overall, cannabis smoking per se was not associated with a significantly increased risk of lung cancer. However, individuals in the highest tertile of use (>10.5 joint-years of exposure) did have significantly increased risk of lung cancer (RR 5.7 [95% CI 1.5-21.6]) after adjustment for age, sex, ethnicity, pack-years of cigarette smoking, and family history of lung cancer. As demonstrated in Table 3, each joint-year of cannabis use increased the risk of lung cancer by 8%, an increase similar in magnitude to the increased risk related to one pack-year of cigarette smoking.

This study demonstrates that the risk of developing lung cancer is higher in a relatively young (<55 years of age) population of cannabis smokers compared with noncannabis smokers matched for cigarette exposure. The authors estimate that the attributable risk for lung cancer related to cannabis smoking in this group is 5%, a risk that is not insubstantial and that might increase if cannabis use were maintained as this population aged. It appears that cannabis should be added to the list of known modifiable risk factors contributing to lung cancer, and that this should be taken into consideration when taking a patient history or when the legal status of cannabis is debated.

**L. T. Tanoue, MD**

*References*

1. Carchman RA, Harris LS, Munson AE. The inhibition of DNA synthesis by cannabinoids. *Cancer Res.* 1976;36:95-100.
2. Wu TC, Tashkin DP, Djahed B, Rose JE. Pulmonary hazards of smoking marijuana as compared with tobacco. *N Engl J Med.* 1988;318:347-351.

---

## Endobronchial Ultrasound-Guided Transbronchial Needle Aspiration of Lymph Nodes in the Radiologically and Positron Emission Tomography-Normal Mediastinum in Patients With Lung Cancer

Herth FJF, Eberhardt R, Krasnik M, et al (Thoraxklinik am Universitätsklinikum Heidelberg, Germany; Gentofte Univ Hosp, Copenhagen, Denmark; et al)
*Chest* 133:887-891, 2008

---

Endobronchial ultrasound-guided transbronchial needle aspiration (EBUS-TBNA) can reliably sample enlarged mediastinal lymph nodes in patients with non-small cell lung cancer (NSCLC), and in practice is mostly used to sample nodes visible on CT or positron emission tomography (PET). Few data are available on the use of endoscopic procedures to stage the mediastinum in clinical stage 1 lung cancer. The aim of the present study was to determine the results of EBUS-TBNA in sampling mediastinal lymph nodes in patients with lung cancer and a radiographically normal mediastinum and no PET activity.

From January 2004 to May 2007, patients highly suspicious for NSCLC with CT scans showing no enlarged lymph nodes (no node > 1 cm) and a negative PET finding of the mediastinum underwent EBUS-TBNA. Identifiable lymph nodes at locations 2r, 2L, 4r, 4L, 7, 10r, 10L, 11r, and 11L were aspirated. All patients underwent subsequent surgical staging. Diagnoses based on aspiration results were compared with those based on surgical results.

One hundred patients (mean age, 52.4 years; 59 men) were included. After surgery, 97 patients (mean age, 52.9 years; 57 men) had NSCLC confirmed and were included in the analysis. In this group, 156 lymph nodes ranging 5 to 10 mm in size were detected and sampled. Malignancy was detected in nine patients but missed in one patient. Mean diameter of the punctured lymph nodes was 7.9 mm. The sensitivity of EBUS-TBNA for detecting malignancy was 89%, specificity was 100%, and the negative predictive value was 98.9%. No complications occurred.

In conclusion, EBUS-TBNA can be used to accurately sample and stage patients with clinical stage 1 lung cancer and no evidence of mediastinal involvement on CT and PET. Potentially operable patients with no signs of mediastinal involvement may benefit from presurgical staging with EBUS-TBNA.

▶ Most studies demonstrating high sensitivity and specificity of endobronchial ultrasound-guided transbronchial needle aspiration (EBUS-TBNA) for mediastinal staging in nonsmall cell lung cancer (NSCLC) have been performed in patients with enlarged mediastinal nodes identified by chest computed tomography (CT) or positron emission tomography (PET) scanning. In such studies, the prevalence of malignancy in imaging-identified abnormal nodes is typically high, which would increase measured sensitivity. This report by Herth and colleagues evaluated the use of EBUS-TBNA in 100 patients suspected of NSCLC and who had no evidence of abnormal mediastinal lymph nodes by CT or PET. Importantly, these patients all underwent surgical resection with complete lymph node dissection, and so the results of EBUS-TBNA, particularly negative findings, could be confirmed. Ninety-seven of the 100 patients had NSCLC at surgery. EBUS-TBNA correctly identified 2 out of 3 patients with metastases in hilar (N1) nodes and 6 out of 6 patients with metastases in ipsilateral (N2) or contralateral (N3) mediastinal nodes. The sensitivity, specificity, and negative predictive value of EBUS-TBNA were 89%, 100%, 99%, respectively.

EBUS-TBNA appears to be highly accurate in mediastinal staging of NSCLC, even in this population of patients with negative CT and PET imaging, in whom the prevalence of mediastinal metastasis was only 9%. It is important to point out that extensive EBUS-TBNA of mediastinal N2 (lymph node stations 2, 4, and 7) and hilar N1 (lymph node stations 10 and 11) was performed, and that these authors are among the most skilled interventional pulmonologists in the world. EBUS procedures require considerable training and more time than usual for bronchoscopy. Generalization to less focused pulmonary practices and less trained hands may not be associated with equal results. However, use of EBUS will surely increase given its widening availability, its minimally invasive features compared with traditional mediastinoscopy, reports that it is useful in the diagnosis of benign diseases such as sarcoidosis,[1] and an accumulation of evidence that it is a highly accurate staging procedure for lung cancer.

**L. T. Tanoue, MD**

*Reference*

1. Tremblay A, Stather DR, Maceachern P, Khalil M, Field SK. A randomized controlled trial of standard vs endobronchial ultrasonography-guided transbronchial needle aspiration in patients with suspected sarcoidosis. *Chest.* 2009;136: 340-346.

## Preoperative Staging of Lung Cancer with Combined PET–CT

Fischer B, Lassen U, Mortensen J, et al (Copenhagen Univ Hosp; et al)
*N Engl J Med* 361:32-39, 2009

*Background.*—Fast and accurate staging is essential for choosing treatment for non–small-cell lung cancer (NSCLC). The purpose of this randomized study was to evaluate the clinical effect of combined positron-emission tomography and computed tomography (PET–CT) on preoperative staging of NSCLC.

*Methods.*—We randomly assigned patients who were referred for preoperative staging of NSCLC to either conventional staging plus PET–CT or conventional staging alone. Patients were followed until death or for at least 12 months. The primary end point was the number of futile thoracotomies, defined as any one of the following: a thoracotomy with the finding of pathologically confirmed mediastinal lymph-node involvement (stage IIIA [N2]), stage IIIB or stage IV disease, or a benign lung lesion; an exploratory thoracotomy; or a thoracotomy in a patient who had recurrent disease or death from any cause within 1 year after randomization.

*Results.*—From January 2002 through February 2007, we randomly assigned 98 patients to the PET–CT group and 91 to the conventional-staging group. Mediastinoscopy was performed in 94% of the patients. After PET–CT, 38 patients were classified as having inoperable NSCLC, and after conventional staging, 18 patients were classified thus. Sixty patients in the PET–CT group and 73 in the conventional-staging group underwent thoracotomy ($P = 0.004$). Among these thoracotomies, 21 in the PET–CT group and 38 in the conventional-staging group were futile ($P = 0.05$). The number of justified thoracotomies and survival were similar in the two groups.

*Conclusions.*—The use of PET–CT for preoperative staging of NSCLC reduced both the total number of thoracotomies and the number of futile thoracotomies but did not affect overall mortality. (ClinicalTrials.gov number, NCT00867412.)

▶ Positron emission tomography (PET) imaging is widely used in the evaluation of lung cancer. State of the art scanners now combine PET with computed tomography (PET-CT), which enables metabolic information derived from PET imaging to be integrated with anatomic information best obtained by CT scanning. Previous studies have demonstrated that PET is both more sensitive and specific than CT for identifying mediastinal lymph node involvement with tumor.[1,2]

The 189 subjects in this study were all felt to have operable disease using conventional procedures; half were randomized to receive PET-CT imaging. Patients underwent invasive diagnostic procedures (mediastinoscopy, endoscopic, or endobronchial ultrasound-guided evaluation) to evaluate the mediastinum and to confirm positive imaging findings. Nearly all (94%) patients had mediastinoscopy for pathologic confirmation. In the PET-CT group, 38 patients were deemed inoperable based on clinical staging, of whom 13 were identified by PET-CT findings alone, 7 by endoscopic ultrasonography and another 16 by mediastinoscopy. In the conventional staging group, 18 patients were deemed inoperable, 7 by endoscopic ultrasonography and 11 by mediastinoscopy. Even after these extensive evaluations, "futile" thoracotomies, defined as the identification of benign, stage IIIA, IIIB, or IV disease, or recurrence or death within 12 months, occurred in 21 of the 98 patients in the PET-CT group (21%) and 38 of the 91 patients in the conventional staging group (42%). The sensitivity of PET-CT and conventional staging in correctly predicting operability were 64% (95% CI, 52 to 75) and 32% (95% CI, 21 to 45), respectively.

What should we learn from this? Clinical staging, including PET-CT imaging, is more sensitive in identifying inoperable lung cancer than staging with CT scanning alone. In this study, PET-CT was associated with fewer futile thoracotomies than conventional staging, though it should be noted that conventional staging performed more poorly than might have been expected based on previous analyses.[1,2] However, this study makes clear that, even with the inclusion of PET-CT, clinical staging is still imperfect. Both false negative, as highlighted in this study, and false-positive findings often occur. Clinicians must remain cognizant of the limitations of new technologies as they become part of routine practice. If anything, recognition of those limitations reinforces the need to maintain a rigorous approach to clinical staging because in most patients with lung cancer it is still the major influence on initial treatment decisions.

**L. T. Tanoue, MD**

*References*


1. Toloza EM, Harpole L, McCrory DC. Noninvasive staging of non-small cell lung cancer: a review of the current evidence. *Chest.* 2003;123:137S-146S.
2. Silvestri GA, Gould MK, Margolis ML, et al. American College of Chest Physicians. Noninvasive staging of non-small cell lung cancer: ACCP evidenced-based clinical practice guidelines (2nd edition). *Chest.* 2007;132:178S-201S.

# 31 Asthma and Cystic Fibrosis

**Racial disparities in asthma-related health outcomes in severe or difficult-to-treat asthma**

Haselkorn T, for the TENOR Study Group (Genentech Inc, South San Francisco, CA; et al)

*Ann Allergy Asthma Immunol* 101:256-263, 2008

*Background.*—The underlying reasons for racial disparities in asthma morbidity are not well understood. Multivariate epidemiologic studies evaluating the presence and extent of racial differences in a large cohort of adults with severe or difficult-to-treat asthma are lacking.

*Objective.*—To analyze an extensive array of clinical and patient-reported outcomes, using multivariate analysis with a sequential approach, to explain racial differences in asthma-related outcomes in one of the largest cohorts of difficult-to-treat asthmatic patients.

*Methods.*—Black and white patients (≥18 years old at baseline) were included (n = 2,128). Differences between the 2 racial groups were assessed using several outcome measures at month 12. Assessments were adjusted for confounding variables using a sequence of statistical models.

*Results.*—Most patients were white (88.6%). Blacks were slightly younger, less educated, and more likely to live in urban areas than whites. Blacks were more likely to have severe asthma and to be treated with 3 or more long-term controllers. Poorer quality of life, more asthma control problems, and higher risk of emergency department visits were observed in blacks compared with whites; differences were not explained by adjustment for broad sets of confounding variables. Differences in asthma-related health outcomes remained statistically significant after adjusting for asthma severity.

*Conclusions.*—Asthma is a serious health problem in blacks and is not explained by differences in demographics, severity, or other health conditions (Fig 2, Table 1).

▶ Prospective, multivariate analysis/observational study of severe or difficult-to-treat white and black asthmatics (TENOR study).[1] Table 1 details differences between white and black subjects enrolled in this study, showing that blacks were younger; more likely to have severe asthma; more likely to be treated with 3 or more long-term controller medications and at higher risk of emergency

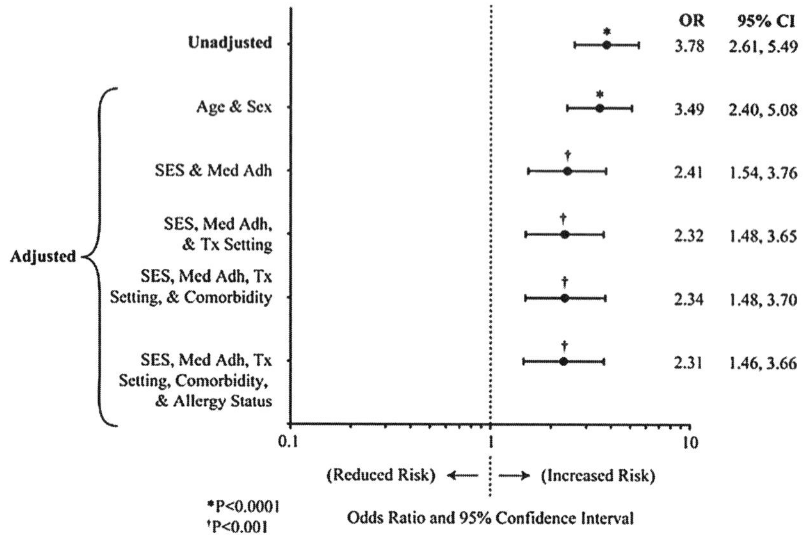


FIGURE 2.—Multivariate regression comparing emergency department visits in the previous 3 months at month 12 (black vs white patients). Allergy measures consist of allergic rhinitis, atopic dermatitis, and IgE; comorbidity of chronic obstructive pulmonary disease, bronchitis, weight, and body mass index; and socioeconomic status (SES) of urban/rural, geographic region, income, education, employment status, and insurance coverage. CI indicates confidence interval; Med Adh, medication adherence; OR, odds ratio; Tx, treatment. (Reprinted from Haselkorn T, for the TENOR Study Group. Racial disparities in asthma-related health outcomes in severe or difficult-to-treat asthma. *Ann Allergy Asthma Immunol.* 2008;101:256-263.)

department visits. Fig 2 details multivariate analysis of factors related to emergency department visits in the final 3 months of the 12-month monitoring period. Despite similar adherence to medications and use of more controller medications, blacks had worse outcomes. These data suggest that factors other than disparities in treatment (specifically undertreatment or suboptimal treatment) and adherence account for worse outcomes and document the need for further study of genetic factors responsible for responsible factors. Genetic studies in blacks related to response to specific asthma controller medications must be given a high priority during the coming years to substantively impact what has been proven to be disparity in response to medications.

**S. K. Willsie, DO**

*Reference*

1. Dolan CM, Fraher KE, Bleecker ER, et al. TENOR study group. Baseline characteristics of the epidemiology and natural history of asthma outcomes and treatment regimens study (TENOR): a large cohort of patients with severe or difficult to treat asthma. *Ann Allergy Asthma Immunol.* 2004;92:32-39.

TABLE 1.—Demographic and Clinical Characteristics of Black and White Patients at Baseline

| Characteristics | White patients (n = 1,885) | Black patients (n = 243) | *P* value |
|---|---|---|---|
| Age, mean (SD), y | 50.7 (14.56) | 46.9 (14.02) | .001 |
| Sex, No. (%) | | | .06 |
| Female | 1,343 (71.2) | 187 (77.0) | |
| Male | 542 (28.8) | 56 (23.0) | |
| Urban/rural, No. (%) | | | <.001 |
| Urban core area | 1,429 (75.8) | 220 (90.5) | |
| Suburban area | 216 (11.5) | 11 (4.5) | |
| Large town area | 113 (6.0) | 6 (2.5) | |
| Small town and isolated rural area | 127 (6.7) | 6 (2.5) | |
| Education, No. (%) | | | <.001 |
| High school or less | 462 (24.5) | 106 (43.6) | |
| Some college/trade school | 656 (34.8) | 85 (35.0) | |
| College graduate or advanced degree | 767 (40.7) | 52 (21.4) | |
| Annual income estimate, mean (SD), $ | 59,691 (20,843) | 44,170 (18,646) | <.001 |
| Health care provider, No. (%) | | | <.001 |
| Commercial/PPO | 877 (46.5) | 72 (29.6) | |
| HMO | 525 (27.9) | 51 (21.0) | |
| Medicaid | 49 (2.6) | 39 (16.0) | |
| Medicare | 322 (17.1) | 58 (23.9) | |
| Other | 112 (5.9) | 23 (9.5) | |
| Treatment setting, No. (%) | | | <.001 |
| Pulmonologist | 465 (24.7) | 108 (44.4) | |
| Allergist | 1,420 (75.3) | 135 (55.6) | |
| Body mass index, mean (SD)[a] | 30.1 (7.42) | 33.9 (8.27) | <.001 |
| Lung function, mean (SD) | | | |
| Postbronchodilator % of predicted $FEV_1$ | 80.5 (23.97) | 68.3 (20.91) | <.001 |
| Postbronchodilator actual $FEV_1$/FVC, % | 71.8 (11.99) | 71.1 (12.44) | .44 |
| Race-adjusted postbronchodilator % of predicted $FEV_1$[b] | 75.7 (20.51) | 77.3 (24.11) | .30 |

Abbreviations: $FEV_1$, forced expiratory volume in 1 second; FVC, forced vital capacity; HMO, health maintenance organization; PPO, preferred provider organization.

[a]Calculated as weight in kilograms divided by height in meters squared.

[b]Predicted values for spirometry measures were race adjusted based on Hankinson reference values.[33] Editor's note: Please check the original article for full references.

## Alendronate Once Weekly for the Prevention and Treatment of Bone Loss in Canadian Adult Cystic Fibrosis Patients (CFOS Trial)

Papaioannou A, Kennedy CC, Freitag A, et al (McMaster Univ, Ontario, Canada; et al)

*Chest* 134:794-800, 2008

*Background.*—Patients with cystic fibrosis (CF) are at risk for early bone loss, and demonstrate increased risks for vertebral fractures and kyphosis. A multicenter, randomized, controlled trial was conducted to assess the efficacy, tolerability, and safety of therapy with oral alendronate (FOSAMAX; Merck; Whitehouse Station, NJ) in adults with CF and low bone mass.

*Methods.*—Participants received placebo or alendronate, 70 mg once weekly, for 12 months. All participants received 800 IU of vitamin D and 1,000 mg of calcium daily. Adults with confirmed CF with a bone mineral density (BMD) T score of < − 1.0 were eligible for inclusion. Participants who had undergone organ transplantation or had other reported contraindications were excluded from the study. The primary outcome measure was the mean (± SD) percentage change in lumbar spine BMD after 12 months. Secondary measures included the percentage change in total hip BMD, the number of new vertebral fractures (grade 1 or 2), and changes in quality of life.

*Results.*—A total of 56 participants were enrolled in the study (mean age, 29.1 ± 8.78 years; 61% male). The absolute percentage changes in lumbar spine and total hip BMDs at follow-up were significantly higher in the alendronate therapy group (5.20 ± 3.67% and 2.14 ± 3.32%, respectively) than those in the control group (− 0.08 ± 3.93% and − 1.3 ± 2.70%, respectively; p < 0.001). At follow-up, two participants (both in the control group) had a new vertebral fracture (not significant), and there were no differences in quality of life or the number of adverse events (including serious and GI-related events).

*Conclusion.*—Alendronate therapy was well tolerated and produced a significantly greater increase in BMD over 12 months compared with placebo (Tables 2 and 3).

▶ This is a small (57 subjects) 12-month long randomized controlled trial (RCT) of weekly alendronate (A) versus placebo (P) in young adult patients with cystic fibrosis (CF) (majority were male subjects) with reduced bone mineral density. Aris and colleagues previously compared demonstrated efficacy of daily A in this population.[1] Study design is reflected in Fig 1 in the original article; subjects received 70 mg of alendronate or placebo weekly for 12 months. Following the treatment phase, statistically significant improvement in bone mineral density (BMD) was observed in the A group versus placebo ($P < .05$); significant persisted when multivariate analyses were applied. No significant reduction occurred in vertebral fractures in the A group. There was no statistically significant difference between adverse events associated with

TABLE 2.—Number of Participants With One or More Adverse Event*

| Variables | Alendronate Group (n = 27) No. | % | Control Group (n = 29) No. | % |
|---|---|---|---|---|
| Any AE | 15 | 56 | 19 | 66 |
| Serious AE | 7† | 26 | 3‡ | 10 |
| Drug-related AE | 8 | 30 | 8 | 28 |

*AE = adverse event.

†In the alendronate group, three patients were classified as having had an exacerbation of CF, one patient was identified as having a bronchial superinfection, one patient was identified as having a hypoglycemic seizure, one patient was identified as having a GI obstruction, and one patient was identified as having an intestinal obstruction.

‡In the control group, all three participants were classified as having an exacerbation of CF, with two of them having additional GI complaints.

TABLE 3.—Total GI-Related AEs*

| AEs | Alendronate Group (n = 27) | Control Group (n = 29) |
|---|---|---|
| Nausea and/or vomiting | 3 | 4 |
| Reflux | 1 | 0 |
| Difficulty swallowing | 1 | 0 |
| Esophagitis | 1 | 0 |
| Constipation | 1 | 1 |
| GI upset | 1 | 0 |
| Intestinal obstruction | 1 | 1 |
| Stomach pain/burn | 1 | 1 |

*More than one event could have occurred per participant. See Table 2 for abbreviation not used in the text.

A versus P (Tables 2 and 3). Patients with CF are living longer and longer, and more often are considered for transplantation. The investigators suggest that therapy with oral bisphosphonates be considered early in the course of CF, before bone loss becomes advanced. The investigators caution clinicians about the use of these agents in women with childbearing potential due to the fact that these drugs are not approved for use during pregnancy.

**S. K. Willsie, DO**

*Reference*

1. Aris RM, Lester GE, Caminiti M, et al. Efficacy of alendronate in adult patients with CF with low bone mineral density. *Am J Resp Crit Care Med.* 2004;169: 77-82.

## Persistent Methicillin-resistant *Staphylococcus aureus* and Rate of $FEV_1$ Decline in Cystic Fibrosis

Dasenbrook EC, Merlo CA, Diener-West M, et al (The Johns Hopkins Univ School of Medicine, Baltimore, MD; The Johns Hopkins Univ Bloomberg School of Public Health, Baltimore, MD)

*Am J Respir Crit Care Med* 178:814-821, 2008

*Rationale.*—Theprevalence in cystic fibrosis (CF) of respiratory cultures with methicillin-resistant *Staphylococcus aureus* (MRSA) has dramatically increased over the last 10 years, but the effect of MRSA on $FEV_1$ decline in CF is unknown.

*Objectives.*—To determine the association between MRSA respiratory infection and $FEV_1$ decline in children and adults with CF.

*Methods.*—This was a 10-year cohort study using the Cystic Fibrosis Foundation patient registry from 1996–2005. We studied individuals who developed new MRSA respiratory tract infection. Repeated-measures regression was used to assess the association between MRSA and $FEV_1$ decline, adjusted for confounders, in individuals aged 8–21 years and adults (aged 22-45 yr). Two different statistical models were used to assess robustness of results.

*Measurements and Main Results.*—The study cohort included 17,357 patients with an average follow-up of 5.3 years. During the study period, 1,732 individuals developed new persistent MRSA infection (≥3 MRSA cultures; average, 6.8 positive cultures) and were subsequently followed foran average of 3.5 years. Even after adjustment for confounders, rate of $FEV_1$ decline in individuals aged 8–21 years with persistent MRSA was more rapid in both statistical models. Their average $FEV_1$ decline of 2.06% predicted/year was 43% more rapid than the 1.44% predicted/year in those without MRSA (difference, −0.62% predicted/yr; 95% confidence interval, −0.70 to −0.54; $P < 0.001$). Effect of MRSA on $FEV_1$ decline in adults was not clinically significant.

*Conclusions.*—Persistent infection with MRSA in individuals with CF between the ages of 8 and 21 years is associated with a more rapid rate of decline in lung function (Table 4).

▶ Despite the increasing frequency of persistent infection of cystic fibrosis patients (CF) with methicillin-resistant *Staphylococcus aureus* (MRSA), little is known about the effects of MRSA infection on rate of pulmonary function decline. This study represents longitudinal analysis of more than 17 000 CF patients over more than 5 years with a focus on 1732 patients who developed new and then persistent infection with MRSA. Fig 2 in the original article demonstrates linear $FEV_1$ decline in patients between the ages of 8- and 21-years who developed persistent MRSA infection. Table 4 shows a model

TABLE 4.—Model 1: Lung Function Decline in Individuals with Cystic Fibrosis Aged 8–21 Years with Persistent Methicillin-Resistant *Staphylococcus Aureus*, Adjusted for Confounders

| | Coefficient | 95% CI | *P* Value |
|---|---|---|---|
| Difference in rate of decline with MRSA* | −0.62 | −0.70 to −0.54 | <0.001 |
| Age, yr | −1.44 | −1.46 to −1.41 | <0.001 |
| Positive for MRSA† | −3.36 | −3.66 to −3.06 | <0.001 |
| Sex, female | −1.52 | −1.97 to −1.08 | <0.001 |
| Pancreatic insufficient‡ | −1.01 | −1.43 to −0.59 | <0.001 |
| CF-related diabetes | −3.61 | −3.86 to −3.36 | <0.001 |
| Positive for Pseudomonas aeruginosa | −0.17 | −0.34 to −0.01 | 0.046 |
| Positive for Burkholderia cepacia complex | −1.42 | −1.89 to −0.95 | <0.001 |
| Baseline $FEV_1$ | 0.76 | 0.75 to 0.77 | <0.001 |

*Definition of abbreviations*: CI = confidence interval; CF = cystic fibrosis; MRSA = methicillin-resistant *Staphylococcus aureus*.

*This coefficient represents the difference between the mean rate of decline of lung function ($FEV_1$% predicted/yr) between those without MRSA and those with persistent MRSA (≥3 MRSA cultures). This interaction term captured the variable of time in years by age. Therefore, those without MRSA had lung function decline of −1.44 $FEV_1$% predicted/year, whereas those with MRSA lost −2.06 $FEV_1$% predicted/year.

†This coefficient represents the difference in mean absolute $FEV_1$% predicted between those without and with persistent MRSA, adjusted for confounders. Those with persistent MRSA averaged an absolute $FEV_1$% predicted that was −3.4% lower.

‡Subjects taking pancreatic enzymes.

of lung function decline, accounting for various confounders, including pancreatic insufficiency, CF-associated diabetes mellitus, gender, infection with *Pseudomonas aeruginosa*, or *Burkholderia cepacia* complex. Fig 3 in the original article demonstrates $FEV_1$ decline before and after acquisition of persistent MRSA infection. Interestingly, persistent infection with MRSA portends a statistically significant and more rapid decline in children ages 8 to 21, but not in adults with CF. These data demonstrate the need to primarily prevent, or, if MRSA infection occurs, to take necessary steps to prevent persistent infection with MRSA to preserve long-term pulmonary function in children with CF.

**S. K. Willsie, DO**

---

**Inhaled Aztreonam Lysine For Chronic Airway *Pseudomonas aeruginosa* In Cystic Fibrosis**

McCoy KS, Quittner AL, Oermann CM, et al (Ohio State Univ, Columbus; Univ of Miami, Coral Gables, FL; Baylor College of Medicine, Houston, TX; et al)
*Am J Respir Crit Care Med* 178:921-928, 2008

---

*Rationale.*—The effectiveness and safety of aztreonam lysine for inhalation (AZLI) in patients with cystic fibrosis (CF) on maintenance treatment for *Pseudomonas aeruginosa* (PA) airway infection was evaluated in this randomized, double-blind, placebo-controlled study.

*Objectives.*—To evaluate the safety and efficacy of inhaled aztreonam lysine in controlling PA infection in patients with CF.

*Methods.*—After randomization and a 28-day course of tobramycin inhalation solution (TIS), patients ($n = 211$; $\geq 6$ yr; $\geq 3$ TIS courses within previous year; $FEV_1 \geq 25\%$ and $\leq 75\%$ predicted values) were treated with 75 mg AZLI or placebo, twice or three times daily for 28 days, then monitored for 56 days. The primary efficacy endpoint was time to need for additional inhaled or intravenous antipseudomonal antibiotics. Secondary endpoints included changes in respiratory symptoms (CF Questionnaire-Revised [CFQ-R] Respiratory Scale), pulmonary function (FEV1), and sputum PA density. Adverse events and minimum inhibitory concentrations of aztreonam for PA were monitored.

*Measurements and Main Results.*—AZLI treatment increased median time to need for additional antipseudomonal antibiotics for symptoms of pulmonary exacerbation by 21 days, compared with placebo (AZLI, 92 d; placebo, 71 d; $P = 0.007$). AZLI improved mean CFQ-R respiratory scores (5.01 points, $P = 0.02$), $FEV_1$ (6.3%, $P = 0.001$), and sputum PA density (−0.66 log 10 cfu/g, $P = 0.006$) compared with placebo; no AZLI dose–response was observed. Adverse events reported for AZLI and placebo were comparable and consistent with CF lung disease. Susceptibility of PA to aztreonam at baseline and end of therapy were similar.

*Conclusions.*—AZLI was effective in patients with CF using frequent TIS therapy. AZLI delayed time to need for inhaled or intravenous antipseudomonal antibiotics, improved respiratory symptoms and pulmonary function, and was well tolerated.

Clinical trial registered with www.clinicaltrials.gov (NCT 00104520).

▶ This is a randomized, placebo-controlled, double-blind controlled trial conducted within 56 cystic fibrosis (CF) centers in United States in patients with chronic *Pseudomonas aeruginosa* (PA) infection. All subjects received aerosolized tobramycin solution bid for 28 days and were then randomized to receive either placebo (P) or aztreonam 75 mg bid (AB) twice a day (AT) for an additional 28 days. Aztreonam data were evaluated according to administration bid versus twice a day and as pooled data (AP). Fig 2 in the original article shows treatment and time to need for inhaled or intravenous antiPA antibiotics to treat respiratory exacerbations. An additional 21 days of time to need for treatment with antibiotics was seen with aztreonam treated (AP) patients versus P ($P = .007$). Antibiotic resistance to aztreonam (AP) did not change from pre- to posttreatment periods. Treatment with A was safe. This study suggests that for patients with chronic CF and chronic PA infection who are already receiving aerosolized tobramycin therapy, addition of aerosolized aztreonam may afford both an efficacious and safe alternative to improve and sustain lung health longer than current therapeutic strategies.

**S. K. Willsie, DO**

---

**Assessing the value of disease management: impact of 2 disease management strategies in an underserved asthma population**

Galbreath AD, Smith B, Wood PR, et al (Univ of Texas Health Science Ctr at San Antonio; Altarum Inst, San Antonio, TX; et al)

*Ann Allergy Asthma Immunol* 101:599-607, 2008

---

*Background.*—The goal of disease management (DM) is to improve health outcomes and reduce cost through decreasing health care utilization. Although some studies have shown that DM improves asthma outcomes, these interventions have not been examined in a large randomized controlled trial.

*Objective.*—To compare the effectiveness of 2 previously successful DM programs with that of traditional care.

*Methods.*—Nine hundred two individuals with asthma (429 adults; 473 children) were randomly assigned to telephonic DM, augmented DM (ADM; DM plus in-home visits by a respiratory therapist), or traditional care. Data were collected at enrollment and at 6 and 12 months. Primary outcomes were time to first asthma-related event, quality of life (QOL), and rates of asthma-related health care utilization. Secondary outcomes included rate of controller medication initiation, number of oral corticosteroid bursts, asthma symptom scores, and number of school days missed.

*Results.*—There were no significant differences between groups in time to first asthma-related event or health care utilization. Adult participants in the ADM group had greater improvement in QOL ($P = .04$) and a decrease in asthma symptoms ($P = .001$) compared with other groups. Of children not receiving controller medications at enrollment (13%), those in the intervention groups were more likely to have controller medications initiated than the control group ($P = .01$). Otherwise, there were no differences in outcomes.

*Conclusions.*—Overall, participation in asthma DM did not result in significant differences in utilization or clinical outcomes. The only significant impact was a higher rate of controller medication initiation in children and improvement in asthma symptoms and QOL in adults who received ADM.

▶ This is an interesting randomized controlled trial evaluating outcomes following implementation of 2 different types of disease management programs versus no intervention in over 900 patients, inclusive of adults and children. Despite improvement in patient-perceived quality of life ($P = .04$), and reduction in asthma symptoms in adults ($P = .001$), as well as an increase in receipt of controller medications by children ($P = .01$), the impact of resource intensive disease management strategies did not change time to first asthma-related event or health care use. In the absence of improved outcomes and a reduction in costs, will this type of focused disease management intervention be the first to be sacrificed with health care reform?

**S. K. Willsie, DO**

---

**Asthma**

Fanta CH (Brigham and Women's Hosp and Harvard Med School, Boston, MA)

*N Engl J Med* 360:1002-1014, 2009

---

According to survey data for which the diagnosis of asthma was based on a physician's assessment, it is estimated that approximately 7% of Americans have current asthma. The disease affects people of all races and ethnic groups worldwide, from infancy to old age, with slightly more boys than girls affected and, after puberty, more women than men. Dramatic increases in the prevalence of atopy and asthma have occurred over the past few decades in Westernized countries and more recently in less-developed nations. Estimates suggest that as many as 300 million persons are affected worldwide.

In the 1970s and 1980s, severe asthmatic exacerbations (as indicated by emergency department visits and hospitalizations for asthma) and asthma-related mortality rose steeply in the United States. Yet despite the persistently high prevalence of disease, the most recently available data indicate improved outcomes, with fewer annual hospitalizations for asthmatic attacks and fewer asthma-related deaths. Among the possible explanations for these favorable trends are the more widespread preventive use of inhaled corticosteroids and the introduction over the past 10 to 15 years of new, highly effective medications and improved medication formulations for the treatment of asthma.

Airway obstruction in asthma and the consequent symptoms of cough, shortness of breath, chest tightness, and wheezing are caused by some combination of airway smooth-muscle constriction and inflammation of the bronchi. The former can be severe, leading to life-threatening narrowing and closure of airways, even in the absence of mucous plugging. Both abnormal smooth-muscle contractility and excess smooth-muscle mass may contribute. Airway inflammation in asthma consists of mucosal, submucosal, and adventitial edema; cellular infiltration, particularly by eosinophils (and in some cases, neutrophils) and activated helper T lymphocytes as well as mast cells that (unlike mast cells in other eosinophilic airway diseases) infiltrate smooth-muscle bundles; increased airway secretions, including secreted mucus, desquamated lining cells, and intraluminal eosinophils; capillary engorgement; hyperplasia of smooth muscle; and deposition of excess collagen, particularly immediately beneath the basement membrane of the epithelium.

Traditionally, drugs used to treat asthma were categorized according to their predominant effect — relaxation of airway smooth muscle (bronchodilators) or suppression of airway inflammation (antiinflammatory drugs). Newer medications (e.g., the leukotriene modifiers) and drug combinations (e.g., inhaled corticosteroids combined with long-acting $\beta$-adrenergic agonists) have dual effects, resisting such traditional dichotomization. Now, asthma medications are classified according to their roles in the overall management of asthma (quick relief or long-term control), a model that is particularly useful when speaking to patients about their asthma medicines.

All patients with asthma should have available a quick-relief bronchodilator for use as needed. Consensus opinion suggests that when quick-acting bronchodilators are needed for symptom relief more than 2 days per week (or more than twice a month for nighttime awakenings caused by asthmatic symptoms), controller medications should be prescribed.

▶ This review article of drug therapy for asthma in *New England Journal of Medicine* presents a succinct and comprehensive review for care providers. Stepped care is discussed, as well as different dosages/formulations of available agents. This is a worthwhile read for all providers.

**S. K. Willsie, DO**

**Prevalence of Low Bone Mass and Deficiencies of Vitamins D and K in Pediatric Patients With Cystic Fibrosis From 3 Canadian Centers**

Grey V, Atkinson S, Drury D, et al (McMaster Children's Hosp, Ontario, Canada; Montreal Children's Hosp, Québec, Canada; et al)

*Pediatrics* 122:1014-1020, 2008

*Objective.*—In this cross-sectional observational study, we assessed both vitamins D and K status and bone health in pancreatic insufficient pediatric patients with cystic fibrosis from 3 Canadian cystic fibrosis centers.

*Methods.*—Eighty-one patients who had cystic fibrosis and were clinically stable for at least 3 months were enrolled. At the time of the clinic visit, anthropometric variables, lung function, pubertal status, intake of calcium and vitamins D and K, and physical activity were assessed. Blood was taken for analysis of biochemical biomarkers of bone turnover and status of vitamins D and K, and a urine sample was obtained for calcium, creatinine, sodium, and deoxypyridoline analyses. Whole-body bone mineral content and lumbar spine (L1–L4) bone mineral density were measured.

*Results.*—The children were relatively well nourished and had moderate to mild lung disease. Low bone mineral mass defined as a z score between −1.0 and −2.0, for gender and age was detected in 38% of the children for whole body and in 28% for lumbar spine. *z* score less than −2.0 was observed in 7 children for both bone measures. Suboptimal vitamin D status occurred in 95% of patients;suboptimal vitamin K status occurred in 82% of patients. Measures of plasma osteocalcin and carboxy-terminal propeptide type 1 procollagen and urinary deoxypyridoline compared with reference values for age, gender, and pubertal status reflected a state of suppressed bone formation and elevated bone resorption in a large proportion of the patients.

*Conclusions.*—Bone mass of the whole body and spine was lower than expected for chronological age in approximately one third of pediatric patients with cystic fibrosis irrespective of gender or age. This may be explained by the observation of low bone turnover for developmental stage as indicated by bone biomarkers. Suboptimal status of vitamins D and K may be key causative factors of the low bone status for age.

▶ Summary:Suboptimal bone health is widespread in patients with cystic fibrosis (CF) secondary to a variety of factors which include vitamin (D and K) and mineral (calcium) malabsorption (resulting from pancreatic insufficiency), malnutrition, inactivity, corticosteroid usage, underlying inflammatory processes. Because of this, a recently published recommendation suggested that plasma 25-hydroxyvitamin D (25-OHD) levels be maintained at ≥75 nmol/L[1] in patients with CF. In this observational study, 81 Canadian pediatric clinically stable patients with CF were assessed for bone mineral density, bone mineral content, vitamin D and K levels, and biochemical biomarkers of bone turnover. Clinical characteristics of study subjects did not differ statistically by gender. Fifty-nine of 78 subjects had mild lung disease, 16/78 had moderate lung disease, and 3/78 had severe lung disease. Two of 81 subjects had a body mass index (BMI) $z$ score less than −2.0, and 14/81 had BMI $z$ score between −1 and −2.0. The status of levels of calcium and vitamin D are reflected in Table 2 in the original article. Ninety-five percent of subjects had suboptimal levels of 25-OHD defined as <75 nmol/L. No seasonal difference was noted. Vitamin K levels were suboptimal in 82% of subjects and 30% had undetectable levels. Parathyroid hormone (PTH) levels were elevated in 10% of subjects, and there was no correlation between PTH and vitamin D levels. Dietary intake of calcium and vitamins D and K exceeded recommended intake for most children (Table 3 in the original article). Whole body bone mass was lower than expected for chronological age in approximately 1 of 3 subjects, irrespective of age or gender. Low bone turnover for developmental age was suggested by bone biomarkers (plasma osteocalcin and carboxy-terminal propeptide type 1 procollagen and urinary deoxypyridoline). The authors state that their observance of low vitamin D and K levels may represent key causative factors for low bone status for age in the CF subjects studied. This study points to the need to regularly monitor vitamin A and K levels in accordance with bone health, even in relatively active and healthy patients with CF. Greater than the recommended supplementation of vitamin D and K may be required in order to maintain optimal levels of vitamin D and K, which should be monitored to ensure optimum levels, particularly in this population. Doing so is exceedingly important, as the life span of patients with CF grows longer and longer, and accordingly, preservation of quality of life is paramount.

**S. K. Willsie, DO**

*Reference*

1. Aris RM, Merkel PA, BAchrach LK, et al. Guide to bone health and disease in cystic fibrosis. *J Clin Endocrinol Metab.* 2005;90:1888-1896.

# 32 Community-Acquired Pneumonia

---

**Epidemiology of Invasive Pneumococcal Disease among Adult Patients in Barcelona Before and After Pediatric 7-Valent Pneumococcal Conjugate Vaccine Introduction, 1997–2007**

Ardanuy C, Tubau F, Pallares R, et al (Hosp Universitari de Bellvitge, Spain; et al)

*Clin Infect Dis* 48:57-64, 2009

---

*Background.*—A dramatic decrease in the incidence of invasive pneumococcal disease (IPD) was observed among children and adults in the United States after the introduction of the 7-valent pneumococcal conjugate vaccine (PCV7). Little is known about the incidence of IPD after PCV7 licensure in Europe. The objective of this study was to examine changes in the prevalence of IPD among adults in the PCV7 era.

*Methods.*—We undertook a prospective study involving adults with IPD who required hospital admission in the southern area of Barcelona, Spain. Three periods were studied: the pre-PCV7 period (1997–2001), the early PCV7 period (2002–2004), and the late PCV7 period (2005–2007).

*Results.*—A total of 1007 episodes of IPD were observed. Rates of IPD among adults increased from 13.9 to 14.6 episodes per 100,000 population between the pre-PCV7 period and the early PCV7 period ($P = .6$) and then to 19.55 episodes per 100,000 population in the late PCV7 period ($P < .001$). The rates of IPD among adults due to non-PCV7 serotypes increased from 8.4 to 9.7 episodes per 100,000 population between the pre-PCV7 period and the early PCV7 period ($P = .15$) and then to 15.3 episodes per 100,000 population in the late PCV7 period ($P < .001$); IPD due to PCV7 serotypes decreased from 5.6 to 4.9 episodes per 100,000 population between the pre-PCV7 period and the early PCV7 period ($P = .3$), then to 4.3 episodes per 100,000 population in the late PCV7 period ($P = .056$). Among people aged ≥65 years, IPD due to PCV7 serotypes decreased from 19.5 to 14.6 episodes per 100,000 population between the pre-PCV7 period and the early PCV7 period ($P = .13$), then to 12.3 episodes per 100,000 population in the late PCV7 period ($P = .02$). A decrease in the prevalence of antibiotic-resistant pneumococci in the late PCV7 period was associated with a decrease in the prevalence of multidrug-resistant PCV7 clones (Spain$^{23F}$-ST81, Spain$^{6B}$-ST90, and ST88$^{19F}$) and an increase in the prevalence of non-PCV7 antibiotic-susceptible clones (ST306$^{1}$, ST191$^{7F}$, ST989$^{12F}$, and ST433$^{22F}$).

*Conclusions.*—Rates of IPD among adults increased in Barcelona in the late PCV7 period, coinciding with a clonal expansion of non-PCV7 serotypes. In contrast, rates of IPD caused by PCV7 serotypes decreased among people aged ≥65 years, which suggests the development of a herd immunity (Fig 1).

▶ When Prevnar (7-valent conjugate pneumococcal vaccine) was introduced in 2000 shortly followed by a universal recommendation into the United States for vaccination of children up to 2 years of age it had a dramatic effect. Within 4 years, not only did it decrease invasive pneumococcal disease by the 7 serotypes in those vaccinated, but also in adults more than 50 years of age.[1] Disease by serotypes not contained either in the conjugate vaccine or in the more

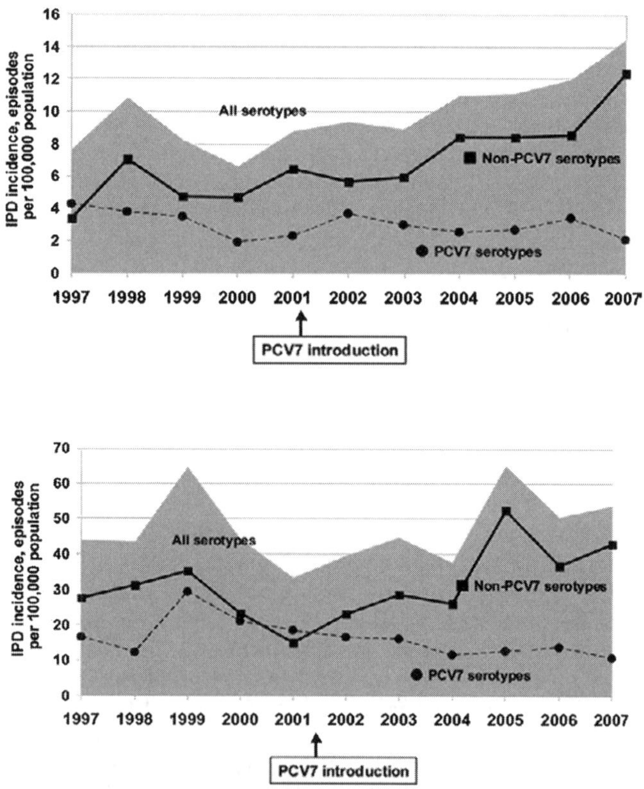


FIGURE 1.—The incidence of invasive pneumococcal disease (IPD) by year and serotype group among adults aged 18–64 years (*top*) and among adults aged ≥65 years (*bottom*). PCV7, 7-valent pneumococcal conjugated vaccine. (Reprinted from Ardanuy C, Tubau F, Pallares R, et al. Epidemiology of invasive pneumococcal disease among adult patients in Barcelona before and after pediatric 7-valent pneumococcal conjugate vaccine introduction, 1997-2007. *Clin Infect Dis*. 2009;48:57-64, with permission from Infectious Diseases Society of America.)

commonly used vaccine for adults, Pneumovax increased slightly during this time period. This article reports on the introduction of 7-valent conjugate vaccine in Spain that occurred in much different fashion than in the United States. After being made available in June 2001, there has been no universal recommendation for vaccination in the target age group. Initially, only high-risk children received the vaccination; gradually the application increased until now approximately 50% of children are covered. Probably not surprisingly, the resultant decrease in invasive pneumococcal disease in children has not been as dramatic as in the United States, and disease from serotypes not covered by the vaccine have risen.[2] However, there has been a great deal of variability of response across Europe and in Spain depending on how the vaccine was introduced. This study addresses the other phenomenon seen in the United States with the introduction of Prevnar: the reduction in adult disease. In Spain there was some reduction in disease from serotypes in the conjugate vaccine late after the introduction, but in the adult population between 18 and 64 there was a marked increase of invasive disease from non-vaccine serotypes (Fig 1). This study (and some other European reports before it) demonstrate that how a vaccine is introduced and used can dramatically affect its impact and, actually, result in unintended consequences.

**J. R. Maurer, MD, MBA**

*References*

1. Lexau CA, Lynfield R, Danila R, et al. Changing epidemiology of invasive pneumococcal disease among older adults in the era of pediatric pneumococcal conjugate vaccine. *JAMA*. 2005;294:2043-2051.
2. Calbo E, Diaz A, Canadell E, et al. Invasive pneumococcal disease among children in a health district of barcelona: early impact of pneumococcal conjugate vaccine. *Clin Microbiol Infect*. 2006;12:867-872.

## Radiologic Progression of Pulmonary Infiltrates Predicts a Worse Prognosis in Severe Community-Acquired Pneumonia Than Bacteremia

Lisboa T, for the Community-Acquired Pneumonia Intensive Care Units Study Investigators (Joan XXIII Univ Hosp & Univ Rovira i Virgili, Ciber Enfermedades Respiratorias, Tarragona, Spain; et al)
*Chest* 135:165-172, 2009

*Background.*—It remains unknown whether bacteremia and rapid radiologic progression of pulmonary infiltrates increase the risk of shock and mortality in ICU patients with community-acquired pneumonia (CAP). The objective of this study was to investigate the relative importance of these two factors in the outcome of patients with severe CAP (sCAP).

*Methods.*—A secondary analysis in a multicenter observational study was conducted in 457 patients with CAP admitted to the ICU. Patients were classified into four groups: group RB, rapid radiographic spread of pulmonary infiltrates and bacteremia (n = 48); group R, rapid radiographic spread but no bacteremia (n = 183); group B, bacteremia but without rapid radiographic spread (n = 39); and group C, neither rapid radiographic spread nor bacteremia (n = 187).

*Results.*—Logistic regression analysis showed that group RB and group R had a greater risk for shock than group C (adjusted odds ratio [aOR], 8.9; 95% confidence interval [CI], 4.0 to 19.7; and aOR, 3.8; 95% CI, 2.5 to 5.9; respectively), while patients in group B had no increased risk. In addition, compared to group C, group RB and group R had an increased risk of ICU death (aOR, 3.4; 95% CI, 1.4 to 8.1; and aOR, 3.1; 95% CI, 1.7 to 5.7, respectively), while patients in group B had none.

*Conclusions.*—In this cohort of patients with severe CAP, radiologic progression of pulmonary infiltrates in the first 48 h is a significant adverse prognostic feature. In contrast, bacteremia does not affect outcomes.

▶ Several tools can be used to help determine risk of morbidity and mortality of patients presenting with community-acquired pneumonia, and can thereby help to determine whether or not the patient requires admission for appropriate care. These instruments typically predict need for ICU management or 30-day mortality. This study looks at a slightly different question. It asks: if a patient requires ICU care, what can be used to predict the short-term course of the patient? Investigators focused on 2 known predictors of worse outcomes: bacteremia and rapid progression of infiltrates. The relative importance of these indicators of severe disease is unknown once a patient is in intensive care. In this study, bacteremia alone was not a predictor of increased mortality independent of the type of organism, but rapid progression of pulmonary infiltrates by 48 hours was (whether alone or in combination with bacteremia) a strong predictor of death. The authors identify several reasons why bacteremia may not be a useful predictor. One explanation is that criteria for patient admission to ICU in Spain (where the study took place) would exclude patients with multiple comorbidities and a strong likelihood of 30-day mortality so that those admitted are generally in better health and more able to survive bacteremia, especially if treated early with antibiotics. However, the prognostic value of finding rapid progression of infiltrates should not be surprising. This likely represents overwhelming infection and/or a systemic inflammatory response that, even in a relatively healthy person, is common in this setting and typically highly lethal.

**J. R. Maurer, MD, MBA**

# 33 Chronic Obstructive Pulmonary Disease

**Effects of Home-Based Pulmonary Rehabilitation in Patients with Chronic Obstructive Pulmonary Disease: A Randomized Trial**

Maltais F, for the Chronic Obstructive Pulmonary Disease Axis of the Respiratory Health Network, Fonds de la recherche en santé du Québec (Hôpital Laval, Centre de pneumologie, Québec, Canada; et al)

*Ann Intern Med* 149:869-878, 2008

*Background.*—Home-based rehabilitation is a promising approach to improve access to pulmonary rehabilitation.

*Objective.*—To assess whether self-monitored, home-based rehabilitation is as effective as outpatient, hospital-based rehabilitation in patients with chronic obstructive pulmonary disease (COPD).

*Design.*—Randomized, multicenter, noninferiority trial.

*Setting.*—10 academic and community medical centers in Canada.

*Patients.*—252 patients with moderate to severe COPD.

*Intervention.*—After a 4-week education program, patients took part in home-based rehabilitation or outpatient, hospital-based rehabilitation for 8 weeks. They were followed for 40 weeks to complete the 1-year study.

*Measurements.*—The primary outcome was the change in Chronic Respiratory Questionnaire dyspnea subscale score at 1 year. The primary analysis took a modified intention-to-treat approach by using all patients who provided data at the specified follow-up time, regardless of their level of adherence. The analysis used regression modeling that adjusted for the effects of center, sex, and baseline level. All differences were computed as home intervention minus outpatient intervention.

*Results.*—Both interventions produced similar improvements in the Chronic Respiratory Questionnaire dyspnea subscale at 1 year: improvement in dyspnea of 0.62 (95% CI, 0.43 to 0.80) units in the home intervention ($n = 107$) and 0.46 (CI, 0.28 to 0.64) units in the outpatient intervention ($n = 109$). The difference between the 2 treatments at 1 year was small and clinically unimportant. The 95% CI of the difference did not exceed the prespecified noninferiority margin of 0.5: difference in dyspnea score of 0.16 (CI, −0.08 to 0.40). Most adverse events were related to COPD exacerbations. No serious adverse event was considered to be related to the study intervention.

*Limitation.*—The contribution of the educational program to the improvement in health status and exercise tolerance cannot be ascertained.

*Conclusion.*—Home rehabilitation is a useful, equivalent alternative to outpatient rehabilitation in patients with COPD.

▶ Pulmonary rehabilitation is widely recognized as a useful adjunct in the management of patients with chronic obstructive pulmonary disease (COPD). A number of recent studies, including a meta-analysis of randomized trials, support its use to improve the functional status and quality of life of these patients.[1] In addition, there is some data to support a lower rate of depression in COPD patients who participate in rehabilitation programs.[2] However, very few patients have access to rehabilitation programs because most are delivered in a hospital or clinic-associated outpatient setting, which are both limited in the number of patients they can accommodate and hard to access by the patients. Thus, the authors sought to compare, in a randomized trial, the results of a traditional outpatient program with that of an in-home, self-monitored program. All patients participated in an educational program that included disease management training and a description of the exercise modules; upon conclusion the patients were randomized. For home programs, a qualified exercise specialist initially came into the home and initiated the program to ensure patient understanding. After that, the only contact throughout the 8-week program was by telephone. Home programs were modified to include a slightly lower level of exercise for safety, but patients exercised for longer time periods. Following the formal programs, maintenance programs were handled similarly for both groups. Patients were encouraged to use exercise equipment and to continue exercising. Telephonic follow-up was conducted every 2 months. Results at 1 year were similar in the 2 programs. These results are very encouraging, as home-based programs that use considerably fewer skilled resources (as described here) would make pulmonary rehabilitation much more widely available to COPD patients. This is a treatment option that shows promise and deserves further investigation.

**J. R. Maurer, MD, MBA**

*References*

1. Lacasse Y, Goldstein R, Lasserson TJ, Martin S. Pulmonary rehabilitation for chronic obstructive pulmonary disease. *Cochrane Database Syst Rev.* 2006; CD003793. [PMID: 17054186].
2. Maurer J, Rebbapragada V, Borson S, et al. Anxiety and depression in COPD: current understanding, unanswered questions, and research needs. *Chest.* 2008; 134:43S-56S.

# 34 Lung Transplantation

---

**Herpes Zoster After Lung Transplantation: Incidence, Timing, and Outcome**

Fuks L, Shitrit D, Fox BD, et al (Pulmonary Inst, Petah Tiqwa, Israel; Tel Aviv Univ, Israel)

*Ann Thorac Surg* 87:423-426, 2009

---

*Background.*—Although herpes zoster is a common complication of lung transplantation, the epidemiologic data are limited. The aims of the present study were to determine the incidence and clinical manifestations of herpes zoster in a large cohort of lung transplant recipients and to identify risk factors associated with its development.

*Methods.*—The files of all adult patients who underwent lung transplantation at a major tertiary medical center from January 2001 to December 2007 were reviewed. Data were extracted on background, transplant-related, and posttransplantation factors. The occurrence and clinical characteristics of all episodes of herpes zoster were recorded.

*Results.*—Of the 198 lung transplant recipients, 23 had a herpes zoster infection, of whom 18 had herpes in a single dermatome. Disseminated cutaneous infection was documented in 4 cases (17%) and visceral involvement in 1. The median duration of follow-up was 34 months (range, 1 to 85 months). There were no recurrent infections. Postherpetic neuralgia was detected in 26% of cases. Antiviral prophylaxis, primarily for cytomegalovirus, was effective (during treatment) against herpes zoster. The incidence of herpes zoster was higher in patients treated with rabbit antithymocyte globulin.

*Conclusions.*—The occurrence of herpes zoster peaks between 12 and 36 months after lung transplantation. Additional immunosuppression may increase the risk. Further studies on preventive strategies against herpes zoster in this population are warranted.

▶ I have included this article on herpes zoster because this is such a common complication following lung transplantation and not much has been written about it. I am surprised at the rate of less than 15% reported in this population, and suspect that if the cohort were to be followed for a few more years the rate would be much higher. The risks, of course, in an immunosuppressed population are life-threatening disseminated cutaneous disease and visceral disease, as are reported in small numbers here. Another really distressing aspect of this disease is postherpetic neuralgia, which can result in such an impairment in quality of life that the sufferer becomes severely depressed. What about Zostavax, the new vaccine that helps prevent or reduce the severity of zoster?

It is a live, attenuated virus, so it cannot be given safely to immunosuppressed patients. It is approved, however, and recommended for most other patients ages 60 and above. Thus, it is appropriate for many people who might become candidates for transplant a few months in the future.

**J. R. Maurer, MD, MBA**

---

**Lung Transplantation in Older Patients With Cystic Fibrosis: Analysis of UNOS Data**

Weiss ES, Allen JG, Modi MN, et al (The Johns Hopkins Med Institutions, Baltimore, MD)

*J Heart Lung Transplant* 28:135-140, 2009

---

*Background.*—The lifespan for patients with cystic fibrosis (CF) is increasing. As a result, greater numbers of older CF patients are presenting for lung transplantation (LTx). The UNOS database provides an opportunity to examine outcomes for this population.

*Methods.*—We retrospectively reviewed UNOS data to identify 1,637 first-time LTx recipients with the indication of CF between 1999 and 2007. Patients were stratified by quartile age. Our primary end-point was all-cause mortality. Post-transplant survival was compared using Cox proportional hazards regression.

*Results.*—Of the patients who met the inclusion criteria, the distribution by age quartile was as follows: Quartile 1 (Q1), age 7 to 20 years, $N = 408$; Q2, 21 to 27, $N = 470$; Q3, 28 to 34, $N = 365$; and Q4,≥35, $N = 394$. Patients in the lowest quartile had the lowest 5-year cumulative survival (43%); 19% lower than for patients in Quartile 4 (age ≥35, cumulative survival = 62%; $p < 0.001$). On multivariable analysis, patients in Q3 and Q4 had a 38% and 32% reduction in cumulative hazard for death, respectively (reference Q1, age 7 to 20) (hazards ratios: Q3, 0.62 [0.46 to 0.85], $p < 0.001$; Q4, 0.68 [0.5 to 0.93], $p = 0.02$). Thirty-day and 1-year cumulative survival were not different among the four quartiles (30-day survival: Q1, 96.4%; Q2, 96.2%; Q3, 96.2%; and Q4, 95.5% [$p = 0.94$]; 1-year survival: Q1, 83.7%; Q2, 83.1%; Q3, 85.4%; and Q4, 83.4% [$p$ 0.88]). Increasing age was associated with decreases in early post-operative infections, reduction in the cumulative hazard of developing bronchiolitis obliterans (BO) syndrome, and decreases in hospitalizations and treatment for rejection.

*Conclusions.*—The UNOS database has provided a large series examining survival after LTx in older CF patients. LTx is safe in this group and older age may be protective against infection, rejection and BO syndrome (Fig 2).

► Cystic fibrosis (CF) has always been a common indication for lung transplantation, and these patients represent one of the youngest groups among

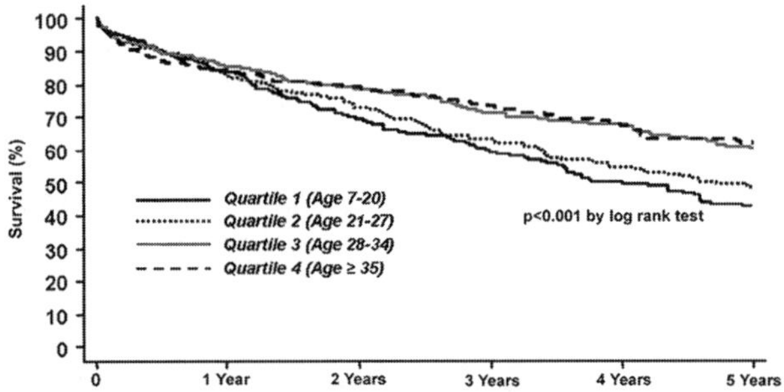


*Number of Patients At Risk Per Follow-Up Year*

| | 0 | 1 Year | 2 Years | 3 Years | 4 Years | 5 Years |
|---|---|---|---|---|---|---|
| Quartile 1 | 408 | 287 | 199 | 139 | 89 | 49 |
| Quartile 2 | 470 | 307 | 225 | 143 | 100 | 62 |
| Quartile 3 | 365 | 261 | 202 | 149 | 111 | 74 |
| Quartile 4 | 394 | 262 | 197 | 146 | 112 | 71 |

FIGURE 2.—Kaplan–Meier models of survival stratified by quartiles of age. Also presented are the numbers of patients at risk per year during the follow-up period. The $p$-value corresponds to Mantel–Cox log-rank test results (based on OPTN data, January 2007). (Reprinted from Weiss ES, Allen JG, Modi MN, et al. Lung transplantation in older patients with cystic fibrosis: analysis of UNOS data. *J Heart Lung Transplant.* 2009;28:135-140.)

adults coming to transplant. Over the years as medical management of cystic fibrosis lung disease has improved, the age of patients reaching end stage has increased so that many transplant candidates are now in their 40s. CF patients in their 40s, however, can have other problems that younger patients do not. In particular, these patients often have significant liver disease, gallbladder disease, and diabetes. They also have significant osteoporosis. Whether these and other comorbidities impact the overall survival of this older group of patients has not previously been specifically addressed. This report that reviews the United Network for Organ Sharing (UNOS) database, the largest repository of lung transplant patients, actually found better survivals up to 5 years in older patients than in younger patients. Not only were survivals better, the older CF recipients experienced fewer posttransplant complications. Physicians treating CF patients should not hesitate to refer their older patients for transplants as the outcomes appear superior to those of younger candidates (Fig 2).

**J. R. Maurer, MD, MBA**

# 35 Sleep Disorders

### Diagnosis of Obstructive Sleep Apnea Syndrome and Its Outcomes With Home Portable Monitoring

de Oliveira ACT, Martinez D, Vasconcelos LFT, et al (Universidade Federal do Rio Grande do Sul, Porto Alegre, RS, Brazil; et al)
*Chest* 135:330-336, 2009

*Background.*—The use of portable respiratory monitoring (PM) has been proposed for the diagnosis of obstructive sleep apnea syndrome (OSAS), but most studies that validate PM accuracy have not followed the best standards for diagnostic test validation. The objective of the present study was to evaluate the accuracy of PM performed at home to diagnose OSAS and its outcomes after first validating PM in the laboratory setting by comparing it to polysomnography (PSG).

*Methods.*—Patients with suspected OSAS were submitted, in random order, to PM at the sleep laboratory concurrently with PSG (lab-PM) or at home-PM. The diagnostic performance was assessed by sensitivity, specificity, positive and negative predictive values, positive likelihood ratio (+LR), negative likelihood ratio (−LR), intraclass correlation coefficients, κ statistic, and Bland-Altman plot.

*Results.*—One hundred fifty-seven subjects (73% men, mean age ± SD, 45 ± 12 yr) with an apnea-hypopnea index (AHI) of 31 (SD ± 29) events/h were studied. Excluding inadequate recordings, 149 valid comparisons with lab-PM and 121 with unattended home-PM were obtained. Compared to PSG for detecting AHI > 5, the lab-PM demonstrated sensitivity of 95.3%, specificity of 75%, +LR of 3.8, and −LR of 0.11; the home-PM exhibited sensitivity of 96%, specificity of 64%, +LR of 2.7, and −LR of 0.05. Kappa statistics indicated substantial correlation between PSG and PM results. Bland-Altman plot showed smaller dispersion for lab-PM than for home-PM. Pearson product moment correlation coefficients among the three AHIs and clinical outcomes were similar, denoting comparable diagnostic ability.

*Conclusions.*—This study used all available comparison methods to demonstrate accuracy of PM in-home recordings similar to that of repeated PSGs. PM increases the possibility of correctly diagnosing and effectively treating OSAS in populations worldwide.

▶ Sleep disordered breathing (SDB) is very common. The Wisconsin Sleep Cohort Study reported that 9% of women and 24% of men have SDB as defined by an apnea-hypopnea index (AHI) > 5. Hence, with longer wait times for in laboratory polysomnography, the field has turned to alternative methods of diagnosis using home portable monitoring. Several types of monitors have been developed, and guidelines for the use of such devices have been set forth by the Portable Monitoring Task Force of the American Academy of Sleep Medicine.[1] However, questions still arise as to the diagnostic accuracy of these devices. This study examines the diagnostic accuracy of a home portable monitor used one night in the home (home-portable respiratory monitoring [PM]) followed by a night in the laboratory in which both the gold standard polysomnography and portable monitor were simultaneously worn (lab-PM). Home-PM is a good tool to use to essentially rule in or out the diagnosis of severe obstructive sleep apnea (OSA), and hence, is useful in screening a population where disease is common. The probability of home-PM to correctly exclude severe OSA was 91.7%, and to correctly diagnose severe OSA was 87.6%.[2] The sensitivity of home-PM to detect AHI < 5 was 96.1% specificity 64.7%.[2] The authors excluded 16% of the home-PM studies due to technical problems and short duration of recording. This number, in my clinical opinion, is somewhat large, but nevertheless is similar to reports from other studies. Based on the findings in this study, using home portable monitoring is an accurate means of diagnosing OSA.

**S. F. Jones, MD, FCCP, DABSM**

*References*

1. Collop NA, Anderson WM, Boehlecke B, et al. Clinical guidelines for the use of unattended portable monitors in the diagnosis of obstructive sleep apnea in adult patients. *J Clin Sleep Med.* 2007;3:737-747.
2. Tonelli de Oliveira AC, Martinez D, Vasconcelos LF, et al. Diagnosis of obstructive sleep apnea syndrome and its outcomes with home portable monitoring. *Chest.* 2009;135:330-336.

**Effectiveness of Pillar palatal implants for snoring management**

Gillespie MB, Smith JE, Clarke J, et al (Med Univ of South Carolina)
*Otolaryngol Head Neck Surg* 140:363-368, 2009

*Objective.*—Determine patient factors associated with the success and complications of using the Pillar palatal implants for snoring management.

*Study Design.*—Retrospective series of 79 consecutive adult patients receiving Pillar implants for snoring management between January 2005 and December 2007. Multiple regression analysis was used to determine factors associated with initial and final bed partner satisfaction with the snoring result, and factors associated with Pillar-related complications.

*Results.*—A total of 64 of 79 (81%) bed partners reported snoring improvement in patients after initial Pillar implantation; however, only 31 (39%) were satisfied with the level of reduction. Following secondary procedures, the number of satisfied bed partners improved to 52 (66%). Factors associated with final bed partner satisfaction included lower initial apnea-hypopnea index (AHI) ($P = 0.029$), Friedman tongue position I or II ($P = 0.008$), and shorter follow-up time ($P = 0.001$). Sixteen patients (20%) experienced procedure-related complications. Factors associated with Pillar complications included female gender ($P = 0.001$) and placement under general anesthesia ($P = 0.009$).

*Conclusions.*—Initial AHI values and tongue position scores are important determinants of final snoring success. Pillar implants placed in women and under general anesthesia may have a higher risk of poor placement and extrusion.

▶ The Pillar palatal implant system is an alternative treatment for patients who snore that has been shown to reduce the level of snoring[1] and improve satisfaction scores of bed partners.[2] It has also been used in mild to moderate obstructive sleep apnea with significant improvement in the apnea-hypopnea index (AHI) in a very small study of 35 subjects.[3] In this particular study, authors performed a retrospective case series of 79 adult patients who underwent Pillar palatal implant for snoring and/or mild to moderate obstructive sleep apnea, examining factors associated with complications and initial and final bed partner snoring satisfaction. While improvement in snoring was reported by 81% of bed partners, only 39% of bed partners were satisfied initially. Satisfaction improved to 66% after additional procedures were performed.

Lower AHI, Friedman tongue position I or II, and follow-up times were associated with final bed partner satisfaction. Follow-up time was also associated with both initial bed partner satisfaction. In the dissatisfied group, mean follow-up time was 14 months compared with 5.4 months in the satisfied group. This may suggest that the efficacy of the device decreases over time. The satisfaction scores from this study are not as impressive as those published by Nordgård et al.[2] This is most likely due to the fact that subjects were not required to undergo polysomnography before Pillar implant procedure, and perhaps some patients classified as snorers actually had obstructive sleep apnea to a significant degree. Because a lower AHI was associated with final bed partner satisfaction, performing polysomnography before Pillar implantation may help with patient selection.

**S. F. Jones, MD, FCCP, DABSM**

*References*

1. Nordgård S, Wormdal K, Bugten V, Stene BK, Skjøstad KW. Palatal implants: a new method for the treatment of snoring. *Acta Otolaryngol.* 2004;124:970-975.
2. Nordgård S, Bugten V, Wormdal K, et al. Palatal implants for the treatment of snoring: long term results. *Otolaryngol Head Neck Surg.* 2006;134:558-564.
3. Nordgård S, Stene BK, Skjøstad KW. Soft palate implants for the treatment of mild to moderate obstructive sleep apnea. *Otolaryngol Head Neck Surg.* 2006;134:565-570.

**The New AASM Criteria for Scoring Hypopneas: Impact on the Apnea Hypopnea Index**

Ruehland WR, Rochford PD, O'Donoghue FJ, et al (Inst for Breathing and Sleep, Austin Health, Heidelberg, Victoria, Australia; et al)
*Sleep* 32:150-157, 2009

*Study Objectives.*—To compare apnea-hypopnea indices (AHIs) derived using 3 standard hypopnea definitions published by the American Academy of Sleep Medicine (AASM); and to examine the impact of hypopnea definition differences on the measured prevalence of obstructive sleep apnea (OSA).

*Design.*—Retrospective review of previously scored in-laboratory polysomnography (PSG).

*Setting.*—Two tertiary-hospital clinical sleep laboratories.

*Patients or Participants.*—328 consecutive patients investigated for OSA during a 3-month period.

*Interventions.*—N/A.

*Measurements and Results.*—AHIs were originally calculated using previous AASM hypopnea scoring criteria ($AHI_{Chicago}$), requiring either > 50% airflow reduction or a lesser airflow reduction with associated > 3% oxygen desaturation or arousal. AHIs using the "recommended" ($AHI_{Rec}$) and the "alternative" ($AHI_{Alt}$) hypopnea definitions of the *AASM Manual for Scoring of Sleep and Associated Events* were then derived in separate passes of the previously scored data. In this process, hypopneas that did not satisfy the stricter hypopnea definition criteria were removed. For $AHI_{Rec}$, hypopneas were required to have ≥ 30% airflow reduction and ≥ 4% desaturation; and for $AHI_{Alt}$, hypopneas were required to have ≥ 50% airflow reduction and ≥ 3% desaturation or arousal. The median $AHI_{Rec}$ was approximately 30% of the median $AHI_{Chicago}$, whereas the median $AHI_{Alt}$ was approximately 60% of the $AHI_{Chicago}$, with large, AHI-dependent, patient-specific differences observed. Equivalent cut-points for $AHI_{Rec}$ and $AHI_{Alt}$ compared to $AHI_{Chicago}$ cut-points of 5, 15, and 30/h were established with receiver operator curves (ROC). These cut-points were also approximately 30% of $AHI_{Chicago}$ using $AHI_{Rec}$ and 60% of $AHI_{Chicago}$ using $AHI_{Alt}$. Failure to adjust cut-points for the new criteria would result in approximately 40% of patients previously classified as positive for OSA using $AHI_{Chicago}$ being negative using $AHI_{Rec}$ and 25% being negative using $AHI_{Alt}$.

*Conclusions.*—This study demonstrates that using different published standard hypopnea definitions leads to marked differences in AHI. These results provide insight to clinicians and researchers in interpreting results obtained using different published standard hypopnea definitions, and they suggest that consideration should be given to revising the current scoring recommendations to include a single standardized hypopnea definition.

▶ The definition of hypopnea has undergone multiple revisions, and with that controversy. This controversy surrounds methods of airflow monitoring (nasal pressure vs thermal devices), degree of desaturation, and amount of airflow reduction. The American Academy of Sleep Medicine (AASM) defined a hypopnea known as "Chicago criteria" on 2 different types: (1) a 50% reduction in the airflow signal. These reductions do not necessarily have associated desaturations or arousals or (2) any discernable reduction in airflow associated with an oxygen desaturation of at least 3%, or an associated arousal. This definition, however, is not used universally by all laboratories. The Centers for Medicare and Medicaid services accepts another definition (also published by the AASM) in which a hypopnea is defined as a 30% reduction in airflow associated with a 4% or greater oxygen desaturation. Recently, the AASM redefined hypopneas as events characterized by a reduction in nasal pressure by at least 30% of baseline for a duration of at least 10 seconds accompanied by an oxygen desaturation ≥4% (this is the recommended definition). In addition, the new AASM criteria offers an alternative definition of hypopnea defined as reduction in nasal pressure signal by ≥50% of baseline for a duration of at least 10 seconds accompanied by a ≥3% desaturation or arousal.

In this particular study, the authors examined the effect of the AHI when each of the above definitions of hypopnea are applied. When the Chicago and alternative definitions of hypopneas are applied using the arousals, the median AHI increases. If the recommended definition is used, the median AHI is decreased. By employing different definitions that affect the AHI, there will be changes to OSA severity, prevalence of disease, etc. This article highlights that it is important to identify which definition of respiratory events are being used not only in the laboratory, but also in the literature.

**S. F. Jones, MD, FCCP, DABSM**

---

**Obstructive Sleep Apnea, Insulin Resistance, and Steatohepatitis in Severe Obesity**

Polotsky VY, Patil SP, Savransky V, et al (Johns Hopkins Bloomberg School of Public Health, Baltimore, MD; et al)

*Am J Respir Crit Care Med* 179:228-234, 2009

---

*Rationale.*—Obstructive sleep apnea is associated with insulin resistance and liver injury. It is unknown whether apnea contributes to insulin resistance and steatohepatitis in severe obesity.

*Objectives.*—To examine whether sleep apnea and nocturnal hypoxemia predict the severity of insulin resistance, systemic inflammation, and steatohepatitis in severely obese individuals presenting for bariatric surgery.

*Methods.*—We performed sleep studies and measured fasting blood glucose, serum insulin, C-reactive protein, and liver enzymes in 90 consecutive severely obese individuals, 75 women and 15 men, without concomitant diabetes mellitus or preexistent diagnosis of sleep apnea or liver disease. Liver biopsies (n = 20) were obtained during bariatric surgery.

*Measurements and Main Results.*—Obstructive sleep apnea with a respiratory disturbance index greater than 5 events/hour was diagnosed in 81.1% of patients. The median respiratory disturbance index was 15 ± 29 events/hour and the median oxygen desaturation during apneic events was 4.6 ± 1.8%. All patients exhibited high serum levels of C-reactive protein, regardless of the severity of apnea, whereas liver enzymes were normal. Oxygen desaturation greater than 4.6% was associated with a 1.5-fold increase in insulin resistance, according to the homeostasis model assessment index. Histopathology data suggested that significant nocturnal desaturation might predispose to hepatic inflammation, hepatocyte ballooning, and liver fibrosis. Fasting blood glucose levels and steatosis scores were not affected by nocturnal hypoxia. There was no relationship between the respiratory disturbance index and insulin resistance or liver histopathology.

*Conclusions.*—Hypoxic stress of sleep apnea may be implicated in the development of insulin resistance and steatohepatitis in severe obesity.

▶ Obstructive sleep apnea (OSA) is associated with insulin resistance, systemic inflammation, liver injury, and glucose intolerance; however, it is unclear whether the mechanism is related to hypoxemia or obesity. By examining an obese population undergoing bariatric surgery, the investigators were able to examine the relationship between OSA and nonalcoholic fatty liver disease (steatosis and steatohepatitis). Not surprisingly, with a mean body mass index of 49 kg/m$^2$, a large portion of subjects (81%) had undiagnosed sleep apnea. Those with more severe degrees of OSA (respiratory disturbance index [RDI] > 15 events per hour) had a greater mean fall in oxyhemoglobin saturation ($\Delta SaO_2$) and had lower daytime $PaO_2$. C-reactive protein, a marker of systemic inflammation, was high for all subjects but did not correlate with OSA. Insulin resistance correlated with the severity of oxyhemoglobin desaturation, even after adjustment for obesity, suggesting an independent effect between intermittent hypoxemia and insulin resistance.

One of the strong factors in this study is the performance of liver biopsies on 20 subjects. The investigators were able to infer possible mechanisms of liver injury. Hypoxemia, rather than the severity of the OSA (defined by number of events), correlated more with liver injury (fibrosis, ballooning, and inflammation on liver biopsy). It may be that hypoxemia is the factor that leads to progressive liver damage and eventually nonalcoholic steatohepatitis, and perhaps even cirrhosis, although no subject had cirrhosis and this was not addressed by the study. This study sheds light on mechanisms and will lead to further studies examining interventions such as continuous positive airway pressure (CPAP) and its effect on liver disease.

**S. F. Jones, MD, FCCP, DABSM**

**Compliance in sleep apnoea therapy: influence of home care support and pressure mode**

Damjanovic D, Fluck A, Bremer H, et al (Univ Hosp Freiburg, Germany)
*Eur Respir J* 33:804-811, 2009

Continuous positive airway pressure (CPAP) is an effective treatment for obstructive sleep apnoea syndrome (OSAS) but therapy adherence is often low. The hypothesis that CPAP-adherence and clinical outcomes can be improved by either using an autoadjusting-CPAP (APAP) device or an intensive support was tested.

A controlled parallel group study was performed with 100 newly diagnosed OSAS patients, randomised into 4 groups (n = 25 each): standard or intensive support plus either APAP or CPAP. Intensive support included education and monthly home visits for 6 months. Clinical outcome was monitored by polysomnography at CPAP initiation and, after 3 and 9 months, compliance data were downloaded from the CPAP devices.

After 9 months, intensively supported patients returned for follow-up in 88 *versus* 68% in the standard-support-group. Daily usage (mean ± SEM 5.7 ± 0.2 for intensive support *versus* 4.6 ± 0.4 h for standard support), percentage of days used (80.4 ± 2.8 *versus* 57.0 ± 5.9%) and proportion of individual sleep time (80.6 ± 3.2 *versus* 64.9 ± 6.2%) were also higher. There was no significant difference between APAP or CPAP, (daily usage 5.2 ± 0.4 *versus* 5.1 ± 0.3 h, percentage of days 67.9 ± 5.0 *versus* 69.2 ± 4.9%, proportion of sleep time 72.5 ± 5.0% *versus* 72.1 ± 5.2%, for APAP and CPAP) but retention rate was higher with CPAP.

In summary, intensive support after continuous positive airway pressure initiation, rather than the application of autoadjusting-continuous positive airway pressure, increased therapy adherence.

▶ It is well known that compliance with continuous positive airway pressure (CPAP) remains a challenging task for both the patient and a frustration for the practitioner. Behavioral interventions such as intensive educational support and technological advances such as autotitration devices have been used to help the CPAP user, each with varying degrees of success. The investigators examined the use of autotitrating CPAP versus standard CPAP plus intensive support, including education and monthly home visits versus standard therapy. The addition of intensive support for a total of 9 months led to increased compliance with CPAP as far as percentage of days used and number of hours used per night compared with the standard therapy group. Over time, compliance with CPAP (both standard and autotitrating) diminishes. Compliance with CPAP using standard therapy also decreases over time. However, this decrement is not seen with intensive support. Perhaps it is because subjects in the intensive support arm benefit from the reminders and motivation that education and counseling gives as well as the optimization of mask fit.

The study does not address the cost-effectiveness of having an intensive support intervention for CPAP users. It would be interesting to see. However, if one factors the enormous economic impact of sleep disorders in our nation, use of intensive support may be financially prudent. In fact, according to this study, to improve compliance we would be better off performing intensive support versus prescribing autotitration CPAP.

**S. F. Jones, MD, FCCP, DABSM**

## Cognitive Behavioral Therapy, Singly and Combined With Medication, for Persistent Insomnia: A Randomized Controlled Trial

Morin CM, Vallières A, Guay B, et al (Université Laval, Québec, Canada; et al)
*JAMA* 301:2005-2015, 2009

*Context.*—Cognitive behavioral therapy (CBT) and hypnotic medications are efficacious for short-term treatment of insomnia, but few patients achieve complete remission with any single treatment. It is unclear whether combined or maintenance therapies would enhance outcome.

*Objectives.*—To evaluate the added value of medication over CBT alone for acute treatment of insomnia and the effects of maintenance therapies on long-term outcome.

*Design, Setting, and Patients.*—Prospective, randomized controlled trial involving 2-stage therapy for 160 adults with persistent insomnia treated at a university hospital sleep center in Canada between January 2002 and April 2005.

*Interventions.*—Participants received CBT alone or CBT plus 10 mg/d (taken at bedtime) of zolpidem for an initial 6-week therapy, followed by extended 6-month therapy. Patients initially treated with CBT attended monthly maintenance CBT for 6 months or received no additional treatment and those initially treated with combined therapy (CBT plus 10 mg/d of zolpidem) continued with CBT plus intermittent use of zolpidem or CBT only.

*Main Outcome Measures.*—Sleep onset latency, time awake after sleep onset, total sleep time, and sleep efficiency derived from daily diaries (primary outcomes); treatment response and remission rates derived from the Insomnia Severity Index (secondary outcomes).

*Results.*—Cognitive behavioral therapy used singly or in combination with zolpidem produced significant improvements in sleep latency, time awake after sleep onset, and sleep efficiency during initial therapy (all $P < .001$); a larger increase of sleep time was obtained with the combined approach ($P = .04$). Both CBT alone and CBT plus zolpidem produced similar rates of treatment responders (60% [45/75] vs 61% [45/74], respectively; $P = .84$) and treatment remissions (39% [29/75] vs 44% [33/74], respectively; $P = .52$) with the 6-week acute treatment, but combined therapy produced a higher remission rate compared with CBT alone during the 6-month extended therapy phase and the 6-month follow-up period (56% [43/74 and 32/59] vs 43% [34/75 and 28/68]; $P = .05$). The best long-term outcome was obtained with patients treated with combined therapy initially, followed by CBT alone, as evidenced by higher remission rates at the 6-month follow-up compared with patients who continued to take zolpidem during extended therapy (68% [20/30] vs 42% [12/29]; $P=.04$).

*Conclusion.*—In patients with persistent insomnia, the addition of medication to CBT produced added benefits during acute therapy, but long-term outcome was optimized when medication is discontinued during maintenance CBT.

*Trial Registration.*—clinicaltrials.gov Identifier: NCT00042146.

▶ The prevalence of insomnia exceeds that of obstructive sleep apnea while the economical impact of insomnia reaches a multibillion dollar level. Cognitive behavioral therapy (CBT), a combined approach involving sleep restrictions and education about appropriate sleep hygiene, aims to change common misconceptions about sleep. It is known that CBT is not a "quick fix" for insomnia and sometimes multiple sessions with trained medical staff are needed. Meanwhile, hypnotics may provide rapid improvement of sleep complaints, but their long-term use raises many questions. The investigators addressed important questions in the treatment of insomnia: Is a combined (CBT with hypnotic) more effective than CBT alone? What is the effectiveness of discontinuing the hypnotic after the initial treatment versus continuing it on an intermittent basis? The investigators used a 4-arm randomization: CBT alone or combined therapy with 10 mg zolpidem nightly. After 6 weeks (termed acute therapy), subjects were then randomized again. Those receiving CBT alone were randomized to either CBT alone for 6 additional months or nothing at all. Those receiving combined therapy were randomized to CBT alone for 6 months or CBT for 6 months with intermittent use zolpidem. The combined treatment was more effective at increasing total sleep time in the short-term (6 weeks). It appears that use of CBT, both singly and in combination, was associated with remission of insomnia, but those who discontinued zolpidem after 6 weeks had the highest remission rates. Futhermore, remission increased over time, suggesting that benefits are sustainable. In this study, the population consisted of predominantly white females with higher levels of education. This may not be applicable to other populations. Furthermore, I question whether this is useful in a real world setting. CBT was conducted by at least a master's level clinical psychologists in this study. Access to CBT remains prohibitive for many. I think repeating some aspects of this study using some of the online CBT modules may further expand its clinical usefulness.

**S. F. Jones, MD, FCCP, DABSM**

# 36 Pleural, Interstitial Lung, and Pulmonary Vascular Disease

**Long-term Anticoagulant Therapy for Idiopathic Pulmonary Embolism in the Elderly: A Decision Analysis**

Haspel J, Bauer K, Goehler A, et al (Harvard Med School, Boston, MA; Massachusetts General Hosp, Boston, MA)

*Chest* 135:1243-1251, 2009

*Background.*—Elderly patients with idiopathic pulmonary embolism (PE) are at high risk for recurrent venous thromboembolic disease and might benefit from long-term anticoagulant therapy. But they are also at higher risk for bleeding complications. Because there have been no clinical trials addressing PE treatment in elderly patients, the balance of therapeutic benefits and risks is unclear.

*Methods.*—We constructed a decision-analytic model to forecast the effects of long-term warfarin therapy for idiopathic PE. We focused on 65- and 80-year-old outpatients, with or without a propensity for falls, who previously had completed 6 to 12 months of anticoagulant therapy without experiencing a major bleed. The model incorporated age-appropriate thromboembolic recurrence rates after PE, major bleeding risks of warfarin use, and the contribution of falls to major bleeding episodes in anticoagulated elderly patients. We used probabilistic sensitivity analysis to model outcomes over ranges of potential thromboembolic and bleeding risks.

*Results.*—In our baseline analysis, long-term warfarin was superior to conventional duration therapy. Depending on the patient subgroup (stratified by age and fall risk), it increased life expectancy by 0.16 to 0.56 years and event-free life expectancy by 0.32 to 0.51 years. Probabilistic sensitivity analysis demonstrated that long-term warfarin therapy was likely to increase life expectancy when compared with conventional-duration therapy (76 to 93% likelihood across all groups).

*Conclusions.*—Extended anticoagulant therapy for idiopathic PE may be beneficial in a subgroup of elderly patients who tolerate the initial 6 to 12 months of therapy without bleeding complications. In this population, advanced age and fall risk were not contraindications to long-term anticoagulation.

▶ The study is interesting because it is always an issue for clinicians to determine the length of anticoagulation, especially in elderly patients with pulmonary embolism (PE). We also know that approximately 50% of PEs are idiopathic, and compared with known precipitants PEs are 2- to 3-fold more likely to recur and carry a higher risk of death.

In this study, a simulated model has shown some interesting findings. It was done in patients ranging from 65 to 80 years of age.

Long-term warfarin therapy reduced venous thromboembolic event (VTE) recurrences by 2- to 3-fold. As the simulation progressed, warfarin usage fell in the long-term arm (because of major bleeding events) and rose in the conventional duration arm (because of recurrent VTE).

Long-term warfarin therapy increased absolute life expectancy by 0.16 to 0.56 years compared with conventional therapy. Event-free life expectancy also increased by 0.32 to 0.51 years.

Long-term warfarin therapy was most beneficial in 65-year-old patients with no history of falls, and was least valuable in 80-year-old patients with a history of falls.

Limitations: The model could only investigate effects on hard end points (such as absolute or event-free survival) and does not speak to the societal cost effectiveness of long-term anticoagulation for PE. It did not include inferior vena cava filters in the model.

By any standards, at the end it is still a simulated assessment; please take it with a grain of salt.

**M. Ali Raza, MD, FCCP, DABSM**

---

**Pulmonary Cement Embolism after Percutaneous Vertebroplasty in Osteoporotic Vertebral Compression Fractures: Incidence, Characteristics, and Risk Factors**

Kim YJ, Lee JW, Park KW, et al (Seoul Natl Univ Bundang Hosp, South Korea; et al)

*Radiology* 251:250-259, 2009

---

*Purpose.*—To prospectively evaluate the incidence of, characteristics of, and risk factors for pulmonary cement embolism after percutaneous vertebroplasty (PVP) in osteoporotic vertebral compression fractures (VCFs).

*Materials and Methods.*—Institutional review board approval and written informed consent were obtained. From June 2006 to September 2007, 75 patients (57 women, 18 men; mean age, 74.78 years; range, 48–93 years) who underwent 78 PVP sessions at 119 levels for osteoporotic VCFs were prospectively enrolled in this study. Computed tomographic (CT) scans of the chest and treated vertebrae were obtained after PVP. The presence, location, involved pulmonary arteries, number, and size of each pulmonary cement embolus were analyzed at CT. Possible risk factors were analyzed as follows: Age, injected cement volumes, and numbers of treated vertebrae were analyzed by using the Mann-Whitney *U* test; operators (radiologist or nonradiologist), level of treated vertebrae, guidance equipment, approach (uni- or bipedicular), presence of intravertebral vacuum clefts, and presence of paravertebral venous leakage were analyzed by using Pearson $\chi^2$ and Fisher exact tests.

*Results.*—Pulmonary cement emboli developed in 18 (23%) of 78 PVP sessions and were detected in the distal to third-order pulmonary arteries. Only cement leakage into the inferior vena cava showed a statistically significant relationship to pulmonary cement embolism ($P = .03$). A higher frequency of pulmonary cement embolism was noted for the absence of intravertebral vacuum clefts, for the bipedicular approach, and for a nonradiologist operator with C-arm fluoroscopy ($P > .05$).

*Conclusion.*—In osteoporotic VCFs, pulmonary cement embolism was detected in 23% of PVP sessions, developed in the distal to third-order pulmonary arteries, and was related to leakage into the inferior vena cava.

▶ This study prospectively evaluates the incidence and risk factor of pulmonary cement embolism after vertebroplasty. Firstly, pulmonary cement embolism occurs more frequently (up to 23%) than previously reported. There are a number of risk factors: 1) Cement leakage into the inferior vena cava. 2) The absence of intravertebral vacuum clefts. 3) The use of a bipedicular approach. 4) Performance by a nonradiologist operator with intraoperative C-arm fluoroscopy.

Percutaneous vertebroplasty (PVP) performed by a radiologist with biplanar digital subtraction angiography (DSA) showed the lowest frequency of pulmonary cement embolism (4 [15.4%] of 26 sessions), but these differences were not statistically significant because of the study's small number.

Pulmonary cement embolism can develop without evidence of paravertebral leakage at intraoperative fluoroscopy and postvertebroplasty CT.

**M. Ali Raza, MD, FCCP, DABSM**

---

**Diagnostic Surgical Lung Biopsies for Suspected Interstitial Lung Diseases: A Retrospective Study**

Sigurdsson MI, Isaksson HJ, Gudmundsson G, et al (Landspitali Univ Hosp, Reykjavik, Iceland; Univ of Iceland, Reykjavik)

*Ann Thorac Surg* 88:227-232, 2009

---

*Background.*—Current guidelines for interstitial lung disease support a surgical biopsy for optimal diagnosis and treatment, yet only a minority of patients undergo such biopsy. Our objectives were to address the properties of a surgical lung biopsy for suspected interstitial lung disease, the diagnostic yield of the procedure, and whether it resulted in changes in diagnosis and treatment.

*Methods.*—A retrospective nationwide study including 73 patients (mean age, 57.3 years; 58% males) who underwent a surgical lung biopsy for suspected interstitial disease in Iceland between 1986 and 2007 was conducted. Patient records and histologic specimens were reviewed. Before the surgical biopsy a transbronchial or computed tomography–guided biopsy had been performed in two thirds of the patients.

*Results.*—The complication rate for surgical lung biopsy was 16%, and 30-day operative mortality was 2.7%, both significantly higher in patients with preoperative respiratory failure. After the procedure, a definite histopathologic diagnosis was obtained in 81% of the patients. Usual interstitial pneumonia was the most common diagnosis (31%). The clinical diagnosis was changed for 73% of the patients, and in 53% of the patients the biopsy resulted in changes in treatment.

*Conclusions.*—Surgical lung biopsy is a powerful tool for diagnosis of suspected interstitial lung disease. It results in a specific diagnosis for the majority of patients and changes in treatment for more than half. Operative morbidity and mortality are low but still significant, so patients should be carefully selected for the procedure, especially those with respiratory failure.

▶ It is mostly a debate among pulmonologists when to send somebody with interstitial lung disease (ILD) to open lung biopsy. It is even harder to decide when the patient is in impending respiratory failure. Most of the trials and observations before Dr Sigurdson's retrospective study have shown that doing open lung biopsy (OLB) has no mortality improvement, changes diagnosis in almost one third of patients, and the treatment is altered in about 20% of those patients.

I think this retrospective trial is more optimistic because it spans 21 years, and a lot of improvement has occurred in the diagnostic modalities in that time period. In my opinion the take home point is: If you think the diagnosis is not sure, and you think an altered and aggressive therapy will save the patient's life, it is reasonable to go for the biopsy. Interestingly, no cutoff of respiratory parameters were found, and the number of biopsies did not matter either, so maybe we don't need an extensive procedure for these patients, and a small video-assisted thoracoscopic surgery (VATS) biopsy is enough. Alternatively bronchoscopy is another technique for sick patients who are not candidates for anesthesia.

A strength of this study is its nationwide design; patients were operated on in a single cardiothoracic center by 6 surgeons.

Main weaknesses are the limited number of patients and the retrospective design. Indications for referring patients for surgical biopsy were not standardized during the whole study period.

**M. Ali Raza, MD, FCCP, DABSM**

**Contrast echocardiography for pulmonary arteriovenous malformations screening: does any bubble matter?**

Gazzaniga P, Buscarini E, Leandro G, et al (Maggiore Hosp, Crema, Italy; IRCCS, Castellana Grotte, Italy; et al)
*Eur J Echocardiogr* 10:513-518, 2009

*Aims.*—To evaluate diagnostic accuracy of contrast echocardiography (CE) as compared with CT, for the screening of pulmonary arteriovenous malformations (PAVMs) in hereditary haemorrhagic telangiectasia (HHT); to evaluate the clinical significance of semi-quantitative analysis of a shunt on CE.

*Methods and Results.*—A blinded prospective study was conducted in 190 consecutive subjects at risk of HHT who underwent screening for PAVMs, including clinical evaluation, pulse oximetry, standard and CE, and chest multirow CT without contrast medium. A semi-quantitative analysis of the shunt size was performed according to the contrast echo opacification of the left-sided chambers: Grade 0, no bubbles; 1, occasional filling with <20 bubbles; 2, moderate filling; 3, complete opacification. The first 100 patients were compared with 100 controls. A total of 119 (63) patients had positive CE (32.2 Grade 1, 13.1 Grade 2, 11 Grade 3, 6.3 with patent foramen ovale). The overall diagnostic performance of CE was sensitivity 1.00, specificity 0.49, positive predictive value (PPV) 0.32, negative predictive value (NPV) 1.00. The PPV for the different grades was 0.00 for Grade 1, 0.56 for Grade 2, 1.00 for Grade 3; the NPV of Grade 0 was 1.00. A significant correlation was found between the CE grading and the number of PAVM, and complications ($P < 0.0001$).

*Conclusion.*—CE is an extremely sensitive procedure for the detection of PAVMs with substantial clinical impact.

▶ This is the first prospective controlled blinded study to evaluate the role of Contrast echo in screening Pulmonary AVMs in HHT.

Grading was done from 0 to 3 as described above. It was then compared with CT angiogram.

The study shows an excellent sensitivity of CE to detect PAVMs. One NPV of CE tells me that CT should only be done in cases with grade 2 or more shunt seen on CE. Of course this means less dye and radiation for the HHT patients, and less bill. I also think that this economical way will also be proven fruitful in following these patients after coiling if ever needed.

CE has its own downside, but minimal, if any, side effects have been reported with this method, even in the large shunts.

One limitation of the study is that patients with CE positive/CT negative were not subject to angiography.

**M. Ali Raza, MD, FCCP, DABSM**

### Is Full Postpleurodesis Lung Expansion a Determinant of a Successful Outcome After Talc Pleurodesis?

Terra RM, Junqueira JJM, Teixeira LR, et al (Univ of São Paulo Med School, Brazil)

*Chest* 136:361-368, 2009

*Study Objectives.*—To analyze and compare radiologic lung expansion after talc pleurodesis performed either by videothoracoscopy or chest tube and correlate it with clinical outcome. Secondary end points evaluated were as follows: clinical efficacy; quality of life; safety; and survival.

*Methods.*—Prospective randomized study that included 60 patients (45 women, 15 men; mean age, 55.2 years) with recurrent malignant pleural effusion between January 2005 and January 2008. They were randomized into the following two groups: video-assisted thoracic surgery (VATS) talc poudrage; and talc slurry (TS) administered through a chest tube. Lung expansion was evaluated through chest CT scans obtained 0, 1, 3 and 6 months after pleurodesis. Complications, drainage time, hospital stay, and quality of life (Medical Outcomes Study 36-item short form and World Health Organization quality-of-life questionnaires) were also analyzed.

*Results.*—There were no significant differences in preprocedure clinical and pathologic variables between groups. The immediate total (*ie*, > 90%) lung expansion was observed in 27 patients (45%) and was more frequent in the VATS group (60% vs 30%, respectively; $p = 0.027$). During follow-up, 71% of the patients showed unaltered or improved lung expansion and 9 patients (15%) needed new pleural procedures (VATS group, 5 recurrences; TS group, 4 recurrences; $p = 0.999$). No differences were found between groups regarding quality of life, complications, drainage time, hospital stay, and survival. Immediate lung expansion did not correlate with radiologic recurrence, clinical recurrence, or complications ($p = 0.60$, 0.15, and 0.20, respectively).

*Conclusion.*—Immediate partial lung expansion was a frequent finding and was more frequent after TS. Nonetheless, no correlation between immediate lung expansion and clinical outcome was found in this study.

*Trial Registration.*—ClinicalTrials.gov Identifier: NTC00789087.

▶ No significant differences in preprocedure clinical and pathologic variables were observed between groups.

Postoperative total lung expansion seen in video-assisted thoracic surgery (VATS) patients was better than talc slurry (TS), but there seemed to be no significant difference between groups regarding quality of life, complications, drainage time, hospital stay, and survival.

The point is that postprocedure complete lung expansion, which makes sense as a marker for better pleurodesis, does not have any bearing on how the patient is going to do. Both the procedures, VATS and TS, are almost equally efficacious. The length of stay was favored in VATS, but did not meet significance.

**M. Ali Raza, MD, FCCP, DABSM**

PART SIX

# HEART AND CARDIOVASCULAR DISEASE

BERNARD J. GERSH, MB, CHB, D.PHIL, FRCP

# 37 Cardiac Arrhythmias, Conduction Disturbances, and Electrophysiology

---

**Effect of Clopidogrel Added to Aspirin in Patients with Atrial Fibrillation**

The ACTIVE Investigators (McMaster Univ, Hamilton, Ontario, Canada)

*N Engl J Med* 360:2066-2078, 2009

---

*Background.*—Vitamin K antagonists reduce the risk of stroke in patients with atrial fibrillation but are considered unsuitable in many patients, who usually receive aspirin instead. We investigated the hypothesis that the addition of clopidogrel to aspirin would reduce the risk of vascular events in patients with atrial fibrillation.

*Methods.*—A total of 7554 patients with atrial fibrillation who had an increased risk of stroke and for whom vitamin K–antagonist therapy was unsuitable were randomly assigned to receive clopidogrel (75 mg) or placebo, once daily, in addition to aspirin. The primary outcome was the composite of stroke, myocardial infarction, non–central nervous system systemic embolism, or death from vascular causes.

*Results.*—At a median of 3.6 years of follow-up, major vascular events had occurred in 832 patients receiving clopidogrel (6.8% per year) and in 924 patients receiving placebo (7.6% per year) (relative risk with clopidogrel, 0.89; 95% confidence interval [CI], 0.81 to 0.98; $P = 0.01$). The difference was primarily due to a reduction in the rate of stroke with clopidogrel. Stroke occurred in 296 patients receiving clopidogrel (2.4% per year) and 408 patients receiving placebo (3.3% per year) (relative risk, 0.72; 95% CI, 0.62 to 0.83; $P < 0.001$). Myocardial infarction occurred in 90 patients receiving clopidogrel (0.7% per year) and in 115 receiving placebo (0.9% per year) (relative risk, 0.78; 95% CI, 0.59 to 1.03; $P = 0.08$). Major bleeding occurred in 251 patients receiving clopidogrel (2.0% per year) and in 162 patients receiving placebo (1.3% per year) (relative risk, 1.57; 95% CI, 1.29 to 1.92; $P < 0.001$).

*Conclusions.*—In patients with atrial fibrillation for whom vitamin K–antagonist therapy was unsuitable, the addition of clopidogrel to aspirin reduced the risk of major vascular events, especially stroke, and increased the risk of major hemorrhage. (ClinicalTrials.gov number, NCT00249873.)

▶ Investigators from the ACTIVE study group continue to better define the role of anticoagulants in atrial fibrillation (AF). The ACTIVE A trial compared therapy with aspirin alone (75-100 mg daily) with dual platelet inhibition with aspirin plus clopidogrel 75 mg daily in patients for whom vitamin K antagonists (VKAs) were considered unsuitable. Reasons for enrollment included physician judgment that VKA was inappropriate in approximately 50%, patient preference in 26%, and specific bleeding risk in 23%. Treatment groups were similar, with mean $CHADS_2$ score of 2.0. Therapy with aspirin plus clopidogrel reduced major vascular events from 7.6% per year to 6.8% per year, with a reduction in stroke from 3.3% per year to 2.4% per year (see Fig 3 in the original article). Major bleeding was increased with dual platelet inhibition from 1.3% per year to 2.0% per year, with a small but significant increase in intracranial hemorrhage (0.2%/y-0.4%/y). There was no difference in mortality between groups. For 1000 patients treated for 1 year, therapy with aspirin plus clopidogrel would prevent 9 strokes and 2 myocardial infarctions at a cost of 7 major bleeding episodes. This study emphasizes the narrow therapeutic window for anticoagulation in this population. It is also important to note that this study only evaluated patients deemed unsuitable for warfarin; so it should not be considered to show that dual antiplatelet therapy is equivalent to warfarin for stroke prophylaxis in high-risk patients with AF.

**E. M. Quin, MD**

---

## Effects of rosuvastatin on atrial fibrillation occurrence: ancillary results of the GISSI-HF trial

Maggioni AP, on behalf of the GISSI-HF Investigators (ANMCO Res Ctr, Florence, Italy; et al)
*Eur Heart J* 30:2327-2336, 2009

---

*Aims.*—This ancillary analysis of the GISSI-HF database aims at assessing the effect of rosuvastatin on the occurrence of atrial fibrillation (AF) in patients with chronic heart failure (HF) who were not in AF at study entry.

*Methods and Results.*—GISSI-HF was a double-blind, placebo-controlled trial testing n-3 PUFA and rosuvastatin vs. corresponding placebos in patients with chronic HF. Atrial fibrillation occurrence was defined as the presence of AF in the electrocardiogram (ECG) performed at each visit during the trial or AF as a cause of worsening HF or hospital admission or as an event during hospitalization. Among the 3690 patients (80.7%) without AF on their baseline ECG, 15.0% developed AF during a median follow-up period of 3.7 years, 258 randomized to rosuvastatin (13.9%) vs. 294 allocated to placebo (16.0%). Although the difference was not significant at unadjusted analysis ($P = 0.097$) and multivariable analysis adjusting for clinical variables ($P = 0.067$), it became significant after adjustment for clinical variables and laboratory examinations ($P = 0.039$), and for clinical variables, laboratory examinations, and background therapies ($P = 0.038$).

*Conclusion.*—This study shows that there is some evidence of a beneficial effect of rosuvastatin in terms of reduction of AF occurrence in patients with HF. Larger populations are needed to provide a definite answer to the question. ClinicalTrials.gov Identifier: NCT00336336 (Fig 2).

▶ Limited data suggest that statin medications reduce the incidence of atrial fibrillation (AF). GISSI-HF randomized a group of congestive heart failure (CHF) patients to rosuvastatin 10 mg daily vs placebo. Primary outcomes were overall mortality and combined all-cause mortality/hospitalization from cardiac causes, both of which were not significantly different between treatment groups. The authors performed a post hoc analysis, focusing on the effect of rosuvastatin on AF incidence. A subset of patients who did not have AF on baseline ECG were evaluated for new appearance of AF on subsequent study ECGs. AF was noted in 13.9% of the rosuvastatin arm vs 16% of the placebo group during the 3.7 year follow-up period ($P = 0.097$, Fig 2). Though this

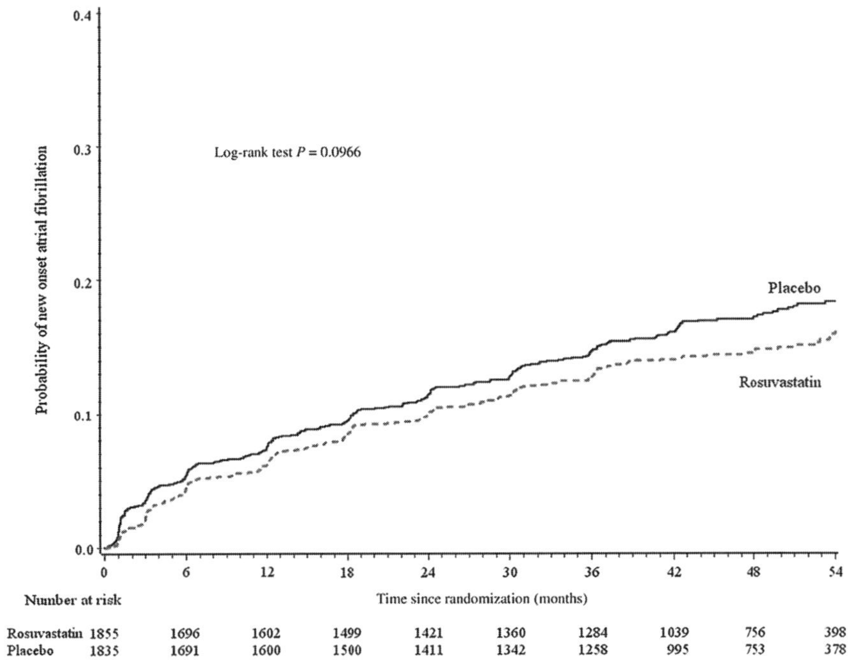


FIGURE 2.—Kaplan–Meier curves for time to new onset of atrial fibrillation. (Reprinted from Maggioni AP, on behalf of the GISSI-HF Investigators. Effects of rosuvastatin on atrial fibrillation occurrence: ancillary results of the GISSI-HF trial. *Eur Heart J*. 2009;30:2327-2336, with permission from The European Society of Cardiology.)

result was not statistically significant, significance was reached after multivariate analysis adjusted for clinical variables and laboratory examinations ($P = 0.039$). Since GISSI-HF was not primarily designed to evaluate for incidence of AF, and because the results rely on complex mathematical models to reach significance, the findings are considered suggestive and not definitive. The results must be reproduced as the primary end point of a randomized, prospective trial before recommending statins routinely for prevention of AF in CHF patients. However, statins may confer modest protection against new AF if being used primarily for standard indications in heart failure.

**C. R. Reynolds, MD**

## Clinical characteristics and in-hospital outcome of patients with end-stage renal disease on dialysis referred for implantable cardioverter-defibrillator implantation

Aggarwal A, for the National Cardiovascular Data Registry (Comprehensive Cardiovascular Med Group, Bakersfield, CA; et al)
*Heart Rhythm* 6:1565-1571, 2009

*Background.*—Little is known about the clinical profile of end-stage renal disease (ESRD) patients who undergo implantable cardioverter-defibrillator (ICD) implantation.

*Objective.*—This study sought to analyze the risk profile of ESRD patients admitted for ICD implantation.

*Methods.*—Patients undergoing first-time device implantation in National Cardiovascular Data Registry/ICD registry from 01/01/06 to 12/31/07 were analyzed (n = 164,069). Patients with ESRD (defined as those requiring dialysis) were compared with patients without ESRD. Primary outcome was in-hospital complications. Because length of hospital stay for ERSD patients was significantly longer (8 vs. 4 days), complications within 2 days of ICD implantation were also examined. The proportion of patients meeting approved indications for ICD implantation was evaluated.

*Results.*—ESRD patients (n = 6,851, 4.4%) had higher rates of comorbid medical conditions, major complications, and total complications, and were less likely to receive an ICD for primary prevention. ESRD patients who received ICD implantation for primary prevention were more likely to meet trial criteria. ESRD patients were less likely to receive beta-blockers and angiotensin inhibitors ($P < .0001$). Unadjusted in-hospital mortality was almost 5-fold among patients with ESRD (1.9% vs. 0.4%, $P < .0001$). Multivariable analysis confirmed that ESRD was independently associated with total in-hospital complications (odds ratio [OR] = 1.38, 95% confidence interval: 1.23 to 1.54, $P < .0001$), and total complications at 2 days (OR = 1.20, 95% confidence interval: 1.05 to 1.36, $P = .006$).

*Conclusion.*—ESRD patients presenting for ICD implantation are sicker, and have higher rates of in-hospital complications even when accounting for overall longer length of hospital stay. Strategies to decrease complications among ESRD patients who undergo ICD implantation need exploration.

▶ Numerous implantable cardioverter-defibrillator (ICD) trials demonstrated improved survival with this therapy in patients at high risk for sudden cardiac death. Patients with end-stage renal disease (ESRD) on chronic hemodialysis have been underrepresented in these trials. Although it is known that approximately 50% of ESRD patients die from cardiac causes and more than half of these deaths are caused by cardiac arrhythmias, little is known regarding the efficacy and potential complications of ICD therapy in this cohort. Aggarwal et al sought to clarify the clinical characteristics and in-hospital outcome of ICD implantation in this challenging population using data derived from the National Cardiovascular Data Registry from 2006 through 2007. More than 164 000 records were analyzed, of which 4.4% were ESRD patients. When compared with non-ESRD patients, ESRD patients had higher rates of comorbid conditions, were less likely to receive ICD therapy as primary prevention, and were less likely to receive beta-blockers or angiotensin inhibitors.

**TABLE 5.**—Unadjusted Rates of In-Hospital Complications (Primary Outcomes)

| | Patients with ESRD (n = 6,851) | Patients without ESRD (n = 157,218) | *P* Value |
|---|---|---|---|
| Any complication (%) | 5.1 | 3.5 | <.0001 |
| Major complication (%)* | 2.2 | 1.3 | <.0001 |
| Minor complication (%)† | 3.0 | 2.3 | .0001 |
| In-hospital death (%) | 1.9 | 0.4 | <.0001 |
| Cardiac arrest (%) | 1.3 | 0.3 | <.0001 |
| Drug reaction (%) | 0.3 | 0.1 | <.0001 |
| Cardiac perforation (%) | 0.04 | 0.08 | .25 |
| Cardiac valve injury (%) | 0 | 3 | .72 |
| Conduction block (%) | 0.04 | 0.04 | .96 |
| Coronary venous dissection (%) | 0.06 | 0.15 | .05 |
| Hematoma (%) | 1.9 | 1.0 | <.0001 |
| Lead dislodgement (%) | 0.9 | 1.1 | .06 |
| Hemothorax (%) | 0.2 | 0.1 | .01 |
| Pneumothorax (%) | 0.4 | 0.5 | .12 |
| Peripheral nerve injury (%) | 0 | 8 | .55 |
| Peripheral embolism (%) | 0.1 | 0.03 | .25 |
| Superficial phlebitis (%) | 0 | 0.1 | .06 |
| Deep phlebitis (%) | 0.01 | 0.03 | .53 |
| Transient ischemic attack (%) | 0.03 | 0.02 | .65 |
| Stroke (%) | 0.1 | 0.1 | .50 |
| Myocardial infarction (%) | 0.06 | 0.03 | .22 |
| Pericardial tamponade (%) | 0.1 | 0.1 | .62 |
| Arteriovenous fistula (%) | 0.01 | 0.01 | .42 |
| Infection related to device (%) | 0.07 | 0.03 | .06 |

ESRD = end-stage renal disease.
*Composite end point of major complications are defined in the text.
†Composite end point of minor complications are defined in the text.

Furthermore, unadjusted in-hospital mortality was significantly higher (1.9% vs 0.4%, $P < .0001$), hospital stays were longer, and multivariate analysis showed an independently associated increase in total complication rate (odds ratio [OR] = 1.38, 95% confidence interval: 1.23-1.54, $P < .0001$, Table 5). Limitations of this study include, primarily, the accuracy and completeness of the database as well as poorly matched control and study groups. Despite these limitations, it is clear from the data analyzed that ICD implantation in the ESRD population carries a higher risk of death or periprocedural complication. These data should be helpful when making decisions about the appropriateness of ICD use in individual subjects.

**J. L. Sturdivant, MD**

## Cardiac-Resynchronization Therapy for the Prevention of Heart-Failure Events

Moss AJ, Hall WJ, Cannom DS, et al (Univ of Rochester Med Ctr, NY; Hosp of the Good Samaritan, CA; et al)
*N Engl J Med* 361:1329-1338, 2009

*Background.*—This trial was designed to determine whether cardiac-resynchronization therapy (CRT) with biventricular pacing would reduce the risk of death or heart-failure events in patients with mild cardiac symptoms, a reduced ejection fraction, and a wide QRS complex.

*Methods.*—During a 4.5-year period, we enrolled and followed 1820 patients with ischemic or nonischemic cardiomyopathy, an ejection fraction of 30% or less, a QRS duration of 130 msec or more, and New York Heart Association class I or II symptoms. Patients were randomly assigned in a 3:2 ratio to receive CRT plus an implantable cardioverter–defibrillator (ICD) (1089 patients) or an ICD alone (731 patients). The primary end point was death from any cause or a nonfatal heart-failure event (whichever came first). Heart-failure events were diagnosed by physicians who were aware of the treatment assignments, but they were adjudicated by a committee that was unaware of assignments.

*Results.*—During an average follow-up of 2.4 years, the primary end point occurred in 187 of 1089 patients in the CRT–ICD group (17.2%) and 185 of 731 patients in the ICD-only group (25.3%) (hazard ratio in the CRT–ICD group, 0.66; 95% confidence interval [CI], 0.52 to 0.84; $P = 0.001$). The benefit did not differ significantly between patients with ischemic cardiomyopathy and those with nonischemic cardiomyopathy. The superiority of CRT was driven by a 41% reduction in the risk of heart-failure events, a finding that was evident primarily in a prespecified subgroup of patients with a QRS duration of 150 msec or more. CRT was associated with a significant reduction in left ventricular volumes and improvement in the ejection fraction. There was no significant difference between the two groups in the overall risk of death, with a 3% annual

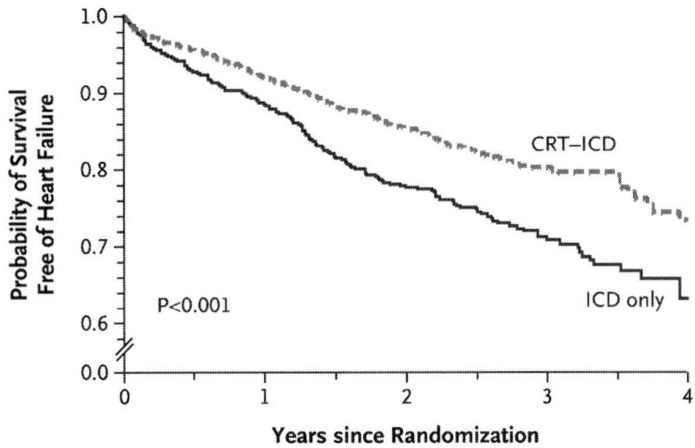


**No. at Risk (Probability of Survival)**

| | | | | | |
|---|---|---|---|---|---|
| ICD only | 731 | 621 (0.89) | 379 (0.78) | 173 (0.71) | 43 (0.63) |
| CRT–ICD | 1089 | 985 (0.92) | 651 (0.86) | 279 (0.80) | 58 (0.73) |

FIGURE 2.—Kaplan–Meier estimates of the probability of survival free of heart failure. There was a significant difference in the estimate of survival free of heart failure between the group that received cardiac-resynchronization therapy plus an implantable cardioverter–defibrillator (CRT–ICD) and the group that received an ICD only (unadjusted $P < 0.001$ by the log-rank test). (Reprinted from Moss AJ, Hall WJ, Cannom DS, et al. Cardiac-resynchronization therapy for the prevention of heart-failure events. *N Engl J Med*. 2009;361:1329-1338. Copyright 2009 Massachusetts Medical Society. All rights reserved.)

mortality rate in each treatment group. Serious adverse events were infrequent in the two groups.

*Conclusions*.—CRT combined with ICD decreased the risk of heart-failure events in relatively asymptomatic patients with a low ejection fraction and wide QRS complex. (ClinicalTrials.gov number, NCT00180271.)

▶ Cardiac resynchronization therapy (CRT) with an implantable cardioverter-defibrillator (ICD) has been proven in numerous clinical trials to reduce heart failure symptoms, hospitalizations, and all-cause mortality in patients with left ventricular dysfunction, moderate-severe congestive heart failure (CHF), and intraventricular conduction delay. The MADIT-CRT trial was a large-scale, randomized, controlled, multi-center trial that was designed to determine if prophylactic CRT-ICD therapy versus ICD therapy alone would reduce the risk of death or non-fatal heart failure events among patients with mild CHF. In this study, the investigators showed that the primary endpoint was met, driven predominantly by a reduction in heart-failure events. Also, the probability of survival free of heart failure was significantly better in the CRT-ICD group (Fig 2). In the subgroup analysis, patients with more severe intraventricular conduction delay (QRS 150ms or greater) had the most benefit. Additionally, the results of Multicenter Automatic Defibrillator Implantation Trial with Cardiac Resynchronization Therapy (MADIT-CRT) support the findings in the recently published REVERSE trial[1] that prophylactic CRT causes positive remodeling including increased systolic function and reduction in left ventricular cavity size in addition to a reduction of hospitalizations. The observation that overall mortality was not statistically different between the CRT-ICD and

ICD groups is not surprising, as these patients had relatively mild CHF and would not be expected to have high risk of mortality from severe CHF; rather it would be expected that the patients in this trial would more likely die secondary to arrhythmia. Because both arms of this study had ICDs implanted, they would not be expected to have markedly different rates of arrhythmic death. Overall, this should be considered a landmark trial for CRT, and it will likely impact the guidelines for implanting CRT devices in patients with less severe CHF.

**M. R. Gold, MD, PhD**

*Reference*

1. Daubert C, Gold MR, Abraham WT, et al. Prevention of disease progression by cardiac resynchronization therapy in patients with asymptomatic or mildly symptomatic left ventricular dysfunction: insights from the European cohort of the REVERSE (Resynchronization Reverses Remodeling in Systolic Left Ventricular Dysfunction) trial. *J Am Coll Cardiol.* 2009;54:1837-1846.

---

## Combined Evaluation of Bedside Clinical Variables and the Electrocardiogram for the Differential Diagnosis of Paroxysmal Atrioventricular Reciprocating Tachycardias in Patients Without Pre-Excitation

González-Torrecilla E, Almendral J, Arenal A, et al (Hosp General Universitario Gregorio Marañón, Madrid, Spain)
*J Am Coll Cardiol* 53:2353-2358, 2009

---

*Objectives.*—The aim of this study was to assess the independent predictive contribution to the electrocardiogram (ECG) of bedside clinical variables to distinguish the major forms of paroxysmal supraventricular tachycardias.

*Background.*—Atrioventricular nodal re-entrant tachycardias (AVNRTs) and orthodromic reciprocating tachycardias (ORTs), through concealed accessory pathways, are major mechanisms of paroxysmal atrioventricular re-entrant tachycardias.

*Methods.*—We prospectively included 370 consecutive patients undergoing an electrophysiologic study for paroxysmal, regular, narrow-QRS complex tachycardias without pre-excitation in sinus rhythm. A diagnostic interpretation of ECG recordings was performed by 2 observers blinded to invasive diagnosis used as gold standard. The independent diagnostic contribution of basic clinical variables from a 7-item questionnaire was analyzed alone and in combination with the ECG interpretation by stepwise logistic regression.

*Results.*—AVNRTs and ORTs were demonstrated in 262 and 108 patients, respectively. Age at symptom onset (odds ratio [OR]: 1.27), presence of palpitations in the neck (OR: 3.54), and female sex (OR: 2.96) (all $p = 0.0001$) were the clinical variables with significant diagnostic power for AVNRT diagnosis. These variables were selected by the logistic model as predictors of the tachycardia diagnosis when the ECG interpretation was included in the analysis (C statistic $= 0.81$ vs. $0.75$ with clinical variables alone; $p = 0.003$). Neck palpitation was the only predictor of AVNRT when positive ECG findings were lacking.

*Conclusions.*—Age at the onset of symptoms, sensation of rapid regular pounding in the neck during tachycardia, and female sex are the only significant clinical variables in the differential diagnosis of paroxysmal atrioventricular reciprocating tachycardias in patients without pre-excitation in sinus rhythm. Their consideration adds significant diagnostic information to the ECG.

▶ Accurate differentiation of atrioventricular nodal reentrant tachycardia (AVNRT) and orthodromic reciprocating tachycardia (ORT) with a concealed bypass tract is key for risk assessment and planning of pharmacologic or ablation strategies. The electrocardiogram during tachycardia has been the cornerstone of diagnosis, aided by clinical factors associated with either arrhythmia. This study evaluates the utility of clinical variables and symptoms during tachycardia in conjunction with the ECG to predict the presence of AVNRT or ORT at electrophysiologic study. A total of 370 patients, 262 with AVNRT and 108 with ORT, were included. In multivariate analysis, only rapid regular palpitations in the neck occurred more frequently in AVNRT than ORT (odds ratio (OR) 3.54). Physiologically, since AVNRT results in simultaneous atrial and ventricular activation, the right atrium contracts on a closed tricuspid valve leading to "cannon" A waves and palpitations in the neck. Patients with AVNRT were also more likely to be female (OR 2.96) and were older (OR 1.27 per 5 year increment in age at onset of symptoms). When combined with standard ECG criteria for AVNRT or ORT, these clinical factors continued to be predictive, with little change in odds ratios (OR 2.6 for female sex, 3.37 for neck palpitations, and 1.25 for each 5 year increment in age). The addition of these simple clinical factors to ECG algorithms differentiating AVNRT from ORT should improve diagnostic accuracy.

**E. M. Quin, MD**

---

**Syncope While Driving: Clinical Characteristics, Causes, and Prognosis**

Sorajja D, Nesbitt GC, Hodge DO, et al (Mayo Clinic, Rochester, MN)

*Circulation* 120:928-934, 2009

---

*Background.*—The risk of syncope occurring while driving has obvious implications for personal and public safety. We aimed to define the clinical characteristics, causes, and prognosis of syncope while driving.

*Methods and Results.*—In this case-control study of consecutive patients evaluated for syncope from 1996 through 1998 at an academic medical center, we documented causes, clinical characteristics, and recurrence of syncope while driving. Of 3877 patients identified, 381 (9.8%) had syncope while driving (driving group). Compared with the 3496 patients (90.2%) who did not have syncope while driving, the driving group was younger ($P = 0.01$) and had higher percentages of male patients ($P < 0.001$) and patients with a history of any cardiovascular disease ($P = 0.01$) and stroke ($P = 0.02$). Syncope while driving was commonly caused by neurally mediated syncope (37.3%) and cardiac arrhythmias (11.8%). Long-term survival in the driving group was comparable to that of an age- and sex-matched cohort from the Minnesota population ($P = 0.15$). Among the driving group, syncope recurred in 72 patients, 35 of whom (48.6%) had recurrence >6 months after the initial evaluation. Recurrences during driving happened in 10 patients in the driving group, 7 of which (70%) were >12 months after the initial evaluation.

*Conclusions.*—In our study, neurally mediated syncope was the most common type of syncope while driving. The causes of syncope, the late recurrences of syncope (during ≥6 months of follow-up), and the overall low incidence of recurrent syncope while driving provide useful information to supplement current recommendations on driving for these patients (Table 3).

▶ Restrictions and guidelines for driving motor vehicles in patients with syncope is an important clinical problem. Previous scientific statements were delineated from little prosective data. This article is the first large case controlled study of this problem. The major cause of syncope was most frequently neurally mediated syncope in both driving and nondriving groups. The causes of syncope while driving are similar to those in patients who were not driving (Table 3). Of the patients who presented with syncope, 9.8% were driving at the time. The recurrence rate in this group was only 0.7% in 6 months and 1.1% at 12 months. In 17-23% of the patients, the etiology of syncope could

TABLE 3.—Causes and Recurrence of Syncope

| Cause of Syncope | Group,* n (%) Driving (n = 381) | Group,* n (%) Nondriving (n = 3496) | *P* | Recurrence of Syncope, n (%) Driving (n = 72) | Recurrence of Syncope, n (%) Nondriving (n = 713) |
|---|---|---|---|---|---|
| Neurally mediated | 142 (37.3) | 1247 (35.7) | 0.54 | 28 (38.9) | 243 (34.1) |
| Bradyarrhythmia | 25 (6.6) | 221 (6.3) | 0.86 | 9 (12.5) | 50 (7.0) |
| Supraventricular tachyarrhythmia | 8 (2.1) | 71 (2.0) | 0.93 | 3 (4.2) | 15 (2.1) |
| Ventricular tachyarrhythmia | 20 (5.2) | 130 (3.7) | 0.14 | 3 (4.2) | 21 (2.9) |
| Structural cardiopulmonary disease | 1 (0.3) | 9 (0.3) | 0.99 | 0 (0) | 3 (0.4) |
| Cerebrovascular disease | 14 (3.7) | 100 (2.9) | 0.37 | 6 (8.3) | 21 (2.9) |
| Carotid sinus hypersensitivity | 12 (3.1) | 100 (2.9) | 0.75 | 1 (1.4) | 30 (4.2) |
| Orthostatic intolerance | 18 (4.7) | 223 (6.4) | 0.20 | 7 (9.7) | 53 (7.4) |
| Others | 87 (22.8) | 1044 (29.9) | 0.004 | 11 (15.3) | 227 (31.8) |
| Unknown | 90 (23.6) | 622 (17.8) | 0.005 | 15 (20.8) | 111 (15.6) |

*Total diagnoses for both the driving and nondriving groups exceed 100% because some patients have >1 presumed diagnosis.

not be elucidated. This population may also include more patients with neurally mediated syncope. The incidence of neurally mediated events triggering syncope while driving is higher than previously suspected. Accordingly, the scientific statement, "Personal and public safety use related to arrhythmias may effect consciousness implications for a physician recommendation," in 1996,[1] considered neurally mediated syncope, but it was a minor cause. Based on previous studies on consensus, the recommendation to limit driving for 3 months was made. The data from this study reveal that such restrictions may not be helpful in eliminating further accidents because recurrence rates are so low. Thus, these data suggest that the current guidelines for driving after syncope should be reassessed.

**R. B. Leman, MD**

*Reference*

1. Epstein AE, Miles WM, Benditt GG, et al. Personal and public safety issues related to arrhythmias that may affect consciousness: implications for regulation and physician recommendations. A medical/scientific statement from the American Heart Association and the North American Society of Pacing and Electrophysiology. *Circulation*. 1996;94:1147-1166.

## Propranolol Decreases Tachycardia and Improves Symptoms in the Postural Tachycardia Syndrome Less Is More

Raj SR, Black BK, Biaggioni I, et al (Vanderbilt Univ, Nashville, TN)
*Circulation* 120:725-734, 2009

*Background.*—Postural tachycardia syndrome (POTS) induces disabling chronic orthostatic intolerance with an excessive increase in heart rate on standing. β-Blockade is an appealing treatment approach, but conflicting preliminary reports are conflicting. We tested the hypothesis that propranolol will attenuate the tachycardia and improve symptom burden in patients with POTS. In protocol 1, a low dose (20 mg) was compared with placebo, and the dose response was assessed in protocol 2.

*Methods and Results.*—In protocol 1, patients with POTS ($n = 54$) underwent acute drug trials of propranolol 20 mg orally and placebo, on separate mornings, in a randomized crossover design. Blood pressure, heart rate, and symptoms were assessed while the patients were seated and after standing for up to 10 minutes before and hourly after the study drug. Supine ($P < 0.001$) and standing ($P < 0.001$) heart rates were significantly lower after propranolol compared with placebo. The symptom burden improvement from baseline to 2 hours was greater with propranolol than placebo (median, −4.5 versus 0 arbitrary units; $P = 0.044$). In protocol 2, 18 patients with POTS underwent similar trials of high-dose (80 mg) versus low-dose (20 mg) propranolol. Although the high dose elicited a greater decrease than the low dose in standing heart rate ($P < 0.001$) and orthostatic tachycardia ($P < 0.001$), the improvement

TABLE 2.—Orthostatic Hemodynamics and Symptoms With Propranolol 20 mg and Placebo (Protocol 1) in Patients With POTS (n = 54)

| | Before | 2 Hours After | 4 Hours After | *P*, Repeated-Measures ANOVA |
|---|---|---|---|---|
| δHR (standing–seated), $min^{-1}$ | | | | |
| Propranolol 20 mg | 27.4 ± 16.1 | 15.4 ± 9.1 | 16.3 ± 9.4 | |
| Placebo | 30.2 ± 15.7 | 25.0 ± 16.3 | 25.0 ± 15.8 | |
| *P* (between drugs) | NS | 0.033 | 0.028 | 0.076 |
| Standing HR, $min^{-1}$ | | | | |
| Propranolol 20 mg | 114.0 ± 16.6 | 86.1 ± 12.2 | 87.3 ± 13.8 | |
| Placebo | 116.7 ± 18.6 | 107.7 ± 19.1 | 108.2 ± 19.3 | |
| *P* (between drugs) | NS | <0.001 | <0.001 | <0.001 |
| Seated HR, $min^{-1}$ | | | | |
| Propranolol 20 mg | 86.7 ± 13.0 | 70.1 ± 11.4 | 71.1 ± 10.6 | |
| Placebo | 86.6 ± 12.4 | 82.8 ± 13.8 | 83.2 ± 12.7 | |
| *P* (between drugs) | NS | <0.001 | <0.001 | <0.001 |
| δSBP (standing–seated), mm Hg | | | | |
| Propranolol 20 mg | 5.4 ± 12.8 | 2.5 ± 9.0 | 6.1 ± 8.2 | |
| Placebo | 3.5 ± 18.3 | 4.6 ± 9.6 | 2.8 ± 12.5 | |
| *P* (between drugs) | NS | NS | NS | 0.057 |
| Standing SBP, mm Hg | | | | |
| Propranolol 20 mg | 109.5 ± 16.9 | 100.3 ± 11.7 | 105.9 ± 12.9 | |
| Placebo | 109.5 ± 17.8 | 111.6 ± 15.5 | 110.3 ± 17.1 | |
| *P* (between drugs) | NS | <0.001 | NS | 0.001 |
| Sitting SBP, mm Hg | | | | |
| Propranolol 20 mg | 104.0 ± 12.5 | 97.8 ± 10.5 | 99.8 ± 10.5 | |
| Placebo | 106.0 ± 14.2 | 107.0 ± 14.5 | 107.5 ± 13.2 | |
| *P* (between drugs) | NS | 0.001 | 0.005 | 0.002 |
| Symptom score, AU (n = 36) | | | | |
| Propranolol 20 mg | 17 (9, 29) | 9.5 (3.75, 16.25) | 10 (4, 16) | |
| Placebo | 16 (7.25, 28.5) | 15 (6, 28.25) | 12.5 (5, 30) | |
| *P* (between drugs) | 0.385 | 0.012 | 0.007 | 0.035 (van Elteren test) |

For hemodynamic parameters, data are presented as mean ± SD. Repeated-measures ANOVA was used to determine the *P* value for the overall change between study drug and placebo, and paired comparisons were made with the use of within-model contrasts. Symptom data are presented as median (25th percentile, 75th percentile) and were analyzed with the van Elteren test overall and with the Wilcoxon signed rank test for paired data. $P < 0.05$ was considered significant. NS indicates not significant.

in symptoms at 2 hours was greater with low-dose propranolol (−6 versus −2 arbitrary units; $P = 0.041$).

*Conclusions.*—Low-dose oral propranolol significantly attenuated tachycardia and improved symptoms in POTS. Higher-dose propranolol did not further improve, and may worsen, symptoms (Table 2).

▶ Postural tachycardia syndrome is a disorder of orthostatic intolerance that is poorly understood. The treatment of this disorder is problematic. However, stroke volume and blood volume seem to effect recurrence. Accordingly, hydration is important for these patients. In this study, patients were hydrated and their diet was appropriately adjusted to avoid hypovolemia before being randomized to treatment. The first protocol (Table 2) compared low-dose propranolol with placebo. As expected, the drug reduced the heart rate and other physiological parameters. It also resulted in a significant improvement in symptoms. The second protocol was a dose-ranging protocol used to assess whether a larger dose of propranolol would be more effective. The hemodynamic effect increased with a larger dose of propranolol, but the clinical response was inconsistent. Some symptoms improved, many did not, and some worsened. Thus, low-dose beta blockade with appropriate volume status and dietary treatments seems to be an effective treatment in these patients. Paradoxically, higher doses are not more effective in symptom control, and should probably be avoided.

**R. B. Leman, MD**

---

**Systematic Assessment of Patients With Unexplained Cardiac Arrest: Cardiac Arrest Survivors With Preserved Ejection Fraction Registry (CASPER)**

Krahn AD, Healey JS, Chauhan V, et al (Univ of Western Ontario, London, Canada; Hamilton Health Sciences Ctr, Ontario, Canada; Univ Health Network, Toronto, Ontario, Canada; et al)

*Circulation* 120:278-285, 2009

---

*Background.*—Cardiac arrest without evident cardiac disease may be caused by subclinical genetic conditions. Provocative testing to unmask a phenotype is often necessary to detect primary electrical disease, direct genetic testing, and perform family screening.

*Methods and Results.*—Patients with apparently unexplained cardiac arrest and no evident cardiac disease (normal cardiac function on echocardiogram, no evidence of coronary artery disease, and a normal ECG) underwent systematic evaluation that included cardiac magnetic resonance imaging, signal-averaged ECG, exercise testing, drug challenge, and selective electrophysiological testing. Diagnostic criteria were based on accepted criteria or provocation of the characteristic clinical features for long-QT syndrome, catecholaminergic polymorphic ventricular tachycardia, Brugada syndrome, early repolarization, arrhythmogenic right ventricular cardiomyopathy, coronary spasm, and myocarditis. Sixty-three patients in 9 centers were enrolled (age 43.0 ± 13.4 years, 29 women). A diagnosis was obtained in 35 patients (56%): Long-QT syndrome in 8, catecholaminergic polymorphic ventricular tachycardia in 8, arrhythmogenic right ventricular cardiomyopathy in 6, early repolarization in 5, coronary spasm in 4, Brugada syndrome in 3, and myocarditis in 1. Targeted genetic testing demonstrated evidence of causative mutations in 9 (47%) of 19 patients. Screening of 64 family members of these patients identified 15 affected individuals who were treated (24%). The remaining 28 patients (44%) were considered to have idiopathic ventricular fibrillation.

*Conclusions.*—Systematic clinical testing, including drug provocation and advanced imaging, results in unmasking of the cause of apparently unexplained cardiac arrest in >50% of patients. This approach assists in directing genetic testing to diagnose genetically mediated arrhythmia syndromes, which results in successful family screening.

▶ Sudden cardiac arrest (SCA) remains one of the leading causes of mortality in western societies. Epidemiologic studies suggest that the decline in SCA is lagging that of other causes of cardiovascular mortality. This suggests that our strategies to prevent SCA are suboptimal. In this regard, most efforts in the prevention of SCA are directed toward medical treatment of coronary artery disease (CAD) and heart failure, and implantable defibrillator therapy for high-risk patients, primarily with left ventricular dysfunction. However, prospective observational studies typically show that most victims of SCA do not have manifest CAD or heart failure. Accordingly, better strategies to identify these subjects are needed. Cardiac Arrest Survivors With Preserved Ejection Fraction Registry (CASPER) was a prospective registry that evaluated the characteristics of a cohort with unexplained SCA in 9 Canadian centers. About 63 patients underwent a comprehensive battery of tests, including MRI, catheterization, provocative drug challenges, and electrophysiology study. As expected, this group was younger (mean age 43 years) than most unselected series of SCA. A putative cause of SCA was identified with this strategy in more than half the subjects, most commonly, long-QT syndrome, right ventricular (RV) dysplasia, short-QT syndrome, catecholaminergic ventricular tachycardia (VT), or coronary artery spasm. This allowed for genetic screening of relatives when appropriate and 15 were identified and treated who were considered at high risk of SCA. This study highlights the utility of a systematic approach to identify the cause of SCA; however, it also demonstrates that a challenge still exists given the diversity of causes identified and that more than 40% of subjects with no etiology were identified, despite extensive testing.

**M. R. Gold, MD, PhD**

# 38 Cardiac Surgery

**Aortic Valve Replacement for Aortic Stenosis in Patients With Left Ventricular Dysfunction**

Halkos ME, Chen EP, Sarin EL, et al (Emory Univ School of Medicine, Atlanta, GA)

*Ann Thorac Surg* 88:746-751, 2009

*Background.*—The purpose of this study was to assess the impact of left ventricular dysfunction and other risk factors on short- and mid-term outcomes after aortic valve replacement for aortic stenosis.

*Methods.*—From January 1, 2002, to December 31, 2007, 773 consecutive patients underwent primary aortic valve replacement for aortic stenosis at a single institution; concomitant coronary artery bypass graft surgery (CABG) was performed in 45.4% (351 of 773). Multivariable regression analysis was used to identify predictors of in-hospital mortality, with ejection fraction (EF) as the primary variable of interest. After discharge, survival status was determined using the Social Security Death Index. A Cox proportional hazards regression model was used to identify predictors of mid-term mortality.

*Results.*—On univariable analysis, EF (odds ratio [OR] 0.979, 95% confidence interval [CI]: 0.960 to 0.999, $p = 0.044$) but not concomitant CABG emerged as a predictor of in-hospital mortality. However, on multivariable analysis, neither EF nor concomitant CABG was associated with increased in-hospital mortality. Multivariable predictors of in-hospital mortality included age, emergent status, and prolonged bypass time. On univariable analysis, mid-term mortality was associated with EF and concomitant CABG (OR 0.979, 95% CI: 0.966 to 0.991, $p = 0.001$, and OR 1.61, 95% CI: 1.11 to 2.36, $p = 0.013$, respectively). However, after multivariable adjustment, only EF was associated with mid-term mortality (adjusted OR 0.985, 95% CI: 0.970 to 1.00, $p = 0.049$). Other multivariable predictors of mid-term mortality included age, dialysis-dependent renal failure, previous stroke, and peripheral vascular disease.

*Conclusions.*—Left ventricular dysfunction, in addition to other patient comorbidities, may negatively impact survival after aortic valve replacement. Careful consideration of the cumulative effect of these multiple risk factors is necessary to optimize patient outcomes.

▶ Dr Halkos and colleagues from Emory University report the results of 773 consecutive patients undergoing primary aortic valve replacement for aortic valve stenosis with or without concomitant coronary artery bypass grafting to determine the effect of preoperative risk factors, particularly preoperative ejection fraction on survival. Forty-five percent of patients had concomitant bypass grafting. They found that while ejection fraction was a univariate predictor of early death, it was not an independent risk factor while age, emergent status, and prolonged bypass times were. Mid-term mortality was predicted by preoperative ejection fraction, age, dialysis-dependent renal failure, previous stroke, and peripheral vascular disease.

The authors undertook the study owing to the fact that there are discrepant results regarding the short- and long-term outcomes of aortic valve replacement with left ventricular dysfunction.[1-3] Although a recent report demonstrated that low ejection fraction may exist in 26% of patients with severe aortic valve stenosis, less than one third are referred for intervention.[4] It is for this reason the influence of ejection fraction on postoperative outcome is important to understand. Patients referred for surgical intervention increasingly have multiple comorbidities, including advanced age, renal insufficiency, coronary disease, and peripheral vascular disease. The novel finding of this study is that short-term survival may not be independently related to ejection fraction alone. This is significant because if the sought after aim of aortic valve replacement in a population in elderly patients with multiple comorbidities is improvement of symptoms, then aortic valve replacement may indeed be an important palliative therapy. While depressed ejection fraction itself may portend a poor mid-term prognosis, the relief of severe aortic valve stenosis at least in the short-term is an important therapeutic aim.

**R. Suri, MD, DPhil**

*References*

1. Carabello BA, Green LH, Grossman W, Cohn LH, Koster JK, Collins JJ Jr. Hemodynamic determinants of prognosis of aortic valve replacement in critical aortic stenosis and advanced congestive heart failure. *Circulation*. 1980;62:42-48.
2. Vaquette B, Corbinau H, Laurent M, et al. Valve replacement in patients with critical aortic stenosis and depressed left ventricular function: predictors of operative risk, left ventricular function recovery, and long-term outcomes. *Heart*. 2005;91: 1324-1329.
3. Connolly H, Oh J, Orszulak T, et al. Aortic valve replacement for aortic stenosis with left ventricular dysfunction: Prognostic indicators. *Circulation*. 1997;95:2395-2400.
4. Pai RG, Varadarajan P, Razzouk A. Survival benefits of aortic valve replacement in patients with severe aortic stenosis with low ejection fraction and low gradient with normal ejection fraction. *Ann Thorac Surg*. 2008;86:1781-1790.

## Coronary Bypass Surgery with or without Surgical Ventricular Reconstruction

Jones RH, for the STICH Hypothesis 2 Investigator (Duke Univ Med Ctr, Durham, NC; et al)
*N Engl J Med* 360:1705-1717, 2009

*Background.*—Surgical ventricular reconstruction is a specific procedure designed to reduce left ventricular volume in patients with heart failure caused by coronary artery disease. We conducted a trial to address the question of whether surgical ventricular reconstruction added to coronary-artery bypass grafting (CABG) would decrease the rate of death or hospitalization for cardiac causes, as compared with CABG alone.

*Methods.*—Between September 2002 and January 2006, a total of 1000 patients with an ejection fraction of 35% or less, coronary artery disease that was amenable to CABG, and dominant anterior left ventricular dysfunction that was amenable to surgical ventricular reconstruction were randomly assigned to undergo either CABG alone (499 patients) or CABG with surgical ventricular reconstruction (501 patients). The primary outcome was a composite of death from any cause and hospitalization for cardiac causes. The median follow-up was 48 months.

*Results.*—Surgical ventricular reconstruction reduced the end-systolic volume index by 19%, as compared with a reduction of 6% with CABG alone. Cardiac symptoms and exercise tolerance improved from baseline to a similar degree in the two study groups. However, no significant difference was observed in the primary outcome, which occurred in 292 patients (59%) who were assigned to undergo CABG alone and in 289 patients (58%) who were assigned to undergo CABG with surgical ventricular reconstruction (hazard ratio for the combined approach, 0.99; 95% confidence interval, 0.84 to 1.17; $P = 0.90$).

*Conclusions.*—Adding surgical ventricular reconstruction to CABG reduced the left ventricular volume, as compared with CABG alone. However, this anatomical change was not associated with a greater improvement in symptoms or exercise tolerance or with a reduction in the rate of death or hospitalization for cardiac causes. (ClinicalTrials.gov number, NCT00023595.)

▶ Surgical ventricular reconstruction (SVR) was initially proposed as a method of decreasing left ventricular size at the time of coronary revascularization to decrease heart failure symptoms and increase ejection fraction.[1-3] The STITCH trial was designed to study the effect of SVR in patients undergoing coronary revascularization. Between September 2002 and January 2006, 1000 patients with an ejection fraction of 35% or less who were candidates for coronary revascularization (CABG) and had left ventricular dysfunction plus ventricular dilation amenable to SVR were randomly assigned to CABG alone (499) or CABG plus SVR (501). The primary outcome was a composite of death and hospitalization for cardiac causes. The median follow-up was 48 months. SVR was better at decreasing end systolic volume (19%) versus CABG (6%). However, cardiac symptoms and exercise tolerance improved to a similar degree in both groups. Importantly, no significant difference was observed in death or cardiac readmission. The authors conclude that the anatomic benefits of SVR did not significantly improve symptoms, exercise tolerance, death, or cardiac hospitalization.

Coronary artery disease is a significant cause of heart failure.[4] Adverse left ventricular remodeling following myocardial ischemia produces left ventricular enlargement leading to less effective ventricular ejection and heart failure symptoms. This study examines "hypothesis 2" in the STITCH trial—that SVR would decrease the rate of death or cardiac-related hospitalization versus CABG alone. The strength of the study includes the fact that it is a multicenter non-blinded randomized trial performed at 127 clinical sites in 26 countries. The authors also excluded patients undergoing aortic valve replacement, PCI, and those with non existing cardiac disease having a life expectancy of less than 3 years. All echocardiograms were examined in a third party core laboratory. The following were increased in the SVR group: operative, intubation, and index hospitalization times.

While the results of this trial are negative, several explanations can be offered. The first possibility is that the patients who were thought to derive definite benefit from SVR may have been excluded from randomization and offered SVR in addition to CABG. This is difficult to determine, however, owing to the broad range of opinions regarding the efficacy of SVR in clinical practice. The second possibility is that SVR might in fact decrease diastolic compliance, thus counteracting the benefits of decreased ventricular volume and increased systolic function. The third possibility is that the inability to blind clinicians may have skewed readmission rates; however, this is hard to determine. In summary, this is an important trial which indicates that SVR in patients undergoing CABG does not significantly influence death or cardiac-related readmission. Whether patients with a distinct area of left ventricular aneurysmal change benefit from SVR with or without coronary revascularization is still unknown, and the answer to this question will hopefully accompany the results of future trials.

**R. Suri, MD, DPhil**

*References*

1. Athanasuleas CL, Stanley AWH Jr, Buckberg GD. Restoration of contractile function in the enlarged left ventricle by exclusion of remodeled akinetic anterior segment: surgical strategy, myocardial protection, and angiographic results. *J Card Surg.* 1998;13:418-428.
2. Athanasuleas C, Buckberg GD, Stanley AWH Jr, et al. Surgical ventricular restoration in the treatment of congestive heart failure due to post-infarction ventricular dilatation. *J Am Coll Cardiol.* 2004;44:1439-1445.
3. Menicanti L, Castelvecchio S, Ranucci M, et al. Surgical therapy for ischemic heart failure: single-center experience with surgical anterior ventricular restoration. *J Thorac Cardiovasc Surg.* 2007;134:433-441.
4. Hunt SA, Abraham WT, Chin MH, et al. American College of Cardiology, American Heart Association Task Force on Practice Guidelines, American College of Chest Physicians, International Society for Heart and Lung Transplantation, Heart Rhythm Society. ACC/AHA 2005 guideline update for the diagnosis and management of chronic heart failure in the adult: a report of the American College of Cardiology/American Heart Association task force on practice guidelines. *Circulation.* 2005;112:e154-e235.

**Evidence for Using *Clopidogrel* Alone or in Addition to *Aspirin* in Post Coronary Artery Bypass Surgery Patients**

Patel JH, Stoner JA, Owora A, et al (Univ of Oklahoma Health Science Ctr; et al)

*Am J Cardiol* 103:1687-1693, 2009

Clopidogrel is recommended with aspirin for patients who undergo coronary artery bypass grafting (CABG) after non–ST elevation myocardial infarctions. Cardiothoracic surgeons widely use clopidogrel in addition to aspirin for post-CABG patients, including those with stable coronary artery disease. The aim of this study was to systematically review the published research to determine whether clopidogrel use after CABG is based on good trial data. Studies reporting safety and/or efficacy data for clopidogrel use with or without aspirin after on- or off-pump CABG were included. Fourteen studies met the inclusion criteria, of which 11 were reported trials and 3 are ongoing trials. Subgroup retrospective analyses of previously reported large trials of patients presenting with acute coronary syndromes (n = 1) or patients with stable coronary artery disease (n = 3) did not show a clear clinical benefit of clopidogrel when given in addition to aspirin after CABG. In contrast, there was a trend toward increased major and minor bleeding after the use of clopidogrel plus aspirin. Two small prospective trials providing data on surrogate end points and 5 small trials involving off-pump CABG patients were not of good quality to draw meaningful conclusions. In conclusion, summarized data based on subgroup analyses, surrogate end points, and observational cohort studies fail to demonstrate a clear beneficial effect of clopidogrel alone or in combination with aspirin on clinical outcomes after CABG.

▶ Dr Patel and colleagues from the University of Oklahoma report on a systematic review of published data to determine the evidence against the use of clopidogrel following coronary artery bypass grafting surgery (CABG). They included studies reporting safety and/or efficacy after on- or off-pump CABG. Of the 14 studies included, 11 trials had been concluded and 3 were ongoing at the time of publication. The subgroup analysis did not show a clear benefit of clopidogrel in addition to standard aspirin therapy following CABG. They did find a trend toward increased major and minor bleeding in those treated with clopidogrel plus aspirin. Two small prospective trials using surrogate end points and other small trials examining off-pump patients were excluded. The authors conclude that the observational cohort studies examined in their analysis were unable to demonstrate a clear beneficial effect of clopidogrel alone or in combination with aspirin following CABG.

Although aspirin is widely used following CABG, the addition of clopidogrel has been suggested by the American College of Chest Physicians in patients who undergo CABG following a non-ST elevation myocardial infarction.[1] Surgeons recognize the bleeding risk associated with preoperative use of Plavix, and therefore discontinuation of the drug at least 5 days before cardiac surgery is recommended.[2,3] This study is an important one in that the use of postoperative clopidogrel has not been justified by double-blind randomized control trials. The existing data is derived from observational cohort trials that do little to convince us that there is a real effect of clopidogrel in decreasing death, myocardial infarction, stroke, unstable angina, or recurrence of angina following CABG compared with aspirin alone postoperatively. Further clarification of this important question will await the completion of placebo controlled randomized trials.

**R. Suri, MD, DPhil**

*References*


1. Stein PD, Schünemann HJ, Dalen JE, Gutterman D. Antithrombotic therapy in patients with saphenous vein and internal mammary artery bypass grafts: the Seventh ACCP Conference on Antithrombotic and Thrombolytic Therapy. *Chest.* 2004;126:600S-608S.
2. Ascione R, Ghosh A, Rogers CA, Cohen A, Monk C, Angelini GD. In-hospital patients exposed to clopidogrel before coronary artery bypass grafting: a word of caution. *Ann Thorac Surg.* 2005;79:1210-1216.
3. Kang W, Theman TE, Reed JF III, Stoltzfus J, Weger N. The effect of preoperative clopidogrel on bleeding after coronary artery bypass surgery. *J Surg Educ.* 2007; 64:88-92.


---

## Comparison of Early Surgery Versus Conventional Treatment in Asymptomatic Severe Mitral Regurgitation

Kang D-H, Kim JH, Rim JH, et al (Univ of Ulsan, Seoul, Korea)
*Circulation* 119:797-804, 2009

---


*Background.*—The optimal timing of surgical intervention in asymptomatic patients with severe mitral regurgitation is unclear. We therefore compared the long-term results of early surgery with a conventional treatment strategy.

*Methods and Results.*—From 1996 to 2005, 447 consecutive asymptomatic patients (253 men, age 50 ± 15 years) with severe degenerative mitral regurgitation and preserved left ventricular function were evaluated prospectively. The end point was defined as the composite of operative mortality, cardiac death, repeat mitral valve surgery, and urgent admission due to congestive heart failure during follow-up. Early surgery was performed on 161 patients (operated group), and the conventional treatment strategy was used for 286 patients (conventional treatment group). There were no significant differences between the 2 groups in terms of age, gender, euroSCORE (European System for Cardiac Operative Risk Evaluation), or ejection fraction. During a median follow-up of 1988 days, there were 2 repeat surgeries and no cardiac deaths or operative mortality in the operated group compared with 12 cardiac deaths, 1 repeat surgery, and 22 admissions for congestive heart failure in the conventional treatment group. The estimated actuarial 7-year cardiac mortality rate was 0% in the operated group and 5 ± 2% in the conventional treatment group

($P = 0.008$), and for 127 propensity score-matched pairs, the estimated actuarial 7-year event-free survival rate was significantly higher in the operated than in the conventional treatment group (99 ± 1% versus 85 ± 4%, $P = 0.007$). In the conventional treatment group, baseline grade of pulmonary hypertension (hazard ratio 1.87, 95% CI 1.22 to 2.87, $P = 0.003$), age (hazard ratio 1.02, 95% CI 1.01 to 1.04, $P = 0.005$), and effective regurgitant orifice area (hazard ratio 2.06, 95% CI 1.11 to 3.82, $P = 0.02$) were independent variables that predicted late development of surgical indications or congestive heart failure on Cox multivariate analysis.

*Conclusions.*—Compared with conservative management, the strategy of early surgery was associated with an improved long-term event rate by decreasing cardiac mortality and congestive heart failure hospitalization more effectively in patients with severe degenerative mitral regurgitation. Early surgery may therefore further improve clinical outcomes in asymptomatic severe mitral regurgitation with preserved left ventricular systolic function and a high likelihood of mitral valve repair.

▶ Dr Kang and colleagues from Asan Medical Center in Seoul, Korea report the results of a retrospective study performed between 1996 and 2005 examining 444 consecutive patients with severe degenerative mitral regurgitation and preserved left ventricular function who were entered into a prospective database. They studied a composite end point, which included operative mortality, cardiac death, repeat mitral valve surgery, or urgent admission due to congestive heart failure during follow-up. Surgery was performed in 161 patients and conventional medical therapy was used in 286 patients. There were no significant differences between the 2 groups in terms of age, gender, euro SCORE, or ejection fraction. Median follow-up was 1988 days, and in the surgical group, there were 2 repeat operations and no early deaths compared with 12 cardiac deaths, 1 repeat surgery in 22 heart failure admissions in the conventional group. The 7-year survival was 0% in the surgical group and 5% in the conventional group ($P = .008$). In order to further account for potential selection bias, the authors established 127 propensity score matched pairs, once again finding that the 7-year event-free survival rate was significantly higher in the operated group (99 vs 85%, $P = .007$). Independent predictors of late surgery or heart failure were pulmonary hypertension and increased effective regurgitant orifice area in the conventional group. The authors concluded that early surgery was associated with improved long-term event rate including decreased cardiac mortality and decreased congestive heart failure. They, therefore, suggest that early surgery may improve clinical outcomes in those with asymptomatic severe mitral regurgitation.

This is an important study, which underlines previous work in the field demonstrating the importance of early mitral valve repair for degenerative leaflet prolapse.[1-5] Although 6% of patients in this series required mitral replacement, which may theoretically alter the long-term outcomes following correction of mitral regurgitation,[6] the effect is likely small in this report. In addition to optimizing the long-term outcomes, the advantage of early mitral valve repair in eliminating the 0.8% per year risk of sudden death associated with a flail leaflet is important.[7] This in association with the facts that the current surgical mortality associated with mitral valve repair is less than 1%,[6] and that mitral valve repair is capable of restoring survival to that expected in age and sex-matched population indicates that deferring surgery is actually associated with higher risk. Larger left ventricular end diastolic and end systolic volumes in patients undergoing late surgery in this study pointing to an increased incidence of adverse left ventricular remodeling in those who are denied the advantages of early surgical intervention. In summary, the data presented within this important report stand on their own in demonstrating that even asymptomatic patients with preserved ejection fraction benefit from early mitral valve repair. Patients should be referred to centers where high likelihood of mitral valve repair exists in order to optimize long-term outcome.

**R. Suri, MD, DPhil**

*References*


1. Bonow RO, Carabello B, de Leon AC Jr, et al. Guidelines for the management of patients with valvular heart disease: executive summary. A report of the American College of Cardiology/American Heart Association Task Force on Practice Guidelines (Committee on Management of Patients with Valvular Heart Disease). *Circulation.* 1998;98:1949-1984.
2. Bonow RO, Carabello BA, Kanu C, et al. ACC/AHA 2006 guidelines for the management of patients with valvular heart disease: a report of the American College of Cardiology/American Heart Association Task Force on Practice Guidelines (writing committee to revise the 1998 Guidelines for the Management of Patients with Valvular Heart Disease): developed in collaboration with the Society of Cardiovascular Anesthesiologists: endorsed by the Society for Cardiovascular Angiography and Interventions and the Society of Thoracic Surgeons. *Circulation.* 2006;114:450-527.
3. Vahanian A, Baumgartner H, Bax J, et al. Guidelines on the management of valvular heart disease: the Task Force on the Management of Valvular Heart Disease of the European Society of Cardiology. *Eur Heart J.* 2007;28:230-268.
4. Enriquez-Sarano M, Avierinos JF, Messika-Zeitoun D, et al. Quantitative determinants of the outcome of asymptomatic mitral regurgitation. *N Engl J Med.* 2005;352:875-883.
5. Rosenhek R, Rader F, Klaar U, et al. Outcome of watchful waiting in asymptomatic severe mitral regurgitation. *Circulation.* 2006;113:2238-2244.
6. Suri RM, Schaff HV, Dearani JA, Sundt TM 3rd, Daly RC, Mullany CJ, Enriquez-Sarano M, Orszulak TA. Survival advantage and improved durability of mitral repair for leaflet prolapse subsets in the current era. *Ann Thorac Surg.* 2006;82:819-826.
7. Grigioni F, Enriquez-Sarano M, Ling LH, et al. Sudden death in mitral regurgitation due to flail leaflet. *J Am Coll Cardiol.* 1999;34:2078-2085.

# 39 Coronary Heart Disease

---

**Declining Severity of Myocardial Infarction From 1987 to 2002: The Atherosclerosis Risk in Communities (ARIC) Study**

Myerson M, for the ARIC Investigators (Natl Insts of Health, Bethesda, MD; et al)

*Circulation* 119:503-514, 2009

---

*Background.*—Death rates for coronary heart disease have been declining in the United States, but the reasons for this decline are not clear. One factor that could contribute to this decline is a reduction in the severity of acute myocardial infarction (MI). We hypothesized that for those patients hospitalized in the Atherosclerosis Risk in Communities (ARIC) Study with acute incident MI, there was a decline in MI severity from 1987 to 2002.

*Methods and Results.*—The community surveillance component of the ARIC Study consisted of tracking residents 35 to 74 years of age with hospitalized MI or fatal coronary heart disease in 4 diverse communities. For incident, hospitalized MI, a probability sample of hospital discharges was validated and an MI classification was assigned according to an algorithm consisting of chest pain, ECG evidence, and cardiac biomarkers. Severity indicators were chosen from abstracted hospital charts validated as a definite or probable MI. With few exceptions, the MI severity indicators suggested a significant decline in the severity of MI during the period of 1987 to 2002. The percent of MI cases with major ECG abnormalities decreased as evidenced by a 1.9%/y ($P = 0.002$) decline in the proportion of those with initial ST-segment elevation, a 3.9%/y ($P < 0.001$) decline in those with subsequent Q-waves, and a 4.5%/y ($P < 0.001$) decline in those with any major Q wave. Maximum creatine kinase and creatine kinase-MB values declined (5.2% and 7.6%; $P < 0.001$, $P < 0.001$ per year, respectively), although in the later years, maximum troponin I values remained stable (1.1%/y decline; $P = 0.66$). The percent with shock declined (5.7%/y; $P < 0.001$), although those with congestive heart failure remained stable. A combined severity score, the Predicting Risk of Death in Cardiac Disease Tool (PREDICT) score, also declined (0.2%/y; $P < 0.001$). Results for blacks paralleled those of the entire group, as did results for women.

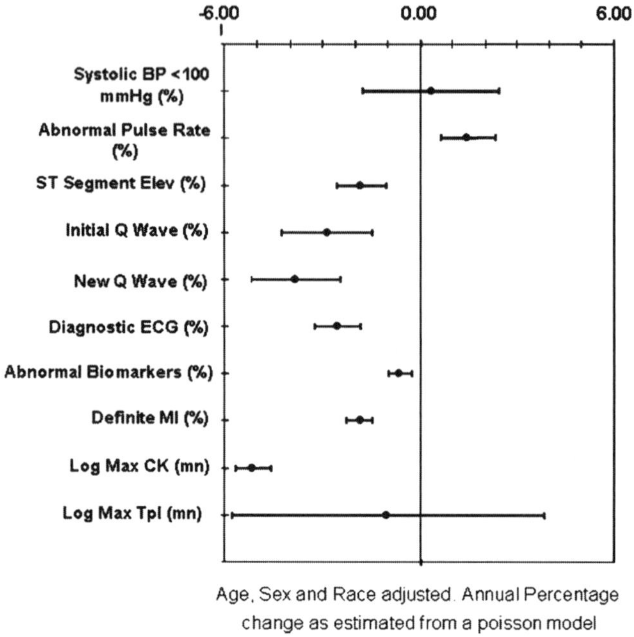


FIGURE 2.—Annual percentage change and 95% CIs for selected indicators of MI severity: ARIC Community Surveillance, 1987 to 2002. BP indicates blood pressure; TpI, troponin I. (Reprinted from Myerson M, for the ARIC Investigators, et al. Declinign severity of myocardial infarction from 1987 to 2002: the Atherosclerosis Risk in Communities (ARIC) Study. *Circulation*. 2009;119:503-51.)

*Conclusions*.—Evidence from ARIC community surveillance suggests that the severity of acute MI has declined among community residents hospitalized for incident MI. This reduction in severity may have contributed, along with other factors, to the decline in death rates for coronary heart disease (Fig 2).

▶ This 15-year survey of patients with hospitalized myocardial infarction or fatal coronary heart disease from the Atherosclerosis Risk in Communities Study (ARIC) is a source of encouragement. The ARIC study was designed to study cardiovascular disease in 4 geographically defined communities with different baseline and socioeconomic characteristics but within the United States.

Several previous epidemiological studies, including Framingham in Olmsted county, Minnesota demonstrated declines in the annual death rates from myocardial infarction over the last 4 decades.[1] One contributory factor could be a decline in the incidence, and although national data are unavailable, a previous study from ARIC showed that the incidence of acute myocardial infarction remained steady with the exception of blacks, who demonstrated an increase.[2]

This study provides another explanation by demonstrating a substantial and significant decline in the severity of myocardial infarction based on a number of indicators, including ST-segment elevation, new Q-waves, major EKG abnormalities, the magnitude of biomarker elevation (specifically creatine kinase [CK] and CK-MB), and the proportion with definite or probable myocardial infarction. Race- and sex-specific results were consistent with the results of the overall patient population.

The extent to which these are influenced by primary prevention versus acute care factors is uncertain. What does not appear to have been a factor is the time of presentation and prehospital delay, which unfortunately and frustratingly appears resistant to improvement.

The widespread chronic use of aspirin, β-blockers, lipid lowering agents, and previous revascularization may be an important contributory factor as are improvements in using evidence-based strategies.

The possibility that these changes in severity are an artifact explained by changes in the use of biomarkers and the shift to the troponins is addressed by the authors and adequately defended. The MI algorithm in ARIC is strongly influenced by the EKG and for troponins to be diagnostic these had to be elevated to twice the upper limit of normal.

These encouraging declines in coronary heart disease death rates are also being found in other parts of the developed world, for example, England and Wales.[3] Whatever the reasons underlying the decline in severity and in mortality, this is good news.

**B. J. Gersh, MB, ChB, DPhil, FRCP**

*References*

1. Gerber Y, Jacobsen SJ, Frye RL, Weston SA, Killian JM, Roger VL. Secular trends in deaths from cardiovascular diseases. *Circulation.* 2006;113:2285-2292.
2. Rosamond WD, Folsom AR, Chambless LE, Wang C-H. Coronary heart disease trends in four United States communities: the Atherosclerosis Risk in Communities (ARIC) study 1987-1996. *Int J Epidemiol.* 2001;30:S17-S22.
3. Unal B, Critchley JA, Capewill S. Explaining the decline in coronary heart disease mortality in England and Wales between 1981 and 2000. *Circulation.* 2004; 1101-1107.

---

**Impact of Blood Transfusion on Short- and Long-Term Mortality in Patients With ST-Segment Elevation Myocardial Infarction**

Shishehbor MH, Madhwal S, Rajagopal V, et al (Cleveland Clinic, OH; Piedmont Heart Inst, Atlanta, GA; et al)

*JACC Cardiovasc Interv* 2:46-53, 2009

---

*Objectives.*—We sought to examine the short- and long-term outcomes of blood transfusion in patients presenting with ST-segment elevation myocardial infarction (STEMI).

*Background.*—The short- and long-term consequences of blood transfusion in anemic patients with recent STEMI remain controversial.

*Methods.*—We evaluated 30-day, 6-month, and 1-year all-cause mortality among 4,131 STEMI patients enrolled in the GUSTO (Global Use of Strategies to Open Occluded Coronary Arteries) IIb trial. Patients were categorized according to whether they received a blood transfusion during hospitalization. Cox proportional hazards survival models with transfusion as a time-dependent covariate were conducted for the whole and for the propensity-matched groups. Additionally, a series of sensitivity analyses assessed the magnitude of hidden bias that would need to be present to explain the associations actually observed.

*Results.*—Death at 30 days (13.7% vs. 5.5%), 6 months (19.7% vs. 6.9%), and 1 year (21.8% vs. 8.7%) was significantly higher for transfused patients than for nontransfused patients, respectively. After adjusting for over 25 baseline characteristics, nadir hemoglobin, and propensity score for transfusion, and using transfusion as a time-dependent covariate, transfusion remained significantly associated with increased risk of mortality at 30 days (hazard ratio [HR]: 3.89, 95% confidence interval [CI]: 2.66 to 5.68, $p < 0.001$), 6 months (HR: 3.63, 95% CI: 2.67 to 4.95, $p < 0.001$), and 1 year (HR: 3.03, 95% CI: 2.25 to 4.08, $p < 0.001$). Similar results were observed in the propensity-matched patients.

*Conclusions.*—Blood transfusion is associated with increased short- and long-term mortality in the setting of STEMI (Fig 1).

▶ A consistent theme in studies of acute coronary syndromes and other cardiovascular diseases is the adverse effect of anemia on prognosis.[1] There are a number of plausible explanations, and some may be correlated with the need for blood transfusions. In addition, there is considerable debate over the use of blood transfusions to correct anemia in otherwise stable patients.[2,3] On one hand, in patients with ST-segment elevation myocardial infarction (STEMI), anemia can exacerbate disparities between myocardial oxygen demand and supply, and this could be improved by transfusion. Alternatively, the increased viscosity and thrombogenicity associated with myocardial infarction may be increased by the transfusion of stored blood leading to poor oxygen delivery.

This is an interesting study, but it does not answer the question as to whether patients with coronary artery disease and anemia who are otherwise stable should be transfused. There are so many confounding variables that this issue would probably only be resolved by a randomized controlled trial. It is not surprising that transfusion is associated with increased mortality of 30 days and at 1 year. The transfused patients are clearly a "sicker group," and the old adage still applies—multivariant analyses adjusts the differences in baseline variables but cannot eliminate the impact of these or the effect of unmeasured confounders.

Bleeding, anemia, and transfusion are all strong adverse prognostic factors in the acute coronary syndrome. There are many potential explanations. Firstly, bleeding may result in hemodynamic derangements and impaired oxygen supply due to a fall in coronary perfusion pressure. Secondly, patients who

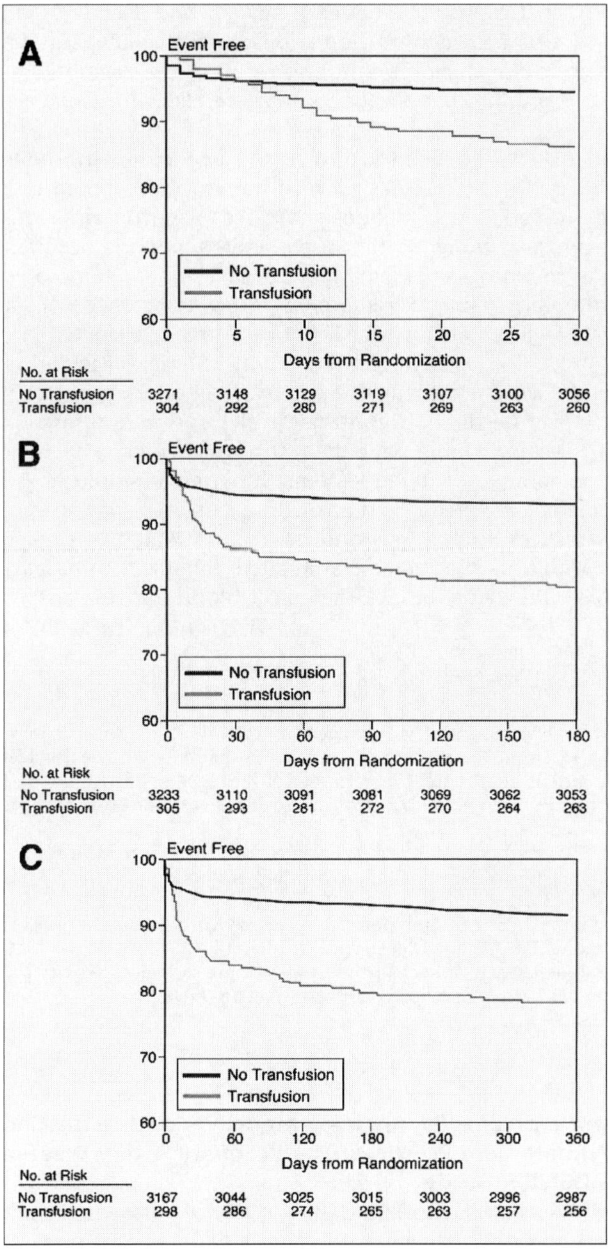


FIGURE 1.—Kaplan-Meier Curves for Mortality in the Overall Population. Kaplan-Meier curves (**A**) for 30-day mortality in the overall population (n = 3,575), (**B**) for 6-month mortality in the overall population (n = 3,538), and (**C**) for 1-year mortality in the overall population (n = 3,465). (Reprinted from Shishehbor MH, Madhwal S, Rajagopal V, et al. Impact of blood transfusion on short-and long-term mortality in patients with ST-segment elevation myocardial infarction. *JACC Cardiovasc Interv.* 2009;2:46-53, with permission from Elsevier.)

require blood transfusions are older and "sicker," and despite multivariant analyses bias cannot be excluded. A third and likely possibility is that bleeding and anemia leading to transfusion might also result in the discontinuation of other antiplatelet and antithrombotic agents that are also anti-ischemia, eg, aspirin and Plavix.

The fourth possibility as discussed in the accompanying editorial[4] is that blood transfusions in themselves may be harmful. This could be the result of structural and biochemical changes that take place during storage and that could affect oxygen affinity so that tissue oxygenation is not improved. There are also the familiar hazards of microbial transmission, immunological reactions, and altered rheology causing tissue plugging of transfused cells at the microvascular level. There is also evidence that the transport of nitric oxide by red blood cells and the release of NO bioactivity to microvascular cells that may be beneficial are significantly affected by storage of erythrocytes.[5]

Although it will be difficult and unethical to perform a randomized trial of blood transfusion in anemic patients with clear evidence of ongoing cardiac ischemia or hemodynamic derangements, it certainly would be possible to do a trial of transfusion versus no transfusion in stable, asymptomatic patients following an acute coronary syndrome. It is difficult to perceive that blood transfusions would be that beneficial in such patients, but at least such a trial would establish the safety or lack thereof of blood transfusions.

**B. J. Gersh, MB, ChB, DPhil, FRCP**

*References*


1. Spencer FA, Moscucci M, Granger CB, et al. GRACE Investigators. Does comorbidity account for the excess mortality in patients with major bleeding in acute myocardial infarction? *Circulation.* 2007;116:2793-2801.
2. Herbert PC, Fergusson DA. Do transfusions get to the heart of the matter? *JAMA.* 2004;292:1610-1612.
3. Wu WC, Rathore SS, Wang Y, Radford MJ, Krumholz HM. Blood transfusion in elderly patients with acute myocardial infarction. *N Engl J Med.* 2001;345:1230-1236.
4. Doyle B. There will be blood. *JACC Cardiovasc Interv.* 2009;2:54-55.
5. Reynolds JD, Ahearn GS, Angelo M, Zhang J, Cobb F, Stamler JS. S-nitrosohemoglobin deficiency: a mechanism for loss of physiological activity in banked blood. *Prox Natl Acad Sci U S A.* 2007;104:17058-17062.


## The Prevalence of Weekly Angina Among Patients With Chronic Stable Angina in Primary Care Practices: The Coronary Artery Disease in General Practice (CADENCE) Study

Beltrame JF, Weekes AJ, Morgan C, et al (Univ of Adelaide, Australia; Pty Ltd, Hawththorn, Victoria, Australia; et al)

*Arch Intern Med* 169:1491-1499, 2009

*Background.*—Angina, the cardinal symptom of coronary artery disease (CAD), is amenable to a range of therapies, and its routine assessment is considered a performance measure of quality. However, the prevalence of frequent angina among outpatients with CAD is unknown.

*Methods.*—The Coronary Artery Disease in General Practice (CADENCE) Study utilized a cluster-stratified, cross-sectional design to examine angina frequency in patients with stable angina attending Australian primary care practices. The 207 participating primary care practitioners recruited 2031 consecutive patients, irrespective of the purpose of their visit. Angina frequency was quantified with the Seattle Angina Questionnaire (SAQ), and weekly angina was defined as having 1 or more episodes per week over the preceding 4 weeks [hereinafter, "weekly (≥1) angina"].

*Results.*—Among primary care practice patients with stable angina, 29% (95% confidence interval [CI], 26%-31%) experienced weekly (≥1) angina, which was associated with greater physical limitations and worse quality of life (24% and 27% lower SAQ scores, respectively; $P < .05$) compared with those with minimal angina (angina less than once a week over the preceding 4 weeks). The proportion of patients with weekly (≥1) angina within a clinic ranged from none (14% of clinics) to more than 50% (18% of clinics). Patient characteristics associated with weekly (≥1) angina included female sex (odds ratio [OR], 1.42; 95% CI, 1.13-1.78), a history of heart failure (OR, 1.59; 95% CI, 1.22-2.08), and peripheral artery disease (OR 1.89; 95% CI, 1.42-2.51; $P < .001$ for all comparisons).

*Conclusions.*—Almost 1 in 3 patients with stable angina attending primary care practices had angina at least once a week, which was associated with worse quality of life. Moreover, weekly (≥1) angina varied considerably across clinics, possibly reflecting variability in the identification and management of angina. The potential role of an angina performance measure to improve patients' outcomes, including symptom control, warrants further consideration.

▶ This prospective study of general practitioners in Australia provides a somewhat different perspective of the problem of chronic stable angina in the community at large. Two thousand and thirty-one consecutive patients recruited from 207 participating primary care practitioners were evaluated for the frequency of angina by the Seattle Angina Questionnaire.[1] Twenty-nine percent of these patients had experienced angina at least once per week during the preceding 4 weeks, and this was associated with a 24% reduction in the quality-of-life and a 27% increase in physical limitation in comparison with those with lesser degrees of angina. Patient characteristics associated with more frequent episodes were female sex, history of congestive heart failure, and peripheral arterial disease—"the usual suspects."

What is interesting and as is illustrated in the accompanying Fig 4 in the original article is the discordance between patients and physicians' perceptions of angina control. From the general practitioner's perspective, 61% of patients had minimal angina-related impediment in physical activity (Canadian Cardiovascular Society class 1), including 12% reporting angina on a daily basis.

Among patients reporting weekly and daily angina, general practitioners felt that 48% and 30% were "optimally controlled." In addition, the frequency of weekly angina varied enormously across the 207 primary care clinics ranging from 0% to 100%.

There are several implications to the studies. Firstly, recurrent angina is a major cause of morbidity, and although coronary revascularization has come under fire recently, we should not underestimate its efficacy in improving symptoms. A key first step, however, is to "optimize" medical therapy, and there is certainly a need for new pharmacologic agents and an appreciation for the intensity of medical therapy required. Given the variability and physician estimates of angina control, the authors make the important point that performance measures for the documentation of angina control and its impact upon symptoms and quality-of-life should be introduced.[2]

In the interim, physicians need to take heed and need to listen to the patient in regard to their perception of their symptoms and the effect that these exert on the quality of their lifestyle.

**B. J. Gersh, MB, ChB, DPhil, FRCP**

*References*

1. Spertus JA, Winder JA, Dewhurst TA, et al. Development and evaluation of the Seattle Angina Questionnaire: a new functional status measure for coronary artery disease. *J Am Coll Cardiol.* 1995;25:333-341.
2. Spertus JA, Eagle KA, Krumholz HM, Mitchell KR, Normand SL. American College of Cardiology/American Heart Association task force on performance measures. American College of Cardiology and American Heart Association methodology for the selection and creation of performance measures for quantifying the quality of cardiovascular care. *J Am Coll Cardiol.* 2005;45:1147-1156.

## Current Use of Beta Blockers in Patients With Reactive Airway Disease Who Are Hospitalized With Acute Coronary Syndromes

Olenchock BA, for the Get With The Guidelines[SM] Steering Committee (Brigham and Women's Hosp, Boston, MA; et al)
*Am J Cardiol* 103:295-300, 2009

Beta blockers have a proven benefit in the management of patients with acute coronary syndromes (ACS) and for secondary prevention of coronary events. Current guidelines list such reactive airway diseases (RADs) such as asthma and chronic obstructive pulmonary disease as relative contraindications to β-blocker use. However, the co-morbid burden of RAD and coronary heart disease is substantial, and data suggest that the treatment benefit of β blockers is shared by patients with RAD. The Get with the Guidelines[SM] (GWTG) database was used to evaluate use of β blockers within 24 hours of admission and at discharge in patients with ACS with (n = 12,967) and without (n = 81,140) a history of RAD. Data were collected in 435 hospitals between January 2000 and

September 2006. A multivariable logistic regression model was used to determine predictors of β-blocker treatment. In patients with no RAD history, β-blocker prescription rates were 78.3% at admission and 88.7% at discharge; in patients with a RAD history, rates were 65.6% at admission and 77.2% at discharge. Compared with patients with no history of RAD, patients with a history of RAD were 42% less likely (odds ratio 0.58, confidence interval 0.54 to 0.62, p <0.0001) to receive a β blocker upon admission and 55% less likely (odds ratio 0.45, confidence interval 0.41 to 0.48, p <0.0001) to receive a β blocker at discharge in multivariable analysis. Among all other clinical factors, RAD history was the most significant predictor of likelihood of not receiving a β blocker at admission or discharge. Receipt of β blockers within 24 hours after admission was associated with a lower in-hospital mortality rate for patients with RAD (odds ratio = 0.52, p <0.001) and for patients without RAD (odds ratio = 0.38, p <0.001). Careful assessment of β-blocker safety and RAD severity by physicians is needed to improve β-blocker prescription rates in this large group of patients with ACS (Table 3).

▶ This large registry study in patients with acute coronary syndromes raises a number of clinical issues that are germane to day-to-day clinical practice; namely, the role of beta blockers in patients with chronic obstructive pulmonary disease (COPD) and reactive airway disease (RAD).

Not surprisingly, the use of beta blockers on admission and at discharge were significantly less in patients with a history of RAD compared with those without a history of RAD. Patients with a history of RAD were 42% less likely to receive a beta blocker on admission and 55% less likely to receive a beta blocker at

TABLE 3.—Clinical Factors Associated with Decision to Prescribe a β Blocker Within 24 Hours of Admission and at Discharge

| | Within 24 h of Admission | | | At Discharge | | |
|---|---|---|---|---|---|---|
| | OR | 95% CI | p Value | OR | 95% CI | p Value |
| RAD history | 0.58 | 0.54–0.62 | <0.001 | 0.45 | 0.42–0.48 | <0.001 |
| Age increase by 10 | 0.90 | 0.88–0.92 | <0.001 | 0.93 | 0.91–0.96 | <0.001 |
| Race: White vs other | 0.97 | 0.91–1.03 | 0.27 | 0.98 | 0.91–1.06 | 0.63 |
| Body mass index increase by 1 | 1.01 | 1.01–1.01 | <0.001 | 1.00 | 1.00–1.01 | 0.07 |
| Insurance: Medicare | 0.86 | 0.79–0.93 | <0.001 | 0.83 | 0.75–0.91 | <0.001 |
| Insurance: Medicaid | 0.80 | 0.71–0.90 | <0.001 | 0.76 | 0.65–0.89 | <0.001 |
| Insurance: Other | 0.94 | 0.86–1.01 | 0.10 | 0.91 | 0.83–1.00 | 0.04 |
| Ejection fraction < 0.4 | 0.96 | 0.91–1.01 | 0.10 | 1.26 | 1.18–1.33 | <0.001 |
| Diabetes history | 0.98 | 0.94–1.02 | 0.34 | 1.06 | 1.00–1.11 | 0.04 |
| Heart failure history | 0.83 | 0.79–0.88 | <0.001 | 0.88 | 0.82–0.95 | 0.001 |
| Hypertension history | 1.24 | 1.19–1.29 | <0.001 | 1.25 | 1.19–1.32 | <0.001 |
| Hyperlipidemia | 1.14 | 1.09–1.20 | <0.001 | 1.22 | 1.16–1.28 | <0.001 |
| Previous MI | 1.14 | 1.08–1.19 | <0.001 | 1.10 | 1.04–1.16 | <0.001 |
| Peripheral vascular disease | 0.97 | 0.92–1.02 | 0.27 | 0.98 | 0.91–1.06 | 0.66 |
| Chronic kidney disease | 0.90 | 0.84–0.96 | <0.001 | 0.95 | 0.89–1.02 | 0.18 |
| Previous stroke | 0.92 | 0.86–0.98 | 0.009 | 0.95 | 0.87–1.02 | 0.16 |
| History of smoking | 0.99 | 0.94–1.06 | 0.86 | 1.03 | 0.98–1.09 | 0.26 |

OR = odds ratio; CI = confidence interval.

discharge. Moreover, among all the other clinical factors determining the use of beta blockers, RAD history was the most significant independent predictor of not receiving a beta blocker both on admission and at discharge. In addition, receipt of beta blockers within 24-hours after admission was associated with a lower hospital mortality rate for patients with and without RAD. Nonetheless, there are a number of other explanations for these associations including the presence of multiple potential confounding variables, and it is unclear whether the administration of beta blockers is actually responsible for the mortality reduction, although this would be a logical premise.

The inclination to withhold beta blockers in patients with RAD is understandable given evidence that beta blockers could precipitate life threatening bronchial constriction.[1] It is now accepted that the risk is higher among noncardiac-selective beta blockers such as propanolol or nadolol, but cardioselectivity is only relative in terms of bronchial responsiveness.[2]

Although frank bronchospasm is a contraindication to beta-blocker use, in patients with either acute or chronic coronary artery disease who have COPD and a history of RAD, beta blockers are usually well tolerated over the long term and cardioselective agents should be used. A recent meta-analysis demonstrated that the chronic use of cardioselective beta blockers in patients with COPD did not result in adverse effects as assessed by changes on FEV1 or respiratory symptoms in comparison with placebo.[3] A subgroup analysis demonstrated no change in results for those participants with severe chronic airway obstruction or for those with a reversible obstructive component. From a clinical standpoint the inpatient setting is ideal for beta-blocker initiation in patients with RAD because adverse effects can be closely monitored, and patients can be stabilized on therapy that might be beneficial after discharge. As pointed out by the authors there is a need for efforts focused upon clinical education and quality improvement to bridge this gap between drugs that are potentially beneficial but underused.

**B. J. Gersh, MB, ChB, DPhil, FRCP**

*References*


1. Kendall MJ, Beeley L. Beta-adrenoceptor blocking drugs: adverse reactions and drug interactions. *Pharmacol Ther.* 1983;21:351-369.
2. van der Woude HJ, Zaagsma J, Postma DS, Winter TH, van Hulst M, Albers R. Detrimental effects of beta-blockers in COPD: a concern for nonselective beta-blockers. *Chest.* 2005;127:818-824.
3. Salpeter S, Ormiston T, Salpeter E. Cardioselective beta-blockers for chronic obstructive pulmonary disease. *Update of Cochran Database Syst Rev.* 2002;19. CD003566.

**Effects of a polypill (Polycap) on risk factors in middle-aged individuals without cardiovascular disease (TIPS): a phase II, double-blind, randomised trial**

The Indian Polycap Study (TIPS) (Hamilton Health Sciences and McMaster Univ, Canada)

*Lancet* 373:1341-1351, 2009

*Background.*—The combination of three blood-pressure-lowering drugs at low doses, with a statin, aspirin, and folic acid (the polypill), could reduce cardiovascular events by more than 80% in healthy individuals. We examined the effect of the Polycap on blood pressure, lipids, heart rate, and urinary thromboxane B2, and assessed its tolerability.

*Methods.*—In a double-blind trial in 50 centres in India, 2053 individuals without cardiovascular disease, aged 45–80 years, and with one risk factor were randomly assigned, by a central secure website, to the Polycap (n=412) consisting of low doses of thiazide (12·5 mg), atenolol (50 mg), ramipril (5 mg), simvastatin (20 mg), and aspirin (100 mg) per day, or to eight other groups, each with about 200 individuals, of aspirin alone, simvastatin alone, hydrochlorthiazide alone, three combinations of the two blood-pressure-lowering drugs, three blood-pressure-lowering drugs alone, or three blood-pressure-lowering drugs plus aspirin. The primary outcomes were LDL for the effect of lipids, blood pressure for antihypertensive drugs, heart rate for the effects of atenolol, urinary 11-dehydrothromboxane B2 for the antiplatelet effects of aspirin, and rates of discontinuation of drugs for safety. Analysis was by intention to treat. This study is registered with ClinicalTrials.gov, number NCT00443794.

*Findings.*—Compared with groups not receiving blood-pressure-lowering drugs, the Polycap reduced systolic blood pressure by 7·4 mm Hg (95% CI 6·1–8·1) and diastolic blood pressure by 5·6 mm Hg (4·7–6·4), which was similar when three blood-pressure-lowering drugs were used, with or without aspirin. Reductions in blood pressure increased with the number of drugs used (2·2/1·3 mm Hg with one drug, 4·7/3·6 mm Hg with two drugs, and 6·3/4·5 mm Hg with three drugs). Polycap reduced LDL cholesterol by 0·70 mmol/L (95% CI 0·62–0·78), which was less than that with simvastatin alone (0·83 mmol/L, 0·72–0·93; p=0·04); both reductions were greater than for groups without simvastatin (p<0·0001). The reductions in heart rate with Polycap and other groups using atenolol were similar (7·0 beats per min), and both were significantly greater than that in groups without atenolol (p<0·0001). The reductions in 11-dehydrothromboxane B2 were similar with the Polycap (283·1 ng/mmol creatinine, 95% CI 229·1–337·0) compared with the three blood-pressure-lowering drugs plus aspirin (350·0 ng/mmol creatinine, 294·6–404·0), and aspirin alone (348·8 ng/mmol creatinine, 277·6–419·9) compared with groups without aspirin. Tolerability of the Polycap was similar to that of other treatments,

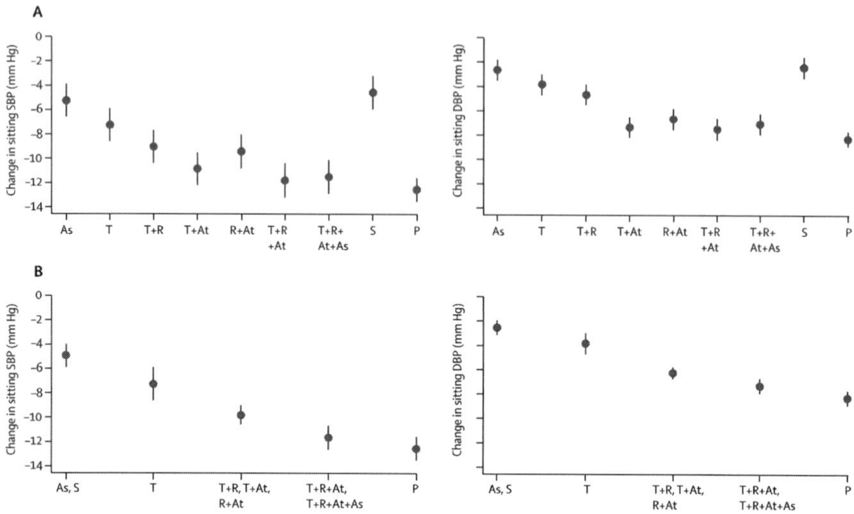


FIGURE 3.—Mean changes in systolic blood pressure (SBP) and diastolic blood pressure (DBP). Error bars indicate 95% CI. Mean changes from baseline in the nine groups (A), and the effects of no blood-pressure-lowering drugs (As, S), one blood-pressure-lowering drug (T), two blood-pressure-lowering drugs (T+R, T+At, or R+At), or three blood-pressure-lowering drugs (T+R+At, T+R+At+S), or the Polycap (B). As=aspirin. T=thiazide. R=ramipril. At=atenolol. S=simvastatin. P=Polycap. (Reprinted from The Indian Polycap Study (TIPS). Effects of a polypill (Polycap) on risk factors in middle-aged individuals without cardiovascular disease (TIPS): a phase II, double-blind, randomised trial. *Lancet.* 2009;373:1341-1351, with permission from Elsevier.)

with no evidence of increasing intolerability with increasing number of active components in one pill.

*Interpretation.*—This Polycap formulation could be conveniently used to reduce multiple risk factors and cardiovascular risk (Fig 3).

▶ This phase II double-blind randomized trial of the effects of a polypill represents a remarkable effort from 50 centers in India. It is possible that this study could be the harbinger of a breakthrough in the primary and secondary prevention of cardiovascular disease in the developing world.

The concept of the polypill was hypothesized by Wald and Law several years ago, and it was proposed that a combination of aspirin, a β blocker, angiotensin-converting enzyme inhibitor, and a statin together with folic acid could reduce cardiovascular disease by more than 80%.[1] Subsequently, homocysteine-lowering has not been shown to reduce cardiovascular disease, whereas the other components of the polypill have been retained and formed the basis of the Polycap pill used in this study.

This trial addressed several crucial questions that need to be answered before large trials can be undertaken. Firstly, can 1 pill or a capsule be formulated that can deliver an effect similar to the additive effects of each component provided separately? Secondly, what would be the magnitude in the reduction in blood pressure and low-density lipoprotein (LDL) cholesterol in patients with normal levels of risk factors? Other issues addressed included tolerability, the potential for interaction, and the possibility that aspirin could reduce the blood pressure lowering effects of the other drugs.

The trial admirably succeeded in its aims and demonstrated both safety and efficacy, and there was no evidence of increasing tolerability with an increasing number of active components in 1 pill. As pointed out by the authors, however, adherence was a problem perhaps because participants deduced that there would be no benefit due to the fact that their risk factors were normal to begin with and therefore refused further participation, and in about 4% of individuals follow-up blood pressure or heart rate readings were unobtainable, and follow-up lipid values were unavailable in 9%. Future trials will need to pay careful attention to retention to adherence and compliance.

Nonetheless, the study has several strengths and in particular by including 9 groups in large numbers of patients they were able to assess the effects of various combinations of drugs on a range of outcomes. The results of this study suggest that the formulation of the Polycap used in this trial could be a suitable preparation for trials examining cardiovascular risks and events in large and long-term studies.

**B. J. Gersh, MB, ChB, DPhil, FRCP**

*Reference*

1. Wald NJ, Law MR. A strategy to reduce cardiovascular disease by more than 80%. *BMJ*. 2003;326:1419-1424.

---

**Aspirin in the primary and secondary prevention of vascular disease: collaborative meta-analysis of individual participant data from randomised trials**

Antithrombotic Trialists' (ATT) Collaboration (Univ of Oxford, UK)

*Lancet* 373:1849-1860, 2009

---

*Background.*—Low-dose aspirin is of definite and substantial net benefit for many people who already have occlusive vascular disease. We have assessed the benefits and risks in primary prevention.

*Methods.*—We undertook meta-analyses of serious vascular events (myocardial infarction, stroke, or vascular death) and major bleeds in six primary prevention trials (95 000 individuals at low average risk, 660 000 person-years, 3554 serious vascular events) and 16 secondary prevention trials (17 000 individuals at high average risk, 43 000 person-years, 3306 serious vascular events) that compared long-term aspirin versus control. We report intention-to-treat analyses of first events during the scheduled treatment period.

*Findings.*—In the primary prevention trials, aspirin allocation yielded a 12% proportional reduction in serious vascular events (0·51% aspirin *vs* 0·57% control per year, p=0·0001), due mainly to a reduction of about a fifth in non-fatal myocardial infarction (0·18% *vs* 0·23% per

| | Events (% per year) | | Ratio (CI) of yearly event rates | |
|---|---|---|---|---|
| | Allocated aspirin | Adjusted control | Aspirin:control | |
| CHD | 372 (0·11) | 393 (0·12) | | 0·95 (0·78–1·15) |
| Stroke | 119 (0·04) | 98 (0·03) | | 1·21 (0·84–1·74) |
| GI or other extracranial haemorrhage | 9 (-) | 20 (-) | | 0·48 (0·17–1·34) |
| Remaining vascular | 119 (0·04) | 126 (0·04) | | 0·96 (0·68–1·35) |
| **Subtotal: any vascular** | **619 (0·19)** | **637 (0·19)** | | **0·97 (0·87–1·09) p=0·7** |
| **Non-vascular** | **913 (0·27)** | **986 (0·30)** | | **0·93 (0·85–1·02) p=0·1** |
| Unknown | 137 (0·04) | 143 (0·04) | | 0·96 (0·70–1·30) |
| **Total: any death** | **1669 (0·50)** | **1766 (0·53)** | | **0·95 (0·88–1·02) p=0·1** |

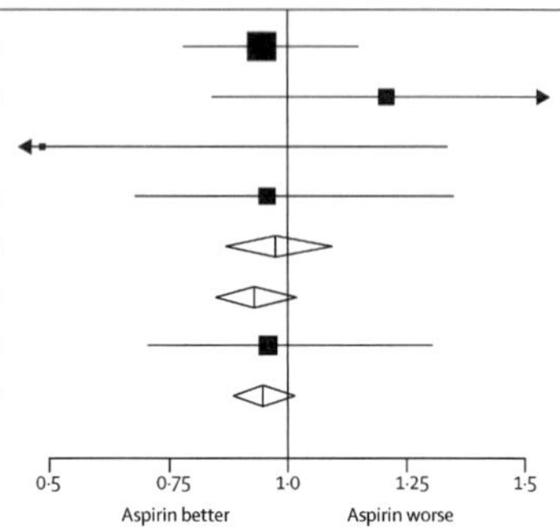


FIGURE 5.—Mortality by cause in primary prevention trials. Actual numbers for aspirin-allocated trial participants, and adjusted numbers for control-allocated trial participants, are presented together with the corresponding mean yearly event rate (in parentheses). Rate ratios (RRs) for all trials are indicated by squares and their 99% CIs by horizontal lies. Subtotals and their 95%CIs are represented by diamonds. Squares or diamonds to the left of the solid line indicate benefit. CHD=coronary heart disease. GI=gastointestinal. (Reprinted from Antithrombotic Trialists' (ATT) Collaboration. Aspirin in the primary and secondary prevention of vascular disease: collaborative meta-analysis of individual participant data from randomised trials. *Lancet*. 2009;373:1849-1860, with permission from Elsevier.)

year, p<0·0001). The net effect on stroke was not significant (0·20% *vs* 0·21% per year, p=0·4: haemorrhagic stroke 0·04% *vs* 0·03%, p=0·05; other stroke 0·16% *vs* 0·18% per year, p=0·08). Vascular mortality did not differ significantly (0·19% *vs* 0·19% per year, p=0·7). Aspirin allocation increased major gastrointestinal and extracranial bleeds (0·10% *vs* 0·07% per year, p<0·0001), and the main risk factors for coronary disease were also risk factors for bleeding. In the secondary prevention trials, aspirin allocation yielded a greater absolute reduction in serious vascular events (6·7% *vs* 8·2% per year, p < 0.0001), with a non-significant increase in haemorrhagic stroke but reductions of about a fifth in total stroke (2·08% *vs* 2·54% per year, p=0·002) and in coronary events (4·3% *vs* 5·3% per year, p<0·0001). In both primary and secondary prevention trials, the proportional reductions in the aggregate of all serious vascular events seemed similar for men and women.

*Interpretation.*—In primary prevention without previous disease, aspirin is of uncertain net value as the reduction in occlusive events needs to be weighed against any increase in major bleeds. Further trials are in progress (Fig 5).

► This is a new meta-analysis that is based upon individual participant data that take into account the benefits and risks of aspirin in specific subgroups, eg, older patients, may certainly create some waves. There is little argument over the benefits of aspirin in the secondary prevention of cardiovascular disease, and the consensus is that in this setting the benefits of aspirin far outweigh the risks of bleeding.[1] This meta-analysis raises doubts about the net value of aspirin in regard to the reduction in ischemic events versus the risk of bleeding in the setting of primary prevention. Current guidelines recommend that aspirin should be used widely for primary prevention in those with a moderately raised risk of coronary heart disease.[2] The major conclusion of this study is that the very patients at higher risk of heart disease are also at a higher risk of bleeding with aspirin. Another factor in recent years are the benefits of cholesterol and blood pressure reduction in lowering the risk of heart disease, and this might tend to dilute or negate the impact of aspirin.

It will be interesting to see whether this meta-analysis will change the guidelines in any way—I suspect not. Decisions should be made on an individual basis. The data from 6 large scale primary prevention trials and their meta-analyses demonstrate that aspirin reduces the risk of a first myocardial infarction by about a quarter to a third, but the data on stroke and cardiovascular death are less conclusive. Serious bleeds are certainly increased. The role of enteric-coated aspirin has not been adequately tested. In addition, the totality of available evidence suggests that there are no differences between men and women.[3]

**B. J. Gersh, MB, ChB, DPhil, FRCP**

*References*

1. Hansson L, Zanchetti A, Carruthers SG, et al. Effects of intensive blood-pressure lowering and low-dose aspirin in patients with hypertension: principal results of the hypertension optimal treatment (HOT) randomised trial. *Lancet.* 1998;351: 1755-1762.
2. US Preventive Services Task Force. Aspirin for the prevention of cardiovascular disease: US preventive services task force recommendation statement. *Ann Intern Med.* 2009;150:396-404.
3. Hennekens CH, Hollar D, Baigent C. Sex-related differences in response to aspirin and cardiovascular disease: an untested hypothesis. *Nat Clin Pract Cardiovasc Med.* 2006;3:4-5.

---

## Statin Adherence and Risk of Accidents: A Cautionary Tale

Dormuth CR, Patrick AR, Shrank WH, et al (Univ of British Columbia, Vancouver, Canada; Harvard Med School, Boston, MA)
*Circulation* 119:2051-2057, 2009

---

*Background.*—Bias in studies of preventive medications can occur when healthier patients are more likely to initiate and adhere to therapy than less healthy patients. We sought evidence of this bias by examining associations between statin exposure and various outcomes that should not be causally affected by statin exposure, such as workplace and motor vehicle accidents.

*Methods and Results.*—We conducted a prospective cohort study of statin patients using data from British Columbia, Canada, a multiethnic society with a population of 4.3 million people. Study subjects were 141 086 patients who initiated statins for primary prevention. We examined the association between adherence and multiple outcomes such as accidents and screening procedures using multivariable-adjusted Cox proportional hazards models. The study population was 49% female and had an average age of 61 years. The results from our multivariable-adjusted models showed that more adherent patients were less likely to have accidents than less adherent patients. This effect was greatest for motor vehicle accidents (hazard ratio, 0.75; 95% confidence interval, 0.72 to 0.79) and workplace accidents (hazard ratio, 0.77; 95% confidence interval, 0.74 to 0.81). More adherent patients had a greater likelihood of using screening services (hazard ratio, 1.17; 95% confidence interval, 1.15 to 1.20) and a lower likelihood of developing other diseases likely to be unrelated to a biological affect of a statin (hazard ratio, 0.87; 95% confidence interval, 0.86 to 0.89).

*Conclusions.*—Our study contributes compelling evidence that patients who adhere to statins are systematically more health seeking than comparable patients who do not remain adherent. Caution is warranted when interpreting analyses that attribute surprising protective effects to preventive medications.

▶ This analysis of statin adherence and the risk of accidents is indeed "a cautionary tale" as stated in the title of the article.

Using a very large database of 141 086 patients in British Columbia who had been prescribed statins for primary prevention, patients were stratified into 2 groups according to the extent to which their prescriptions were filled. Patients were categorized according to whether they were "more adherent" or "less adherent." The results show that more adherent patients were less likely to have accidents, particularly in regard to motor vehicle accidents and accidents in the workplace. In addition, more adherent patients had a greater likelihood of using screening services, including fecal occult blood testing, bone mineral density testing, regular eye examinations, and prosthetic-specific antigen testing. They also had a lower likelihood of developing other diseases most likely unrelated to the biological effects of the statins.The lesson is important in regard to how we interpret the results of observational studies that report benefits for drug therapies, particularly if the magnitude of benefit is larger than expected, in that adherence to drug therapy and other health behaviors are enormously susceptible to various sources of bias, including the so-called healthy-user and healthy-adherence bias.[1] Examples of such confounding effects include studies on the "apparent" benefits of long-term estrogen therapy[2] and vitamin E.[3] In this study, the approximate magnitude of the effect was 15%, but in addition patients who follow the advice of their physicians in regard to drug compliance appear to also be more likely to have other healthy behaviors. We, therefore, need to maintain a healthy skepticism in regard to the observational studies, which demonstrate benefits of a particular drug or lifestyle modification, particularly if these benefits are somewhat unexpected or the magnitude is larger than expected.

**B. J. Gersh, MB, ChB, DPhil, FRCP**

*References*

1. Simpson SH, Eurich DT, Majumdar SR, et al. A meta-analysis of the association between adherence to drug therapy and mortality. *BMJ.* 2006;333:15.

2. Barrett-Connor E, Grade D. Hormone replacement therapy, heart disease, and other considerations. *Annu Rev Public Health*. 1998;19:55-72.
3. Redberg RF. Vitamin E and cardiovascular health: does sex matter? *JAMA*. 2005; 294:107-109.

**Effect of fish oil on arrhythmias and mortality: systematic review**

León H, Shibata MC, Sivakumaran S, et al (Epidemiology Coordinating and Res (EPICORE) Centre, Edmonton, Alberta, Canada; et al)
*BMJ* 338:a2931, 2009

*Objective.*—To synthesise the literature on the effects of fish oil—docosahexaenoic acid (DHA) and eicosapentaenoic acid (EPA)—on mortality and arrhythmias and to explore dose response and formulation effects.

*Design.*—Systematic review and meta-analysis.

*Data Sources.*—Medline, Embase, the Cochrane Library, PubMed, CINAHL, IPA, Web of Science, Scopus, Pascal, Allied and Complementary Medicine, Academic OneFile, ProQuest Dissertations and Theses, Evidence-Based Complementary Medicine, and LILACS.

*Studies Reviewed.*—Randomised controlled trials of fish oil as dietary supplements in humans.

*Data Extraction.*—The primary outcomes of interest were the arrhythmic end points of appropriate implantable cardiac defibrillator intervention and sudden cardiac death. The secondary outcomes were all cause mortality and death from cardiac causes. Subgroup analyses included the effect of formulations of EPA and DHA on death from cardiac causes and effects of fish oil in patients with coronary artery disease or myocardial infarction.

*Data Synthesis.*—12 studies totalling 32 779 patients met the inclusion criteria. A neutral effect was reported in three studies (n = 1148) for appropriate implantable cardiac defibrillator intervention (odds ratio 0.90, 95% confidence interval 0.55 to 1.46) and in six studies (n = 31 111) for sudden cardiac death (0.81, 0.52 to 1.25). 11 studies (n = 32 439 and n = 32 519) provided data on the effects of fish oil on all cause mortality (0.92, 0.82 to 1.03) and a reduction in deaths from cardiac causes (0.80, 0.69 to 0.92). The dose-response relation for DHA and EPA on reduction indeaths fromcardiac causeswas not significant.

*Conclusions.*—Fish oil supplementation was associated with a significant reduction in deaths from cardiac causes but had no effect on arrhythmias or all cause mortality. Evidence to recommend an optimal formulation of EPA or DHA to reduce these outcomes is insufficient. Fish oils are a heterogeneous product, and the optimal formulations for DHA and EPA remain unclear (Figs 2 and 3).

▶ There has been considerable interest in the possibility that fish oils reduce deaths from cardiac causes and in particular sudden arrhythmic death. The

| Study and subcategory | Fish oil (No with event/No in group) | Placebo (No with event/No in group) | Weight (%) | Odds ratio (random) (95% CI) |
|---|---|---|---|---|
| **Implantable cardiac defibrillator intervention** | | | | |
| Leaf et al 2005[w3] | 44/200 | 66/202 | 33.86 | 0.58 (0.37 to 0.91) |
| Raitt et al 2005[w2] | 51/100 | 41/100 | 26.75 | 1.50 (0.86 to 2.62) |
| Brouwer et al 2006[w4] | 75/273 | 81/273 | 39.39 | 0.90 (0.62 to 1.30) |
| Total (95% CI) | 573 | 575 | 100.00 | 0.90 (0.55 to 1.46) |
| Total events: 170 (fish oil), 188 (placebo) | | | | |
| Test for heterogeneity: $\chi^2$=6.81, df=2, P=0.03, $I^2$=70.6% | | | | |
| Test for overall effect: z=0.43, P=0.67 | | | | |
| **Sudden cardiac death** | | | | |
| Singh et al 1997[w11] | 2/122 | 8/118 | 6.47 | 0.23 (0.05 to 1.10) |
| GISSI-Prevenzione 1999[w1] | 122/5666 | 164/5658 | 60.77 | 0.74 (0.58 to 0.93) |
| Nilsen et al 2001[w9] | 0/150 | 1/150 | 1.66 | 0.33 (0.01 to 8.19) |
| Leaf et al 2005[w3] | 3/200 | 1/202 | 3.24 | 3.06 (0.32 to 29.68) |
| Raitt et al 2005[w2] | 2/100 | 0/100 | 1.83 | 5.10 (0.24 to 107.62) |
| JELIS 2007[w5] | 18/9326 | 17/9319 | 26.02 | 1.06 (0.55 to 2.05) |
| Total (95% CI) | 15 564 | 15 547 | 100.00 | 0.81 (0.52 to 1.25) |
| Total events: 147 (fish oil), 191 (placebo) | | | | |
| Test for heterogeneity: $\chi^2$=6.45, df=5, P=0.26, $I^2$=22.5% | | | | |
| Test for overall effect: z=0.97, P=0.33 | | | | |

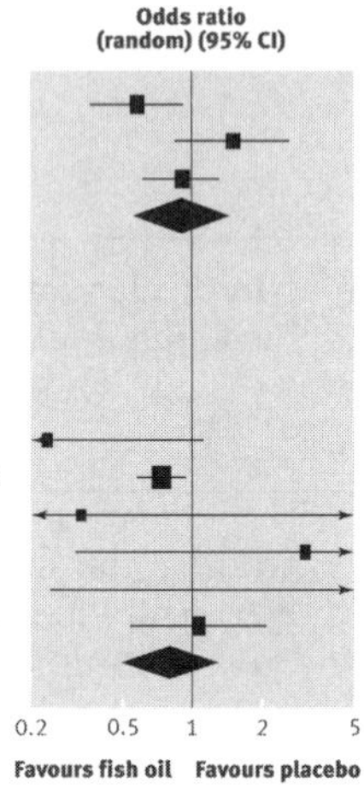


FIGURE 2.—Effect of fish oil on appropriate implantable cardiac defibrillator intervention and sudden cardiac death. (Reprinted from León H, Shibata MC, Sivakumaran S, et al. Effect of fish oil on arrhythmias and mortality: systematic review. *BMJ*. 2009;338:a2931. Reproduced with permission from the BMJ Publishing Group Ltd.)

| Study | Fish oil (No with event/No in group) | Placebo (No with event/No in group) | Weight (%) | Odds ratio (random) (95% CI) |
|---|---|---|---|---|
| Sacks et al 1995[w10] | 0/41 | 1/39 | 0.20 | 0.31 (0.01 to 7.82) |
| Singh et al 1997[w11] | 14/122 | 26/118 | 4.10 | 0.46 (0.23 to 0.93) |
| GISSI-Prevenzione 1999[w1] | 291/5666 | 348/5658 | 79.77 | 0.83 (0.70 to 0.97) |
| Johansen et al 1999[w8] | 1/250 | 3/250 | 0.40 | 0.33 (0.03 to 3.20) |
| Von Shacky et al 1999[w12] | 0/111 | 1/112 | 0.20 | 0.33 (0.01 to 8.27) |
| Durrington et al 2001[w7] | 0/30 | 1/29 | 0.20 | 0.31 (0.01 to 7.96) |
| Nilsen et al 2001[w9] | 8/150 | 8/150 | 2.02 | 1.00 (0.37 to 2.74) |
| Leaf et al 2005[w3] | 9/200 | 9/202 | 2.29 | 1.01 (0.39 to 2.60) |
| Raitt et al 2005[w2] | 2/100 | 5/100 | 0.74 | 0.39 (0.07 to 2.05) |
| Brouwer et al 2006[w4] | 6/273 | 13/273 | 2.12 | 0.45 (0.17 to 1.20) |
| JELIS 2007[w5] | 29/9326 | 31/9319 | 7.96 | 0.93 (0.56 to 1.55) |
| Total (95% CI) | 16 269 | 16 250 | 100.00 | 0.80 (0.69 to 0.92) |
| Total events: 360 (fish oil), 446 (placebo) | | | | |
| Test for heterogeneity: $\chi^2$=6.90, df=10, P=0.74, $I^2$=0% | | | | |
| Test for overall effect: z=3.08, P=0.002 | | | | |

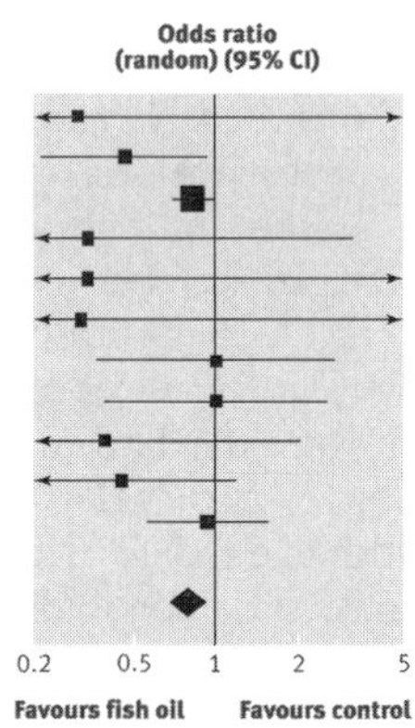


FIGURE 3.—Effect of fish oil on death from cardiac causes. (Reprinted from León H, Shibata MC, Sivakumaran S, et al. Effect of fish oil on arrhythmias and mortality: systematic review. *BMJ*. 2009;338:a2931. Reproduced with permission from the BMJ Publishing Group Ltd.)

evidence to support this comes from multiple sources, including epidemiologic studies of populations who consume large amounts of fish oil;[1] one large randomized trial in postinfarct patients,[2] plus some evidence that fish oil supplements may reduce the risk of restenosis after percutaneous transluminal coronary angioplasty (PTCA); and a number of experimental and mechanistic studies suggesting a variety of potentially beneficial cardioprotective effects.

These include cardiac myocyte membrane stabilization and an effect on ion channels, a favorable effect on the lipid profile, a reduction platelet aggregation, and prothrombotic effects.[3] There is also evidence that fish oils may favorably stabilize atherosclerotic plaques by multiple mechanisms that include anti-inflammatory properties, inhibition of lipoprotein lipase in the plaque, modification of matrix metalloproteinases and chemokines, and reduction of monocyte adhesion and migration—an important role in the process of atherogenesis.

This meta-analysis of 32 779 patients (92% of whom were enrolled in the 2 largest trials) provides some good and also some discouraging news. In regard to the latter, there is no apparent benefit on sudden cardiac death or implantable cardiac defibrillator (ICD) discharges, which perhaps is not surprising given the presence of a fixed arrhythmogenic substrate characterized by scar, ischemia, and a border zone in many patients with implanted devices. Nonetheless, the confidence intervals were wide and do not exclude an approximately 45% relative risk reduction. However, there was a significant (20%) reduction in cardiac deaths, due mainly to a reduction in deaths due to coronary events—could this be due to plaque stabilization?

Limitations of the analysis include marked heterogeneity between studies, a wide variability in the dose, and in the type of fish oil supplements that were used. Nonetheless, the overall benefit in death due to cardiac causes superimposed on a background of relatively minor adverse effects[4] does in my opinion favor continuation of fish oil supplements. The effects on arrhythmias are however inconclusive and warrant further study, and there was no obvious benefit on all cause mortality, although the upper confidence interval was 1.03, which suggests a trend.

**B. J. Gersh, MB, ChB, DPhil, FRCP**

*References*

1. Bang HO, Dyerberg J, Hjoome N. The composition of food consumed by Greenland Eskimos. *Acta Med Scand.* 1976;200:69-73.
2. Dietary supplementation with n-3 polyunsaturated fatty acids and vitamin E after myocardial infarction: results of the GISSI-Prevenzione trial. GISSI-Prevenzione Investigators Gruppo Italiano per lo Studio della Sopravvivenza nell'Infarto miocardico. *Lancet.* 1999;354:447-455.
3. Prichard BN, Smith CC, Ling KL, Betteridge DJ. Fish oils and cardiovascular disease [editorial]. *BMJ.* 1995;310:819-820.
4. Davidson MH, Stein EA, Bays HE, et al. COMBination of prescription Omega-3 with Simvastatin (COMBOS) Investigators. Efficacy and tolerability of adding prescription omega-3 fatty acids for 4 g/d to simvastatin 40 mg/d in hypertriglyceridemic patients: an 8-week, randomized, double-blind, placebo-controlled study. *Clin Ther.* 2007;28:1354-1367.

## On-Pump Versus Off-Pump Coronary-Artery Bypass Surgery

Shroyer AL, for the Veteras Affairs Randomized On/Off Bypass (ROOBY) Study Group (Northport Veterans Affairs (VA) Med Ctr, NY; et al)

*N Engl J Med* 361:1827-37, 2009

*Background.*—Coronary-artery bypass grafting (CABG) has traditionally been performed with the use of cardiopulmonary bypass (on-pump CABG). CABG without cardiopulmonary bypass (off-pump CABG) might reduce the number of complications related to the heart–lung machine.

*Methods.*—We randomly assigned 2203 patients scheduled for urgent or elective CABG to either on-pump or off-pump procedures. The primary short-term end point was a composite of death or complications (reoperation, new mechanical support, cardiac arrest, coma, stroke, or renal failure) before discharge or within 30 days after surgery. The primary long-term end point was a composite of death from any cause, a repeat revascularization procedure, or a nonfatal myocardial infarction within 1 year after surgery. Secondary end points included the completeness of revascularization, graft patency at 1 year, neuropsychological outcomes, and the use of major resources.

*Results.*—There was no significant difference between off-pump and on-pump CABG in the rate of the 30-day composite outcome (7.0% and 5.6%, respectively; $P = 0.19$). The rate of the 1-year composite outcome was higher for off-pump than for on-pump CABG (9.9% vs. 7.4%, $P = 0.04$). The proportion of patients with fewer grafts completed than originally planned was higher with off-pump CABG than with on-pump CABG (17.8% vs. 11.1%, $P < 0.001$). Follow-up angiograms in 1371 patients who underwent 4093 grafts revealed that the overall rate of graft patency was lower in the off-pump group than in the on-pump group (82.6% vs. 87.8%, $P < 0.01$). There were no treatment-based differences in neuropsychological outcomes or short-term use of major resources.

*Conclusions.*—At 1 year of follow-up, patients in the off-pump group had worse composite outcomes and poorer graft patency than did patients in the on-pump group. No significant differences between the techniques were found in neuropsychological outcomes or use of major resources. (ClinicalTrials.gov number, NCT00032630) (Table 2).

▶ This large and important trial from the Veterans Administration system in the United States is consistent with previous trials demonstrating no significant difference in regard to the early outcomes of death or complications from the performance of off-pump coronary artery bypass surgery (OPCAB) as opposed to conventional bypass surgery.[1,2] In this trial, however, 1-year composite outcomes, completeness of revascularization, and graft patency were significantly worse with OPCAB than with conventional Coronary-artery bypass grafting (CABG). Somewhat surprisingly, there were no significant difference in neurocognitive function. Since the individual surgeon's experience may be

TABLE 2.—Short-Term and Long-Term Primary End Points According to Treatment Group*

| Primary End Point | Off-Pump Group (N = 1104) *no. (%)* | On-Pump Group (N = 1099) *no. (%)* | Absolute Percentage-Point Difference (95% CI) | Relative Risk (95% CI) | P Value† |
|---|---|---|---|---|---|
| Short-term | | | | | |
| 30-Day composite‡ | 77 (7.0) | 61 (5.6) | 1.4 (−0.6 to 3.5) | 1.26 (0.91 to 1.74) | 0.19 |
| Death within 30 days after surgery or before discharge | 18 (1.6) | 13 (1.2) | 0.4 (−0.5 to 1.4) | 1.38 (0.68 to 2.80) | 0.47 |
| Complications within 30 days after surgery or before discharge | | | | | |
| Cardiac arrest | 20 (1.8) | 12 (1.1) | 0.7 (−0.3 to 1.7) | 1.66 (0.82 to 3.38) | 0.21 |
| Renal failure requiring dialysis | 9 (0.8) | 10 (0.9) | −0.1 (−0.9 to 0.7) | 0.90 (0.37 to 2.20) | 0.82 |
| Stroke | 14 (1.3) | 8 (0.7) | 0.5 (−0.3 to 1.4) | 1.75 (0.74 to 4.14) | 0.28 |
| Coma | 4 (0.4) | 3 (0.3) | 0.1 (−0.4 to 0.6) | 1.33 (0.30 to 5.93) | 1.00 |
| Repeat cardiac surgery | 8 (0.7) | 8 (0.7) | −0.0 (−0.7 to 0.7) | 1.00 (0.38 to 2.65) | 1.00 |
| Reoperation for bleeding | 30 (2.7) | 23 (2.1) | 0.6 (−0.7 to 1.9) | 1.30 (0.76 to 2.22) | 0.40 |
| New mechanical support | 17 (1.5) | 9 (0.8) | 0.7 (−0.2 to 1.6) | 1.88 (0.84 to 4.21) | 0.17 |
| Mediastinitis | 11 (1.0) | 14 (1.3) | −0.3 (−1.1 to 0.6) | 0.78 (0.36 to 1.72) | 0.55 |
| Tracheostomy | 5 (0.5) | 7 (0.6) | −0.2 (−0.8 to 0.4) | 0.71 (0.23 to 2.24) | 0.58 |
| Long-term | | | | | |
| 1-Yr composite§ | 105 (9.9) | 78 (7.4) | 2.5 (0.1 to 4.9) | 1.33 (1.01 to 1.76) | 0.04 |
| 1-Yr composite with death from cardiac causes rather than from any cause | 93 (8.8) | 62 (5.9) | 2.9 (0.6 to 5.1) | 1.48 (1.09 to 2.02) | 0.01 |
| 1-Yr composite with all end points from time of CABG | 155 (14.6) | 104 (9.9) | 4.7 (1.9 to 7.5) | 1.47 (1.17 to 1.86) | 0.001 |
| Nonfatal myocardial infarction between 30 days and 1 yr after surgery | 21 (2.0) | 23 (2.2) | −0.2 (−1.4 to 1.0) | 0.90 (0.50 to 1.62) | 0.76 |
| Revascularization between 30 days and 1 yr after surgery | 49 (4.6) | 36 (3.4) | 1.2 (−0.5 to 2.9) | 1.35 (0.88 to 2.05) | 0.18 |
| Death from any cause within 1 yr | 43 (4.1) | 30 (2.9) | 1.2 (−0.4 to 2.8) | 1.41 (0.90 to 2.24) | 0.15 |
| Death from cardiac causes within 1 yr | 29 (2.7) | 14 (1.3) | 1.4 (0.2 to 2.6) | 2.05 (1.09 to 3.86) | 0.03 |

*CABG denotes coronary-artery bypass grafting, and CI confidence interval. There were 1061 patients in the off-pump group and 1050 in the on-pump group for analyses of all long-term end points except death.

†P values are based on statistical-test comparisons with missing data excluded.

‡The primary short-term composite end point was death, reoperation, new mechanical support, cardiac arrest, coma, stroke, or renal failure requiring dialysis before discharge or within 30 days after surgery.

§The primary long-term composite end point was death from any cause within 1 year after surgery, nonfatal myocardial infarction between 30 days and 1 year, and any revascularization procedure between 30 days and 1 year.

a factor, it is important to note that a sensitivity analysis based on greater than 50 or less pre-study cases showed no significant difference in outcome.

Whether these results can be explained on the basis of less complete revascularization in the OPCAB group is uncertain, and it should be emphasized that there is still no consensus on the benefit of CR versus IR in the presence of a patent graft to the left anterior descending coronary artery. Nonetheless, completeness of revascularization may be a factor in certain patient subsets.

An accompanying editorial points out that the technical experience of these study surgeons may have been limited.[3] Nonetheless, it should be acknowledged that the number of grafts successfully placed in the OPCAB group as well as 1-year graft patency rates and rates of peri-procedural complications were consistent with those reported in the literature.

Enthusiasm for the OPCAB has waned over the last years and has now plateaued, although there is wide spread variability in utilization rates. Despite this important trial, the debate is likely to continue because the major benefactors of the OPCAB may be women, the elderly, and patients with comorbidities – the very patients who are underrepresented in all of these trials.

**B. J. Gersh, MB, ChB, DPhil, FRCP**

*References*


1. van Dijk D, Diephuis JC, Nierich AP, Keizer AM, Kalkman CJ. Beating heart versus conventional cardiopulmonary bypass: the Octopus experience: a randomized comparison of 281 patients undergoing coronary artery bypass surgery with or without cardiopulmonary bypass. *Semin Cardiothorac Vasc Anesth.* 2006;10: 167-170.
2. Widimsky P, Straka Z, Stros P, et al. One-year coronary bypass graft patency: a randomized comparison between off-pump and on-pump surgery angiographic results of the PRAGUE-4 trial. *Circulation.* 2004;110:3418-3423.
3. Peterson ED. Innovation and comparative-effectiveness research in cardiac surgery. *N Eng J Med.* 2009;361:8097-8099.


## Safety of Short-Term Discontinuation of Antiplatelet Therapy in Patients With Drug-Eluting Stents

Eisenberg MJ, Richard PR, Libersan D, et al (Jewish General Hosp/McGill Univ, Montreal, Quebec, Canada)

*Circulation* 119:1634-1642, 2009

*Background.*—Antiplatelet therapy is often discontinued in patients with drug-eluting stents who are undergoing surgical procedures. However, discontinuation of antiplatelet therapy is an important risk factor for late stent thrombosis. Our objective was to examine the safety of short-term discontinuation of antiplatelet therapy.

*Methods and Results.*—We systematically searched Medline for reported cases of late stent thrombosis and very late stent thrombosis published between January 2001 and July 2008. We restricted our search to Academic Research Consortium–defined definite cases. We identified 161 cases of late stent thrombosis or very late stent thrombosis from 84 articles (79 from case reports, 61 from registries, and 21 from randomized clinical trials). Patients had a mean age of 58.4 ± 13.4 years, and 88% were male. A total of 19 cases occurred in patients who were receiving dual antiplatelet therapy at the time of the event. If patients stopped both antiplatelet agents simultaneously, the median time to event was 7 days. If patients had previously stopped a thienopyridine with no ill effect and subsequently stopped acetylsalicylic acid, the median time to event was also 7 days from the time of acetylsalicylic acid cessation. If the thienopyridine was stopped but acetylsalicylic acid was maintained, the median time to event was 122 days. Among the 48 patients who stopped both agents, 36 cases (75%) occurred within 10 days. Among the 94 patients who discontinued a thienopyridine but continued acetylsalicylic acid, only 6 cases (6%) occurred within 10 days.

*Conclusion.*—If acetylsalicylic acid therapy is maintained, short-term discontinuation of a thienopyridine may be relatively safe in patients with drug-eluting stents.

▶ This is a highly topical and controversial area. Late and very late stent thrombosis in patients with drug-eluting stents (DES), and for that matter bare-metal stents is an infrequent or rare event, but its consequences are often catastrophic. An association with the discontinuation of antiplatelet therapy has been well demonstrated, leading to the recommendation that antiplatelet therapy be continued for at least 12 months.[1] These recommendations are reasonable with the caveat that definitive data are not available. Nonetheless, an increasingly common clinical scenario is the patient with DES in whom a surgical procedure requiring discontinuation of antiplatelet therapy is planned. The risk associated with the short-term discontinuation of antiplatelet therapy remains highly controversial.[2]

This modified, case-only design study is probably the most comprehensive study to date, and provides some guidance and reassurance in an area in which randomized trial data are absent. The choice of study design merits some discussion, and the authors do address this in detail, and despite the lack of control subjects, this design appears to be feasible in regard to addressing an important question. Of the 161 cases of late or very late stent thrombosis that were identified, only 19 occurred in patients receiving dual antiplatelet therapy. The shortest time to an event was in patients stopping both agents simultaneously or in patients in whom the thienopyridine was stopped with no ill effects but subsequently aspirin was discontinued. Among patients who discontinued thienopyridine but remained on aspirin, only 6% of cases occurred within 10 days. It is therefore somewhat reassuring to note the discontinuation of thienopyridine in patients with DES may be relatively safe in the short-term, providing patients continue taking aspirin. This may be helpful in guiding the decision to operate in patients with a high risk of bleeding in which the risk of benefit ratio of discontinuing the thienopyridine may be outweighed by the risk of bleeding. What this study does not answer is the optimal duration of dual antiplatelet therapy and whether these drugs should be used indefinitely. Unfortunately, long-term results from various trials and cohort studies suggest that the risk of late stent thrombosis does not necessarily decline over time. An ongoing trial will hopefully address this particular issue.

Previous studies have identified a number of risk factors associated with late stent thrombosis including inadequate stent expansion and deployment, the presence of bifurcation lesions, reduced ejection fraction, and persistent platelet reactivity while on antiplatelet therapy. Nonetheless, it appears that the cessation of antiplatelet therapy is by far the most significant risk factor and the apparent benefit of maintaining aspirin in this context is consistent with the concept of rebound platelet activation.

**B. J. Gersh, MB, ChB, DPhil, FRCP**

*References*

1. King SB III, Smith SC Jr, Hirshfeld JW Jr, et al. 2007 Focused update of the ACC/AHA/SCAI 2005 guideline update for percutaneous coronary intervention: a report of the American College of Cardiology/American Heart Association Task Force on Practice Guidelines. *J Am Coll Cardiol*. 2008;51:172-209.
2. Jaffe R, Strauss BH. Late and very late thrombosis of drug-eluting stents: evolving concepts and perspectives. *J Am Coll Cardiol*. 2007;50:119-127.

---

## Routine Early Angioplasty after Fibrinolysis for Acute Myocardial Infarction

Cantor WJ, for the TRANSFER-AMI Trial Investigators (Univ of Toronto, Ontario; et al)

*N Engl J Med* 360:2705-2718, 2009

---

*Background.*—Patients with a myocardial infarction with ST-segment elevation who present to hospitals that do not have the capability of performing percutaneous coronary intervention (PCI) often cannot undergo timely primary PCI and therefore receive fibrinolysis. The role and optimal timing of routine PCI after fibrinolysis have not been established.

*Methods.*—We randomly assigned 1059 high-risk patients who had a myocardial infarction with ST-segment elevation and who were receiving fibrinolytic therapy at centers that did not have the capability of performing PCI to either standard treatment (including rescue PCI, if required, or delayed angiography) or a strategy of immediate transfer to another hospital and PCI within 6 hours after fibrinolysis. All patients received aspirin, tenecteplase, and heparin or enoxaparin; concomitant clopidogrel was recommended. The primary end point was the composite of death, reinfarction, recurrent ischemia, new or worsening congestive heart failure, or cardiogenic shock within 30 days.

*Results.*—Cardiac catheterization was performed in 88.7% of the patients assigned to standard treatment a median of 32.5 hours after randomization and in 98.5% of the patients assigned to routine early PCI a median of 2.8 hours after randomization. At 30 days, the primary end point occurred in 11.0% of the patients who were assigned to routine early PCI and in 17.2% of the patients assigned to standard treatment (relative risk with early PCI, 0.64; 95% confidence interval, 0.47 to 0.87; $P = 0.004$). There were no significant differences between the groups in the incidence of major bleeding.

*Conclusions.*—Among high-risk patients who had a myocardial infarction with ST-segment elevation and who were treated with fibrinolysis, transfer for PCI within 6 hours after fibrinolysis was associated with significantly fewer ischemic complications than was standard treatment. (ClinicalTrials.gov number, NCT00164190.)

▶ Fibrinolytic drugs have undoubtedly revolutionized the management of acute myocardial infarction. Nonetheless, in addition to the risk of bleeding, pharmacologic reperfusion is suboptimal in 45% to 50% of patients, and the risk of reocclusion is high. Although primary percutaneous coronary intervention (PPCI) is the best form of reperfusion therapy, a limiting factor is the time it takes to transport patients, particularly in rural areas, to hospitals with PPCI capabilities.

In an attempt to combine the best of both therapies, the combination of lytic therapy followed by routine PCI has been the subject of multiple trials. Initial trials in the late 1980s demonstrated a lack of benefit, but this was attributed to the use of outdated fibrinolytic and antithrombotic regimens in addition to obsolete PCI strategies, including the nonuse of stents.[1]

Nonetheless, subsequent trials which took place in the current era of routine emergency PCI after lytics ("facilitated PCI") were also neutral with a trend towards harm in some trials. This was attributed to bleeding and perhaps the disadvantages of balloon angioplasty and stenting in a vessel, which is the site of the "thrombolytic milieu," which could perhaps lead to complications such as intraplaque hemorrhage.

Other trials, including the Trial of Routine Angioplasty and Stenting after Fibrinolysis to Enhance Reperfusion in Acute Myocardial Infarction (TRANSFER-AMI) trial, have evaluated the role of routine PCI after a longer interval between the administration of lytic drugs and PCI. This not only reduces the risk of bleeding, but enables a strategy of transferring patients from centers without catheterization facilities—the pharmacoinvasive approach. The accompanying editorial addresses the efficacy of this strategy both in this and in the other 4 smaller trials.[2] The intervals between lytic drugs and PCI in these trials range from 2 to 17 hours, and I agree with the editorialist that the former interval should be considered to be the shortest that is acceptable, but PCI should be performed within 24 hours, given the risks of reocclusion.[3] It would appear, therefore, that in areas with the logistical capabilities for prompt transfer, if initial reperfusion therapy consists of fibrinolytic drugs, this should be followed by an invasive approach on a routine basis within 3 to 24 hours and as an emergency "rescue procedure" in those in whom it is felt that fibrinolytic drugs have failed to achieve complete reperfusion.

**B. J. Gersh, MB, ChB, DPhil, FRCP**

*References*

1. Keeley EC, Boura JA, Grines CL. Comparison of primary and facilitated percutaneous coronary interventions for ST-elevation myocardial infarction: quantitative review of randomised trials. *Lancet.* 2006;367:579-588.
2. Verheugt FWA. Routine angioplasty after fibrinolysis – how early should "early" be? *N Engl J Med.* 2009;360:2779-2781.
3. Verheugt FWA, Meijer A, Lagrand WK, et al. Reocclusion: the flip side of coronary thrombolysis. *JACC.* 1996;27:766-773.

**Coronary artery bypass surgery compared with percutaneous coronary interventions for multivessel disease: a collaborative analysis of individual patient data from ten randomised trials**

Hlatky MA, Boothroyd DB, Bravata DM, et al (Stanford Univ School of Medicine, CA; et al)

*Lancet* 373:1190-1197, 2009

*Background.*—Coronary artery bypass graft (CABG) and percutaneous coronary intervention (PCI) are alternative treatments for multivessel coronary disease. Although the procedures have been compared in several randomised trials, their long-term effects on mortality in key clinical subgroups are uncertain. We undertook a collaborative analysis of data from randomised trials to assess whether the effects of the procedures on mortality are modified by patient characteristics.

*Methods.*—We pooled individual patient data from ten randomised trials to compare the effectiveness of CABG with PCI according to patients' baseline clinical characteristics. We used stratified, random effects Cox proportional hazards models to test the effect on all-cause mortality of randomised treatment assignment and its interaction with clinical characteristics. All analyses were by intention to treat.

*Findings.*—Ten participating trials provided data on 7812 patients. PCI was done with balloon angioplasty in six trials and with bare-metal stents in four trials. Over a median follow-up of 5·9 years (IQR 5·0–10·0), 575 (15%) of 3889 patients assigned to CABG died compared with 628 (16%) of 3923 patients assigned to PCI (hazard ratio [HR] 0·91, 95% CI 0·82–1·02; p=0·12). In patients with diabetes (CABG, n=615; PCI, n=618), mortality was substantially lower in the CABG group than in the PCI group (HR 0·70, 0·56–0·87); however, mortality was similar between groups in patients without diabetes (HR 0·98, 0·86–1·12; p=0·014 for interaction). Patient age modified the effect of treatment on mortality, with hazard ratios of 1·25 (0·94–1·66) in patients younger than 55 years, 0·90 (0·75–1·09) in patients aged 55–64 years, and 0·82 (0·70–0·97) in patients 65 years and older (p=0·002 for interaction). Treatment effect was not modified by the number of diseased vessels or other baseline characteristics.

*Interpretation.*—Long-term mortality is similar after CABG and PCI in most patient subgroups with multivesselcoronary artery disease, so choice of treatment should depend on patient preferences for other outcomes. CABG might be a better option for patients with diabetes and patients aged 65 years or older because we found mortality to be lower in these subgroups (Figs 3A and 4).

▶ This is a topic that has been subjected to multiple analyses, but this particular meta-analysis is perhaps the most comprehensive, although I suspect it does not tell us much more than we already know. Nonetheless, the methodology is sound, and the interactions with age and diabetes are interesting, in that

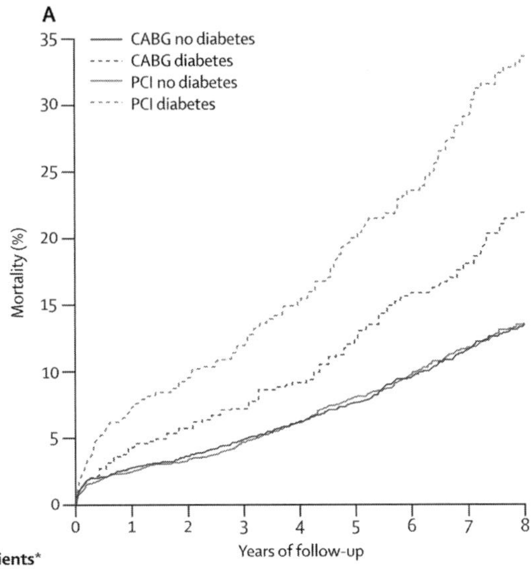


| **Number of patients*** | | | | | | | | | |
|---|---|---|---|---|---|---|---|---|---|
| CABG no diabetes | 3263 | 3169 | 3089 | 2877 | 2677 | 2267 | 1592 | 1380 | 1274 |
| CABG diabetes | 615 | 587 | 575 | 532 | 498 | 421 | 257 | 225 | 200 |
| PCI no diabetes | 3298 | 3217 | 3148 | 2918 | 2725 | 2281 | 1608 | 1393 | 1288 |
| PCI diabetes | 618 | 574 | 555 | 508 | 475 | 373 | 218 | 179 | 160 |

FIGURE 3.—Mortality in patients assigned to coronary artery bypass graft or percutaneous coronary intervention by diabetes status. CABG=coronary artery bypass graft. PCI=percutaneous coronary intervention. *Number of patients available for follow-up. Data show overall unadjusted mortality rates for patients with diabetes and without diabetes. Panel A includes patients from all ten trials. (Reprinted from Hlatky MA, Boothroyd DB, Bravata DM, et al. Coronary artery bypass surgery compared with percutaneous coronary interventions for multivessel disease: a collaborative analysis of individual patient data from ten randomised trials. *Lancet.* 2009;373:1190-1197, with permission from Elsevier.)

coronary bypass surgery appears superior to percutaneous coronary intervention (PCI) in older patients and diabetics.

It needs to be emphasized that trials of revascularization are subject to entry bias in that patients included are a selected subgroup undergoing revascularization who are considered equally amenable to both forms of therapy.[1] Registry studies, however, are more generalizable to clinical practice at large, but conversely are subject to selection bias.

In this respect the patients entered into the trials comprising this meta-analysis had predominantly double-vessel disease (approximately two-thirds), only 50% approximately had involvement of the proximal left anterior descending coronary artery, abnormal left ventricular function was present in only 16% to 18% and congestive heart failure in 2% to 4%—this is not representative of most patients undergoing bypass surgery in current practice.

The other limitation of this meta-analysis is the use of percutaneous transluminal coronary angioplasty (PTCA) alone (plain old balloon angioplasty) in 6 of the trials and bare metal stents in 4 trials. The recent SYNTAX trial was not included, but inclusion would not have altered the conclusions regarding primary outcomes since at 1 year there was no difference in death and

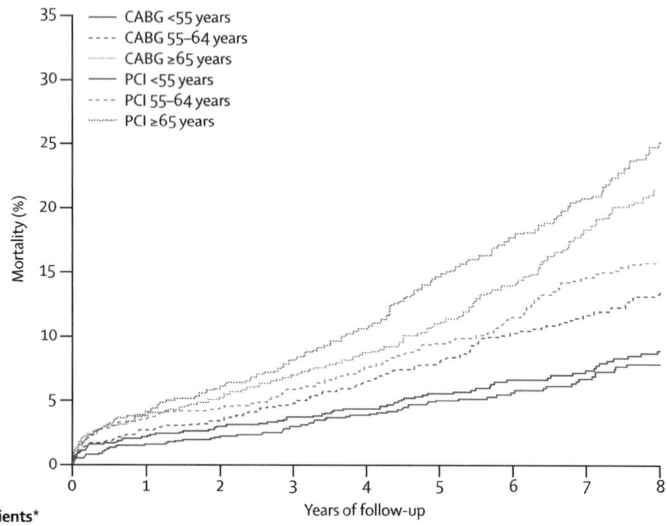


| Number of patients* | 0 | 1 | 2 | 3 | 4 | 5 | 6 | 7 | 8 |
|---|---|---|---|---|---|---|---|---|---|
| CABG <55 years | 1063 | 1039 | 1016 | 938 | 891 | 774 | 556 | 507 | 468 |
| CABG 55–64 years | 1477 | 1434 | 1400 | 1308 | 1206 | 1017 | 711 | 634 | 585 |
| CABG ≥65 years | 1347 | 1292 | 1257 | 1167 | 1082 | 902 | 586 | 468 | 424 |
| PCI <55 years | 1122 | 1104 | 1087 | 1013 | 955 | 817 | 561 | 500 | 466 |
| PCI 55–64 years | 1456 | 1404 | 1371 | 1262 | 1177 | 989 | 705 | 614 | 578 |
| PCI ≥65 years | 1341 | 1286 | 1247 | 1154 | 1072 | 852 | 562 | 462 | 408 |

FIGURE 4.—Mortality in patients assigned to coronary artery bypass graft or percutaneous coronary intervention by age. CABG=coronary artery bypass graft. PCI=percutaneous coronary intervention. *Number of patients available for follow-up. Data show overall unadjusted mortality rates for patients aged less than 55 years, 55–64 years, and 65 years or older. (Reprinted from Hlatky MA, Boothroyd DB, Bravata DM, et al. Coronary artery bypass surgery compared with percutaneous coronary interventions for multivessel disease: a collaborative analysis of individual patient data from ten randomised trials. *Lancet.* 2009;373:1190-1197, with permission from Elsevier.)

myocardial infarction in that trial, and the 5-year follow-up is ongoing.[2] In regard to diabetes, we need to await the results of the ongoing FREEDOM trial, which will not be available for several years.

The decision for coronary artery bypass graft (CABG) or percutaneous coronary intervention (PCI) needs to be individualized, and factors to be taken into account are the coronary anatomy including the diffuseness of disease and the technical suitability for PCI versus CABG, left ventricular function, patient's age, expectations, and comorbidities. Patient preference will certainly play a role in the decision, and in many cases the cardiac surgeon should be part of the decision-making process. The first decision, however, is whether revascularization is necessary in the first place as opposed to a trial of medical therapy. Irrespective of which procedure is chosen, aggressive secondary prevention is a crucial aspect of management.

**B. J. Gersh, MB, ChB, DPhil, FRCP**

*References*


1. Brown ML, Gersh BJ, Holmes DR, Bailey KR, Sundt TM 3rd. From randomized trials to registry studies: translating data into clinical information. *Nat Clin Pract Cardiovasc Med.* 2008;10:613-620.
2. Serruys PW, Morice MC, Kappetein AP, et al. Percutaneous coronary intervention versus coronary artery bypass grafting for severe coronary artery disease. *N Engl J Med.* 2009;360:961-972.


**Cardiovascular Effect of Bans on Smoking in Public Places: A Systematic Review and Meta-Analysis**

Meyers DG, Neuberger JS, He J (Univ of Kansas School of Medicine)

*J Am Coll Cardiol* 54:1249-1255, 2009


*Objectives.*—A systematic review and a meta-analysis were performed to determine the association between public smoking bans and risk for hospital admission for acute myocardial infarction (AMI).

*Background.*—Secondhand smoke (SHS) is associated with a 30% increase in risk of AMI, which might be reduced by prohibiting smoking in work and public places.

*Methods.*—PubMed, EMBASE, and Google Scholar databases plus bibliographies of relevant studies and reviews were searched for peer-reviewed original articles published from January 1, 2004, through April 30, 2009, using the search terms "smoking ban" and "heart" or "myocardial infarct." Investigators supplied additional data. All published peer-reviewed original studies identified were included. Incidence rates of AMI per 100,000 person-years before and after implementation of the smoking bans and incidence rate ratios (IRRs) with 95% confidence intervals (CIs) were calculated. Random effects meta-analyses estimated the overall effect of the smoking bans. Funnel plot and meta-regression assessed heterogeneity among studies.

*Results.*—Using 11 reports from 10 study locations, AMI risk decreased by 17% overall (IRR: 0.83, 95% CI: 0.75 to 0.92), with the greatest effect among younger individuals and nonsmokers. The IRR incrementally decreased 26% for each year of observation after ban implementation.

*Conclusions.*—Smoking bans in public places and workplaces are significantly associated with a reduction in AMI incidence, particularly if enforced over several years (Fig 1).


▶ The risk of acute coronary syndromes (ACSs) from secondhand smoke (SHS) to nonsmokers is well established,[1,2] as is the the physiologic basis for this increased risk, in that SHS enhances platelet activation, endothelial dysfunction, increases arterial stiffness, decreases high-density lipoproteins, increases markers of inflammation, increases intimal-media thickening, increases infarct size, causes mitochondrial damage and oxidative stress, decreases heart rate variability, thus increasing the risk of malignant

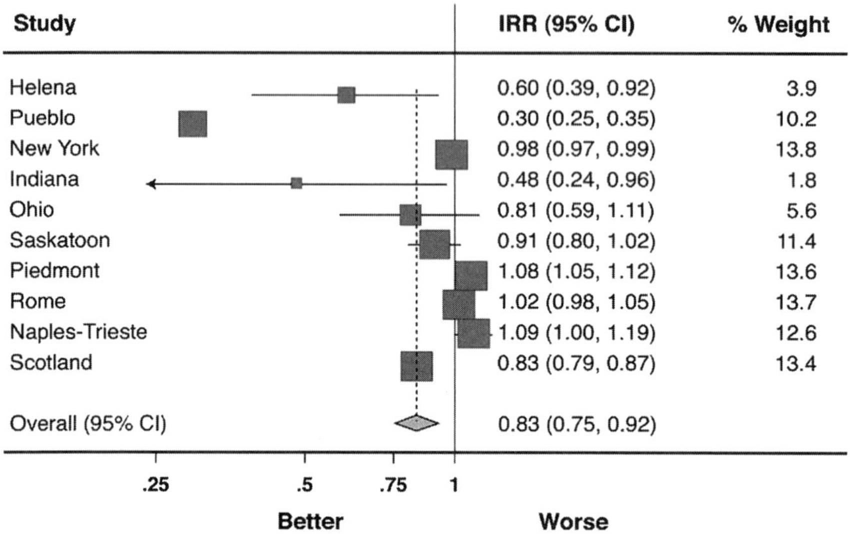


FIGURE 1.—Effects of Community Smoking Bans on Incident Acute Myocardial Infarction (Person-Year Approach). Meta-analysis results for 11 studies in 10 geographic locations. CI = confidence interval; IRR = incidence rate ratio (incidence rate after/before the ban on SHS). (Reprinted from Cardiovascular effect of bans on smoking in public places: a systematic review and meta-analysis. *J Am Coll Cardiol.* 2009;54:1249-1255, with permission from the American College of Cardiology Foundation.)

arrhythmias, and increases insulin resistance.[2] There have been at least 8 published studies demonstrating the effect of smoke-free policies on hospital admission rates for acute myocardial infarction (AMI)[3] since the first drop in rates reported by Sargent et al in 2004 in a relatively small study from Helena, Montana.[4] Stanton Glantz reported a meta-analysis of these 8 studies in 2008.[3] The present study is that of a meta-analysis of 11 studies, including the previous 8 studies, but this time using incidence rates (new cases/100 000 person-years). This type of analysis takes into account the population size as well as the duration of observation, and also allows comparison of the incidence rates between areas where smoke-free laws were in place with control areas without smoke-free laws. There is also the comparison of incidence rates before and after these laws were in place. In the Helena, Montana study, comparison of the incidence rates in the same place with and after the suspension of these smoke-free laws showed a return to pre-ban rates. Although in most of these studies the duration of the smoke-free period is short, all of these studies are consistent with a decrease in the incidence rate of hospital admissions for AMI overall by 17%. Further, the longer the duration of the ban on smoking in public spaces, the greater the drop in incidence rate of AMI. Since the smoking ban was for 1 year or less in many studies, it is probable that the effect on AMI incidence of a longer duration in smoke-free environment will be greater. The problem of assigning cause for the drop in incidence rates of AMI to banning SHS is difficult because in those areas where smoke-free laws were passed, there is frequently also a drop in cigarette use.[5] Also, where the percent of population who are smokers is greatest, the effect of SHS on AMI incidence will be less evident. The effect of creating a smoke-free environment on the incidence rate of AMI will be most powerful in the nonsmoking population.

**M. D. Cheitlin, MD**

*References*

1. He J, Vupputuri S, Allen K, Prerost MR, Hughes J, Whelton PK. Passive smoking and the risk of coronary heart disease—a meta-analysis of epidemiologic studies. *N Engl J Med.* 1999;340:920-926.
2. Barnoya J, Glantz SA. Cardiovascular effects of secondhand smoke: nearly as large as smoking. *Circulation.* 2005;111:2684-2689.
3. Glantz SA. Meta-analysis of the effects of smoke-free laws on acute myocardial infarction: an update. *Prev Med.* 2008;47:452.
4. Sargent RP, Shepard RM, Glantz SA. Reduced incidence of admissions for myocardial infarction associated with public smoking ban: before and after study. *BMJ.* 2004;328:977-980.
5. Gallus S, Zuccare P, Colombo P, et al. Smoking in Italy 2005–2006: effects of a comprehensive national tobacco regulation. *Prev Med.* 2007;45:198-201.

## Adherence to Healthy Lifestyle Habits in US Adults, 1988-2006

King DE, Mainous AG III, Carnemolla M, et al (Med Univ of South Carolina, Charleston)
*Am J Med* 122:528-534, 2009

*Background.*—Lifestyle choices are associated with cardiovascular disease and mortality. The purpose of this study was to compare adherence to healthy lifestyle habits in adults between 1988 and 2006.

*Methods.*—Analysis of adherence to 5 healthy lifestyle trends ($\geq$5 fruits and vegetables/day, regular exercise >12 times/month, maintaining healthy weight [body mass index 18.5-29.9 kg/m$^2$], moderate alcohol consumption [up to 1 drink/day for women, 2/day for men] and not smoking) in the National Health and Nutrition Examination Survey 1988-1994 were compared with results from the National Health and Nutrition Examination Survey 2001-2006 among adults aged 40-74 years.

*Results.*—Over the last 18 years, the percent of adults aged 40-74 years with a body mass index $\geq$30 kg/m$^2$ has increased from 28% to 36% ($P < .05$); physical activity 12 times a month or more has decreased from 53% to 43% ($P < .05$); smoking rates have not changed (26.9% to 26.1%); eating 5 or more fruits and vegetables a day has decreased from 42% to 26% ($P < .05$), and moderate alcohol use has increased from 40% to 51% ($P < .05$). Adherence to all 5 healthy habits has gone from 15% to 8% ($P < .05$). Although adherence to a healthy lifestyle was lower among minorities, adherence decreased more among non-Hispanic Whites over the period. Individuals with a history of

TABLE 1.—Characteristics of Adult Men and Women Ages 40-74 Years

| | NHANES III | | | | NHANES 2001-2006 | | | |
|---|---|---|---|---|---|---|---|---|
| | Men | Women | Totals | $\chi^2$ *P*-Value* | Men | Women | Totals | $\chi^2$ *P*-Value* |
| BMI (kg/m$^2$) (%) | | | | <.01 | | | | .02 |
| <30 | 74.8 | 70.2 | 72.4 | | 66.2 | 61.8 | 64.0 | |
| ≥30 | 25.2 | 29.8 | 27.6 | | 33.8 | 38.2 | 36.0 | |
| Physical activity (%) | | | | <.01 | | | | .02 |
| None | 10.5 | 19.5 | 15.2 | | 34.0 | 38.1 | 36.1 | |
| 1-12 times/month | 32.5 | 31.5 | 31.9 | | 22.7 | 18.6 | 20.6 | |
| >12 times/month | 57.0 | 49.0 | 52.8 | | 43.3 | 43.2 | 43.3 | |
| Smoking (%) | | | | <.01 | | | | <.01 |
| Yes | 32.3 | 22.0 | 26.9 | | 31.0 | 21.1 | 26.0 | |
| No | 67.7 | 78.0 | 73.1 | | 69.0 | 78.9 | 74.0 | |
| Fruit/Veg (%) | | | | <.01 | | | | .44 |
| <5 servings/day | 54.8 | 61.0 | 58.0 | | 73.5 | 75.2 | 74.4 | |
| ≥5 servings/day | 45.2 | 39.0 | 42.0 | | 26.4 | 24.8 | 25.6 | |
| Alcohol (%) | | | | <.01 | | | | <.01 |
| None | 40.0 | 61.9 | 51.5 | | 32.6 | 47.4 | 40.1 | |
| Moderate | 49.8 | 31.5 | 40.2 | | 57.2 | 45.9 | 51.5 | |
| Exceeds moderate | 10.2 | 6.6 | 8.3 | | 10.1 | 6.7 | 8.4 | |
| Healthy habits (%) | | | | .16 | | | | .09 |
| None | 0.4 | 0.2 | 0.3 | | 0.9 | 0.3 | 0.6 | |
| One | 4.0 | 4.1 | 4.0 | | 8.2 | 6.0 | 7.1 | |
| Two | 19.2 | 19.7 | 19.4 | | 26.9 | 27.4 | 27.1 | |
| Three | 29.2 | 32.4 | 30.9 | | 31.4 | 32.6 | 32.0 | |
| Four | 31.4 | 28.9 | 30.1 | | 24.5 | 24.8 | 24.6 | |
| Five | 15.8 | 14.6 | 15.2 | | 8.2 | 8.8 | 8.5 | |

NHANES = National Health and Nutrition Examination Survey; BMI = body mass index.
*Males vs females.

hypertension/diabetes/cardiovascular disease were no more likely to be adherent to a healthy lifestyle than people without these conditions.

*Conclusions.*—Generally, adherence to a healthy lifestyle pattern has decreased during the last 18 years, with decreases documented in 3 of 5 healthy lifestyle habits. These findings have broad implications for the future risk of cardiovascular disease in adults (Table 1).

▶ This makes for interesting but depressing reading. Numerous studies have suggested that approximately 45% to 72% of the decline in mortality from cardiovascular disease in the United States and other high-income countries are attributable to a reduction in the traditional risk factors.[1] The association between a healthy lifestyle, which combines a prudent diet, regular physical activity, maintaining a healthy weight, moderate alcohol consumption, and not smoking and a decreased risk of cardiovascular disease is strong and independent.[2] Moreover, recent studies have demonstrated that a switch to a healthy lifestyle even after the age of 45 years can substantially reduce cardiovascular events within a short space of time of only 4 years.[3] Unfortunately, it would appear that these lifestyle modifications are followed by only a small population of adults, at least in the United States.

This analysis of the NHANES (National Health and Nutrition Examination Survey) in 1988 to 1994 and again in 2001 to 2008 is discouraging. Over the 18-year period, obesity had increased, regular physical activity and the regular consumption of fruits and vegetables had decreased, and the overall adherence to all 5 healthy habits had declined from 15% to 8% ($P < .05$). In other words, it had declined from bad to worse. Moreover, the results were similar in patients with preexisting diseases such as hypertension, diabetes, and hypercholesterolemia.

This study has important implications for public health and raises the possibility that the steady decline in cardiovascular mortality over the last 40 years could flatten out or even trend upward.[4] Solutions are not that easy, but it is obvious that the emphasis upon lifestyle modification in the current system of health care in the United States is inadequate. New approaches to increase motivation are needed, and the benefits for the individual and the public good are self-evident.

**B. J. Gersh, MB, ChB, DPhil, FRCP**

*References*

1. Ford ES, Ajani UA, Croft JB, et al. Explaining the decrease in US deaths from coronary disease, 1980-2000. *N Engl J Med.* 2007;356:2388-2398.
2. Stampfer MJ, Hu FB, Manson JE, Rimm EB, Willett WC. Primary prevention of coronary heart disease in women through diet and lifestyle. *N Engl J Med.* 2000;343:16-22.
3. King DE, Mainous AG III, Geesey M. Turning back the clock: adopting a healthy lifestyle in middle-age. *Am J Med.* 2007;120:598-603.
4. Ford ES, Capewell S. Coronary heart disease mortality among young adults in the US from 1980 through 2002, concealed leveling of mortality rates. *J Am Coll Cardiol.* 2007;50:2128-2132.

---

## Cardiac Outcomes After Screening for Asymptomatic Coronary Artery Disease in Patients With Type 2 Diabetes The DIAD Study: A Randomized Controlled Trial

Young LH, for the DIAD Investigators (Yale Univ School of Medicine, New Haven, CT; et al)

*JAMA* 301:1547-1555, 2009

---

*Context.*—Coronary artery disease (CAD) is the major cause of mortality and morbidity in patients with type 2 diabetes. But the utility of screening patients with type 2 diabetes for asymptomatic CAD is controversial.

*Objective.*—To assess whether routine screening for CAD identifies patients with type 2 diabetes as being at high cardiac risk and whether it affects their cardiac outcomes.

*Design, Setting, and Patients.*—The Detection of Ischemia in Asymptomatic Diabetics (DIAD) study is a randomized controlled trial in which 1123 participants with type 2 diabetes and no symptoms of CAD were randomly assigned to be screened with adenosine-stress radionuclide myocardial perfusion imaging (MPI) or not to be screened. Participants were recruited from diabetes clinics and practices and prospectively followed up from August 2000 to September 2007.

*Main Outcome Measure.*—Cardiac death or nonfatal myocardial infarction (MI).

*Results.*—The cumulative cardiac event rate was 2.9% over a mean (SD) follow-up of 4.8 (0.9) years for an average of 0.6% per year. Seven nonfatal MIs and 8 cardiac deaths (2.7%) occurred among the screened group and 10 nonfatal MIs and 7 cardiac deaths (3.0%) among the not-screened group (hazard ratio [HR], 0.88; 95% confidence interval [CI], 0.44-1.88; $P=.73$). Of those in the screened group, 409 participants with normal results and 50 with small MPI defects had lower event rates than the 33 with moderate or large MPI defects; 0.4% per year vs 2.4% per year (HR, 6.3; 95% CI, 1.9-20.1; $P=.001$). Nevertheless, the positive predictive value of having moderate or large MPI defects was only 12%. The overall rate of coronary revascularization was low in both groups: 31 (5.5%) in the screened group and 44 (7.8%) in the unscreened group (HR, 0.71; 95% CI, 0.45-1.1; $P=.14$). During the course of study there was a significant and equivalent increase in primary medical prevention in both groups.

*Conclusion.*—In this contemporary study population of patients with diabetes, the cardiac event rates were low and were not significantly reduced by MPI screening for myocardial ischemia over 4.8 years.

*Trial Registration.*—clinicaltrials.gov Identifier: NCT00769275.

▶ The results of this trial come perhaps as a surprise and are certainly interesting, and given the magnitude of the epidemic of diabetes could have a significant influence upon clinical practice. Although the current standard of cardiovascular care for type 2 diabetes emphasizes the control of risk factors, there has been considerable interest in the screening of asymptomatic patients for cardiovascular disease using noninvasive stress testing and imaging techniques.[1,2]

This is the first large-scale prospective trial of patients with type 2 diabetes with no symptoms of coronary artery disease who were randomized to screening for inducible ischemia using adenosine-stress radionuclide imaging or nonscreening and followed for clinical outcomes. Overall cardiac event rates in both groups were lower than expected, and outcomes were similar in both groups. A minority of patients had significant myocardial perfusion imaging (MPI) abnormalities and correspondingly higher event rates, but revascularization rates were low in both groups.

The data certainly suggest that routine screening for inducible ischemias among asymptomatic patients is not necessary. Perhaps the low event rates reflect in part the impact of aggressive-based control of risk factors and as such this reflects contemporary practice.[3] Previous studies among patients referred to nuclear laboratories, particularly those with peripheral vascular disease or undergoing preoperative testing before noncardiac surgery had higher event rates, a higher incidence of MPI abnormalities, and as such screening might have been more helpful in these patients.[4] This is a classic example of Bayesian principles.

A limitation of this trial as recognized by the authors is the low event rate, which reduced the power of the study to detect differences between the 2 groups. Another limitation is the subsequent quite high use of stress testing in both groups. The bottom line, however, is that a policy of aggressive risk factor reduction, close follow-up, and appropriate diagnostic evaluation in the event that the patients subsequently develop symptoms will suffice for most type 2 diabetics in the contemporary era.

**B. J. Gersh, MB, ChB, DPhil, FRCP**

*References*

1. Bax JJ, Young LH, Frye RL, Bonow RO, Steinberg HO, Barrett EJ. American Diabetes Association. Screening for coronary artery disease in patients with diabetes. *Diabetes Care*. 2007;30:2729-2736.
2. Raggi P, Shaw LJ, Berman DS, Callister TQ. Prognostic value of coronary artery calcium screening in subjects with and without diabetes. *J Am Coll Cardiol*. 2004;43:1663-1669.
3. Gaede P, Vedel P, Larsen N, Jensen GV, Parving HH, Pedersen O. Multifactorial intervention and cardiovascular disease in patients with type 2 diabetes. *N Engl J Med*. 2003;348:383-393.
4. Zellweger MJ, Hachamovitch R, Kang X, et al. Prognostic relevance of symptoms versus objective evidence of coronary artery disease in diabetic patients. *Eur Heart J*. 2004;25:543-550.

# 40 Hypertension

**Antihypertensive Medication Use During Pregnancy and the Risk of Cardiovascular Malformations**

Caton AR, for the National Birth Defects Prevention Study (Univ at Albany, Rensselaer, NY; et al)

*Hypertension* 54:63-70, 2009

We used data from the National Birth Defects Prevention Study, a population-based, case-control study, to examine whether previously reported associations between antihypertensive medications and cardiovascular malformations could be confirmed and to explore whether new associations might be identified. Cases (n = 5021) were ascertained through birth defects surveillance systems from 1997 through 2003 in 10 US states. Controls (n = 4796) were live births without birth defects selected randomly from birth certificates or hospital discharge listings in the same geographic regions. Logistic regression was used to examine the relationship between antihypertensive medication treatment and the occurrence of cardiovascular malformations while controlling for confounding variables. First-trimester treatment with antihypertensive medication was associated with pulmonary valve stenosis (odds ratio [OR]: 2.6; 95% CI: 1.3 to 5.4), Ebstein malformation (crude OR: 11.4; exact 95% CI: 2.8 to 34.1), coarctation of the aorta (OR: 3.0; 95% CI: 1.3 to 6.6), and secundum atrial septal defects (OR: 2.4; 95% CI: 1.3 to 4.4). Treatment initiated after the first trimester was associated with pulmonary valve stenosis (OR: 2.4; 95% CI: 1.1 to 5.4), perimembranous ventricular septal defects (OR: 2.3; 95% CI: 1.2 to 4.6), and secundum atrial septal defects (OR: 2.4; 95% CI: 1.3 to 4.4). Untreated hypertension was associated with Ebstein malformation (OR: 2.1; 95% CI: 1.0 to 4.3) and secundum atrial septal defects (OR: 1.3; 95% CI: 1.0 to 1.6). Antihypertensive medication use and/or the underlying hypertension might increase the risk of having an infant with specific left and right obstructive and septal defects. Additional studies with adequate power will be needed to confirm these findings.

▶ The potential teratogenic effects of antihypertensive drugs has become a much more important issue since the 2006 publication linking congenital heart defects (especially atrial septal defect, in 7 of 18 cases; and patent ductus arteriosus, in 5 of 18 cases) with angiotensin-converting enzyme (ACE)-inhibitors, even when given during the first trimester.[1] This changed medical practice, and these medications are no longer considered "safe" during the first trimester.

A recent survey of the Swedish national database (consisting of 1418 non-diabetic women who took antihypertensive drugs during early pregnancy) has since suggested that such birth defects are associated with maternal hypertension, and are not specific to ACE-inhibitors.[2,3]

This article may be the largest United States effort to link antihypertensive medications with subsequent birth defects; it collected data from 10 states over 7 years to identify 5021 cases of babies born with cardiovascular anomalies, and compare their mothers' antihypertensive drug use patterns with those of 4796 controls (mothers of babies without birth defects). Unfortunately, the National Birth Defects Prevention Study does not track patent ductus arteriosus, so these authors were unable to confirm the conclusions of Cooper et al[1] regarding this anomaly. They did confirm that atrial septal defects were the most common congenital heart defect (23% of the cases). Presumably because of the ACE-inhibitor data, the authors specifically examined their dataset for those babies who were exposed during the first trimester (n = 162), of which only 8 were exposed to ACE-inhibitors (compared with 3 controls), which led to an adjusted odds ratio of 1.9 (95% CI: 0.5-7.2). Interestingly, the adjusted odds ratio for calcium antagonist use in the first trimester was exactly 1.0 (8 cases, 6 controls); otherwise the point estimates for all antihypertensive drug classes exceeded unity. Interestingly, methlydopa use (which is usually recommended as first-line antihypertensive therapy by most obstetricians and current guidelines[3,4]) at any time during pregnancy was associated with a non-significantly increased risk of congenital cardiovascular malformations.

These data are helpful in trying to understand the risks of antihypertensive drugs during pregnancy, but they tend to implicate hypertension itself, and no particular type of antihypertensive drugs in rare cardiovascular anomalies in babies. It is clear that studying this rare problem is a major challenge, which is good news, since many physicians are now more aware of the potential adverse effects of some of these drugs during pregnancy, and use them less, if at all, compared to years past.

**W. J. Elliott, MD, PhD**

*References*

1. Cooper WO, Hernandez-Diaz S, Arbogast PG, et al. Major congenital malformations after first-trimester exposure to ACE inhibitors. *N Engl J Med.* 2006;354: 2443-2451.
2. Lennestal R, Otterblad Olausson P, Kallen P. Maternal use of antihypertensive drugs in early pregnancy and delivery outcome, notably the presence of congenital heart defects in the infants. *Eur J Clin Pharmacol.* 2009;65:615-625.
3. Report of the National High Blood Pressure Education Program working group on high blood pressure in pregnancy. *Am J Obstet Gynecol.* 2000;183:S1-S22.
4. Chobanian AV, Bakris GL, Black HR, et al. Seventh report of the Joint National Committee on Prevention, Detection, Evaluation and Treatment of High Blood Pressure. National High Blood Pressure Education Program Coordinating Committee. *Hypertension.* 2003;42:1206-1252.

**A multifaceted intervention to improve blood pressure control: The Guideline Adherence for Heart Health (GLAD) study**

Bonds DE, Hogan PE, Bertoni AG, et al (Univ of Virginia School of Medicine, Charlottesville; Wake Forest Univ Health Sciences, Winston-Salem, NC)

*Am Heart J* 157:278-284, 2009

*Background.*—Although high blood pressure is associated with significant morbidity and mortality, the proportion reaching the goal blood pressures as outlined in the Seventh Report of the Joint National Committee on Prevention, Detection, Evaluation, Treatment of High Blood Pressure (JNC 7) is low. We conducted a randomized trial in primary care practices of a multifactorial intervention targeted to improve providers' adherence to hypertension guidelines.

*Method.*—A total of 61 primary care practices in North Carolina were randomized to receive either a multifactorial intervention (guideline dissemination via a continuing medical education session, academic detailing sessions, audit and feedback on preintervention rates of adherence, and automated blood pressure machines) or an attention control of similar magnitude but targeted at a different guideline. Outcomes were determined through review of patient charts conducted by an independent masked quality assurance organization.

*Results.*—We found no difference between the 2 groups in any of the adherence measures including no difference in the percentage of patients at goal (intervention 49.2%, control 50.6%), with undiagnosed hypertension (18.1% vs 13.6%), average systolic (126 vs 125.1 mm Hg), or diastolic blood pressure (73.1 vs 73.4 mm Hg). Similarly, there was no difference in provider adherence to treatment recommendations (use of thiazide-type diuretic as first-line therapy: 32% vs 29.5%; use of 2-drug therapy in stage 2 hypertension: 11.3% vs 10.4%).

*Conclusion.*—An intensive, multifactorial intervention did not improve adherence to national hypertension guidelines among community-based primary care. Efforts should be focused on other types of interventions to improve rates of control of hypertension.

► This relatively large and expensive study attempted to improve blood pressure control rates, through an intervention that included an initial hour-long didactic presentation to providers and staff, 4 in-person visits to providers' offices over 2 years to provide information, feedback and advice, written educational materials for patients, medical record flowsheets, exercise prescription pads, automated blood pressure measuring devices (1 issued per 3 providers per office), and feedback regarding the percentage of patients whose blood pressure was diagnosed or under control.

There are a few unusual features of the study that merit comment. The unit of randomization was the medical office, whereas the unit of analysis was the patient; this therefore qualifies as a "cluster-randomization" trial, which has its own challenges in design and analysis. The intervention on hypertension was apparently cobbled onto the main trial, which was focused on improving control of dyslipidemia (which is presumably the origin of the "D" in the acronym, for "GuideLine Adherence in Dyslipidemia").[1] No data are provided in this report about the control of dyslipidemia in each randomized arm of the trial; presumably, the control clinics for the hypertension intervention would have had better control of the low density lipoprotein (LDL)-cholesterol levels in their clinics. If they did not, perhaps the interventions used in both arms of the study were insufficient to show improvements in the patients studied. A third concern is that they reviewed primary medical records for 2111 patients, but only 35% had evidence of a diagnosis of hypertension. It might have been more efficient to pre-select charts based on diagnosis codes for a visit, as this would have nearly tripled the number of subjects to use as a denominator for hypertension control rather than wasting the time and efforts of the blinded chart abstractors on cases that did not have hypertension. One wonders about the generalizability of the findings when 13 823 clinics were initially invited to participate, but only 59 participated in the final chart review.[2] Lastly, the authors indicate that they based their "academic detailing" or "educational outreach visits" on practices of pharmaceutical companies, but 1 semi-annual visit to an office would likely result in unemployment of most pharmaceutical representatives.

The authors suggest that such programs are not useful, and suggest moving to "patient activation," point-of-care computerized decision support (now available at most Department of Veterans' Affairs Medical Centers), "pay for performance"(soon to be implemented nationwide for all physicians), wider use of "polypills" (perhaps similar to the 3-component antihypertensive medication approved by the United States Food and Drug Administration (FDA) this year), and more techniques to improve patients' adherence to medications.[3]

**W. J. Elliott, MD, PhD**

*References*

1. Bertoni AG, Bonds DE, Chen H, et al. Impact of decision support intervention on cholesterol management in primary care practices: results from the Guideline Adherence for Heart trial. *Circulation*. 2008;117:e414.
2. Ellis SD, Bertoni AG, Bonds DE, et al. Value of recruitment strategies used in a primary care practice-based clinical trial. *Contemp Clin Trials*. 2007;28: 258-267.
3. Green BB, Cook AJ, Ralston JD, et al. Effectiveness of home blood pressure monitoring, web communication, and pharmacist care on hypertension control: a randomized controlled trial. *JAMA*. 2008;299:2857-2867.

**Effects of Dietary Sodium Reduction on Blood Pressure in Subjects With Resistant Hypertension: Results From a Randomized Trial**

Pimenta E, Gaddam KK, Oparil S, et al (Univ of Queensland School of Medicine, Brisbane, Australia; Univ of Alabama at Birmingham, UK)

*Hypertension* 54:475-481, 2009

Observational studies indicate a significant relation between dietary sodium and level of blood pressure. However, the role of salt sensitivity in the development of resistant hypertension is unknown. The present study examined the effects of dietary salt restriction on office and 24-hour ambulatory blood pressure in subjects with resistant hypertension. Twelve subjects with resistant hypertension entered into a randomized crossover evaluation of low (50 mmol/24 hours × 7 days) and high sodium diets (250 mmol/24 hours × 7 days) separated by a 2-week washout period. Brain natriuretic peptide; plasma renin activity; 24-hour urinary aldosterone, sodium, and potassium; 24-hour ambulatory blood pressure monitoring; aortic pulse wave velocity; and augmentation index were compared between dietary treatment periods. At baseline, subjects were on an average of 3.4 ± 0.5 antihypertensive medications with a mean office BP of 145.8 ± 10.8/83.9 ± 11.2 mm Hg. Mean urinary sodium excretion was 46.1 ± 26.8 versus 252.2 ± 64.6 mmol/24 hours during low- versus high-salt intake. Low- compared to high-salt diet decreased office systolic and diastolic blood pressure by 22.7 and 9.1 mm Hg, respectively. Plasma renin activity increased whereas brain natriuretic peptide and creatinine clearance decreased during low-salt intake, indicative of intravascular volume reduction. These results indicate that excessive dietary sodium ingestion contributes importantly to resistance to antihypertensive treatment. Strategies to substantially reduce dietary salt intake should be part of the overall treatment of resistant hypertension.

▶ Resistant hypertension is a formidable clinical challenge, despite the large array of drugs available to lower blood pressure.[1,2] Among the nondrug methods of lowering blood pressure that are being studied in this setting are device-guided breathing,[3] renal arterial denervation by radiofrequency ablation,[4] and carotid sinus baroreflex stimulation.[5] Previous studies have shown that dietary sodium restriction is followed by a significant reduction of blood pressure in all stages of hypertension[6] and outcomes data demonstrating a significant reduction in cardiovascular morbidity and mortality compared with control interventions.[7] This small crossover trial involved 12 patients with resistant hypertension and showed a surprisingly large change in blood pressure when they were switched from the 250- to 50-mEq/d dietary sodium intake.

The strengths of the study include the use of ambulatory blood pressure monitoring (to reduce expectation bias and the number of subjects necessary to see a significant difference), which provided very similar results to the office blood pressure difference between the high- and low-sodium dietary sodium treatment periods, the use of the research kitchen to prepare and serve all meals for the two 4-week treatment periods, and a plethora of measurements of serum markers, all of which point to volume reduction during the low-sodium dietary period.

Potential challenges to the importance of the results were the small sample size, the lack of much description of the population from which the patients were drawn, the dropping of one patient because his blood pressure was considered "too high" to participate in the high-sodium diet part of the protocol, the lack of baseline sodium excretion data before the feeding periods, and the lack of statistical significance of the office diastolic blood pressure differences, after correction for the multiple comparisons performed between the low- and high-sodium diet periods. The generalizability of the conclusions to all patients with resistant hypertension is uncertain, particularly since preparing standardized sodium diets in research kitchens is expensive, and the low-sodium diet containing only 50 mEq/d of sodium is difficult to sustain and/or tolerate, over periods longer than 4 to 6 weeks.

Nonetheless, these data suggest that efforts should be taken to implement low-sodium diets in patients with resistant hypertension. The conclusions are not all that much different from those of a study of patients with resistant hypertension done more than 25 years ago,[8] but the take-home message is the same: more efforts to limit dietary sodium are generally warranted in patients with hypertension or those likely to develop it. Sadly, visits to nutritionists to help educate patients about such dietary changes and to help them maintain such efforts are generally not currently reimbursed by US governmental insurance plans and are unlikely to be paid for after the implementation of "health care reform."

**W. J. Elliott, MD, PhD**

*References*


1. Calhoun DA, Jones D, Textor S, et al. Resistant hypertension: diagnosis, evaluation, and treatment. A scientific statement from the American Heart Association Professional Education Committee of the Council for High Blood Pressure Research. *Hypertension.* 2008;51:1403-1419.
2. Moser M, Setaro JF. Refractory or difficult-to-control hypertension. *N Engl J Med.* 2006;355:385-392.
3. Viskoper R, Shapira I, Priluck R, et al. Non-pharmacological treatment of resistant hypertensives by device-guided slow-breathing exercises. *Am J Hypertens.* 2003;16:484-487.
4. Krum H, Schlaich M, Whitbourne R, et al. Catheter-based renal sympathetic denervation for resistant hypertension: a multicentre safety and proof-of-principle cohort study. *Lancet.* 2009;373:1275-1281.
5. Appel LJ. Another major role for dietary sodium reduction: Improving blood pressure control in patients with resistant hypertension [editorial]. *Hypertension.* 2009;54:444-446.
6. Appel LJ, Brands MW, Daniels SR, Karanja N, Elmer PJ, Sacks FM, American Heart Association. Dietary approaches to prevent and treat hypertension: a scientific statement from the American Heart Association. *Hypertension.* 2006;47:296-308.
7. Cook NR, Cutler JA, Obarzanek E, et al. Long term effects of dietary sodium reduction on cardiovascular disease outcomes: observational follow-up of the trials of hypertension prevention (TOHP). *BMJ.* 2007;334:885.

8. Gavras H, Waeber B, Kershaw GR, et al. Role of reactive hyperreninemia in blood pressure changes induced by sodium depletion in patients with ractory hypertension. *Hypertension.* 1981;3:441-447.

**Effect of lowering blood pressure on cardiovascular events and mortality in patients on dialysis: a systematic review and meta-analysis of randomised controlled trials**

Lambers Heerspink HJ, Ninomiya T, Zoungas S, et al (Univ of Sydney, Australia; et al)

*Lancet* 373:1009-1015, 2009

*Background.*—Patients undergoing dialysis have a substantially increased risk of cardiovascular mortality and morbidity. Although several trials have shown the cardiovascular benefits of lowering blood pressure in the general population, there is uncertainty about the efficacy and tolerability of reducing blood pressure in patients on dialysis. We did a systematic review and meta-analysis to assess the effect of blood pressure lowering in patients on dialysis.

*Methods.*—We systematically searched Medline, Embase, and the Cochrane Library database for trials reported between 1950 and November, 2008, without language restriction. We extracted a standardised dataset from randomised controlled trials of blood pressure lowering in patients on dialysis that reported cardiovascular outcomes. Meta-analysis was done with a random effects model.

*Findings.*—We identified eight relevant trials, which provided data for 1679 patients and 495 cardiovascular events. Weighted mean systolic blood pressure was 4·5 mm Hg lower and diastolic blood pressure 2·3 mm Hg lower in actively treated patients than in controls. Blood pressure lowering treatment was associated with lower risks of cardiovascular events (RR 0·71, 95% CI 0·55–0·92; p=0·009), all-cause mortality (RR 0·80, 0·66–0·96; p=0·014), and cardiovascular mortality (RR 0·71, 0·50–0·99; p=0·044) than control regimens. The effects seem to be consistent across a range of patient groups included in the studies.

*Interpretation.*—Treatment with agents that lower blood pressure should routinely be considered for individuals undergoing dialysis to reduce the very high cardiovascular morbidity and mortality rate in this population.

▶ At first glance, it is a bit surprising that the authors should have had to perform this systematic review and meta-analysis. There are abundant data to show,[1-3] and accepted national and international guidelines that recommend[4-6] that individuals with chronic kidney disease should have lower blood pressures, whether hypertensive or not, than the general population. It is likely that a trial that denied antihypertensive drug therapy to individuals on dialysis in the United States would not be allowed to enroll patients by the supervising institutional review board. It is important to remember in this context that diastolic hypotension, especially, immediately after dialysis is associated with a poor prognosis[7] and that many dialysis sessions end early because the intradialytic blood pressures were too low to continue. This is presumably the reason that the ethics committees of the 6 reported studies done outside the United States allowed these randomized trials to be performed.

There are a number of technical challenges with the reports summarized in this article. The primary outcome of cardiovascular events was nonstandard across studies; the authors merely accepted the numbers of affected patients from each study and performed sensitivity analyses for these. For example, heart failure hospitalization was included in 4 of 8 studies' primary end point, for which there was subsequent evidence of heterogeneity of the results in univariate analyses. Excluding 1 study that included only patients on peritoneal (rather than hemo) dialysis (in which the immediate blood pressure lowering effect of randomized antihypertensive treatment would be expected to be less) seemed to have little impact on the overall results. The authors acknowledge the small number of studies (n = 8), included patients (n = 1679), patients with primary cardiovascular end points (n = 495), fatalities (n = 481), the limited statistical power of methods based on tabulated data for investigations related to inhomogeneity of the results, and the inability to access all data from each study.

Nonetheless, the conclusion is clear: drug treatment of high blood pressure in dialysis patients is beneficial. Despite the scarcity of data on the point, it is now likely that further investigation of this hypothesis will be considered unethical, worldwide.

**W. J. Elliott, MD, PhD**

*References*


1. Pohl MA, Blumenthal S, Cordonner DJ, et al. Independent and additive effect of blood pressure control and angiotensin II receptor blockade on renal outcomes in the irbesartan diabetic nephropathy trial: clinical implications and limitations. *J Am Soc Nephrol.* 2005;16:3027-3037.
2. Sarnak MJ, Greene T, Wang X, et al. The effect of a lower target blood pressure on the progression of kidney disease: long-term follow-up of the modification of diet in renal disease study. *Ann Intern Med.* 2005;142:342-351.
3. Jafar TH, Stark PC, Schmid CH, et al. Progression of chronic kidney disease: the role of blood pressure control, proteinuria, and angiotensin-converting enzyme inhibition: a patient-level meta-analysis. *Ann Intern Med.* 2003;139:244-252.
4. Levey AS, Rocco MV, Anderson S, et al. K/DOQI clinical practice guidelines on hypertension and antihypertensive agents in chronic kidney disease. *Am J Kidney Dis.* 2004;43:S1-S290.
5. Chobanian AV, Bakris GL, Black HR, et al. National High Blood Pressure Education Program Coordinating Committee. Seventh report of the Joint National Committee on Prevention, Detection, Evaluation and Treatment of High Blood Pressure. *Hypertension.* 2003;42:1206-1252.
6. Mancia G, De Backer G, Dominiczak A, et al. 2007 Guidelines for the Management of Arterial Hypertension. Task Force for the Management of Arterial Hypertension of the European Society of Hypertension and the European Society of Cardiology. *J Hypertens.* 2007;25:1105-1187.

7. Klassen PS, Lowrie EG, Reddan DN, et al. Association between pulse pressure and mortality in patients undergoing maintenance hemodialysis. *JAMA*. 2002;287: 1548-1555.

**Reappraisal of European guidelines on hypertension management: a European Society of Hypertension Task Force document**

Mancia G, Laurent S, Agabiti-Rosei E, et al (Univ of Milano-Bicocca, Italy; Hopital Europeen Georges Pompidou, Paris, France; Univ of Brescia, Italy; et al)

*J Hypertens* 27:2121-2158, 2009

*Background.*—The European Society of Hypertension's most recent guidelines were issued in 2007, in conjunction with the European Society of Cardiology. Since then, a number of issues have arisen that were the rationale for this update.

*Methods.*—A committee of the European Society of Hypertension met to review areas in which new guidelines might provide information useful to practitioners.

*Results and Conclusions.*—Stratification of a hypertensive person by his/her absolute risk of cardiovascular disease (particularly involving assessment of target organ damage) is desirable, and supported by much research, but most proposed tests are expensive, complex, and have limited availability. Much controversy, but little clinical trial data, exists about the appropriate blood pressure level at which to initiate drug therapy, or the most appropriate target blood pressure during treatment. All the major antihypertensive drug classes seem to lower blood pressure and cardiovascular risk, so choice of antihypertensive drug therapy should be limited by contraindications, rather than guidelines recommendations. Combination antihypertensive therapy can be recommended, except for diuretic + beta-blocker and ACE-inhibitor + angiotensin receptor blocker. Elderly patients generally benefit from antihypertensive drugs, but treatment should be individualized. Despite decades of progress, many unanswered questions remain about hypertension that should be addressed by simple clinical trials.

▶ This update on the European hypertension guidelines was meant to highlight some of the important areas that the committee feels should be addressed in the next edition of the European Society of Hypertension/European Society of Cardiology guidelines. It serves as a useful stepping-off point for further discussion, and will likely serve as good background reading for those charged with writing the Eighth Report of the Joint National Committee on Prevention, Detection, Evaluation, and Treatment of High Blood Pressure (JNC 8) here in the United States. The European guidelines have always been a little more expansive than American guidelines regarding classification of hypertension, choice of initial therapy, and identification of appropriate blood pressure targets[1,2]; this discussion document suggests that will remain the case.

One of the more interesting aspects of this document is the attention paid to the J-shaped curve, the concern that lowering blood pressure too much may be harmful.[3] This has been widely debated on both sides of the Atlantic, with European guideline writers being more concerned than those in the Americas. Another area highlighted here is the lack of evidence for the target blood pressure in diabetics to be <130/80 mm Hg;[4] sadly, little mention is made of the studies showing benefit to a "lower-than-usual" blood pressure target in the United Kingdom Prospective Diabetes Study[5] and the diabetics in the Hypertension Optimal Treatment Trial.[6] This document also suggests that recommending a "hierarchy" of drugs to use in sequence is unnecessary, which is unlikely to be the opinion of JNC 8.

This article outlines many of the important questions that remain controversial in hypertension and forms a nice outline for further discussion by guidelines committees. It is more likely that more agreement with these concepts will be found in the next set of European guidelines, compared to JNC 8.

**W. J. Elliott, MD, PhD**

*References*


1. Mancia G, De Backer G, Dominiczak A, et al. 2007 Guidelines for the management of arterial hypertension. Task Force for the Management of Arterial Hypertension of the European Society of Hypertension and the European Society of Cardiology. *J Hypertens*. 2007;25:1105-1187.
2. Chobanian AV, Bakris GL, Black HR, et al. Seventh report of the Joint National Committee on Prevention, Detection, Evaluation and Treatment of High Blood Pressure. National High Blood Pressure Education Program Coordinating Committee. *Hypertension*. 2003;42:1206-1252.
3. Messerli FH, Mancia G, Conti CR, et al. Dogma disputed: can aggressively lowering blood pressure in hypertensive patients with coronary artery disease be dangerous? *Ann Intern Med*. 2006;144:884-893.
4. Arguedas JA, Perez MI, Wright JM. Treatment blood pressure targets for hypertension. *Cochrane Database Syst Rev*. 2009;CD004349. 10.1002/14651858.CD004349.pub2.
5. Tight blood pressure control and risk of macrovascular and microvascular complications in type 2 diabetes: UKPDS 38. UK Prospective Diabetes Study Group. *BMJ*. 1998;317:703-713.
6. Hansson L, Zanchetti A, Carruthers SG, et al. Effects of intensive blood pressure lowering and low-dose aspirin in patients with hypertension: principal results of the Hypertension Optimal Treatment (HOT) randomised trial: HOT Study Group. *Lancet*. 1998;351:1755-1762.


## Do COX-2 inhibitors raise blood pressure more than nonselective NSAIDs and placebo? An updated meta-analysis

Chan CC, Reid CM, Aw T-J, et al (Alfred Hosp, Australia; Monash Univ, Australia; et al)

*J Hypertens* 27:2332-2341, 2009

*Background.*—Both COX-2 selective inhibitors (coxibs) and nonselective (ns)-NSAIDs elevate blood pressure (BP) and this may contribute to excess cardiovascular (CV) events. A number of recent large-scale randomized clinical trials (RCTs) comparing coxibs (including newer agents, lumiracoxib and etoricoxib) to both ns-NSAIDs and placebo have been reported, permitting an update to earlier BP analyses of these agents.

*Data Sources/Synthesis.*—Our search yielded 51 RCTs involving coxibs published before April 2008 with a total of 130 541 participants in which BP data were available. The Der Simonian and Laird random effects method for dichotomous variables was used to produce risk ratios (RR) for development of hypertension.

*Results.*—For coxibs versus placebo, there was a RR of 1.49 (1.18–1.88, $P = 0.04$) in the development of new hypertension. For coxibs versus ns-NSAIDs, the RR was 1.12 (0.93–1.35, $P = 0.23$). These results were mainly driven by rofecoxib, with a RR of 1.87 (1.63–2.14, $P = 0.08$) versus placebo, and etoricoxib, with a RR of 1.52 (1.39–1.66, $P = 0.01$) versus ns-NSAID.

*Conclusion.*—On the basis of this updated meta-analysis, coxibs appear to produce greater hypertension than either ns-NSAIDs or placebo. However, this response was heterogeneous, with markedly raised BP associated with rofecoxib and etoricoxib, whereas celecoxib, valdecoxib and lumiracoxib appeared to have little BP effect. The relationship of this increased risk of hypertension to subsequent adverse CV outcomes requires further investigation and prospective RCTs.

▶ These authors have updated their previous meta-analysis[1] that included trials in arthritis patients, which concluded that COX-2 selective inhibitors led to significant increases in blood pressure of about 3.9/1.1 and 2.8/1.3 mm Hg, compared with placebo or nonselective nonsteroidal anti-inflammatory drugs (NSAIDs), respectively. They also found significant inhomogeneity of the effects across the COX-2 inhibitors, with rofecoxib raising blood pressure the most, with etoricoxib somewhat less, with celecoxib's effect being not significant.[1] Since then, many more trials have been completed in different disease states, using many more COX-2 inhibitors, so they repeated their search strategy and have now meta-analyzed 51 trials using 5 different COX-2 inhibitors. They found 13 trials with information about blood pressure changes with different doses of COX-2 inhibitors (which may be especially important for rofecoxib and celecoxib); 43 trials provided the numbers of subjects that became hypertensive after taking the assigned therapies.

Their overall results are similar to those published in 2005.[1] The average increase in blood pressure with any COX-2 inhibitor was 3.2/1.3 or 0.9/0.4 mm Hg, compared with placebo or nonselective NSAID. As before, there was some evidence, mainly from analyses of the risk of developing hypertension, that rofecoxib and (to a slightly lesser extent) etoricoxib were more likely than the other COX-2 inhibitors to raise blood pressure, particularly when compared with other NSAIDs (especially naproxen). In these analyses, rofecoxib was significantly more likely to be associated with incident hypertension than either placebo or nonselective NSAIDs; etoricoxib was not significantly different than placebo, but was significantly different from nonselective NSAIDs;

celecoxib, valdecoxib, and lumiracoxib were not significantly different from either comparator. They also report that naproxen appears to have a slightly greater effect in raising blood pressure than diclofenac or ibuprofen, based on these drugs' use as comparators in the head-to-head COX-2 versus NSAID trials.

The more challenging question is how much of the increased risk of cardiovascular events seen with COX-2 inhibitors, especially rofecoxib,[2-5] can be attributed to this increase in blood pressure. Since its removal from the worldwide market on September 30, 2004, no further studies have been done with this compound, and the answer may never be known. The very large Prospective Randomized Evaluation of Celecoxib Integrated Safety versus Ibuprofen or Naproxen (PRECISION) trial will enroll 20 000 arthritis patients with a high risk of cardiovascular disease, but blood pressure differences are likely to be minimized because "extra" treatment for those whose blood pressure increases are offered as part of the study protocol.[6]

**W. J. Elliott, MD, PhD**

*References*


1. Aw TJ, Haas SJ, Liew D, Krum H. Meta-analysis of cyclooxygenase-2 inhibitors and their effects on blood pressure. *Arch Intern Med.* 2005;165:490-496.
2. Jüni P, Nartey L, Reichenbach S, Sterchi R, Dieppe PA, Egger M. Risk of cardiovascular events and rofecoxib: cumulative meta-analysis. *Lancet.* 2004;364: 2021-2029.
3. Bresalier RS, Sandler RS, Quan H, et al. Cardiovascular events associated with rofecoxib in a colorectal adenoma chemoprevention trial. *N Engl J Med.* 2005; 352:1092-1102.
4. Weir MR, Sperling RS, Reicin Agertz BJ. Selective COX-2 inhibition and cardiovascular effects: a review of the rofecoxib development program. *Am Heart J.* 2003;146:591-604.
5. White WB, Faich G, Borer JS, Makuch RW. Cardiovascular thrombotic events in arthritis trials of the cyclooxygenase-2 inhibitor, celecoxib. *Am J Cardiol.* 2003;92: 411-418.
6. Becker MC, Wang TH, Wisniewski L, et al. Rationale, design, and governance of the Prospective Randomized Evaluation of Celecoxib Integrated Safety versus Ibuprofen Or Naproxen (PRECISION), a cardiovascular end point trial of nonsteroidal antiinflammatory agents in patients with arthritis. *Am Heart J.* 2009;157: 606-612.


## The Misdiagnosis of Hypertension: The Role of Patient Anxiety

Ogedegbe G, Pickering TG, Clemow L, et al (Columbia Univ/New York)
*Arch Intern Med* 168:2459-2465, 2009

*Background.*—The white coat effect (defined as the difference between blood pressure [BP] measurements taken at the physician's office and those taken outside the office) is an important determinant of misdiagnosis of hypertension, but little is known about the mechanisms underlying this phenomenon. We tested the hypothesis that the white coat effect may be a conditioned response as opposed to a manifestation of general anxiety.

*Methods.*—A total of 238 patients in a hypertension clinic wore ambulatory blood pressure monitors on 3 separate days 1 month apart. At each clinic visit, BP readings were manually triggered in the waiting area and the examination room (in the presence and absence of the physician) and were compared with the mercury sphygmomanometer readings taken by the physician in the examination room. Patients completed trait and state anxiety measures before and after each BP assessment.

*Results.*—A total of 35% of the sample was normotensive, and 9%, 37%, and 19% had white coat, sustained, and masked hypertension, respectively.The diagnostic category was associated with the state anxiety measure ($F_{3,237} = 6.4$, $P < .001$) but not with the trait anxiety measure. Patients with white coat hypertension had significantly higher state anxiety scores ($t = 2.67$, $P < .01$), with the greatest difference reported during the physician measurement. The same pattern was observed for BP changes, which generally paralleled the changes in state anxiety ($t = 4.86$, $P < .002$ for systolic BP; $t = 3.51$, $P < .002$ for diastolic BP).

*Conclusions.*—These findings support our hypothesis that the white coat effect is a conditioned response. The BP measurements taken by physicians appear to exacerbate the white coat effect more than other means. This problem could be addressed with uniform use of automated BP devices in office settings.

▶ These interesting data support many previous hypotheses about white-coat hypertension. Originally described in Milan, Italy (when only physicians measured blood pressure),[1] the phenomenon was soon thereafter found NOT to be present when trained nurses measured blood pressure (which is now standard practice in many locales).[2] This team of physicians and psychologists designed this study to correlate scores on standardized psychological questionnaires regarding anxiety to the blood pressure responses in patients visiting a physician's office, with the background hypothesis that the white-coat effect is a conditioned response.

Their data support their original hypothesis, primarily because the anxiety scores were higher among those with white-coat hypertension in the presence of the physician and not across individuals (ranked according to their anxiety trait scores). This hypothesis suggests that (1) people with white-coat hypertension ought not to have hypertensive responses to other stressors, outside the medical office setting; (2) it may be possible to decondition people with white-coat hypertension by having them spend more time chronically in the physician's office; and (3) the probability of sustained hypertension and its sequelae ought to be lower in people with white-coat hypertension than masked hypertension, presuming they spend similar, small proportions of time in the physician's office. These hypotheses are probably already being tested by this productive research group.

The authors complete their discussion with an impassioned plea for the use of objective, calibrated, and automated devices for measuring blood pressure in the physician's office. This is clearly a less expensive alternative to the method used in this study (24-hour ambulatory blood pressure monitoring). As mercury-containing sphygmomanometers have recently been banned from nearly all health care workplaces by the Occupational Safety and Health Administration, this offers an opportunity to replace a potentially toxic, but lifesaving device, with one that is less prone to error than most human measurements. It will be interesting to see if the next set of American Heart Association guidelines, formerly chaired by one of these coauthors, will recommend automated devices for office blood pressure measurements.[3]

**W. J. Elliott, MD, PhD**

*References*

1. Mancia G, Bertinieri G, Grassi G, et al. Effects of blood pressure measurement by the doctor on patients' blood pressure and heart rate. *Lancet*. 1983;2:695-697.
2. Mancia G, Parati G, Pomidossi G, Grassi G, Casadei R, Zanchetti A. Alerting reaction and rise in blood pressure during measurement by physician and nurse. *Hypertension*. 1987;9:209-215.
3. Pickering TG, Hall JE, Appel LJ, et al. Recommendations for blood pressure measurement in humans and experimental animals: Part 1: blood pressure measurement in humans: a statement for professionals from the Subcommittee of Professional and Public Education of the American Heart Association Council on High Blood Pressure Research. *Hypertension*. 2005;45:142-161.

# 41 Non-Coronary Heart Disease in Adults

**B-CONVINCED: Beta-blocker CONtinuation Vs. INterruption in patients with Congestive heart failure hospitalizED for a decompensation episode**

Jondeau G, for the B-CONVINCED Investigators (Hôpital Bichat, Paris, France; et al)

*Eur Heart J* 30:2186-2192, 2009

*Aims.*—Whether or not beta-blocker therapy should be stopped during acutely decompensated heart failure (ADHF) is unsure.

*Methods and Results.*—In a randomized, controlled, open labelled, non-inferiority trial, we compared beta-blockade continuation vs. discontinuation during ADHF in patients with LVEF below 40% previously receiving stable beta-blocker therapy. 169 patients were included, among which 147 were evaluable. Mean age was 72 ± 12 years, 65% were males. After 3 days, 92.8% of patients pursuing beta-blockade improved for both dyspnoea and general well-being according to a physician blinded for therapy vs. 92.3% of patients stopping beta-blocker. This was the main endpoint and the upper limit for unilateral 95% CI (6.6%) is lower that of the pre-defined upper limit (12.5%), indicating non-inferiority. Similar findings were obtained at 8 days and when evaluation was made by the patient. Plasma BNP at Day 3, length of hospital stay, re-hospitalization rate, and death rate after 3 months were also similar. Beta-blocker therapy at 3 months was given to 90% of patients vs. 76% ($P < 0.05$).

*Conclusion.*—In conclusion, during ADHF, continuation of beta-blocker therapy is not associated with delayed or lesser improvement, but with a higher rate of chronic prescription of beta-blocker therapy after 3 months, the benefit of which is well established (Figs 1 and 2).

▶ Prospective, randomized, controlled trials in patients with chronic heart failure (HF) with reduced left ventricular ejection fraction (LVEF) have consistently shown that β-blocker therapy, starting with a low dose and gradually increasing the dose over time improves survival, quality of life, and decreases HF rehospitalization rate.[1-4] However, patients admitted for acute decompensated HF (ADHF) not on β-blockers if started on the usual dose of β-blocker can exacerbate the symptoms and become worse hemodynamically because the β-blockers antagonize the compensatory positive inotropic effect of sympathetic and adrenergic activation.[5] In patients with HF, both cardiac output and

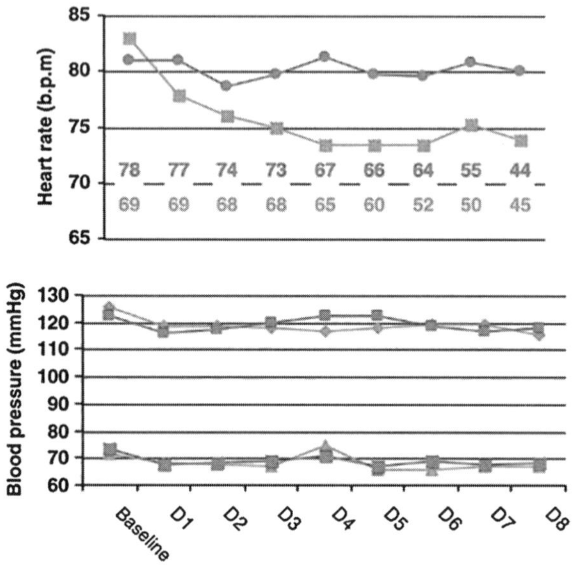


FIGURE 1.—Evolution of heart rate (top) and systolic and diastolic blood pressure (bottom) in the two groups. The 'group keep' is depicted in green, the 'group stop' in red. No difference in blood pressure was observed, whereas significant interaction was observed between time and group for heart rate ($P < 0.001$), indicating that heart rate decrease was significantly more in the group continuing with beta-blocker therapy. For interpretation of the references to color in this figure legend, the reader is referred to web version of this article. (Reprinted from Jondeau G, for the B-CONVINCED Investigators. B-CONVINCED: Beta-blocker CONtinuation Vs. INterruption in patients with Congestive heart failure hospitalizED for a decompensation episode. *Eur Heart J.* 2009;30:2186-2192, with permission from The European Society of Cardiology.)

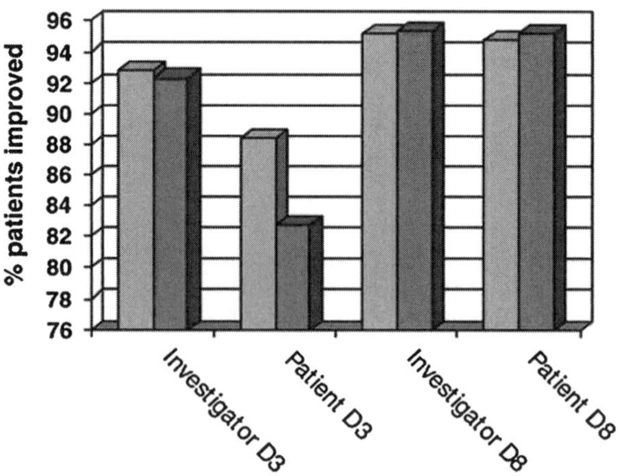


FIGURE 2.—Percentage of patients improved for both general well-being and dyspnoea according to the fact that they keep (green) or stop (red) beta-blocker therapy, evaluated by a blinded investigator (investigator) or the patient (patient), at Day 3 and at Day 8. See text for statistics. For interpretation of the references to color in this figure legend, the reader is referred to web version of this article. (Reprinted from Jondeau G, for the B-CONVINCED Investigators. B-CONVINCED: Beta-blocker CONtinuation Vs. INterruption in patients with Congestive heart failure hospitalizED for a decompensation episode. *Eur Heart J.* 2009;30:2186-2192, with permission from The European Society of Cardiology.)

blood pressure drops and brain natriuretic peptide (BNP) plasma levels increase after the first dose of β-blockers [8, 9]. Further, if inotopic support is needed, β-blockers alter the effectiveness of intravenous dobutamine.[6] When a patient is hospitalized with ADHF already taking β-blockers, there is concern about continuing the β-blockers for fear of exacerbating the symptoms and worsening the HF. The present randomized, controlled, open-labeled non-inferiority study compares the evolution of clinical symptoms of patients hospitalized for an episode of ADHF, and a LVEF < 40% who had been receiving β-blockers for > 1 month before admission, randomized to continue or stop the β-blockers on hospital admission. The patients were representative of the severely ill patients seen in clinical practice with a mean age of 72 years, a mean LVEF of 32%, a mean plasma BNP of 1200 pg/ml, and a rehospitalization rate of 40% at 3 months. The results of the study clearly show that the clinical improvement in dyspnea and feeling of well-being was similar in both groups at 3 and 8 days after admission. Also similar were the duration of hospital stay, the HF rehospitalization rate at 3 months, and the death rate. The major difference between continuing the β-blockers and stopping them on admission was that if the β-blockers were continued, at 3 months a higher percentage of patients were taking β-blockers than if they were stopped on admission. Clearly, it is to the patient's advantage that with chronic HF, β-blockers be given chronically.

**M. D. Cheitlin, MD**

*References*


1. Packer M, Bristow MR, Cohn JN, et al. The effect of carvedilol on morbidity and mortality in patients with chronic heart failure. U.S. Carvedilol Heart Failure Study Group. *N Engl J Med.* 1996;334:1349-1355.
2. CIBIS Investigators and Committees. The Cardiac Insufficiency Bisoprolol Study II (CIBIS-II): a randomised trial. *Lancet.* 1999;353:9-13.
3. Hjalmarson A, Goldstein S, Fagerberg B, et al. Effects of controlled-release metoprolol on total mortality, hospitalizations, and well-being in patients with heart failure: the Metoprolol CR/XL Randomized Intervention Trial in congestive heart failure (MERIT-HF). MERIT-HF Study Group. *JAMA.* 2000;283: 1295-1302.
4. Flather MD, Shibata MC, Coats AJ, et al. for the SENIORS Investigators Randomized trial to determine the effect of nebivolol on mortality and cardiovascular hospital admission in elderly patients with heart failure (SENIORS). *Eur Heart J.* 2005;26:215-225.
5. Dickstein K, Cohen-Solal A, Filippatos G, et al. ESC Guidelines for the diagnosis and treatment of acute and chronic heart failure 2008: the Task Force for the Diagnosis and Treatment of Acute and Chronic Heart Failure 2008 of the European Society of Cardiology. Developed in collaboration with the Heart Failure Association of the ESC (HFA) and endorsed by the European Society of Intensive Care Medicine (ESICM). *Eur Heart J.* 2008;29:2388-2442.
6. Metra M, Nodari S, D'Aloia A, et al. Beta-blocker therapy influences the hemodynamic response to inotropic agents in patients with heart failure: a randomized comparison of dobutamine and enoximone before and after chronic treatment with metoprolol or carvedilol. *J Am Coll Cardiol.* 2002;40:1248-1258.

### Clinical Characteristics and Four-Year Outcomes of Patients in the Rhode Island Takotsubo Cardiomyopathy Registry

Regnante RA, Zuzek RW, Weinsier SB, et al (Warren Alpert Med School of Brown Univ, Providence, RI)

*Am J Cardiol* 103:1015-1019, 2009

The aim was to establish a registry of patients with a diagnosis of Takotsubo cardiomyopathy (TC) to help learn more about the characteristics, treatment strategies, and natural history of this disease. Data for patients with TC diagnosed from July 2004 to April 2008 at 2 major hospitals in Rhode Island were obtained. A data set was created that included baseline demographics and characteristics, hospital, course, and clinical outcomes. TC was diagnosed in 70 patients during the study period. Postmenopausal women comprised 95% of the cohort. Six patients presented with cardiogenic shock, 9 required intubation, 3 experienced sustained ventricular arrhythmias, and 1 patient died of cardiac causes. Average ejection fraction was 37% at cardiac catheterization. Troponin-I was increased in all except 1 patient. Follow-up echocardiography showed full recovery of wall motion abnormalities, with an average ejection fraction of 59%. Most patients were treated using standard cardiovascular medications for acute coronary syndrome, and 43% were discharged on warfarin therapy because of severe apical wall motion abnormalities. Univariate analysis suggested that long-term use of angiotensin-converting enzyme inhibitors before the onset of TC was protective against cardiogenic shock, sustained ventricular arrhythmia, and death. Consecutive cases grouped into different seasons showed a statistically significant spike in the occurrence of TC during the summer months. In conclusion, the acute phase of this condition may lead to critical illness and death, and use of an angiotensin-converting enzyme inhibitor may have a protective effect. Overall long-term prognosis and recovery of left ventricular function were excellent.

▶ This registry of patients with Takotsubo disease from 2 hospitals in Rhode Island has a promise of yielding more insight into this strange disease. Because they have found only 70 patients so far, the findings are limited and for the most part similar to other accounts of patients with this disease.[1,2] Postmenopausal women comprised 95% of the case. What is interesting is that two thirds of these women had either emotional or physical stress as precipitators of the disease and one third had neither. Another unique finding was that over a 3-year period, the highest number of cases appeared during the summer months, from June to August, ($P = .001$) compared to the rest of the year (Fig 2). This is opposite of the peak incidence of acute myocardial infarction, which is during the winter months.[3]

Although the patient is stabilized during the first 48 hours the prognosis is excellent, the disease is not benign. There were 11 patients who had critical complications early on admission, death, cardiogenic shock, ventricular fibrillation, or sustained ventricular tachycardia (Table 3). On univariate analysis, if the

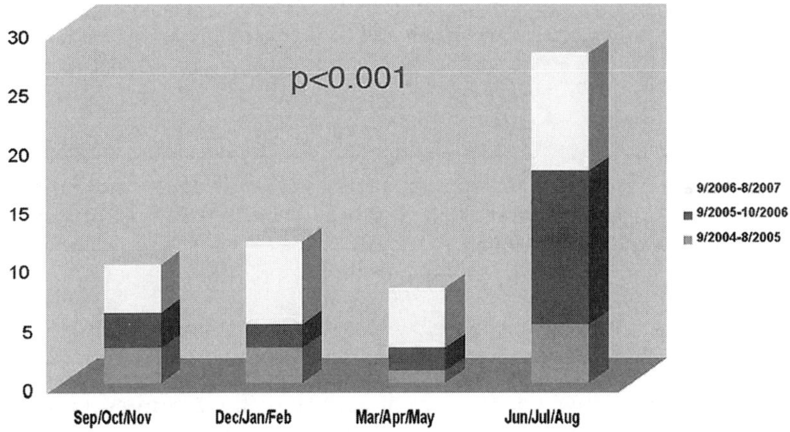


FIGURE 2.—Number of cases of TC by season. (Reprinted from Regnante RA, Zuzek RW, Weinsier SB, et al. Clinical characteristics and four-year outcomes of patients in the Rhode Island Takotsubo Cardiomyopathy Registry. *Am J Cardiol.* 2009;103:1015-1019, with permission from Elsevier.)

TABLE 3.—Clinical Outcomes

| | |
|---|---|
| Intubated | 9 (13%) |
| Shock/vasopressors/intra-aortic balloon pump | 6 (9%) |
| Sustained ventricular arrhythmias | 3 (4%) |
| Mean peak troponin-I | 6.9 ng/ml ± 6 |
| Median length of stay (d) | 4 days |
| Follow-up ejection fraction using echocardiography (%) | 59 ± 7% |
| TC recurrence | 2 |
| Death | 3 (1 cardiac, 2 noncardiac) |
| Thromboembolic events | 0 |

patient was taking an ACE inhibitor (ACEI) before admission, none had a critical illness ($P = .026$). If the patient needed intubation at the time of presentation, there was a high incidence of critical complications. The patients were discharged on the same medications as patients with acute coronary syndromes. The only possible clue as to a medication that might decrease severity if the syndrome recurs is that ACEI seems to be protective of the occurrence of critical complications.

**M. D. Cheitlin, MD**

*References*

1. Abe Y, Kondo M, Matsuoka R, Araki M, Dohyama K, Tanio H. Assessment of clinical features in transient left ventricular apical ballooning. *J Am Coll Cardiol.* 2003;41:737-742.
2. Elesber AA, Prasad A, Lennon RJ, Wright RS, Lerman A, Rihal CS. Four-year recurrence rate and prognosis of the apical ballooning syndrome. *J Am Coll Cardiol.* 2007;50:448-452.

3. Spencer F, Goldberg R, Becker R, Gore J. Seasonal distribution of acute myocardial infarction in the Second Registry of Myocardial Infarction. *J Am Coll Cardiol.* 1996;31:1226-1233.

---

**Association between degenerative aortic valve disease and long-term exposure to cardiovascular risk factors: results of the longitudinal population-based KORA/MONICA survey**

Stritzke J, for the MONICA/KORA Investigators (Univ of Lübeck, Germany; et al)

*Eur Heart J* 30:2044-2053, 2009

---

*Aims.*—Degenerative aortic valve disease (DAVD), a common finding in the elderly, is associated with an increased risk of death due to cardiovascular causes. Taking advantage of its longitudinal design, this study evaluates the prevalence of DAVD and its temporal associations with long-term exposure to cardiovascular risk factors in the general population.

*Methods and Results.*—We studied 953 subjects (aged 25–74 years) from a random sample of German residents. Risk factors had been determined at a baseline investigation in 1994/95. At a follow-up investigation, 10 years later, standardized echocardiography determined aortic valve morphology and aortic valve area (AVA) as well as left ventricular geometry and function. At the follow-up study, the overall prevalence of DAVD was 28%. In logistic regression models adjusting for traditional cardiovascular risk factors at baseline age (OR 2.0 [1.7–2.3] per 10 years, $P < 0.001$), active smoking (OR 1.7 [1.1–2.4], $P = 0.009$) and elevated total cholesterol levels (OR 1.2 [1.1–1.3] per increase of 20 mg/dL, $P < 0.001$) were significantly related to DAVD at follow-up. Furthermore, age, baseline status of smoking, and total cholesterol level were significant predictors of a smaller AVA at follow-up study. In contrast, hypertension and obesity had no detectable relationship with long-term changes of aortic valve structure.

*Conclusions.*—In the general population we observed a high prevalence of DAVD that is associated with long-term exposure to elevated cholesterol levels and active smoking. These findings strengthen the notion that smoking cessation and cholesterol lowering are promising treatment targets for prevention of DAVD (Figs 1, 4, and 5).

▶ Degenerative aortic valve disease (DVAD) is common in the elderly and reported to be 21% to 31%[1-3] and commonly is a precursor of hemodynamically significant aortic stenosis. It is also associated with a high incidence of death from cardiovascular (CV) causes, predominantly coronary artery disease (CAD).[1] This article is from the WHO-MONICA study, a population-based longitudinal study over 10 years that had evaluated baseline cardiovascular risk factors. They defined DVAD echocardiographically as thickening or increased echogenicity with or without reduced systolic opening. The study

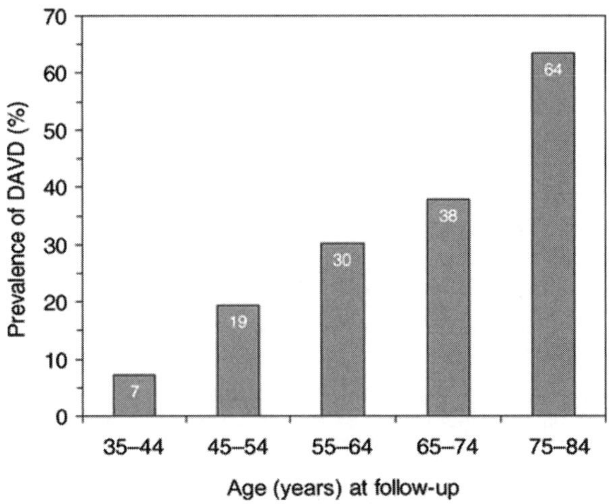


FIGURE 1.—Prevalence of degenerative aortic valve disease by age groups. (Reprinted from Stritzke J, for the MONICA/KORA Investigators. Association between degenerative aortic valve disease and long-term exposure to cardiovascular risk factors: results of the longitudinal population-based KORA/MONICA survey. *Eur Heart J*. 2009;30:2044-2053, with permission from The European Society of Cardiology.)

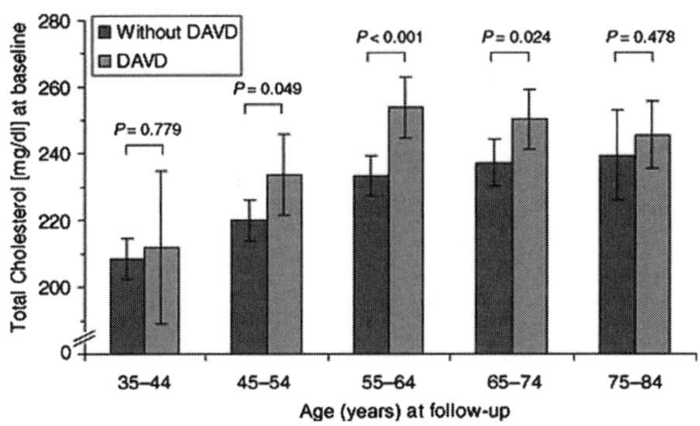


FIGURE 4.—Total cholesterol levels in individuals without and with degenerative aortic valve disease. Adjusted mean values with 95% confidence interval as estimated with univariate variance analysis, adjusted for gender; *P*-values for comparison of individuals presenting without and with degenerative aortic valve disease. (Reprinted from Stritzke J, for the MONICA/KORA Investigators. Association between degenerative aortic valve disease and long-term exposure to cardiovascular risk factors: results of the longitudinal population-based KORA/MONICA survey. *Eur Heart J*. 2009;30:2044-2053, with permission from The European Society of Cardiology.)

showed that long-term exposure to risk factors such as increased cholesterol and active smoking are associated with the development of DAVD and coronary disease. Also, in the absence of significant aortic stenosis, the afterload burden on the left ventricle was increased as detected by a higher relative wall thickness (the ratio of the septal and posterior wall thickness over the left ventricular [LV] end-diastolic diameter). The message of this study is the possibility that early

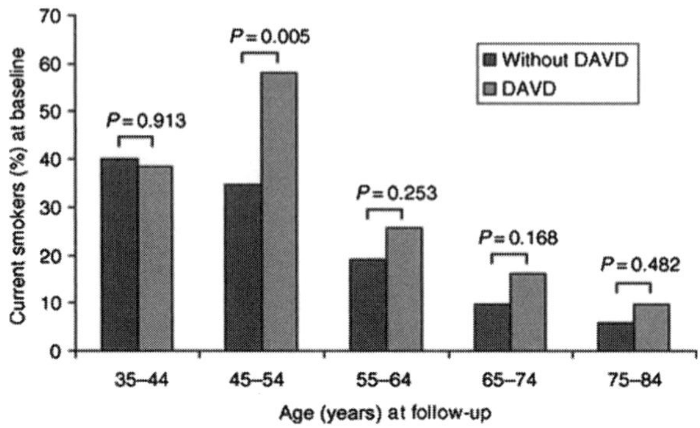


FIGURE 5.—Proportion of active smokers in individuals without and with degenerative aortic valve disease. *P*-values for comparison of individuals presenting without and with degenerative aortic valve disease were obtained using the $\chi^2$-test. (Reprinted from Stritzke J, for the MONICA/KORA Investigators. Association between degenerative aortic valve disease and long-term exposure to cardiovascular risk factors: results of the longitudinal population-based KORA/MONICA survey. *Eur Heart J.* 2009;30:2044-2053, with permission from The European Society of Cardiology.)

control of CV risk factors could decrease the incidence of DAVD in the elderly and even significant aortic stenosis.

Although most studies of statin's influence on the progression of aortic stenosis have been negative, it is probable that the subjects selected have been late in the course of their obstructive disease. A study by Antonini-Canterin and colleagues[4] reported a large series of patients with long-term follow-up showing progression only in those with DAVD and mild stenosis and not in those with moderate stenosis. Since statins are effective in altering the progression of coronary artery disease, it is logical to believe that they should decrease the progression of DAVD to significant aortic stenosis if started early in the course of the disease.

**M. D. Cheitlin, MD**

*References*

1. Otto CM, Lind BK, Kitzman DW, Gersh BJ, Siscovick DS. Association of aortic-valve sclerosis with cardiovascular mortality and morbidity in the elderly. *N Engl J Med.* 1999;341:142-147.
2. Lindroos M, Kupari M, Heikkila J, Tilvis R. Prevalence of aortic valve abnormalities in the elderly: an echocardiographic study of a random population sample [Abstract]. *J Am Coll Cardiol.* 1993;21:1220-1225.
3. Stewart BF, Siscovick D, Lind BK, et al. Clinical factors associated with calcific aortic valve disease. Cardiovascular Health Study. *J Am Coll Cardiol.* 1997;29: 630-634.
4. Antonini-Canterin F, Hirsu M, Popescu BA, et al. Stage-related effect of statin treatment on the progression of aortic valve sclerosis and stenosis. *Am J Cardiol.* 2008;102:738-742.

# 42 Pediatric Cardiovascular Disease

**Burden of Coronary Artery Disease in Adults With Congenital Heart Disease and Its Relation to Congenital and Traditional Heart Risk Factors**

Giannakoulas G, Dimopoulos K, Engel R, et al (Royal Brompton Hosp, London, UK)

*Am J Cardiol* 103:1445-1450, 2009

As adult patients with congenital heart disease (CHD) grow older, the risk of developing coronary artery disease (CAD) increases. We sought to estimate the prevalence of CAD in adult patients with CHD, the safety of coronary angiography in this setting, and the potential relation of CAD to clinical and hemodynamic parameters. Two hundred fifty adult patients with CHD (mean age 51 ± 15 years; 53% men) underwent selective coronary angiography in our center for reasons other than suspected CAD. Clinical and hemodynamic data were retrieved retrospectively from medical records and echocardiographic and angiographic databases, respectively. Significant CAD using quantitative coronary angiography was found in 9.2% of adult patients with CHD. No patient with cyanosis or age <40 years had significant CAD. Systolic and diastolic systemic ventricular dimensions were significantly higher in patients with CAD, even after adjustment for age (odds ratio [OR] for 10-mm increase 2.59, 95% confidence interval [CI] 1.29 to 5.21, $p = 0.007$; OR 2.31, 95% CI 1.24 to 4.31, $p = 0.008$, respectively). Systemic arterial hypertension and hyperlipidemia were strong predictors of CAD (OR 4.54, 95% CI 1.82 to 12.0, $p = 0.001$; OR 9.08, 95% CI 3.56 to 24.54, $p < 0.0001$, respectively), whereas no relation to chest pain was found. Only 1 major adverse event was recorded during coronary angiography. In conclusion, the prevalence of significant CAD in a hospital adult CHD cohort was similar to that in the general population. This study supported the performance of selective coronary angiography in patients >40 years referred for cardiac surgery, with low risk of major complications. Traditional cardiovascular risk factors for CAD also applied to adult patients with CHD, in whom primary prevention of CAD was as important as in the general population.

▶ This interesting article indicates that coronary artery disease (CAD) is present in a similar prevalence to patients without congenital heart disease (CHD). An exception to this finding is that cyanotic patients appear to have a lower incidence of CAD despite having dilated and tortuous arteries. Risk factors for CAD follow the usual pattern seen in patients without CHD. These data support the performance of coronary angiography in all patients with CHD 40 or more years before cardiac surgery.

**T. P. Graham, Jr, MD**

---

### The Natural History of Asymptomatic Ventricular Pre-Excitation. A Long-Term Prospective Follow-Up Study of 184 Asymptomatic Children

Santinelli V, Radinovic A, Manguso F, et al (San Raffaele Scientific Inst, Milan, Italy)

*J Am Coll Cardiol* 53:275-280, 2009

---

*Objectives.*—The aim of this study was to describe the natural history of asymptomatic ventricular pre-excitation in children and to determine predictors of potentially life-threatening arrhythmic events.

*Background.*—Sudden death can be the first clinical manifestation in asymptomatic children with ventricular pre-excitation, but reduction of its incidence by prophylactic ablation requires the identification of subjects at high risk.

*Methods.*—Between 1995 and 2005 we prospectively collected clinical and electrophysiologic data from 184 children (66% male; median age 10 years; range 8 to 12 years) with asymptomatic ventricular pre-excitation on the electrocardiogram. After electrophysiologic testing, subjects were followed as outpatients taking no medications. The primary end point of the study was the occurrence of arrhythmic events. Predictors of potentially life-threatening arrhythmias were analyzed.

*Results.*—Over a median follow-up of 57 months (min/max 32/90 months) after electrophysiologic testing, 133 children (mean age 10 years; range 8 to 12 years) did not experience arrhythmic events, remaining totally asymptomatic, while 51 children had within 20 months (min/max 8/60 months) a first arrhythmic event, which was potentially life-threatening in 19 of them (mean age 10 years; range 10 to 14 years). Life-threatening tachyarrhythmias resulted in cardiac arrest (3 patients), syncope (3 patients), atypical symptoms (8 patients), or minimal symptoms (5 patients). Univariate analysis identified tachyarrhythmia inducibility ($p < 0.001$), anterograde refractory period of accessory pathways (APERP) $\leq$240 ms ($p < 0.001$), and multiple accessory pathways ($p < 0.001$) as risk factors for potentially life-threatening arrhythmic events. Independent predictors by multivariate analysis were APERP ($p = 0.001$) and multiple accessory pathway ($p = 0.001$).

*Conclusions.*—These findings are potentially relevant in terms of early identification of high-risk asymptomatic children with ventricular pre-excitation. Subjects with short APERPs and multiple pathways are at higher risk of developing life-threatening arrhythmic events and are the best candidates for prophylactic ablation.

▶ This study clearly indicates that Wolff-Parkinson-White (WPW) on EKG in an asymptomatic child or adolescent is not always a benign condition. There is a definite indication for EP testing and RFA in patients when the risk factors shown in this study are found. Questions remain such as, eg, can the AERP change with time? Does inducibility change with time? If so, shouldn't one go ahead with RFA while the patient is being studied? Hopefully, these questions can be answered in the future.

**T. P. Graham, Jr, MD**

---

**Prevalence of severe congenital heart disease after folic acid fortification of grain products: time trend analysis in Quebec, Canada**

Ionescu-Ittu R, Marelli AJ, Mackie AS, et al (McGill Univ, Montreal, Canada; Univ of Alberta, Edmonton, Canada; et al)

*BMJ* 338:b1673, 2009

---

*Objective.*—To investigate whether the 1998 government policy for mandatory fortification of flour and pasta products with folate was followed by a reduction in the prevalence of severe congenital heart defects.

*Design.*—Time trend analysis.

*Setting.*—Province of Quebec, Canada.

*Participants.*—Infants born in 1990-2005 identified with severe congenital heart defects (tetralogy of Fallot, endocardial cushion defects, univentricular hearts, truncus arteriosus, or transposition complexes) in Quebec administrative databases.

*Methods.*—Data analysed in two time periods (before and after fortification). Birth prevalence measured annually as infants (live and stillbirths) with severe congenital heart defects per 1000 births in Quebec. Changes in the birth prevalence from the period before to the period after fortification were estimated with Poisson regression.

*Results.*—Among the 1 324 440 births in Quebec in 1990-2005 there were 2083 infants born with severe congenital heart defects, corresponding to an average birth prevalence of 1.57/1000 births. Time trend analysis showed no change in the birth prevalence of severe birth defects in the nine years before fortification (rate ratio 1.01, 95% confidence interval 0.99 to 1.03), while in the seven years after fortification there was a significant 6% decrease per year (0.94, 0.90 to 0.97).

*Conclusions.*—Public health measures to increase folic acid intake were followed by a decrease in the birth prevalence of severe congenital heart defects. These findings support the hypothesis that folic acid has a preventive effect on heart defects.

▶ This is potentially exciting news, particularly if future studies document this trend. If the elective termination became higher during the study period, then these results may not have been the cause of the decline in severe congenital heart defects (CHD). Hopefully, such is not the case and the increase in dietary folate may be one of the first public health measures to actually prevent severe CHD.

**T. P. Graham, Jr, MD**

PART SEVEN

# THE DIGESTIVE SYSTEM

NICHOLAS J. TALLEY, MD, PHD

# 43 Esophagus

---

**Medications (NSAIDs, Statins, Proton Pump Inhibitors) and the Risk of Esophageal Adenocarcinoma in Patients With Barrett's Esophagus**

Nguyen DM, Richardson P, El-Serag HB (Veterans Affairs Med Ctr, Houston, TX)

*Gastroenterology* 138:2260-2266, 2010

---

*Background & Aims.*—Limited evidence suggests that proton pump inhibitors (PPI), nonsteroidal anti-inflammatory drugs (NSAID)/aspirin, and statins may be associated with a low risk of esophageal neoplasia. However, the possible effect these medications may have on the risk of esophageal adenocarcinoma (EAC) in patients with existing Barrett's esophagus (BE) is unclear.

*Methods.*—We conducted a nested case-control study in a cohort of patients with BE identified in the national Department of Veterans' Affairs computerized databases. Cases with incident EAC were matched by incidence density sampling to controls with BE who remained without EAC at the date of the EAC diagnosis for the corresponding case. We identified prescriptions for PPI, NSAIDs/aspirin, and statins that were filled between BE diagnosis and EAC diagnosis. Incidence density ratios were calculated using conditional logistic regression models that adjusted for race, outpatient encounters, a disease comorbidity index, and socioeconomic status.

*Results.*—In a cohort of 11,823 patients with first-time BE diagnosis, we examined 116 EAC cases and 696 matched controls. Most cases and controls had at least one filled PPI prescription (95% vs 94%; $P = .5$). In this setting of almost universal PPI use, filled NSAID/aspirin prescriptions were associated with a reduced risk of EAC (adjusted incidence density ratio, 0.64; 95% confidence interval, 0.42–0.97). Filled statin prescriptions also were associated with a reduction in EAC risk (0.55; 95% confidence interval, 0.36–0.86), with a significant trend toward greater risk reduction with longer duration of statin use. However, the strong inverse associations with even short periods of use raise concerns of uncontrolled confounding.

*Conclusions.*—This observational study indicates that in patients with BE using PPI, NSAID/aspirin, or statin therapy might reduce the risk of developing EAC.

▶ These authors have performed a nested case-control study to evaluate the role of several medications in the outcome of patients with Barrett's esophagus. From a database of 11 000 patients, they identified 116 cancer cases and 696 matched controls. Almost all patients were on acid suppression, and the use of nonsteroidal anti-inflammatory drugs, such as aspirin or long-term statins, was associated with a reduction in the risk of developing esophageal adenocarcinoma.

Most patients identified with Barrett's esophagus did not develop cancer, but a subset of patients developed dysplasia, which will develop into cancer. Short-term placebo-controlled trials have suggested a decrease in malignant markers when patients with Barrett's esophagus are treated with aspirin or nonsteroidal agents. To my knowledge, similar data from humans have not been reported with statins. There are several ongoing clinical trials looking at aspirin in Barrett's esophagus. It will be several years before convincing data from these trials are available. For now, the use of aspirin in a patient with Barrett's esophagus who is already on a proton pump inhibitor presents a very low risk of an adverse event and should be considered. The correct dose of aspirin is not clear, but pulmonary data suggest that a full dose (325 mg) may be needed.

**K. R. DeVault, MD**

**Efficacy of Venlafaxine for Symptomatic Relief in Young Adult Patients With Functional Chest Pain: A Randomized, Double-Blind, Placebo-Controlled, Crossover Trial**

Lee H, Kim JH, Min B-H, et al (Sungkyunkwan Univ School of Medicine, Seoul, Korea; Konkuk Univ School of Medicine, Seoul, Korea; et al)

*Am J Gastroenterol* 105:1504-1512, 2010

*Objectives.*—Esophageal hypersensitivity is currently believed to have a crucial role in the pathogenesis of functional chest pain (FCP). The aim of this study was to evaluate the clinical efficacy of venlafaxine, a serotonin–norepinephrine reuptake inhibitor (SNRI), for FCP in young adult patients.

*Methods.*—Patients diagnosed with FCP were randomized to either an extended-release formulation of venlafaxine (75 mg hora somni) or a placebo for 4 weeks. After a washout period of 2 weeks, patients crossed over to the other arm of the study. The primary efficacy variable was the number of patients with > 50% improvement in symptom scores. The secondary efficacy variables were (i) the symptom intensity score during each week, (ii) quality of life (QOL), (iii) the Beck Depression Inventory (BDI) score, and (iv) side effects.

*Results.*—A total of 43 patients (37 men, mean age 23.5 ± 1.9 years) completed the study. A positive response was observed in 52.0% of patients during venlafaxine treatment; 4.0% had a positive response with placebo treatment as assessed by the intention-to-treat analysis (venlafaxine vs. placebo: odds ratio 26.0; 95% confidence interval 5.7–118.8; $P < 0.001$). Results of Short-Form 36 (SF-36) indicated that patients who received venlafaxine treatment had a significantly greater improvement in body pain and emotional role compared with those who received placebo treatment ($P = 0.002$ and $P = 0.002$, respectively). No significant change was noted in the depression score after venalafaxine or placebo treatment. One patient withdrew from the study because of sleep disturbance and loss of appetite while receiving venlafaxine.

*Conclusions.*—Venlafaxine, an SNRI antidepressant, significantly improved symptoms in young adult patients with FCP.

▶ This trial compared a serotonin-norepinephrine reuptake inhibitor antidepressant with placebo in young patients with functional chest pain. The authors found a positive response in 52% of treated patients compared with only 4% of placebo, although complete response was less than 20% on therapy and did not occur at all on placebo. The response in this study did not seem to be related to baseline or any improvement in questionnaire monitored depression. Many health care providers currently treat functional gastrointestinal (GI) disorders, such as functional chest pain, with antidepressants, despite relatively limited data from well-designed trials. This crossover trial provides additional support for that practice. There are several limitations to wide application of these results. This was a very young population (20-29 years), and it is unclear whether similar results could be expected in older patients. The authors also carefully selected the patients by excluding reflux and esophageal dysmotility with endoscopy, pH testing, and manometry, which is reasonable but perhaps different from empirically treating patients who may or may not have been through a similar evaluation. The placebo response rate in this study was also lower than in most studies of functional GI disorders, with the reason for this difference being unclear.

Despite those differences, it is becoming increasingly clear that antidepressants are beneficial in functional GI disorders. In chest pain for example, trazodone, imipramine, and other antidepressants have demonstrated efficacy. Venlafaxine is now another agent that can be tried to help in these often frustrated patients. Gastroenterologists should take time to learn about the indications, dosage, and potential side effects of this class of agents in order to use them safely and effectively in their practices.

**K. R. DeVault, MD**

## Iatrogenic Gastric Acid Suppression and the Risk of Nosocomial *Clostridium difficile* Infection

Howell MD, Novack V, Grgurich P, et al (Beth Israel Deaconess Med Ctr, Boston, MA; Harvard Clinical Res Inst, Boston, MA; Froedtert Hosp, Milwaukee, WI)

*Arch Intern Med* 170:784-790, 2010

*Background.*—The incidence and severity of *Clostridium difficile* infections are increasing. Acid-suppressive therapy has been suggested as a risk factor for *C difficile*, but this remains controversial.

*Methods.*—We conducted a pharmacoepidemiologic cohort study, performing a secondary analysis of data collected prospectively on 101 796 discharges from a tertiary care medical center during a 5-year period. The primary exposure of interest was acid suppression therapy, classified by the most intense acid suppression therapy received (no acid suppression, histamine$_2$-receptor antagonist [$H_2RA$] therapy, daily proton pump inhibitor [PPI], and PPI more frequently than daily).

*Results.*—As the level of acid suppression increased, the risk of nosocomial *C difficile* infection increased, from 0.3% (95% confidence interval [CI], 0.21%-0.31%) in patients not receiving acid suppressive therapy to 0.6% (95% CI, 0.49%-0.79%) in those receiving $H_2RA$ therapy, to 0.9% (95% CI, 0.80%-0.98%) in those receiving daily PPI treatment, and to 1.4% (1.15%-1.71%) in those receiving more frequent PPI therapy. After adjustment for comorbid conditions, age, antibiotics, and propensity score–based likelihood of receipt of acid-suppression therapy, the association persisted, increasing from an odds ratio of 1 (no acid suppression [reference]) to 1.53 (95% CI, 1.12-2.10) ($H_2RA$), to 1.74 (95% CI, 1.39-2.18) (daily PPI), and to 2.36 (95% CI, 1.79-3.11) (more frequent PPI). Similar estimates were found with a matched cohort analysis and with nested case-control techniques.

*Conclusions.*—Increasing levels of pharmacologic acid suppression are associated with increased risks of nosocomial *C difficile* infection. This evidence of a dose-response effect provides further support for the potentially causal nature of iatrogenic acid suppression in the development of nosocomial *C difficile* infection.

▶ There have been several metabolic and infectious complications recently associated with long-term proton pump inhibitor (PPI) therapy. One of these is *Clostridium difficile* infection. This article is a large retrospective analysis of over 100 000 hospital discharges at a single institution. These data once again support the association between PPI therapy and *C difficile*. There was a clear dose response with a rate of 0.3% in patients not on acid suppression and up to 1.4% in patients treated with greater than once daily PPI. After adjusting for comorbidities, a statistical increase in odds ratio was noted to be present, and the odds ratio increased as treatment moved from histamine$_2$-receptor antagonist (1.53) to daily PPI (1.74) to high-dose PPI (2.36).

How should providers react to studies like this, which suggest a small but statistically significant risk with PPI therapy? First, this study and others confirm that *C difficile* is not only associated with antibiotic therapy, older age, and multiple comorbidities but also associated with PPI use. Interestingly, high-dose PPI had an odds ratio (2.36) intermediate between low-risk antibiotics (1.82) and high-risk antibiotics (3.37). Secondly, up to 60% of the population is exposed to acid suppression medication, and over 15% of PPI prescriptions are for greater than once daily dosing, despite minimal evidence of improved efficacy at higher doses. Finally, *C difficile* infection is increasing and becoming a greater public health issue.

The authors made several valid conclusions. Each patient should have their acid suppression tailored to control symptoms or mucosal disease at the minimally effective dose. Also, not all hospitalized patients need stress ulcer prophylaxis. Finally, this issue needs continued study to develop better cost-benefit ratios in both the outpatient and inpatient environments.

**K. R. DeVault, MD**

# 44 Gastrointestinal Cancers and Benign Polyps

**Low Risk of Colorectal Cancer and Advanced Adenomas More Than 10 Years After Negative Colonoscopy**

Brenner H, Haug U, Arndt V, et al (German Cancer Res Ctr, Heidelberg, Germany; et al)

*Gastroenterology* 138:870-876, 2010

*Background & Aims.*—Screening colonoscopy is an effective method to reduce the incidence of and mortality from colorectal cancer (CRC). There is little empirical evidence available about the optimal interval for screening, making this a subject of debate. We associated the prevalence of advanced colorectal neoplasms with time since negative colonoscopies.

*Methods.*—In a study of participants in the German colonoscopy screening program, we determined the prevalence of colorectal neoplasias detected at screening colonoscopy among subjects who had undergone a previous colonoscopy without detection of polyps (negative colonoscopy). Data were compared with that from subjects who had not received colonoscopies.

*Results.*—No CRCs were detected in participants who had a previous negative colonoscopy an average of 11.9 years previously (n = 553), compared with the 8.4 CRC cases expected based on age- and gender-specific prevalences among participants who had not received a colonoscopy (n = 2701; standardized prevalence ratio [SPR] = 0.00; 95% confidence interval [CI]: 0.00–0.55). Prevalence of advanced adenoma was also much lower among subjects who had previous colonoscopies (SPR = 0.42; 95% CI: 0.25–0.68). Adjusted prevalence ratios (95% CIs) for detecting an advanced adenoma were 0.38 (95% CI: 0.16–0.90), 0.34 (95% CI: 0.15–0.74), 0.38 (95% CI: 0.16–0.90), and 0.53 (95% CI: 0.27–1.04) among participants with a negative colonoscopy conducted 1–5, 6–10, 11–15, and >16 years ago, respectively, compared to participants with no previous colonoscopy.

TABLE 2.—Findings at Screening Colonoscopy According to History of Previous Colonoscopy

| Previous Colonoscopy | Colorectal Cancer n | Colorectal Cancer % | Advanced Adenoma[a] n | Advanced Adenoma[a] % | Other Adenoma n | Other Adenoma % | Hyperplastic Polyp n | Hyperplastic Polyp % | Unspecified Polyp n | Unspecified Polyp % | None n | None % |
|---|---|---|---|---|---|---|---|---|---|---|---|---|
| | Most Advanced Finding at Screening Colonoscopy | | | | | | | | | | | |
| No (n = 2701) | 41 | 1.5 | 267 | 9.9 | 494 | 18.3 | 281 | 10.4 | 54 | 2.0 | 1564 | 57.9 |
| Yes, no polyps detected | | | | | | | | | | | | |
| 1+ y ago (n = 533) | 0 | 0.0 | 25 | 4.7 | 86 | 16.1 | 33 | 6.2 | 5 | 0.9 | 384 | 72.0 |
| 1–5 y ago (n = 115) | 0 | 0.0 | 5 | 4.4 | 13 | 11.3 | 9 | 7.8 | 1 | 0.9 | 87 | 75.7 |
| 6–10 y ago (n = 166) | 0 | 0.0 | 6 | 3.6 | 31 | 18.7 | 6 | 3.6 | 1 | 0.6 | 122 | 73.5 |
| 11–15 y ago (n = 117) | 0 | 0.0 | 5 | 4.3 | 23 | 19.7 | 9 | 7.7 | 0 | 0.0 | 80 | 68.4 |
| 16+ y ago (n = 135) | 0 | 0.0 | 9 | 6.7 | 19 | 14.1 | 9 | 6.7 | 3 | 2.2 | 95 | 70.4 |

[a]Defined as presence of at least 1 adenoma with at least 1 of the following features: >1 cm in size, tubulovillous or villous components, high-grade dysplasia.

*Conclusions.*—The low risk of CRC and advanced adenomas after a negative colonoscopy supports suggestions that screening intervals be extended to ≥10 years (Table 2).

▶ Colonoscopy is considered the gold standard for screening for colorectal cancer (CRC) because the removal of premalignant adenomatous polyps has been demonstrated to lower the risk of future CRC.[1] Considerable effort has been expended to establish the appropriate interval between surveillance colonoscopy procedures due to the expense and risk of this modality.

The National Polyp Study established high-risk cohorts needing surveillance examinations at 3 years. However, the timing of surveillance after a negative colonoscopy has been more problematic due to the lack of data. A recent prospective study of more than 1200 participants demonstrated very low rates of CRC or advanced neoplasia 5 years after a negative colonoscopy. However, there are few studies to help policy makers determine how far surveillance can be pushed beyond 5 years.

In this cohort study from a small state located in Germany, participants presenting for screening colonoscopy filled out a standardized questionnaire that included whether a previous examination had been performed and if polyps were identified. Outcomes of the colonoscopy were compared between those with a previous negative examination versus first-time examinees. This methodology had been previously validated as accurate in this population.

Table 2 shows that patients with a previous negative colonoscopy up to 16 years before had no cancers and a statistically and clinically significant reduction in advanced adenomas. Not surprisingly, the rate of small polyps was similar in the 2 groups. The authors conclude that surveillance intervals after a negative colonoscopy could be extended to 10 years and possibly beyond.

This well-designed but relatively small study (n = 533 subjects in the negative examination cohort) is unlikely to quell the controversy or need for prospective studies to address surveillance intervals. This is especially true in light of recent studies indicating a relative lack of protection in larger population studies from right-sided colon cancer.

**R. K. Pearson, MD**

*Reference*

1. Winawer SJ, Zauber AG, Ho MN, et al. Prevention of colorectal cancer by colonoscopic polypectomy. The National Polyp Study Workgroup. *N Engl J Med.* 1993;329:1977-1981.

---

**Once-only flexible sigmoidoscopy screening in prevention of colorectal cancer: a multicentre randomised controlled trial**

Atkin WS, UK Flexible Sigmoidoscopy Trial Investigators (Imperial College London, UK; et al)

*Lancet* 375:1624-1633, 2010

---

*Background.*—Colorectal cancer is the third most common cancer worldwide and has a high mortality rate. We tested the hypothesis that only one flexible sigmoidoscopy screening between 55 and 64 years of age can substantially reduce colorectal cancer incidence and mortality.

*Methods.*—This randomised controlled trial was undertaken in 14 UK centres. 170 432 eligible men and women, who had indicated on a previous questionnaire that they would accept an invitation for screening, were randomly allocated to the intervention group (offered flexible sigmoidoscopy screening) or the control group (not contacted). Randomisation by sequential number generation was done centrally in blocks of 12, with stratification by trial centre, general practice, and household type. The primary outcomes were the incidence of colorectal cancer, including prevalent cases detected at screening, and mortality from colorectal cancer. Analyses were intention to treat and per protocol. The trial is registered, number ISRCTN28352761.

*Findings.*—113 195 people were assigned to the control group and 57 237 to the intervention group, of whom 112 939 and 57 099, respectively, were included in the final analyses. 40 674 (71%) people underwent flexible sigmoidoscopy. During screening and median follow-up of 11·2 years (IQR 10·7–11·9), 2524 participants were diagnosed with colorectal cancer (1818 in control group *vs* 706 in intervention group) and 20 543 died (13 768 *vs* 6775; 727 certified from colorectal cancer [538 *vs* 189]). In intention-to-treat analyses, colorectal cancer incidence in the intervention group was reduced by 23% (hazard ratio 0·77, 95% CI 0·70–0·84) and mortality by 31% (0·69, 0·59–0·82). In per-protocol analyses, adjusting for self-selection bias in the intervention group, incidence of colorectal cancer in people attending screening was reduced by 33% (0·67, 0·60–0·76) and mortality by 43% (0·57, 0·45–0·72). Incidence of distal colorectal cancer (rectum and sigmoid colon) was reduced

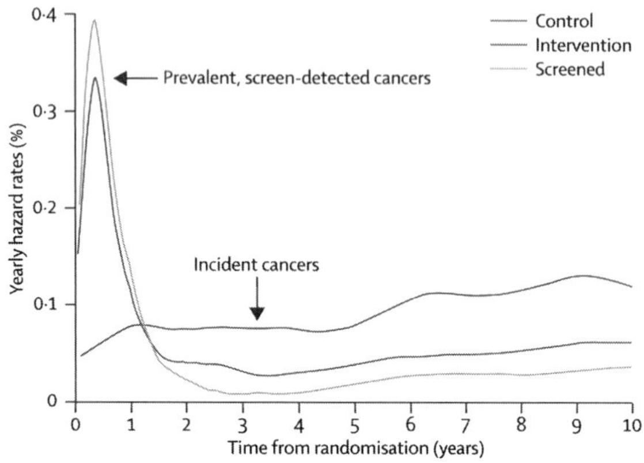


FIGURE 3.—Smoothed yearly hazard rates for distal cancer (rectum and sigmoid colon). Curves are truncated at 10 years of follow-up because of incomplete ascertainment of cancers in the final calendar year of the study. Reprinted from Atkin WS, UK Flexible Sigmoidoscopy Trial Investigators. Once-only flexible sigmoidoscopy screening in prevention of colorectal cancer: a multicentre randomised controlled trial. *Lancet*. 2010;375:1624-1633, with permission from Elsevier.

by 50% (0·50, 0·42–0·59; secondary outcome). The numbers needed to be screened to prevent one colorectal cancer diagnosis or death, by the end of the study period, were 191 (95% CI 145–277) and 489 (343–852), respectively.

*Interpretation.*—Flexible sigmoidoscopy is a safe and practical test and, when offered only once between ages 55 and 64 years, confers a substantial and longlasting benefit (Fig 3).

▶ While assumptions are made about the value of colonoscopy screening in reducing colorectal cancer (CRC) incidence and mortality, it is important to recognize the limitations of the evidence to date. The often-cited report by Atkin and colleagues[1] on 60% to 70% reduction of CRC incidence within the reach of sigmoidoscopy screening is based on a case-control study. The even higher protection afforded by colonoscopic polypectomy (76%-90%) reported in the National Polyp Study used historical controls.[2] Definitive evidence from a sufficiently powered randomized controlled trial has been lacking until this report in *The Lancet*.

Atkin and colleagues from the United Kingdom followed up their influential case-control study reported in the 1990s with this highly anticipated large-scale, randomized, multicenter trial of once-only flexible sigmoidoscopy in preventing CRC. Advocates of colonoscopy screening will be pleased with the results. Table 3 in the original article summarizes the important outcomes: a 50% reduction in incidence and a 43% reduction in mortality in patients receiving sigmoidoscopy compared with a control group. This result is large for any cancer screening test and compares favorably with mammography and prostate-specific antigen testing for prostate cancer.

This study used a prerandomization questionnaire to improve compliance in the sigmoidoscopy group; only potential participants indicating willingness to undergo sigmoidoscopy were enrolled in the intervention group. The 71% enrollment rate even with this prescreening methodology points out one of the challenges with endoscopic screening—patient acceptance.

One of the reasons for the less than 70% to 80% expected reduction of CRC incidence within the reach of sigmoidoscopy is the impact of the detection of prevalent cancers demonstrated in Fig 3. Prevalent CRCs dilute the impact of polypectomy on the reduction of incident cancers. While the follow-up of 11 years in this study is impressive, longer follow-up will likely continue to show additional benefits from the sigmoidoscopy and polyp removal. It is also important to acknowledge that this study was once-only sigmoidoscopy; other large-scale trials that include serial examinations are underway.

Not surprisingly, the rate and mortality from right-sided cancer were not influenced by this study. This is particularly true given the restrictions placed on colonoscopy screening; only patients with advanced or multiple (> 3) adenomas were referred. This represented only 5% of the subjects. A randomized trial of colonoscopy has been started in Europe, but there is concern that in the current climate of enthusiasm for CRC screening, enrollment will suffer.

In the meantime, this important study provides the first-tier[1] evidence that endoscopic screening with polypectomy protects against CRC.

**R. K. Pearson, MD**

*References*

1. Atkin W, Morson B, Cuzick J. Long-term risk of colorectal cancer after excision of rectosigmoid adenomas. *N Engl J Med.* 1992;326:658-662.
2. Winawer SJ, Zauber AG, Ho MN, et al. Prevention of colorectal cancer by colonoscopic polypectomy. The National Polyp Study Workgroup. *N Engl J Med.* 1993;329:1977-1981.

## Medications (NSAIDs, Statins, Proton Pump Inhibitors) and the Risk of Esophageal Adenocarcinoma in Patients With Barrett's Esophagus

Nguyen DM, Richardson P, El-Serag HB (Veterans Affairs Med Ctr, Houston, TX)

*Gastroenterology* 138:2260-2266, 2010

*Background & Aims.*—Limited evidence suggests that proton pump inhibitors (PPI), nonsteroidal anti-inflammatory drugs (NSAID)/aspirin, and statins may be associated with a low risk of esophageal neoplasia. However, the possible effect these medications may have on the risk of esophageal adenocarcinoma (EAC) in patients with existing Barrett's esophagus (BE) is unclear.

*Methods.*—We conducted a nested case-control study in a cohort of patients with BE identified in the national Department of Veterans' Affairs computerized databases. Cases with incident EAC were matched by incidence density sampling to controls with BE who remained without EAC at the date of the EAC diagnosis for the corresponding case. We identified prescriptions for PPI, NSAIDs/aspirin, and statins that were filled between BE diagnosis and EAC diagnosis. Incidence density ratios were calculated using conditional logistic regression models that adjusted for race, outpatient encounters, a disease comorbidity index, and socioeconomic status.

*Results.*—In a cohort of 11,823 patients with first-time BE diagnosis, we examined 116 EAC cases and 696 matched controls. Most cases and controls had at least one filled PPI prescription (95% vs 94%; $P = .5$). In this setting of almost universal PPI use, filled NSAID/aspirin prescriptions were associated with a reduced risk of EAC (adjusted incidence density ratio, 0.64; 95% confidence interval, 0.42–0.97). Filled statin prescriptions also were associated with a reduction in EAC risk (0.55; 95% confidence interval, 0.36–0.86), with a significant trend toward greater risk reduction with longer duration of statin use. However, the strong inverse associations with even short periods of use raise concerns of uncontrolled confounding.

*Conclusions.*—This observational study indicates that in patients with BE using PPI, NSAID/aspirin, or statin therapy might reduce the risk of developing EAC (Table 3).

▶ The Veterans Affairs (VA) system of health care delivery is a national integrated system that approximates the national databases that Canadian and European investigators exploit for large-scale epidemiological studies. The VA system largely included male patients and has limitations. However, Barrett's esophagus (BE) and the risk of esophageal adenocarcinoma (EAC) is predominantly a disease of older men, making this database an acceptable resource for this association.

Chemoprevention for BE would be an attractive development, given that EAC has increased by 6-fold over the past 3 decades.[1] Aspirin or nonsteroidal anti-inflammatory drug (NSAID) is a recognized protective agent for colorectal cancer, and observational studies have suggested a protective effect in EAC. These studies have been limited by the lack of information on the presence or the absence of BE in the control groups. Thus, it's not clear whether the protective effect is because of the prevention of BE or the progression of BE to EAC. Several studies have also suggested that inhibitors of 3-hydroxy-3-methylgluaryl coenzyme A reductase (statins) used commonly in patients with coronary artery disease protect against the development of cancer; studies specific for EAC complicating BE are lacking.

In this large-scale (11 823 patients with a first-time BE diagnosis) study, 116 cases of EAC complicating this large cohort were compared (1:6) with controls without a cancer diagnosis for the use of proton pump inhibitors, aspirin/NSAIDs, and statins. The strengths of the study are the large cohort and the accuracy of the database that measures prescriptions filled or dispensed (not prescribed), increasing the likelihood that the data represent drug usage. As Table 3 demonstrates, NSAIDs/aspirin and statin usage was protective against the development of EAC in a linear dose-dependent fashion, strengthening the possibility of a true chemopreventive effect of these agents.

**TABLE 3.**—The Association Between Duration of Filled Prescriptions and the Risk of EAC

| Duration of Filled Prescriptions, mo | Cases n (%) | Controls n (%) | Incidence Density Ratio (95% CI) | Cochrane–Armitage Trend Test, *P* Value |
|---|---|---|---|---|
| Number of patients | 116 | 696 | | |
| PPI | | | | |
| 0 | 6 (5.2) | 43 (6.2) | Reference | |
| >0 to 12 | 62 (53.5) | 328 (47.1) | 1.39 (0.33–3.41) | |
| >12 to 24 | 31 (26.7) | 219 (31.5) | 0.89 (0.33–2.36) | |
| >24 | 17 (14.7) | 106 (15.2) | 1.00 (0.33–3.00) | |
| NSAIDs/aspirin[a] | | | | .30 |
| 0 | 59 (50.9) | 285 (41.0) | Reference | |
| >0 to 12 | 43 (37.1) | 295 (42.4) | 0.70 (0.46–1.07) | |
| >12 | 14 (12.1) | 116 (16.6) | 0.55 (0.29–1.06) | |
| Statins[a] | | | | .02 |
| 0 | 75 (64.7) | 360 (51.7) | Reference | |
| >0 to 12 | 23 (19.8) | 175 (25.1) | 0.63 (0.38–1.06) | |
| >12 | 18 (15.5) | 161 (23.2) | 0.52 (0.30–0.91) | |

NOTE. Cases were patients with BE and EAC, and controls were patients with BE and no EAC at the time of diagnosis or corresponding case.

[a]More than 24 months was not examined because <5% of patients were in this category.

There are several limitations to this study, including the restricted population studied (VA health care system) and prescriptions abstracted from the VA Pharmacy Benefit Management database; prescriptions filled outside this system would have escaped capture. However, previous studies have shown a 64% capture rate among Medicare-covered veterans. Similar to most nested case-control studies involving prescription medications, lifestyle habits linked to the use of preventive medication could not be accounted for. Statin and NSAID/aspirin use could be functioning as a surrogate for these behaviors (eg, tobacco, alcohol use, obesity).

Cohort studies such as these often generate hypotheses that lead to clinical trials, the cyclooxygenase inhibitor trials in colorectal cancer prevention being 1 important example. While the authors recommend caution when interpreting an observational study such as this, these findings warrant additional studies to evaluate the potential for statins in the prevention of esophageal cancer.

**R. K. Pearson, MD**

### *Reference*

1. Pera M. Trends in incidence and prevalence of specialized intestinal metaplasia, Barrett's esophagus, and adenocarcinoma of the gastroesophageal junction. *World J Surg*. 2003;27:999-1008.

## Antidiabetic Therapies Affect Risk of Pancreatic Cancer

Li D, Yeung S–CJ, Hassan MM, et al (The Univ of Texas M. D. Anderson Cancer Ctr, Houston)

*Gastroenterology* 137:482-488, 2009

*Background & Aims.*—Antidiabetic drugs have been found to have various effects on cancer in experimental systems and in epidemiologic studies, although the association between these therapeutics and the risk of human pancreatic cancer has not been explored. We investigated the effect of antidiabetic therapies on the risk of pancreatic cancer.

*Methods.*—A hospital-based case-control study was conducted at M. D. Anderson Cancer Center from 2004 to 2008 involving 973 patients with pancreatic adenocarcinoma (including 259 diabetic patients) and 863 controls (including 109 diabetic patients). Information on diabetes history and other risk factors was collected by personal interview. The frequencies of use of insulin, insulin secretagogues, metformin, and other antidiabetic medications among diabetic patients were compared between cases and controls. The risk of pancreatic cancer was estimated using unconditional logistic regression analysis.

*Results.*—Diabetic patients who had taken metformin had a significantly lower risk of pancreatic cancer compared with those who had not taken metformin (odds ratio, 0.38; 95% confidence interval, 0.22–0.69; $P = .001$), with adjustments for potential confounders. This difference remained statistically significant when the analysis was restricted to patients with a duration of diabetes >2 years or those who never used insulin. In contrast, diabetic patients who had taken insulin or insulin secretagogues had a significantly higher risk of pancreatic cancer compared with diabetic patients who had not taken these drugs.

*Conclusions.*—Metformin use was associated with reduced risk, and insulin or insulin secretagogue use was associated with increased risk of pancreatic cancer in diabetic patients.

▶ Pancreatic cancer (PC) has the poorest prognosis among primary gastrointestinal (GI) malignancies and is the fourth leading cause of cancer death. Established risk factors for PC include smoking, obesity, chronic pancreatitis, and a family history. The relationship between type 2 diabetes mellitus (DM2) and PC is a complex one. Recent evidence indicates that even early, subclinical PC induces diabetes, probably through a mechanism of insulin resistance.[1,2] In these studies, PC appears to be the cause of new onset glucose intolerance in adults approximately 1% of the time (1 in 125).[1] Alternatively, long-standing DM2 has been associated with an increased risk of PC. Furthermore, hyperinsulinemia associated with the metabolic syndrome can be proposed as a mechanism for the observed increased risk of PC and other malignancies in obesity.

Insulin is a growth-promoting hormone and the exocrine pancreas could be chronically exposed to high local concentrations of this mitogenic factor in hyperinsulinemic states. Therapies for DM2 include agents that both increase

TABLE 4.—Duration of Antidiabetic Therapy and Risk of Pancreatic Cancer

| | All Subjects | | Diabetes Duration >2 Years | |
|---|---|---|---|---|
| Duration of Use (*y*) | No. of Cases/No. of Controls | OR (95% CI)[a]/*P* Value | No. of Cases/No. of Controls | OR (95% CI)[a]/*P* Value |
| Insulin | | | | |
| Never use | 147/88 | 1.0 | 58/63 | 1.0 |
| ≤2 | 70/4 | 11.3 (3.86–33.3)/<.001 | 36/1 | 33.5 (4.26–264)/.001 |
| 3–5 | 9/0 | — | 9/0 | — |
| >5 | 17/9 | 1.30 (0.52–3.23)/.572 | 17/9 | 2.78 (1.00–7.73)/.049 |
| Metformin | | | | |
| Never use | 138/32 | 1.0 | 62/24 | 1.0 |
| ≤2 | 63/35 | 0.34 (0.18–0.63)/.001 | 11/14 | 0.26 (0.09–0.74)/.012 |
| 3–5 | 23/10 | 0.44 (0.18–1.09)/.076 | 23/10 | 0.89 (0.33–2.42)/.816 |
| >5 | 29/27 | 0.18 (0.09–0.38)/<.001 | 29/27 | 0.30 (0.13–0.69)/.005 |
| Insulin secretagogues | | | | |
| Never use | 171/84 | 1.0 | 78/57 | 1.0 |
| ≤2 | 50/6 | 4.94 (1.90–12.8)/.001 | 14/4 | 1.91 (0.54–6.76)/.314 |
| 3–5 | 16/7 | 1.05 (0.40–2.77)/.924 | 16/7 | 1.68 (0.61–4.67)/.317 |
| >5 | 16/8 | 0.71 (0.27–1.90)/.498 | 16/8 | 1.01 (0.35–2.93)/.987 |

[a]OR was adjusted for age, sex, race, smoking, alcohol, BMI, and family history of cancer.

circulating insulin (eg, exogenous insulin, sulfonylureas) or reduce insulin resistance (biguanides, including metformin). Recent epidemiological studies showed that long-term use of metformin was associated with a reduction in the risk of dying from cancer.[3]

To further explore this provocative hypothesis, this well-designed case-control study from M. D. Anderson examined the relationship between antidiabetic therapies and risk of PC. Metformin use was associated with a significant reduction in PC risk and as shown in Table 4, using the agent for more than 5 years resulted in an 80% risk reduction. The study also suggests that therapies associated with higher insulin levels have a higher-than-average risk of PC. The authors openly acknowledge the potential limitations of this case-control study, including recall bias, limited sample size (973 PC subjects), and the single, tertiary referral hospital sample. These observations require confirmation from other centers and in larger populations. However, this remarkable study suggests that this strategy may provide primary chemoprevention for patients with DM2 against this dreadful disease.

**R. K. Pearson, MD**

*References*


1. Chari ST, Leibson CL, Rabe KG, et al. Pancreatic cancer-associated diabetes mellitus: prevalence and temporal association with diagnosis of cancer. *Gastroenterology.* 2008;134:95-101.
2. Pannala R, Leiness JB, Bamlet WR, Basu A, Petersen GM, Chari ST. Prevalence and clinical profile of pancreatic cancer-associated diabetes mellitus. *Gastroenterology.* 2008;134:981-987.
3. Evans JMM, Donnelly LA, Emslie-Smith AM, Alessi DR, Morris AD. Metformin and reduced risk of cancer in diabetic patients. *BMJ.* 2005;330:1304-1305.

# 45 Gastrointestinal Motility Disorders

**Medical records documentation of constipation preceding Parkinson disease: A case-control study**

Savica R, Carlin JM, Grossardt BR, et al (Mayo Clinic, Rochester, MN)

*Neurology* 73:1752-1758, 2009

*Objective.*—Parkinson disease (PD) may affect the autonomic nervous system and may cause constipation; however, few studies have explored constipation preceding the motor onset of PD. We investigated constipation preceding PD using a case-control study design in a population-based sample.

*Methods.*—Using the medical records-linkage system of the Rochester Epidemiology Project, we identified 196 subjects who developed PD in Olmsted County, MN, from 1976 through 1995. Each incident case was matched by age (±1 year) and sex to a general population control. We reviewed the complete medical records of cases and controls in the medical records-linkage system to ascertain the occurrence of constipation preceding the onset of PD (or index year).

*Results.*—Constipation preceding PD or the index year was more common in cases than in controls (odds ratio [OR] 2.48; 95% confidence interval [CI] 1.49 to 4.11; $p = 0.0005$). This association remained significant after adjusting for smoking and coffee consumption (ever vs never), and after excluding constipation possibly induced by drugs. In addition, the association remained significant in analyses restricted to constipation documented 20 or more years before the onset of motor symptoms of PD. Although the association was stronger in women than in men and in patients with PD with rest tremor compared with patients with PD without rest tremor, these differences were not significant.

*Conclusions.*—Our findings suggest that constipation occurring as early as 20 or more years before the onset of motor symptoms is associated with an increased risk of Parkinson disease.

▶ The concept that Parkinson disease, a neurodegenerative disorder, may first manifest with symptoms of constipation before the classical diagnostic neurological symptoms and signs is supported by this well-done medical records linkage case-control study. Surprisingly, constipation could be experienced 20 or more years before the first onset of the symptoms of Parkinson disease. The results are biologically plausible because the neuropathology of Parkinson disease include changes in the autonomic nervous system, which clearly can alter gastrointestinal tract function. Of course, there are other potential explanations for the association, including the fact that there may be a third unknown causal factor that manifests with both constipation and later Parkinson's disease. Such a causal factor might represent for example a genetic susceptibility to both conditions. Gastroenterologists should be aware of this association and be on the lookout in their patients with long-standing constipation for early signs of Parkinson's disease.

**N. J. Talley, MD, PhD**

---

**High Incidence of Mortality and Recurrent Bleeding in Patients With *Helicobacter pylori*–Negative Idiopathic Bleeding Ulcers**

Wong GL-H, Wong VW-S, Chan Y, et al (The Chinese Univ of Hong Kong, China; Hong Kong SAR, China)

*Gastroenterology* 137:525-531, 2009

---

*Background & Aims.*—The long-term prognosis of peptic ulcers associated with neither *Helicobacter pylori* nor nonsteroidal anti-inflammatory drugs (NSAIDs) is unknown.

*Methods.*—This 7-year prospective cohort study recruited patients with bleeding ulcers from January to December 2000. *H pylori*–negative idiopathic bleeding ulcers were defined as having tested negative for *H pylori*, having no exposure to aspirin or analgesics within 4 weeks before endoscopy, and having no other identifiable causative factors. After ulcers healed, patients were divided into 2 groups: patients with prior *H pylori*–negative idiopathic bleeding ulcers (*H pylori*–negative idiopathic ulcer cohort; n = 120) and those with *H pylori*–positive, NSAID-negative bleeding ulcers who received eradication therapy (*H pylori* ulcer cohort; n = 213). Both groups were followed for ≤7 years without gastroprotective therapy. The primary endpoints were recurrent ulcer bleeding and mortality.

*Results.*—The 7-year cumulative incidence of recurrent ulcer bleeding was 42.3% (95% CI, 36.5%–48.1%) in the *H pylori*–negative idiopathic ulcer cohort and 11.2% (95% CI, 8.8%–13.6%) in the *H pylori* ulcer cohort (a difference of 31.1%; 95% CI, 27.7%–34.5%; $P < .0001$). Significantly more patients died in the *H pylori*–negative idiopathic ulcer cohort (87.6%; 95% CI, 83.0%–92.2%) than in the *H pylori* ulcer cohort (37.3%; 95% CI, 34.0%–40.6%) with a difference of 50.3% (95% CI, 49.0%–51.6%; $P < .0001$).

*Conclusions.*—Patients with history of *H pylori*–negative idiopathic bleeding ulcers have a high risk of recurrent ulcer bleeding and mortality.

▶ Since the recognition that *Helicobacter pylori* is causally linked to peptic ulcer disease (PUD), it has become standard practice to ensure *H pylori* is eradicated in all patients with a current or past history of peptic ulcer whether or not they have had upper gastrointestinal bleeding. However, there is a well-recognized group of patients with PUD who have no obvious evidence of *H pylori* infection and have no known exposure to nonsteroidal anti-inflammatory drugs (NSAIDs). In these patients with an idiopathic ulcer who have experienced an upper gastrointestinal bleed, the natural history is unknown and currently long-term acid-suppression therapy is not routinely recommended.

In this large well-conducted cohort study from Hong Kong, 120 patients with *H pylori*-negative idiopathic ulcer bleeding were followed for up to 7 years as was a control cohort with *H pylori*-related ulcer bleeding who underwent *H pylori* eradication therapy. The investigators observed that those with *H pylori*-negative idiopathic bleeding ulcers were about 4 times more likely to have a recurrent ulcer bleed; these data are consistent with observations from Denmark in albeit a much smaller cohort.[1]

The causes of ulcer disease in this *H pylori*-negative cohort are unknown. It may be that there is occult infection that has been missed, although this seems unlikely in most cases. Surreptitious use of NSAIDs is also possible, although the authors meticulously tried to exclude this possibility short of measuring serum salicylate levels. Overall, these data strongly suggest that *H pylori*-negative bleeding ulcer patients need life-long acid-suppression therapy to prevent ulcer recurrence, and this should become the standard of care.

**N. J. Talley, MD, PhD**

*Reference*

1. Bytzer P, Teglbjaerg PS. Danish Ulcer Study Group. *Helicobacter pylori*-negative duodenal ulcers: prevalence, clinical characteristics, and prognosis–results from a randomized trial with 2-year follow-up. *Am J Gastroenterol*. 2001;96: 1409-1416.

---

**Proton pump inhibitors and risk of gastric cancer: a population-based cohort study**

Poulsen AH, Christensen S, McLaughlin JK, et al (Inst of Cancer Epidemiology, Copenhagen, Denmark; Aarhus Univ Hosp, Denmark; International Epidemiology Inst, Rockville MD)

*Br J Cancer* 100:1503-1507, 2009

---

Proton pump inhibitor (PPI) use leads to hypergastrinaemia, which has been associated with gastrointestinal neoplasia. We evaluated the association between PPI use and risk of gastric cancer using population-based health-care registers in North Jutland, Denmark, during 1990–2003. We compared incidence rates among new users of PPI ($n = 18\,790$) or histamine-2-antagonists (H2RAs) ($n = 17\,478$) and non-users of either drug. Poisson regression analysis was used to estimate incidence rate ratios (IRRs) adjusted for multiple confounders. We incorporated a 1-year lag time to address potential reverse causation. We identified 109 gastric cancer cases among PPI users and 52 cases among H2RA users. After incorporating the 1-year lag time, we observed IRRs for gastric cancer of 1.2 (95% CI: 0.8–2.0) among PPI users and 1.2 (95% CI: 0.8–1.8) among H2RA users compared with non-users. These estimates are in contrast to significant overall IRRs of 9.0 and 2.8, respectively, without the lag time. In lag time analyses, increased IRRs were observed among PPI users with the largest number of prescriptions or the longest follow-up compared with H2RA users or non-users. Although our results point to a major influence of reverse causation and confounding by indication on the association between PPI use and gastric cancer incidence, the finding of increased incidence among PPI users with most prescriptions and longest follow-up warrants further investigation.

▶ Gastrin is a well-known trophic hormone, and hypergastrinaemia is associated with an increased risk of gastric carcinoids and adenocarcinoma. While proton pump inhibitors (PPIs) elevate gastrin levels moderately, the association between PPIs and gastric cancer is controversial. In this Danish population-based cohort study, new uses of PPIs and new uses of H2-receptor antagonists were identified to determine whether gastric cancer rates were increased. A 1-year lag time was incorporated to adjust for confounding by indication; there was no significant association between any of the acid-suppressing drug classes and gastric cancer. The finding of gastric cancer was largely confined to those who had no history of *Helicobacter pylori* eradication supporting an effect of confounding by indication. The data support other epidemiological studies that have failed to find an association of PPI use with gastric cancer once confounding was taken into account.[1] Although these data are not definitive, it appears reasonable for clinicians to reassure their patients that there is no risk of gastric cancer from long-term PPI use based on the best available evidence.

**N. J. Talley, MD, PhD**

*Reference*

1. García Rodríguez LA, Lagergren J, Lindblad M. Gastric acid suppression and risk of oesophageal and gastric adenocarcinoma: a nested case control study in the UK. *Gut*. 2006;55:1538-1544.

---

## A Treatment Trial of Acupuncture in IBS Patients

Lembo AJ, Conboy L, Kelley JM, et al (The Beth Israel Deaconess Med Ctr, Boston, MA; Harvard Med School, Boston, MA; Massachusetts General Hosp, Boston; et al)

*Am J Gastroenterol* 104:1489-1497, 2009

---

*Objectives.*—This study aimed to compare the effects of true and sham acupuncture in relieving symptoms of irritable bowel syndrome (IBS).

*Methods.*—A total of 230 adult IBS patients (75% females, average age: 38.4years) were randomly assigned to 3 weeks of true or sham acupuncture (6 treatments) after a 3-week "run-in" with sham acupuncture in an "augmented" or "limited" patient–practitioner interaction. A third arm of the study included a waitlist control group. The primary outcome was the IBS Global Improvement Scale (IBS-GIS) (range: 1–7); secondary outcomes included the IBS Symptom Severity Scale (IBS-SSS), the IBS Adequate Relief (IBS-AR), and the IBS Quality of Life (IBS-QOL).

*Results.*—Although there was no statistically significant difference between acupuncture and sham acupuncture on the IBS-GIS (41 vs. 32%, $P = 0.25$), both groups improved significantly compared with the waitlist control group (37 vs. 4%, $P = 0.001$). Similarly, small differences that were not statistically significant favored acupuncture over the other three outcomes: IBS-AR (59 vs. 57%, $P = 0.83$), IBS-SSS (31 vs. 21%, $P = 0.18$), and IBS-QOL (17 vs. 13%, $P = 0.56$). Eliminating responders during the run-in period did not substantively change the results. Side effects were generally mild and only slightly greater in the acupuncture group.

*Conclusions.*—This study did not find evidence to support the superiority of acupuncture compared with sham acupuncture in the treatment of IBS.

▶ Alternative therapies are commonly sought by patients with irritable bowel syndrome (IBS) as conventional therapy is considered unsatisfactory by many sufferers. In this high quality National Institutes of Health (NIH) funded trial, acupuncture was compared with sham acupuncture. There were 2 types of sham acupuncture: one with a limited patient practitioner encounter and one where there was an augmented patient-practitioner encounter, which included a warm, friendly, and supportive patient practitioner interaction. In the present report, those who received sham acupuncture were rerandomized to either acupuncture or sham acupuncture, and these results were reported to be completely negative. The addition of a supportive patient-physician relationship did not improve the responder rate with acupuncture. These results strongly suggest that acupuncture is not an option that should be considered for patients with IBS.

The trial design included the removal of patients who had responded to sham acupuncture before the rerandomization process. The authors had hoped that removing these sham responders would increase the gap between active treatment and control but found the exact opposite. These data support the view that the removal of placebo responders in a clinical trial (eg, by doing a run-in study) may actually impair finding real differences if they exist (supporting the current Rome III clinical trial design recommendations).

**N. J. Talley, MD, PhD**

### Fecal Incontinence in US Adults: Epidemiology and Risk Factors

Whitehead WE, Borrud L, Goode PS, et al (Univ of North Carolina at Chapel Hill; Ctrs for Disease Control and Prevention, Hyattsville, MD; Veterans Affairs Med Ctr, Birmingham, AL; et al)
*Gastroenterology* 137:512-517, 2009

*Background & Aims.*—The study aims were to estimate the prevalence of different types and frequencies of fecal incontinence (FI), describe demographic factors, and identify risk factors.

*Methods.*—The National Health and Nutrition Examination Survey (NHANES) assesses health status in the civilian noninstitutionalized US population. The validated Fecal Incontinence Severity Index was added to NHANES in 2005–2006. Participants were 2229 women and 2079 men aged 20 years or older. FI was defined as accidental leakage of solid, liquid, or mucus at least once in the preceding month. Sampling weights were used to obtain prevalence estimates for the national population. Multivariate logistic regression identified independent risk factors.

*Results.*—The estimated prevalence of FI in noninstitutionalized US adults is 8.3% (95% confidence interval, 7.1–9.5) and consists of liquid stool in 6.2%, solid stool in 1.6%, and mucus in 3.1%. It occurs at least weekly in 2.7%. Prevalence is similar in women (8.9%) and men (7.7%) and increases with age from 2.6% in 20 to 29 year olds up to 15.3% in participants aged 70 years and older. FI is not significantly associated with race/ethnicity, education, income, or marital status after adjusting for age. Independent risk factors in women are advancing age, loose or watery stools, more than 21 stools per week, multiple chronic illnesses, and urinary incontinence. Independent risk factors in men are age, loose or watery stools, poor self-rated health, and urinary incontinence.

*Conclusions.*—FI is a prevalent age-related disorder. Chronic diarrhea is a strong modifiable risk factor that may form the basis for prevention and treatment.

▶ More data on the illness burden of fecal incontinence are welcome, as this malady is often hidden by those afflicted because of embarrassment. At least in noninstitutionalized adults, around about 8% of the population report at least one episode of fecal incontinence monthly, 3% report an episode at least weekly, and nearly 1% having daily fecal incontinence.

A few of the other observations are worthy of emphasis. First, urinary incontinence often coexists with fecal incontinence as confirmed by these data; it is important to take the history for both disorders as this may alter management. Second, fecal incontinence is often associated with coexistent diarrhea, and based on clinical experience, effectively treating the diarrhea appears to be critically important for the management of the fecal incontinence in many cases. The identification of diarrhea and effectively managing it is likely to reduce the illness burden of fecal incontinence in the population, which is remarkably high.

**N. J. Talley, MD, PhD**

**Soluble or insoluble fibre in irritable bowel syndrome in primary care? Randomised placebo controlled trial**

Bijkerk CJ, de Wit NJ, Muris JWM, et al (Univ Med Ctr Utrecht, Netherlands; Maastricht Univ, Netherlands; et al)

*BMJ* 339:b3154, 2009

*Objective.*—To determine the effectiveness of increasing the dietary content of soluble fibre (psyllium) or insoluble fibre (bran) in patients with irritable bowel syndrome.

*Design.*—Randomised controlled trial.

*Setting.*—General practice.

*Participants.*—275 patients aged 18-65 years with irritable bowel syndrome.

*Interventions.*—12 weeks of treatment with 10 g psyllium (n = 85), 10 g bran (n = 97), or 10 g placebo (rice flour) (n = 93).

*Main Outcome Measures.*—The primary end point was adequate symptom relief during at least two weeks in the previous month, analysed after one, two, and three months of treatment to assess both short term and sustained effectiveness. Secondary end points included irritable bowel syndrome symptom severity score, severity of abdominal pain, and irritable bowel syndrome quality of life scale.

*Results.*—The proportion of responders was significantly greater in the psyllium group than in the placebo group during the first month (57% *v* 35%; relative risk 1.60, 95% confidence interval 1.13 to 2.26) and the second month of treatment (59% *v* 41%; 1.44, 1.02 to 2.06). Bran was more effective than placebo during the third month of treatment only (57% *v* 32%; 1.70, 1.12 to 2.57), but this was not statistically significant in the worst case analysis (1.45, 0.97 to 2.16). After three months of treatment, symptom severity in the psyllium group was reduced by 90 points, compared with 49 points in the placebo group (P = 0.03) and 58 points in the bran group (P = 0.61 versus placebo). No differences were found with respect to quality of life. Fifty four (64%) of the patients allocated to psyllium, 54 (56%) in the bran group, and 56 (60%) in the placebo group completed the three month treatment period. Early dropout was most common in the bran group; the main reason was that the symptoms of irritable bowel syndrome worsened.

*Conclusions.*—Psyllium offers benefits in patients with irritable bowel syndrome in primary care.

*Trial Registration.*—Clinical trials NCT00189033.

▶ This is a high-quality randomized trial that further explores the potential benefits of fiber in the irritable bowel syndrome (IBS), an approach that has become controversial.[1] Although it is common practice to prescribe fiber for patients with IBS, the recommendation has been called into question by work showing that many patients started on fiber actually can have worse symptoms, especially bloating. This excellent research conducted in primary care clearly demonstrates that psyllium (a soluble fiber product) improves global IBS symptoms and reduces the severity of IBS symptoms. A subtype analysis of the constipation-dominant group showed that psyllium was still better than placebo; while the clinical trial included patients with constipation, diarrhea, or mixed bowel habit, the results are not presented for the diarrhea and alternating groups separately to determine whether psyllium was beneficial here (and the study was not powered to look at such differences). Psyllium was compared with insoluble fiber (bran) that failed to show any efficacy in the first 2 months of treatment, although in the third month bran then appeared to be more efficacious than placebo. It was notable that the bran was more likely to worsen symptoms, especially at the beginning of treatment. The trial did not test whether starting with a very small amount of fiber and slowly building it up would be a better approach than just adding in the supplementation at full dose. However, in clinical practice prescribing fiber with a "start low, go slow" approach appears to be optimal. Overall, these data support the view that psyllium rather than bran represents reasonable first-line therapy for IBS, particularly in the constipation subtype and may be worth trying regardless of subtype.

**N. J. Talley, MD, PhD**

*Reference*

1. Ford AC, Talley NJ, Spiegel BM, et al. Effect of fibre, antispasmodics, and peppermint oil in the treatment of irritable bowel syndrome: systematic review and meta-analysis. *BMJ*. 2008;337:a2313.

# 46 Gastrointestinal Motility Disorders/ Neurogastroenterology

**Ischemic Colitis and Complications of Constipation Associated With the Use of Alosetron Under a Risk Management Plan: Clinical Characteristics, Outcomes, and Incidences**

Chang L, Tong K, Ameen V (David Geffen School of Medicine at UCLA, Los Angeles, CA; Prometheus Laboratories Inc, San Diego, CA)

*Am J Gastroenterol* 105:866-875, 2010

*Objectives.*—Alosetron is a potent, selective 5-$HT_3$ receptor antagonist prescribed for women with severe diarrhea-predominant irritable bowel syndrome (IBS-D) under a risk management plan (RMP). The RMP was implemented following cases of ischemic colitis (IC) and complications of constipation (CoC) associated with the use of alosetron. The Objectives of this study were to characterize IC and CoC clinical features, outcomes, and incidence rates in the new restricted patient population to evaluate the effectiveness of the RMP in the prevention of serious outcomes.

*Methods.*—Safety data from adverse event reporting from November 2002 through June 2008 were reviewed for probable and possible IC and CoC using the US Food and Drug Administration/sponsor-defined criteria and definitions. Evidence for IC included medical documentation, colonoscopy, and sigmoidoscopy ± biopsy. Evidence for CoC included medical history and confirmation from health-care professionals.

*Results.*—Within the inclusion dates, 29,072 patients received 203,939 alosetron prescriptions. Although the absolute numbers of IC and CoC cases have declined, the incidence rates for IC and CoC (0.95 and 0.36 cases per 1,000 patient-years, respectively) were similar to rates during the postmarketing cycle before alosetron withdrawal. In patients with severe IBS-D receiving alosetron ($n = 998$) or placebo ($n = 411$) in clinical trials since reintroduction, incidence rates for IC were 4 and 2 cases per 1,000 patients, respectively. Rates for CoC were 2 and 0 cases per 1,000 patients in the alosetron and placebo groups, respectively. No mesenteric ischemia, surgeries, transfusions, or deaths occurred in patients with IC and no cases of CoC were associated with toxic megacolon, perforation, surgeries, transfusions, or deaths. IC and CoC cases were typically of short duration and all improved on prompt withdrawal of alosetron.

*Conclusions.*—Serious outcomes associated with IC and CoC appear to be mitigated since introduction of alosetron under the RMP.

▶ This is a timely and very important clinical article that all gastroenterologists should review. Lotronex (alosetron hydrochloride) is a selective 5-HT, receptor antagonist that is used for the treatment of women with severe, diarrhea-predominant irritable bowel syndrome. This article reviews the safety data from adverse events reported from 2002-2008. Specifically, the data review cases of ischemic colitis and constipation. Over 29 000 patients were studied. The results of this study have shown that the incidence rates for ischemic colitis (IC) and complications of constipation (CoC) have remained stable in the first 5 years since the introduction of alosetron. Most patients with ulcerative colitis (UC) and CoC had comorbid conditions, and there were no cases of death reported. This is a very important article that clinicians and patients who may be treated should review.

**J. S. Scolapio, MD**

---

**Proton-Pump Inhibitor Use Is Not Associated With Osteoporosis or Accelerated Bone Mineral Density Loss**

Targownik LE, Lix LM, Leung S, et al (Univ of Manitoba, Winnipeg, Canada; Univ of Saskatchewan, Saskatoon, Canada; et al)

*Gastroenterology* 138:896-904, 2010

---

*Backgrounds & Aims.*—Recent studies have shown an association between proton-pump inhibitor use (PPI) and hip fracture. The mechanism by which PPI use promotes the development of hip fracture is uncharacterized. Therefore, we sought to determine whether PPI use is associated with osteoporosis or accelerated bone mineral density (BMD) loss.

*Methods.*—We used the Manitoba Bone Mineral Density Database to determine the relationship between chronic PPI use and osteoporosis on an initial assessment of BMD and on BMD loss between successive assessments of BMD. In the cross-sectional study, cases with osteoporosis at the hip or lumbar vertebrae (T-score $\leq -2.5$) were matched to 3 controls with normal BMD (T-score $\geq -1.0$). In the longitudinal analysis, the change in BMD among PPI users and nonusers between successive BMD assessments was assessed. Conditional logistic regression and multivariate linear regression were used to obtain estimates of the association between PPI use and osteoporosis and of the annualized change in BMD associated with PPI use.

*Results.*—PPI use was not associated with having osteoporosis at either the hip (OR, 0.84; 95% CI, 0.55–1.34) or the lumbar spine (OR, 0.79; 95% CI, 0.59–1.06) for PPI use >1500 doses over the previous 5 years.

In the longitudinal study no significant decrease was observed in BMD at either site attributable to PPI use.

*Conclusions.*—PPI use does not appear to be associated with either the presence of osteoporosis or accelerated BMD loss. The association between PPI use and hip fracture is probably related to factors independent of osteoporosis.

▶ This is an important study that suggests that previous reports linking proton-pump inhibitors (PPIs) with osteopenia or osteoporosis may have been misleading. Both a cross-sectional and longitudinal study were done to investigate the association of PPI use with osteoporosis. In the cross-sectional study 2193 subjects with osteoporosis of the hip were matched to 5527 controls with normal hip measurements. In this analysis, PPI use was actually associated with a lower risk of osteoporosis of the lumbar spine and of the hip. A longitudinal study identified 2549 subjects who had 2 separate bone mineral assessments with a mean interval between assessments of 2.3 years. Again, there was no association between PPI use and osteoporosis. It is conceivable that previous studies of the association may have been biased by the presence of unmeasured confounders, but unfortunately, the jury must remain out regarding this association based on the conflicting data. At this stage, clinicians still need to plot a cautious course when advising patients about the pros and cons of long-term use of PPIs. However, the data here do provide some reassurance. It is not unreasonable to continue to ensure that patients on long-term PPIs are receiving adequate amounts of calcium and vitamin D.

**N. J. Talley, MD, PhD**

# 47 Inflammatory Bowel Disease

---

**Adjunctive Antibiotic Therapy with Rifaximin May Help Reduce Crohn's Disease Activity**

Shafran I, Burgunder P (Shafran Gastroenterology Ctr, Winter Park, FL)
*Dig Dis Sci* 55:1079-1084, 2010

---

*Aims.*—Enteric bacteria are thought to contribute to the pathogenesis of Crohn's disease, and antibiotics may be an effective therapy. This study examines the efficacy of the nonsystemic (<0.4% absorbed) antibiotic rifaximin for inducing remission in patients with Crohn's disease.

*Methods.*—Data from charts of patients with Crohn's disease who received rifaximin between 2001 and 2005 and had a Crohn's disease activity index score ≥220 at the time of rifaximin initiation were analyzed. The use of concomitant medications (e.g., steroids, anti-inflammatory agents) was allowed.

*Results.*—In the 68 patient charts analyzed, the median duration of rifaximin treatment was 16.6 weeks, and the majority of patients (94%) received rifaximin 600 mg/day. Eighteen patients (26%) received rifaximin monotherapy, and 31 patients (46%) received concomitant steroids. The median baseline Crohn's disease activity index score at the time of rifaximin initiation was 265 (range, 220–460), and the mean duration of Crohn's disease was 17 years (range, 1–50 years). Crohn's disease remission occurred in 65% of patients. A 70% remission rate was achieved in patients who did not receive steroids, versus 58% in patients who received steroids. Clinical improvements continued 4 months after rifaximin initiation. Remission was achieved in 67% of patients who received rifaximin monotherapy.

*Conclusions.*—Rifaximin therapy was associated with clinical improvement in patients with Crohn's disease and may be a useful treatment option to consider for inducing and maintaining remission.

▶ Antibiotic therapies have long been studied as treatments for Crohn's disease (CD). Metronidazole and ciprofloxacin have received the most attention and have had variable results. There may be a role for antibiotics in patients with colonic or ileocolonic disease, especially after surgery to prevent recurrence. Metronidazole has been the most studied and, while showing some efficacy, is often poorly tolerated by patients because of significant side effects.

Rifaximin is an attractive alternative given its broad spectrum of activity and minimal systemic absorption. In this article, the authors suggest that rifaximin may be a treatment option among patients with active CD. Unfortunately, significant problems exist with the study that limited any conclusions that were made. The study was retrospective, and while all patients had a CD activity index score suggesting moderate disease, there may be other factors that influence treatment assignment with rifaximin that cannot be determined. Unfortunately, one cannot understand the impact of rifaximin because of a lack of a comparison group. We cannot determine the effect of other therapies on reported remission rates. Patient characteristics seemingly did not influence remission rates, and while a higher rate of remission was seen in those who did not receive steroids, the difference was small and, given the sample size, unlikely to be statistically significant. If this difference were significant, it might simply reflect a higher disease severity among those taking corticosteroids. High placebo rates in other studies among patients with IBD and the retrospective open-label study design further limit conclusions regarding the use of rifaximin as monotherapy in this article. The limited experience reported by the authors is of value in that it suggests the need to perform randomized clinical studies testing this nonabsorbable antibiotic in the management of CD.

**M. F. Picco, MD, PhD**

---

**Fecal Calprotectin Correlates More Closely With the Simple Endoscopic Score for Crohn's Disease (SES-CD) than CRP, Blood Leukocytes, and the CDAI**

Schoepfer AM, Beglinger C, Straumann A, et al (McMaster Univ, Hamilton, Ontario, Canada; Univ Hosp Basel, Switzerland; et al)

*Am J Gastroenterol* 105:162-169, 2010

---

*Objectives.*—Studies evaluating the correlation between the widely used Simple Endoscopic Score for Crohn's disease (SES-CD) and noninvasive markers are scarce. The aim of this study was to evaluate the correlation between the SES-CD and fecal calprotectin, C-reactive protein (CRP), blood leukocytes, and the Crohn's disease activity index (CDAI).

*Methods.*—Crohn's disease patients undergoing complete ileocolonoscopy were prospectively enrolled and scored independently according to the SES-CD and the CDAI. SES-CD was defined as follows: inactive 0–3; mild 4–10; moderate 11–19; and high ≥20.

*Results.*—Values in CD patients ($n = 140$ ileocolonoscopies) compared with controls ($n = 43$) are as follows: calprotectin, $334 \pm 322$ vs. $18 \pm 5$ μg/g; CRP, $26 \pm 29$ vs. $3 \pm 2$ mg/l; and blood leukocytes, $9.1 \pm 3.4$ vs. $5.4 \pm 1.9$ g/l (all $P < 0.001$). The SES-CD correlated closest with calprotectin (Spearman's rank correlation coefficient $r = 0.75$), followed by CRP ($r = 0.53$), blood leukocytes ($r = 0.42$), and the CDAI ($r = 0.38$). Calprotectin was the only marker that could discriminate inactive endoscopic disease from mild activity (104 ± 138 vs. 231 ± 244 μg/g, $P < 0.001$), mild from moderate activity (231 ± 244 vs. 395 ± 256 μg/g, $P < 0.008$), and moderate from high activity (395 ± 256 vs. 718 ± 320 μg/g, $P < 0.001$). The overall accuracy for the detection of endoscopically active disease was 87% for calprotectin (cutoff 70 μg/g), 66% for elevated CRP, 54% for blood leukocytosis, and 40% for the CDAI ≥150.

*Conclusions.*—Fecal calprotectin correlated closest with SES-CD, followed by CRP, blood leukocytes, and the CDAI. Furthermore, fecal calprotectin was the only marker that reliably discriminated inactive from mild, moderate, and highly active disease, which underlines its usefulness for activity monitoring.

▶ A reliable noninvasive method to assess activity in Crohn's disease (CD) is sorely needed. Endoscopy is costly and invasive. Fecal calprotectin has been shown in some studies to correlate with disease activity in CD. However, the appropriate use of fecal calprotectin in the management of patients with CD remains unsettled. In this study, the authors show a significant correlation of this marker with endoscopic disease severity among a population of patients with CD involving the colon, ileum, or both. Unfortunately, the study does suffer from problems that limit the application of this test for the assessment of disease activity in practice. It is not clear why patients with CD were compared with healthy controls except to provide data of specificity for the fecal calprotectin. The best group of patients to test specificity would be patients with CD and endoscopic quiescent disease who would likely be from a surveillance population. This would establish a fecal calprotectin level for true endoscopically negative patients. A larger population of these patients would lead to better comparisons, especially patients mildly active disease. While accuracy is important, sensitivity and specificity should also have been reported with a receiver operator characteristic curve. As threshold levels of fecal calprotectin increase, sensitivity is likely to go down and specificity likely to increase. This relationship is important to assess the validity of the test. It is not surprising that predictive values for the test were high, given the high prevalence of active disease in the patients tested. The accuracy reported is for distinction between active and inactive disease only. Most patients with active disease had moderate or high disease activity. Patients with moderate or high activity are probably less likely to be confused with irritable bowel syndrome. The role of fecal calprotectin in distinguishing mild from quiescent disease is not addressed in the study. Furthermore, endoscopic activity may not correlate with clinical improvement. Overall, the study does provide useful information on the correlation of endoscopic findings with fecal calprotectin, but more studies are needed to identify the role of this test in practice.

**M. F. Picco, MD, PhD**

## Immunomodulators Are Associated With a Lower Risk of First Surgery Among Patients With Non-Penetrating Non-Stricturing Crohn's Disease

Picco MF, Zubiaurre I, Adluni M, et al (Mayo Clinic, Jacksonville, FL)

*Am J Gastroenterol* 104:2754-2759, 2009

*Objectives.*—Early immunomodulator therapy may alter the natural history of Crohn's disease in certain patients. We determined whether immunomodulator use was associated with a lower risk of first surgery among patients with non-stricturing non-penetrating Crohn's disease.

*Methods.*—A total of 159 consecutive patients with non-penetrating non-stricturing Crohn's disease from 1994 to 2005 were retrospectively identified and followed from diagnosis to either first surgery (surgery group) or last clinic follow-up (medication group) in a historical cohort analysis. Immunomodulator use, duration, disease location, age at diagnosis, smoking, family history, and decade of diagnosis were compared. Cox proportional hazards models were adjusted for propensity score to determine whether immunomodulator use lasting >6 months decreased the risk of first surgery and whether duration of therapy affected risk.

*Results.*—The median duration of follow-up was similar (6.0 vs. 5.5 years), age at diagnosis 10 years earlier, and isolated colonic disease three times less common (18 vs. 49%) in the surgery group as compared with the medication group. Immunomodulator use increased with time but overall was less common in the surgical group (24 vs. 48%). In the multivariate Cox proportional hazards model immunomodulator use was associated with a lower risk of surgery (hazard ratio, 0.41; 95% confidence interval 0.21–0.81) after adjustment for propensity score. Similarly, risk of surgery declined with duration of use.

*Conclusions.*—Immunomodulator use is associated with a decreased risk of first surgery among patients with non-stricturing non-penetrating CD. Early immunomodulator therapy may be beneficial in preventing first surgery in this population that has yet to develop penetrating or fistulizing complications.

▶ Current therapeutic goals in Crohn's disease (CD) have gone beyond induction or remission and now focus on altering natural history. Biologic therapies have been shown to reduce long-term complications. Unfortunately, despite their wide use, there is little evidence that immunomodulator therapies alter the course of CD. In fact, the evidence is conflicting. In this study from our group, we confined our analysis to patients with nonstricturing, nonpenetrating CD. These patients had yet to develop more aggressive behavior and might benefit most from immunomodulator therapy. In our analysis we showed that immunomodulator use (azathioprine or 6-mercaptopurine) did reduce the risk of first surgery. A drawback of the study is that while it was a cohort study, it was a retrospective or historical cohort. While we were careful to account for potential factors that might influence immunomodulator use or surgery leading to a biased result, the potential does remain. We used the propensity score method to adjust for these other factors that may have been associated with immunomodulator therapy independent of the need for surgery and showed that immunomodulator therapy still resulted in a lower risk. Ideally, a prospective randomized trial would answer the question as to whether these agents alter natural history. Unfortunately, such a trial would require significant time and cost, making it unlikely. This study supports the role of immunomodulator therapy in nonstricturing, nonpenetrating CD to alter natural history by reducing the risk of first surgery.

**M. F. Picco, MD, PhD**

---

**Efficacy of Ceftriaxone or Meropenem as Initial Therapies in Whipple's Disease**

Feurle GE, Junga NS, Marth T (DRK Krankenhaus, Neuwied, Germany; St Josef Krankenhaus, Braunau, Austria; Krankenhaus Maria Hilf, Daun, Germany)

*Gastroenterology* 138:478-486, 2010

---

*Background & Aims.*—Whipple's disease is a chronic infection caused by the actinomycete *Tropheryma whipplei*. We conducted a randomized controlled trial of the efficacy of antimicrobials that are able to cross the blood-brain barrier and to which *T whipplei* is susceptible.

*Methods.*—Patients from central Europe with previously untreated Whipple's disease (n = 40) were assigned randomly to groups given daily infusions of either ceftriaxone (1 × 2 g, 20 patients) or meropenem (3 × 1 g, 20 patients) for 14 days, followed by oral trimethoprim-sulfamethoxazole for 12 months. The primary outcome measured was maintenance of remission for 3 years, determined by a composite index of clinical and laboratory data as well as histology.

*Results.*—All patients were observed for the entire follow-up period (median, 89 mo; range, 71–128 mo); all achieved clinical and laboratory remission. Remission was maintained in all patients during the time of observation, except for 2 who died from unrelated causes. A single patient with asymptomatic cerebrospinal infection who was resistant to both treatments responded to chloroquine and minocycline. The odds ratio for the end point (remission for at least 3 years) was 0.95 (95% confidence interval, 0.05–16.29; $P = 1.0$).

*Conclusions.*—This was a randomized controlled trial to show that treatment with ceftriaxone or meropenem, followed by trimethoprim–sulfamethoxazole, cures patients with Whipple's disease. One asymptomatic individual with infection of the cerebrospinal fluid required additional therapy.

▶ Whipple's disease is rare but very important not to miss, as it is otherwise uniformly fatal. Typical presenting clinical features include migratory arthralgias, weight loss, diarrhea, abdominal pain, hyperpigmentation, and neurological symptoms; small bowel biopsy is diagnostic (if periodic acid-Schiff [PAS]-positive macrophages are present). Tetracycline used to be the primary therapy, but there is a high relapse rate with its use. Thus, treatment of this disease can be difficult and has evolved.

This pivotal randomized controlled trial suggests that either intravenous ceftriaxone or meropenem for 2 weeks followed by trimethoprim-sulfamethoxazole for 1 year is efficacious in terms of curing most patients with Whipple's disease. However, as patients with this rare disease may have an immune defect, regular follow-up of them for life (with annual small bowel biopsy) is recommended once therapy is complete to ensure that there has been no disease relapse. It is important to use antibiotics that will cross the blood-brain barrier in order to potentially cure the disease, and this trial suggests that the microbiological approach used was successful in doing this. Another important point from this study is that a lumbar puncture with examination of the cerebrospinal fluid should be part of the workup for *Tropheryma whipplei*.

Appropriate treatment of this potentially fatal disease is critical, and this research provides additional important information for gastroenterologists faced with these rare patients.

**N. J. Talley, MD, PhD**

## Continuation of Low-Dose Aspirin Therapy in Peptic Ulcer Bleeding: A Randomized Trial

Sung JJY, Lau JYW, Ching JYL, et al (Chinese Univ of Hong Kong, Sha Tin, New Territories)

*Ann Intern Med* 152:1-9, 2010

*Background.*—It is uncertain whether aspirin therapy should be continued after endoscopic hemostatic therapy in patients who develop peptic ulcer bleeding while receiving low-dose aspirin.

*Objective.*—To test that continuing aspirin therapy with proton-pump inhibitors after endoscopic control of ulcer bleeding was not inferior to stopping aspirin therapy, in terms of recurrent ulcer bleeding in adults with cardiovascular or cerebrovascular diseases.

*Design.*—A parallel randomized, placebo-controlled noninferiority trial, in which both patients and clinicians were blinded to treatment assignment, was conducted from 2003 to 2006 by using computer-generated numbers in concealed envelopes. (ClinicalTrials.gov registration number: NCT00153725).

*Setting.*—A tertiary endoscopy center.

*Patients.*—Low-dose aspirin recipients with peptic ulcer bleeding.

*Intervention.*—78 patients received aspirin, 80 mg/d, and 78 received placebo for 8 weeks immediately after endoscopic therapy. All patients received a 72-hour infusion of pantoprazole followed by oral pantoprazole. All patients completed follow-up.

*Measurements.*—The primary end point was recurrent ulcer bleeding within 30 days confirmed by endoscopy. Secondary end points were all-cause and specific-cause mortality in 8 weeks.

*Results.*—156 patients were included in an intention-to-treat analysis. Three patients withdrew from the trial before finishing follow-up. Recurrent ulcer bleeding within 30 days was 10.3% in the aspirin group and 5.4% in the placebo group (difference, 4.9 percentage points [95% CI, −3.6 to 13.4 percentage points]). Patients who received aspirin had lower all-cause mortality rates than patients who received placebo (1.3% vs. 12.9%; difference, 11.6 percentage points [CI, 3.7 to 19.5 percentage points]). Patients in the aspirin group had lower mortality rates attributable to cardiovascular, cerebrovascular, or gastrointestinal complications than patients in the placebo group (1.3% vs. 10.3%; difference, 9 percentage points [CI, 1.7 to 16.3 percentage points]).

*Limitations.*—The sample size is relatively small, and only low-dose aspirin, 80 mg, was used. Two patients with recurrent bleeding in the placebo group did not have further endoscopy.

*Conclusion.*—Among low-dose aspirin recipients who had peptic ulcer bleeding, continuous aspirin therapy may increase the risk for recurrent bleeding but potentially reduces mortality rates. Larger trials are needed to confirm these findings.

▶ In clinical practice, patients presenting with peptic ulcer bleeding are usually treated endoscopically to stop the bleeding, provided effective antisecretory therapy (with a proton pump inhibitor [PPI]), and advised to discontinue aspirin or other antiplatelet agents until ulcer healing has occurred. However, patients taking aspirin or antiplatelet agents for major cardiovascular and cerebrovascular disease may have a very unfavorable risk-to-benefit ratio if the aspirin is stopped.

This trial aimed to determine how safe the continuation of low-dose aspirin is in those who present with acute peptic ulcer bleeding. The study was a relatively small randomized controlled trial but was elegantly designed. The authors observed that approximately 10% of patients had recurrent ulcer bleeding who were continued on low-dose aspirin (81 mg per day) compared with a rate of 5% in those on placebo. However, more striking was the observation that mortality rates were actually significantly higher in the placebo group overall. Patients who received aspirin had more gastrointestinal complications but lower cardiovascular and cerebrovascular mortality rates, and indeed the mortality rates from the gastrointestinal complications were still lower on aspirin than placebo.

The patients in this population studied here were relatively ill; they had multiple comorbid conditions and were elderly, and therefore, these results may not apply to younger patients or patients who receive aspirin for inappropriate reasons. Notably, all patients in the trial received a PPI, which is the current standard practice. The results cannot be extrapolated to higher doses of aspirin, although presumably most patients should not receive higher doses for cardiovascular or cerebrovascular prophylaxis.

This important study suggests that early resumption of low-dose aspirin should be strongly considered for all patients who need the medication, although due diligence in terms of follow-up is required to ensure recurrent bleeding is not occurring.

**N. J. Talley, MD, PhD**

---

**Lymphoproliferative disorders in patients receiving thiopurines for inflammatory bowel disease: a prospective observational cohort study**

Beaugerie L, for the CESAME Study Group (Université Pierre et Marie Curie Paris-VI, France; et al)

*Lancet* 374:1617-1625, 2009

---

*Background.*—Reports of an increased risk of lymphoproliferative disorders in patients receiving thiopurines for inflammatory bowel disease are controversial. We assessed this risk in a prospective observational cohort study.

*Methods.*—19 486 patients with inflammatory bowel disease, of whom 11 759 (60·3%) had Crohn's disease and 7727 (39·7%) had ulcerative colitis or unclassified inflammatory bowel disease, were enrolled in a nationwide French cohort by 680 gastroenterologists, who reported details of immunosuppressive therapy during the observation period, cases of cancer, and deaths. The risk of lymphoproliferative disorder was assessed according to thiopurine exposure. Median follow-up was 35 months (IQR 29–40).

*Findings.*—At baseline, 5867 (30·1%) of patients were receiving, 2809 (14·4%) had discontinued, and 10 810 (55·5%) had never received thiopurines. 23 new cases of lymphoproliferative disorder were diagnosed, consisting of one case of Hodgkin's lymphoma and 22 cases of non-Hodgkin lymphoproliferative disorder. The incidence rates of lymphoproliferative disorder were 0·90 per 1000 (95% CI 0·50–1·49) patient-years in those receiving, 0·20/1000 (0·02–0·72) patient-years in those who had discontinued, and 0·26/1000 (0·10–0·57) patient-years in those who had never received thiopurines (p=0·0054). The multivariate-adjusted hazard ratio of lymphoproliferative disorder between patients receiving thiopurines and those who had never received the drugs was 5·28 (2·01–13·9, p=0·0007). Most cases associated with thiopurine exposure matched the pathological range of post-transplant disease.

*Interpretation.*—Patients receiving thiopurines for inflammatory bowel disease have an increased risk of developing lymphoproliferative disorders.

► Previously disputed, the link of thiopurines to malignancy is now becoming very clear. This is one of several recent studies that have linked malignancy, particularly lymphoproliferative disorders, to thiopurine use among patients with inflammatory bowel disease (IBD). A particular advantage of this study is that it is a prospective study identifying a cohort of patients with IBD followed over time. The patients who had received thiopurines were similar to what one would expect in clinical practice. They tended to have Crohn's disease, were younger, and had a longer disease duration. The association of thiopurines with lymphoproliferative disorders was dramatic even after adjustment for the potential confounding factors of advanced age, male sex, and longer duration of IBD. Unfortunately, information regarding thiopurine therapy prior to study entry and thiopurine dose during the follow-up period was not available. Finally, as with other similar studies, the authors cannot separate whether the thiopurine use led to malignancy or was just a marker of more severe inflammatory disease, which alone may be a risk factor. Overall, the results are important and lead to a growing body of literature pointing out the potential hazards of these drugs. The incidence rate of 1/1000 is higher than other studies and is concerning. However, the rate remains low and needs to be interpreted correctly. The risk-benefit ratio still favors the use of these medications in the appropriate patient, particularly as steroid-sparing agents. Physicians must discuss the risks and benefits of all potential therapies to help their patients make informed decisions.

**M. F. Picco, MD, PhD**

---

**Venous thromboembolism during active disease and remission in inflammatory bowel disease: a cohort study**

Grainge MJ, West J, Card TR (Univ of Nottingham, UK)

*Lancet* 375:657-663, 2010

---

*Background.*—Patients with inflammatory bowel disease who develop deep vein thrombosis or pulmonary embolism often have active disease at the time of thromboembolism. We therefore aimed to quantify the risk of venous thromboembolism prospectively during different activity phases of inflammatory bowel disease.

*Methods.*—From the General Practice Research Database, we matched patients with prospectively recorded inflammatory bowel disease from November, 1987, until July, 2001 with up to five controls by age, sex, and general practice. A flare was defined as the period 120 days after a new corticosteroid prescription. We used Cox regression analysis with time-varying covariates to accommodate changes in the state of inflammatory bowel disease, and whether patients were at high risk of venous thromboembolism after hospitalisation.

*Findings.*—13 756 patients with inflammatory bowel disease and 71 672 matched controls were included in the analysis, and of these 139 patients and 165 controls developed venous thromboembolism. Overall, patients with inflammatory bowel disease had a higher risk of venous thromboembolism than did controls (hazard ratio 3·4, 95% CI 2·7–4·3; $p<0·0001$; absolute risk 2·6 per 1000 per person-years). At the time of a flare, however, this increase in risk was much more prominent (8·4, 5·5–12·8; p<0·0001; 9·0 per 1000 person-years). This relative risk at the time of a flare was higher during non-hospitalised periods (15·8, 9·8–25·5; p<0·0001; 6·4 per 1000 person-years) than during hospitalised periods (3·2, 1·7–6·3; p=0·0006; 37·5 per 1000 person-years).

*Interpretation.*—Trials of primary prophylaxis of venous thromboembolism are warranted to find out whether this important complication can be prevented.

▶ The results of this well-done cohort study are sobering. The authors were careful to separate risk of thromboembolism in acute and chronic inflammatory bowel disease (IBD) and also account for hospitalization, which alone is a risk factor for this complication. However, while the relative risk of thromboembolism is high compared with controls, the absolute risk among all nonhospitalized patients was a maximum rate of 6.4/1000 person-years. This highest risk was for outpatients experiencing an acute flare requiring corticosteroids. Unadjusted rates in hospitalized patients, as would be expected, were higher likely because of both increased severity of disease and immobility issues. As the authors admit, it's possible that some of the increased risk is because of bias in detection. Clinicians may be more likely to look for thromboembolism among IBD patients compared with controls, given the known association. This may have led to artificially increased rates. Also, because disease flare was defined as corticosteroid use, results apply to significant flares that may have higher thromboembolism rates overall. Flares treated with biologic therapies may also have been missed. Given the magnitude of the association, it is unlikely that these biases were responsible for the findings. A strength of this study is the consideration of acute and chronic IBD risk, with exclusion of hospitalized patients. While some comfort can be taken in relatively low absolute risks, the overall impact of thromboembolism on this group of patients is significant. While low, individual risk is high compared with risks with other accepted consequences of IBD and IBD therapies.

**M. F. Picco, MD, PhD**

---

### Clinical Outcomes of Patients with Ulcerative Colitis and Co-existing *Clostridium difficile* Infection

Jodorkovsky D, Young Y, Abreu MT (Inflammatory Bowel Disease Ctr, NY)
*Dig Dis Sci* 55:415-420, 2010

---

*Background.*—The incidence of *Clostridium difficile* infection is increasing in the United States. The aim of our investigation is to compare short-term and long-term outcomes of patients admitted with an ulcerative colitis (UC) flare and co-existent *C. difficile* infection to those of non-infected patients.

*Methods.*—A historical cohort study was undertaken examining admissions at Mount Sinai Hospital between June 2004 and June 2005 using ICD-9 criteria for UC. Charts were abstracted for those patients for whom *C. difficile* testing was performed.

*Results.*—Of 288 admissions, 99 charts met the inclusion criteria. Fifty-two patients were *C. difficile*-negative and 47 were positive. Demographic data and laboratory values upon admission did not differ between the two groups. Patients who were *C. difficile*-positive had significantly more UC-related hospitalizations and emergency room visits in the year following initial admission (58 visits vs. 27, $P = 0.001$ and eight visits vs. 1 visit ($P = 0.012$), respectively). One year following the index admission, *C. difficile* patients had significantly higher rates of colectomy compared to *C. difficile*-negative patients (44.6% vs. 25%, $P = 0.04$). Length of hospitalization (11.7 vs. 11 days), use of cyclosporine therapy during index admission (48% vs. 47% of patients), and percentage requiring colectomy at initial admission (23.4% vs. 13.5%) did not reach statistical significance.

*Conclusions.*—Our data suggest that patients presenting with a UC flare who are infected with *C. difficile* have worse long-term clinical outcomes than those that are *C. difficile*-negative. *C. difficile* testing should be performed for all patients presenting with UC flare. Further studies are warranted to elucidate how infection can alter the natural history of UC.

▶ *Clostridium difficile* infection is a growing concern among patients with inflammatory bowel disease (IBD) presenting with signs and symptoms of disease activity. Rates of infection are higher among IBD patients even in the absence of recent antibiotic use or hospitalization. In-hospital mortality and length of hospitalization are also higher. In this study, among a series of hospitalized patients with active ulcerative colitis (UC) and *C difficile* infection, long-term complications, including colectomy, were higher in the year following hospital admission. Unfortunately, problems in study methodology limit the generalizability of these conclusions. Patients included were those who had a test for *C difficile*, with the assumption made that this would lead to comparisons of similar patients with the key difference being the presence or absence of this infection. Clinician practices regarding which patients and when they were tested during their admission were not given and may have varied. Cyclosporine usage between the 2 groups was similar as were other lab parameters, suggesting that they may have been of similar severity, but this cannot be confirmed. Treatment practices among physicians may have varied. Subsequent hospitalization after initial admission was higher in the *C difficile* group, but the proportion hospitalized for recurrent infection is not known. Recurrence rates for *C difficile* infection are high, and this may explain a large part of the difference in hospitalization rates. Finally, reasons for colectomy were not given and may vary based on the patient and the physician practice. Overall, the findings are interesting and do underscore the need to check for *C difficile* infection among all patients with IBD presenting with diarrhea. More studies are needed to better understand the role of this pathogen in the natural history of IBD.

**M. F. Picco, MD, PhD**

**Hemolytic Uremic Syndrome and Death in Persons with *Escherichia coli* O157:H7 Infection, Foodborne Diseases Active Surveillance Network Sites, 2000–2006**

Gould LH, the Emerging Infections Program FoodNet Working Group (Ctrs for Disease Control and Prevention, Atlanta, GA)

*Clin Infect Dis* 49:1480-1485, 2009

*Background.*—Hemolytic uremic syndrome (HUS) is a life-threatening illness usually caused by infection with Shiga toxin–producing *Escherichia coli* O157 (STEC O157). We evaluated the age-specific rate of HUS and death among persons with STEC O157 infection and the risk factors associated with developing HUS.

*Methods.*—STEC O157 infections and HUS cases were reported from 8 sites participating in the Foodborne Diseases Active Surveillance Network during 2000–2006. For each case of STEC O157 infection and HUS, demographic and clinical outcomes were reported. The proportion of STEC O157 infections resulting in HUS was determined.

*Results.*—A total of 3464 STEC O157 infections were ascertained; 218 persons (6.3%) developed HUS. The highest proportion of HUS cases (15.3%) occurred among children aged <5 years. Death occurred in 0.6% of all patients with STEC O157 infection and in 4.6% of those with HUS. With or without HUS, persons aged ≥60 years had the highest rate of death due to STEC O157 infection. Twelve (3.1%) of 390 persons aged ≥60 years died, including 5 (33.3%) of 15 persons with HUS and 7 (1.9%) of 375 without. Among children aged <5 years, death occurred in 4 (3.0%) of those with HUS and 2 (0.3%) of those without.

*Conclusions.*—Young children and females had an increased risk of HUS after STEC O157 infection. With or without HUS, elderly persons had the highest proportion of deaths associated with STEC O157 infection. These data support recommendations for aggressive supportive care of young children and the elderly early during illness due to STEC O157.

▶ This is an interesting article for all physicians, including gastroenterologists. Shiga toxin-producing *Escherichia coli* O157 (STEC O157) infection is the leading cause of hemolytic uremic syndrome (HUS). HUS is characterized by hemolytic anemia, thrombocytopenia, and renal failure. This article specifically applies to the gastroenterologist when it comes to ordering stool cultures. All stool specimens submitted for the diagnosis of community-acquired diarrhea should be cultured for O157 STEC on selective and differential agar and assayed for O157 STEC. Positive O157 STEC should be reported to public health authorities as well. I think it is important from reading this article that we all make sure our local laboratory has the necessary culture media to perform this test. If not diagnosed, life-threatening cases may be missed.

**J. S. Scolapio, MD**

**Immunosuppression Impairs Response to Pneumococcal Polysaccharide Vaccination in Patients with Inflammatory Bowel Disease**

Melmed GY, Agarwal N, Frenck RW, et al (Univ of California, Los Angeles; Univ of California, Los Angeles, Torrance)

*Am J Gastroenterol* 105:148-154, 2010

*Objectives.*—The treatment of inflammatory bowel disease (IBD) often includes immunosuppressive medications, which may increase the risk of vaccine-preventable illnesses. We aimed to assess the impact of immunosuppression on immune responses to pneumococcal vaccination in patients with IBD.

*Methods.*—The study design consists of a prospective controlled clinical trial. This study was carried out at a tertiary-care IBD clinic. The subjects for the study belonged to one of the following three groups: adult patients with IBD on combination TNF-blockers and immunomodulators (Group A), those without immunosuppressive therapy (Group B), and age-matched healthy controls (Group C). The treatment consisted of immunization with 23-valent pneumococcal polysaccharide vaccines (PSVs). The main outcome was immune response for five serotypes defined as a twofold or greater increase from pre-vaccination titers and $\geq 1$ μg post-vaccination titer.

*Results.*—Sixty-four subjects participated in the study: 20 in Group A, 25 in Group B, and 19 in Group C. Pre-vaccination titers were similar among the three groups. Vaccine responses were lower in Group A than in Group B ($P \leq 0.01$ for four out of five antigens) and Group C ($P < 0.01$ for all five antigens). Overall vaccine response was seen in 45, 80, and 85% of Groups A, B, and C ($P = 0.01$), respectively.

*Conclusions.*—Immune response to PSV-23 is impaired in Crohn's disease (CD) patients on combination immunosuppressive therapy but is normal among non-immunosuppressed patients. Given the unpredictable likelihood for immunosuppressive therapy, newly diagnosed patients with IBD should undergo vaccination before the initiation of immunosuppressive therapy.

▶ Among patients with inflammatory bowel disease (IBD), vaccination is often overlooked. Preventable infections that occur may be more likely to be severe or fatal when patients are taking immunomodulatory or biologic therapy. Vaccination options among patients on immunosuppressive therapies are limited because live vaccines must be avoided.[1] In this study, response to pneumococcal vaccine among patients with IBD on combined immunomodulatory and biologic therapy was significantly lower than patients not taking these medications or healthy controls. It is important to note that nearly half of the immunosuppressed patients responded to the vaccine suggesting that it is still worthwhile among this group. Unfortunately, only those patients on combined immunosuppression could be studied; therefore, neither the effect of monotherapy nor the role of specific therapies could be determined. Also, in the combined immunosuppression group more patients had Crohn's disease (CD). Overall responses in patients with CD were lower, suggesting that vaccine response may also be influenced by the type of IBD and that the study may not be generalizable to patients with ulcerative colitis. Despite these limitations, the message of the study is important. Vaccination of patients with IBD before they require immunomodulatory or biologic therapy results in similar response rates as controls. Patients taking immunomodulatory and/or biologic therapy should be vaccinated with pneumococcal and other dead vaccines and, wherever possible, should have their response measured because of anticipated low response rates.

**M. F. Picco, MD, PhD**

*Reference*

1. Sand BE, Cuffari C, Katz J, et al. Guidelines for immunization in patients with inflammatory bowel disease. *Inflamm Bowel Dis.* 2004;10:677-692.

---

**Maintenance Treatment With Azathioprine in Ulcerative Colitis: Outcome and Predictive Factors After Drug Withdrawal**

Cassinotti A, Actis GC, Duca P, et al ("Luigi Sacco" Univ Hosp, Milano, Italy; "Gradenigo" Hosp, Torino, Italy; Univ of Milano, Italy; et al)
*Am J Gastroenterol* 104:2760-2767, 2009

---

*Objectives.*—Whether the duration of maintenance treatment with azathioprine (AZA) affects the outcome of ulcerative colitis (UC) is unclear. We investigated clinical outcomes and any predictive factors after withdrawal of AZA in UC.

*Methods.*—In this multicenter observational retrospective study, 127 Italian UC patients, who were in steroid-free remission at the time of withdrawal of AZA, were followed-up for a median of 55 months or until relapse. The frequency of clinical relapse or colectomy after AZA withdrawal was analyzed according to demographic, clinical, and endoscopic variables.

*Results.*—After drug withdrawal, a third of the patients relapsed within 12 months, half within 2 years and two-thirds within 5 years. After multivariable analysis, predictors of relapse after drug withdrawal were lack of sustained remission during AZA maintenance (hazard ratio, HR 2.350, confidence interval, CI 95% 1.434–3.852; $P = 0.001$), extensive colitis (HR 1.793, CI 95% 1.064–3.023, $P = 0.028$ vs. left-sided colitis; HR 2.024, CI 95% 1.103–3.717, $P = 0.023$ vs. distal colitis), and treatment duration, with short treatments (3–6 months) more disadvantaged than >48-month treatments (HR 2.783, CI 95% 1.267–6.114, $P = 0.008$). Concomitant aminosalicylates were the only predictors of sustained remission during AZA therapy ($P = 0.009$). The overall colectomy rate was 10%. Predictors of colectomy were drug-related toxicity as the cause of AZA withdrawal ($P = 0.041$), no post-AZA drug therapy ($P = 0.031$), and treatment duration ($P < 0.0005$).

*Conclusions.*—Discontinuation of AZA while UC is in remission is associated with a high relapse rate. Disease extent, lack of sustained remission during AZA, and discontinuation due to toxicity could stratify relapse risk. Concomitant aminosalicylates were advantageous. Prospective randomized controlled trials are needed to confirm whether treatment duration is inversely associated with outcome.

▶ Once in remission, patients with inflammatory bowel disease (IBD) maintained on immunomodulatory therapy are often anxious about discontinuing these medications because of the fear of toxicity. This study provides further evidence for maintaining azathioprine therapy among these patients with ulcerative colitis (UC). Patients who attained remission for at least 3 months taking azathioprine and then discontinued the medication had a disturbingly high rate of disease relapse. While shorter duration of therapy increased risk of relapse, high rates of recurrence were also seen among patients who stopped the medication after 48 months. In this retrospective noncontrolled study, the true role of disease duration is difficult to determine because patients who remained in remission on medication longer may have had a better prognosis prior to starting therapy. Other associations found with relapse make sense clinically, but in the absence of controlled data, it is difficult to draw firm conclusions. Regardless, the main finding of this study and others on UC and Crohn's disease should give clinicians pause before stopping azathioprine among patients with IBD in established remission.

**M. F. Picco, MD, PhD**

## Mucosal Healing Predicts Sustained Clinical Remission in Patients With Early-Stage Crohn's Disease

Baert F, for the Belgian Inflammatory Bowel Disease Research Group and the North-Holland Gut Club (H.–Hartziekenhuis Roeselare–Menen vzw, Belgium; et al)

*Gastroenterology* 138:463-468, 2010

*Background & Aims.*—Few prospective data are available to support the clinical relevance of mucosal healing in patients with Crohn's disease.

This study examined whether complete healing, determined by endoscopy, predicts a better outcome in Crohn's disease.

*Methods.*—One-hundred thirty-three newly diagnosed and treatment-naïve Crohn's disease patients were given either a combination of immunosuppressive therapy (azathioprine) and 3 infusions of infliximab or treatment with conventional corticosteroids. Patients given azathioprine were given repeated doses of infliximab for relapses, patients given corticosteroids were given azathioprine in cases of corticosteroid dependency and infliximab only if azathioprine failed. A representative subset of 49 patients from the initially randomized cohort underwent ileocolonoscopy after 2 years of therapy. Correlation analysis was performed between different clinical parameters including endoscopic activity (Simple Endoscopic Score) and clinical outcome 2 years after this endoscopic examination. Data were available from 46 patients 3 and 4 years after therapy began.

*Results.*—Complete mucosal healing, defined as a simple endoscopic score of 0 after 2 years of therapy, was the only factor that predicted sustained, steroid-free remission 3 and 4 years after therapy was initiated; it was observed in 17 of 24 patients (70.8%) vs 6 of 22 patients with lesions detected by endoscopy (27.3%, Simple Endoscopic Score >0) ($P$=.036; odds ratio = 4.352; 95% confidence interval, 1.10–17.220). Fifteen of 17 patients with mucosal healing at year 2 maintained in remission without further infliximab infusions during years 3 and 4 ($P$=.032; odds ratio = 4.883; 95% confidence interval, 1.144–20.844).

*Conclusions.*—Complete mucosal healing in patients with early-stage Crohn's disease is associated with significantly higher steroid-free remission rates 4 years after therapy began.

▶ This study is a follow-up to the previously published work by the same group on the use of early combined immunosuppression (top-down) therapy in newly diagnosed patients with Crohn's disease.[1] This study illustrates the importance of mucosal healing among this newly diagnosed treatment-naïve group. Mucosal healing was the only factor that predicted steroid-free remission. The study was small with mucosal healing only assessed in 49 patients. Endoscopic activity did not correlate with clinical disease activity (CDAI). In fact only half of the patients in clinical remission by CDAI had mucosal healing. Comparisons of efficacy between medications could not be performed primarily because of the small number of patients. The study was conducted from 2001 to 2004 with infliximab used as induction and rescue therapy, unlike how it is currently used as continued maintenance therapy. Continued scheduled infliximab maintenance therapy would have probably led to higher mucosal healing rates. This study adds to the growing body of literature illustrating the importance of mucosal healing after medical and surgical therapy. Assessment of clinical activity is not enough to adequately determine the likelihood of subsequent disease flares or complications. Endoscopy may be necessary among patients with good clinical response but poor predicted long-term outcome. Other noninvasive methods could aid in evaluating mucosal healing. Accurate assessment of both clinical and endoscopic response may become the standard for the future and lead to better long-term outcomes among patients with Crohn's disease. More research is needed.

**M. F. Picco, MD, PhD**

*Reference*

1. D'Haens G, Baert F, van Assche G, et al. Early combined immunosuppression or conventional management in patients with newly diagnosed Crohn's disease: an open randomised trial. *Lancet*. 2008;371:660-667.

---

**Once-Daily Dosing of Delayed-Release Oral Mesalamine (400-mg Tablet) Is as Effective as Twice-Daily Dosing for Maintenance of Remission of Ulcerative Colitis**

Sandborn WJ, Korzenik J, Lashner B, et al (Mayo Clinic, Rochester, MN; Massachusetts General Hosp, Boston; Cleveland Clinic, OH; et al)
*Gastroenterology* 138:1286-1296, 2010

---

*Background & Aims.*—The practice of dosing mesalamines in divided doses for the treatment of ulcerative colitis (UC) began with sulfasalazine and was driven by sulfapyridine toxicity. This convention and the assumption that dosing multiple times a day is necessary to treat UC had not been challenged until recently. This study was conducted to determine the efficacy and safety of once-daily dosing of delayed-release mesalamine (Asacol 400-mg tablets) compared with twice-daily dosing for maintaining remission in UC patients.

*Methods.*—A multicenter, randomized, investigator-blinded, 12-month, active-control trial was conducted to assess the noninferiority of delayed-release mesalamine 1.6–2.4 g/day administered once daily compared with twice daily in patients with mild-to-moderate UC currently in clinical remission. The primary end point was maintenance of clinical remission at month 6.

*Results.*—A total of 1023 patients were randomized and dosed. The primary objective of noninferiority was met. At month 6, 90.5% of patients receiving once-daily dosing had maintained clinical remission, compared with 91.8% of patients receiving twice-daily dosing (95% confidence interval for twice daily - once daily, −2.3 to 4.9). At month 12, 85.4% of patients receiving once-daily dosing had maintained clinical remission, compared with 85.4% of patients receiving twice-daily dosing (95% confidence interval for twice daily - once daily, −4.6 to 4.7). Both regimens had low rates of withdrawals as a result of adverse events and serious adverse events.

*Conclusions.*—Once-daily dosing of delayed-release mesalamine at doses of 1.6–2.4 g/day was shown to be as effective as twice-daily dosing for maintenance of clinical remission in patients with UC.

▶ Among patients with ulcerative colitis (UC) in remission, mesalamine remains the mainstay of therapy. Compliance is a major issue and is improved by once-daily regimens. Newer preparations such as Lialda and Apriso are marketed with this advantage. Drug delivery systems from these newer medications are thought to be important in allowing once-daily dosing. However, this notion is challenged in this article that compared Asacol (standard preparation) once daily to twice-daily dosing among patients with UC in remission on current maintenance mesalamine. The cumulative daily dose was the same and the efficacy of the regimens was similar. Furthermore, the overall efficacy was similar to the newer preparations. These newer preparations may be more costly than older preparations. This cost may not be justified. The newer preparations do allow for fewer tablets daily, which may be an advantage in compliance, but once-daily dosing regardless of the preparation is probably sufficient in the maintenance of remission among patients with UC. While it is appealing to suggest that once-daily dosing of older preparation such as Asacol may be effective for active disease, more studies are necessary to definitively answer this question.

**M. F. Picco, MD, PhD**

---

## Increased Short- and Long-Term Risk of Inflammatory Bowel Disease After *Salmonella* or *Campylobacter* Gastroenteritis

Gradel KO, Nielsen HL, Schønheyder HC, et al (Aarhus Univ Hosp, Aalborg, Denmark)

*Gastroenterology* 137:495-501, 2009

---

*Background & Aims.*—Various commensal enteric and potentially pathogenic bacteria may be involved in the pathogenesis of inflammatory bowel diseases (IBD). We compared the risk of IBD between a cohort of patients with documented *Salmonella* or *Campylobacter* gastroenteritis and an age- and gender-matched control group from the same population in Denmark.

*Methods.*—We identified 13,324 patients with *Salmonella/Campylobacter* gastroenteritis from laboratory registries in North Jutland and Aarhus counties, Denmark, from 1991 through 2003, and 26,648 unexposed controls from the same counties. Of these, 176 exposed patients with IBD before the infection, their 352 unexposed controls, and 80 unexposed individuals with IBD before the *Salmonella/Campylobacter* infection were excluded. The final study cohort of 13,148 exposed and 26,216 unexposed individuals were followed for up to 15 years (mean, 7.5 years).

*Results.*—A first-time diagnosis of IBD was reported in 107 exposed (1.2%) and 73 unexposed individuals (0.5%). By age, gender, and comorbidity adjusted Cox proportional hazards regression analysis, the hazard ratio (95% confidence interval) for IBD was 2.9 (2.2–3.9) for the whole period and 1.9 (1.4–2.6) if the first year after the *Salmonella*/*Campylobacter* infection was excluded. The increased risk in exposed subjects was observed throughout the 15-year observation period. The increased risk was similar for *Salmonella* (n = 6463) and *Campylobacter* (n = 6685) and for a first-time diagnosis of Crohn's disease (n = 47) and ulcerative colitis (n = 133).

*Conclusions.*—In our population-based cohort study with complete follow-up, an increased risk of IBD was demonstrated in individuals notified in laboratory registries with an episode of *Salmonella*/*Campylobacter* gastroenteritis.

▶ The role of bacteria in the development of inflammatory bowel disease (IBD) has been the subject of intense interest and extensive study. Specific pathogenic bacteria have been implicated, but convincing proof is lacking. In this population-based study from Denmark, the authors conclude that a previous episode of *Salmonella* or *Campylobacter* gastroenteritis is associated with a higher risk of development of IBD. While an intriguing idea, the authors do acknowledge the significant limitations of their data. Patients were retrospectively identified by a national registry, and the association of these infections was demonstrated by comparing the risk of IBD in those with infection (exposed) to those without infection (unexposed). The study design, a population-based cohort study with 15 years of follow-up, strengthens their conclusions. The analysis presenting overall risk and risk after exclusion of the first year of follow-up is important because it addresses the limitations of the article. Exclusion of patients who were diagnosed with IBD within 1 year of infection probably eliminates those with mild existing IBD that was exacerbated by *Salmonella* or *Campylobacter* infection. This is suggested by the finding of a large number of hospitalized exposed patients diagnosed with IBD in the first 2 months after infection. Furthermore, patients with severe symptoms may be more likely to have a stool specimen checked and undergo endoscopy leading to higher rates of diagnosis of IBD. Exclusion of the first year after infection still resulted in an elevated risk strengthening the authors' conclusions. Surveillance bias, as defined by the potential for more stool samples being taken among patients with IBD because of more severe symptoms, was also addressed. This may have led to a higher rate of detection of infection in IBD patients. No such bias was found with most patients being diagnosed with these infections after 1 sample. In summary, the nearly 2-fold increase in risk of IBD among patients with previous *Salmonella* or *Campylobacter* infection is supported by the data with careful methods of data analysis. This provides support for the role of these pathogenic bacteria in the development of IBD.

**M. F. Picco, MD, PhD**

# 48 Liver Disease

**High Dose Ursodeoxycholic Acid for the Treatment of Primary Sclerosing Cholangitis**

Lindor KD, Kowdley KV, Luketic VAC, et al (Mayo Clinic Rochester, MN; Virginia Mason Med Ctr, Seattle, WA; Virginia Commonwealth Univ School of Medicine, Richmond; et al)

*Hepatology* 50:808-814, 2009

*Background.*—Previous controlled trials are inconclusive regarding the efficacy of ursodeoxycholic acid (UDCA) for treating primary sclerosing cholangitis (PSC).

*Methods.*—One hundred fifty adult patients with PSC were enrolled in a long-term, randomized, double-blind controlled trial of high-dose UDCA (28–30 mg/kg/day) versus placebo. Liver biopsy and cholangiography were performed before randomization and after 5 years. The primary outcome measure was development of cirrhosis, varices, cholangiocarcinoma, liver transplantation or death.

*Results.*—The study was terminated after six years because of futility. At enrollment, the UDCA (n=76) and placebo (n=74) groups were similar with respect to gender, age, duration of disease, serum aspartate aminotransferase (AST) and alkaline phosphatase (AP) levels, liver histology and Mayo risk score. During therapy, AST and AP levels decreased more in the UDCA than the placebo group ($p<0.01$) but improvements in liver tests were not associated with decreased endpoints. By the end of the study, 30 patients in the UDCA group (39%) versus 19 patients in the placebo group (26%) had reached one of the pre-established clinical endpoints. After adjustment for baseline stratification characteristics, the risk of a primary endpoint was 2.3 times greater for patients on UDCA than for those on placebo ($p<0.01$) and 2.1 times greater for death, transplantation, or minimal listing criteria ($p=0.038$). Serious adverse events were more common in the UDCA than placebo group (63% vs 37%: $p<0.01$).

*Conclusions.*—Long-term high-dose UDCA therapy is associated with improvement in serum liver tests in PSC but does not improve survival and was associated with higher rates of serious adverse events.

▶ Primary sclerosing cholangitis (PSC) is a chronic cholestatic liver disease of unknown etiology characterized by fibrosing inflammation and destruction of the extrahepatic and/or intrahepatic bile ducts. No effective medical therapy exists for people with PSC. An earlier published pilot study had demonstrated the potential benefit of higher dose ursodeoxycholic acid (UDCA) in the treatment of these patients and provided the basis of this randomized, double-blind, placebo-controlled trial of high-dose UDCA (28-30 mg/kg/d) in PSC. The results of this trial surprised many within the field of hepatology. Serious adverse events including death, transplantation, or meeting minimal listing criteria were more common in the UDCA group versus placebo. Though patients on therapy had improvement in serum liver levels, survival was not improved and a greater number of adverse events were seen in the higher dose UDCA group. At this time, high-dose (28-30 mg/kg/d) UDCA therapy is not recommended for patients with PSC.

**D. M. Harnois, DO**

## Randomized Controlled Trial of Carvedilol Versus Variceal Band Ligation for the Prevention of the First Variceal Bleed

Tripathi D, Ferguson JW, Kochar N, et al (Royal Infirmary, Edinburgh, UK; et al)
*Hepatology* 50:825-833, 2009

Current therapy for preventing the first variceal bleed includes beta-blocker and variceal band ligation (VBL). VBL has lower bleeding rates, with no differences in survival, whereas beta-blocker therapy can be limited by side effects. Carvedilol, a non-cardioselective vasodilating beta-blocker, is more effective in reducing portal pressure than propranolol; however, there have been no clinical studies assessing the efficacy of carvedilol in primary prophylaxis. The goal of this study was to compare carvedilol and VBL for the prevention of the first variceal bleed in a randomized controlled multicenter trial. One hundred fifty-two cirrhotic patients from five different centers with grade II or larger esophageal varices were randomized to either carvedilol 12.5 mg once daily or VBL performed every 2 weeks until eradication using a multibander device. Seventy-seven patients were randomized to carvedilol and 75 to VBL. Baseline characteristics did not differ between the groups (alcoholic liver disease, 73%; median Child-Pugh score, 8; median age, 54 years; median follow-up, 20 months). On intention-to-treat analysis, carvedilol had lower rates of the first variceal bleed (10% versus 23%; relative hazard 0.41; 95% confidence interval 0.19-0.96 [$P = 0.04$]), with no significant differences in overall mortality (35% versus 37%, $P = 0.71$), and bleeding-related mortality (3% versus 1%, $P = 0.26$). Six patients in the VBL group bled as a result of banding ulcers. Per-protocol analysis revealed no significant differences in the outcomes.

*Conclusion.*—Carvedilol is effective in preventing the first variceal bleed. Carvedilol is an option for primary prophylaxis in patients with high-risk esophageal varices.

▶ In previous studies, nonselective beta blockers (NSBB), namely propranolol and nadolol, have been demonstrated in carefully conducted randomized control trials to be highly effective in decreasing the risk of bleeding from portal hypertensive gastropathy. Many studies have also shown NSBB therapy to be beneficial in the prevention of variceal bleeding. However, drug side effects often result in dose reduction or discontinuation. In this study, carvedilol, a drug combination of propranolol and prazosin, was effective in preventing the first variceal bleeding when compared with variceal band ligation (VBL) every 2 weeks, with no significant differences in overall mortality or bleeding-related mortality. This is the first study to demonstrate effectiveness of this therapy against a trial of band ligation for the prevention of variceal bleeding.

**D. M. Harnois, DO**

**Rifaximin Treatment in Hepatic Encephalopathy**

Bass NM, Mullen KD, Sanyal A, et al (Univ of California, San Francisco; Case Western Reserve Univ, Cleveland, OH; Virginia Commonwealth Univ, Richmond; et al)

*N Engl J Med* 362:1071-1081, 2010

*Background.*—Hepatic encephalopathy is a chronically debilitating complication of hepatic cirrhosis. The efficacy of rifaximin, a minimally absorbed antibiotic, is well documented in the treatment of acute hepatic encephalopathy, but its efficacy for prevention of the disease has not been established.

*Methods.*—In this randomized, double-blind, placebo-controlled trial, we randomly assigned 299 patients who were in remission from recurrent hepatic encephalopathy resulting from chronic liver disease to receive either rifaximin, at a dose of 550 mg twice daily (140 patients), or placebo (159 patients) for 6 months. The primary efficacy end point was the time to the first breakthrough episode of hepatic encephalopathy. The key secondary end point was the time to the first hospitalization involving hepatic encephalopathy.

*Results.*—Rifaximin significantly reduced the risk of an episode of hepatic encephalopathy, as compared with placebo, over a 6-month period (hazard ratio with rifaximin, 0.42; 95% confidence interval [CI], 0.28 to 0.64; $P<0.001$). A breakthrough episode of hepatic encephalopathy occurred in 22.1% of patients in the rifaximin group, as compared with 45.9% of patients in the placebo group. A total of 13.6% of the patients in the rifaximin group had a hospitalization involving hepatic encephalopathy, as compared with 22.6% of patients in the placebo group, for a hazard ratio of 0.50 (95% CI, 0.29 to 0.87; $P=0.01$). More than 90% of patients received concomitant lactulose therapy. The incidence of adverse events reported during the study was similar in the two groups, as was the incidence of serious adverse events.

*Conclusions.*—Over a 6-month period, treatment with rifaximin maintained remission from hepatic encephalopathy more effectively than did placebo. Rifaximin treatment also significantly reduced the risk of hospitalization involving hepatic encephalopathy. (ClinicalTrials.gov number, NCT00298038.)

▶ The number of persons within the United States with cirrhosis is currently estimated at 5.5 million. This number is expected to significantly increase over the next 2 decades. Hepatic encephalopathy is a complication of cirrhosis with significant life-altering effects. In 2004, 50 000 patients were hospitalized with hepatic encephalopathy.

The current standard of care for patients with hepatic encephalopathy is treatment with a nonabsorbable disaccharide lactulose. All antibiotics, such as neomycin, vancomycin, paromomycin, and metronidazole are not recommended for long-term use because of significant toxicity.

Rifaximin is a minimally absorbed oral antimicrobial agent that is concentrated in the gastrointestinal tract. In this phase 3 randomized, double-blind, placebo-controlled trial, patients received either rifaximin at a dose of 550 mg twice daily or placebo. Rifaximin significantly reduced the risk of an episode of hepatic encephalopathy as compared with placebo and resulted in less breakthrough episodes. The drug was well tolerated with a low side effect profile. It must be noted that more than 90% of patients received concomitant lactulose therapy. This study confirms the efficacy of rifaximin in reducing the complications of hepatic encephalopathy associated with liver failure secondary to cirrhosis.

**D. M. Harnois, DO**

---

**Simvastatin Lowers Portal Pressure in Patients With Cirrhosis and Portal Hypertension: A Randomized Controlled Trial**

Abraldes JG, Albillos A, Bañares R, et al (Univ of Barcelona, Spain; Centro de Investigación Biomédica en Red de Enfermedades Hepáticas y Digestivas, Spain)

*Gastroenterology* 136:1651-1658, 2009

---

*Background & Aims.*—Simvastatin improves liver generation of nitric oxide and hepatic endothelial dysfunction in patients with cirrhosis, so it could be an effective therapy for portal hypertension. This randomized controlled trial evaluated the effects of continuous simvastatin administration on the hepatic venous pressure gradient (HVPG) and its safety in patients with cirrhosis and portal hypertension.

*Methods.*—Fifty-nine patients with cirrhosis and portal hypertension (HVPG >12 mm Hg) were randomized to groups that were given simvastatin 20 mg/day for 1 month (increased to 40 mg/day at day 15) or placebo in a double-blind clinical trial. Randomization was stratified according to whether the patient was being treated with $\beta$-adrenergic blockers. We studied splanchnic and systemic hemodynamics and variables of liver function and safety before and after 1 month of treatment.

*Results.*—Simvastatin significantly decreased HVPG (−8.3%) without deleterious effects in systemic hemodynamics. HVPG decreases were observed in patients who were receiving β-adrenergic blockers (−11.0%; $P$ =.033) and in those who were not (−5.9%; $P$ =.013). Simvastatin improved hepatic, fractional, and intrinsic clearance of indocyanine green, showing an improvement in effective liver perfusion and function. No significant changes in HVPG and liver function were observed in patients receiving placebo. The number of patients with adverse events did not differ significantly between groups. No patient was withdrawn from the study based on adverse events.

*Conclusions.*—Simvastatin decreased HVPG and improved liver perfusion in patients with cirrhosis. These effects were additive with those of β-adrenergic blockers. The beneficial effects of simvastatin should be confirmed in long-term clinical trials for portal hypertension.

▶ This is a randomized, placebo-controlled, double-blind clinical trial showing the beneficial effects of simvastatin in lowering portal pressures in individuals with portal hypertension. Simvastatin has been shown to improve liver generation of nitric oxide (NO) and hepatic endothelial dysfunction in patients with cirrhosis. Experimental data in humans and animal models have suggested that statin therapy can decrease intrahepatic vascular resistance and improve flow-mediated vasodilation of liver vasculature in the cirrhotic liver through up-regulation of NO production. This study demonstrates that 1 month of simvastatin administration significantly decreased hepatic venous portal gradient (HVPG) in some patients with cirrhosis and severe portal hypertension. Thirty-two percent of patients achieved an HVPG reduction of 20% or greater (> 12 mm Hg). This level of reduction has been shown in previous studies to reduce portal hypertension complications and mortality and is the standard goal for any therapy in the treatment of portal hypertension. This trial was conducted without the use of β-blocker therapy, and it suggests that the combination of simvastatin and nonselective β-blocker therapy may be of even greater benefit. Simvastatin may also provide benefits for those patients intolerant of β-blocker therapy.

**D. M. Harnois, DO**

## Early Laparoscopic Cholecystectomy Improves Outcomes After Endoscopic Sphincterotomy for Choledochocystolithiasis

Reinders JSK, Goud A, Timmer R, et al (St Antonius Hosp, Nieuwegein, The Netherlands; et al)

*Gastroenterology* 138:2315-2320, 2010

*Background & Aims.*—Patients with choledochocystolithiasis generally undergo endoscopic sphincterotomy (ES) followed by laparoscopic cholecystectomy (LC). However, many patients receive this surgery 6–8 weeks after ES. There is a high conversion rate of elective LC after ES, and patients can develop recurrent biliary events during the waiting period. We investigated whether the timing of surgery influences outcome.

*Methods.*—We performed a randomized trial of patients with choledochocystolithiasis who underwent successful ES. Patients were randomly assigned to groups that received early LC (within 72 hours after ES, n = 49) or delayed LC (after 6–8 weeks, n = 47), based on an expected difference in conversion rate of 25% vs 5%, respectively. Conversion rate, biliary events during follow-up, duration and difficulty of surgeries, postoperative morbidity, and hospital stay were scored. Intention-to-treat analyses were performed.

*Results.*—Groups were comparable in age, sex, and comorbidity. There was no difference between groups in conversion rate (4.3% in early vs 8.7% in delayed group) nor were there differences in operating times and/or difficulties or hospital stays. During the waiting period for LC, 17 patients in the delayed group (36.2%) developed recurrent biliary events compared with 1 patient in the early group ($P < .001$).

*Conclusions.*—In a randomized trial to evaluate timing of LC after ES, recurrent biliary events occurred in 36.2% of patients whose LC was delayed for 6–8 weeks. Early LC (within 72 hours) appears to be safe and might prevent the majority of biliary events in this period following sphincterotomy.

▶ Randomized controlled trials have demonstrated superior outcome in laparoscopic cholecystectomy (LC) after endoscopic sphincterotomy (ES) for choledochocystolithiasis rather than a wait-and-see approach. Patients in these trials who were allocated to surgery underwent LC 4 to 6 weeks after ES. There has been a retrospective study, which showed a lower conversion rate to open procedures in patients who underwent LC within 2 weeks after ES versus those who had LC 4 to 6 weeks after ES. This is the first randomized trial to look at the outcome of LC within 72 hours after ES or delayed LC after 6 to 8 weeks. In the delay to surgery, 36.2% of the patients developed a recurrent biliary event compared with 1 patient in the early group. There were no differences in conversion rate, complications, or length of stay. This study concluded that early LC is safe and may prevent recurrent biliary events.

**D. M. Harnois, DO**

---

**Pioglitazone, Vitamin E, or Placebo for Nonalcoholic Steatohepatitis**

Sanyal AJ, for the NASH CRN (Virginia Commonwealth Univ, Richmond; et al)
*N Engl J Med* 362:1675-1685, 2010

---

*Background.*—Nonalcoholic steatohepatitis is a common liver disease that can progress to cirrhosis. Currently, there is no established treatment for this disease.

*Methods.*—We randomly assigned 247 adults with nonalcoholic steatohepatitis and without diabetes to receive pioglitazone at a dose of 30 mg daily (80 subjects), vitamin E at a dose of 800 IU daily (84 subjects), or placebo (83 subjects), for 96 weeks. The primary outcome was an improvement in histologic features of nonalcoholic steatohepatitis, as assessed with the use of a composite of standardized scores for steatosis, lobular inflammation, hepatocellular ballooning, and fibrosis. Given the two planned primary comparisons, P values of less than 0.025 were considered to indicate statistical significance.

*Results.*—Vitamin E therapy, as compared with placebo, was associated with a significantly higher rate of improvement in nonalcoholic steatohepatitis (43% vs. 19%, $P = 0.001$), but the difference in the rate of improvement with pioglitazone as compared with placebo was not significant (34% and 19%, respectively; $P = 0.04$). Serum alanine and aspartate aminotransferase levels were reduced with vitamin E and with pioglitazone, as compared with placebo ($P<0.001$ for both comparisons), and both agents were associated with reductions in hepatic steatosis ($P = 0.005$ for vitamin E and $P<0.001$ for pioglitazone) and lobular inflammation ($P = 0.02$ for vitamin E and $P = 0.004$ for pioglitazone) but not with improvement in fibrosis scores ($P = 0.24$ for vitamin E and $P = 0.12$ for pioglitazone). Subjects who received pioglitazone gained more weight than did those who received vitamin E or placebo; the rates of other side effects were similar among the three groups.

*Conclusions.*—Vitamin E was superior to placebo for the treatment of nonalcoholic steatohepatitis in adults without diabetes. There was no benefit of pioglitazone over placebo for the primary outcome; however, significant benefits of pioglitazone were observed for some of the secondary outcomes. (ClinicalTrials.gov number, NCT00063622.)

▶ Nonalcoholic steatohepatitis (NASH) is characterized histologically by hepatic steatosis and lobular inflammation with hepatocellular ballooning. The progression to cirrhosis in these individuals is 15%. There are no current effective therapies. The disease is associated with insulin resistance providing the basis for looking at pioglitazone and vitamin E in the treatment of NASH.

This was a multicenter, randomized, placebo-controlled, double-blind clinical trial conducted by the NASH Clinical Research Network (CRN) established by the National Institute of Diabetes and Digestive and Kidney Diseases (NIDDK) in the treatment of patients with NASH without diabetes mellitus. A total of 83 patients received placebo, 84 received vitamin E (800 IU daily), and 80 received pioglitazone (30 mg daily). While there was improvement noted in serum liver tests and inflammation in the pioglitazone-treated patients, the study demonstrated no benefit of pioglitazone over placebo in the primary outcome of improvement in histologic findings and the established targets for reduction in activity score. In addition, the patients treated with pioglitazone had a significant gain in weight. Vitamin E at a dose of 800 IU daily did appear to demonstrate improvement over placebo.

The Pioglitazone versus Vitamin E versus Placebo for the Treatment of Nondiabetic Patients with Nonalcoholic Steatohepatitis (PIVENS) trial demonstrated some improvement in certain outcomes in the treatment of NASH, but unfortunately, it still leaves us short of a proven truly effective therapy for these patients.

**D. M. Harnois, DO**

**Efficacy and Safety of Peginterferon Alfa-2a (40KD) Plus Ribavirin in Hepatitis C Patients with Advanced Fibrosis and Cirrhosis**

Bruno S, Shiffman ML, Roberts SK, et al (AO Fatebenefratelli e Oftalmico, Milan, Italy; Virginia Commonwealth Univ Med Ctr, Blacksburg; The Alfred Hosp, Melbourne, Australia; et al)

*Hepatology* 51:388-397, 2010

The objective of this study is to determine the efficacy and safety of peginterferon alfa-2a (40KD)/ribavirin in patients with advanced fibrosis. Data from 341 genotype 1/4 patients (99 with bridging fibrosis/cirrhosis) treated for 48 weeks and 1547 genotype 2/3 patients (380 with bridging fibrosis/cirrhosis) treated for 16 or 24 weeks enrolled in three randomized international studies were analyzed. Sustained virological response (SVR) rates decreased progressively from 60% in genotype 1/4 patients without advanced fibrosis to 51% in those with bridging fibrosis and 33% in those with cirrhosis (trend test $P = 0.0028$); and from 76% to 61% and 57%, respectively, in genotype 2/3 patients treated for 24 weeks (trend test $P < 0.0001$). Irrespective of genotype, patients without advanced fibrosis were more likely to have an earlier response to treatment that was associated with higher SVR rates and lower relapse rates during untreated follow-up. Among patients with or without a diagnosis of advanced fibrosis, rates of SVR and relapse were similar for patients with similar responses in the first 12 weeks.

*Conclusion.*—Compared with patients with less severe disease, SVR rates are significantly lower in patients with advanced fibrosis. However, irrespective of genotype and degree of fibrosis, the time to become hepatitis C virus (HCV) RNA undetectable was the strongest predictor of SVR.

▶ This study was an important contribution to our understanding of the treatment of hepatitis C in patients because it is one of only a small number of trials that have looked at treatment of patients with hepatitis C virus (HCV) with advanced fibrosis and cirrhosis with peginterferon and ribavirin. The vast majority of all trials in HCV treatment have excluded patients with more advanced disease. Patients in this trial were eligible for enrollment if they had quantifiable HCV RNA in the serum (> 600 IU/mL), had elevated alanine aminotransferase (ALT) levels, and a liver biopsy confirming a diagnosis of chronic hepatitis C. The patients were grouped according to the fibrosis score on the baseline liver biopsy. It is important to note that all cases with cirrhosis were well compensated with a Child-Pugh score of <7 (Child's A). The primary efficacy outcome in the study was sustained virology response (SVR) defined as undetectable HCV RNA by qualitative polymerase chain reaction (PCR) assay (<50 IU/mL) at the end of a 24-week untreated follow-up period. Rapid virological response (RVR) was defined as undetectable HCV RNA by qualitative assay after 4 weeks of treatment. Early virological response (EVR) was defined at week 12 on treatment. In this analysis, patients without an RVR at 4 weeks but who achieved an EVR at 12 weeks were divided into 2 groups: those with a complete EVR defined as undetectable HCV RNA by qualitative assay at 12 weeks and those with a slow response at week 12 defined as a detectable level of >50 IU/mL but a 2-log or more decline in serum HCV RNA level. In addition to the primary efficacy outcome, several secondary efficacy outcomes were evaluated, including assessing the impact of RVR and EVR on achievement of SVR.

**D. M. Harnois, DO**

**Entecavir treatment for up to 5 years in patients with hepatitis B e antigen-positive chronic hepatitis B**

Chang T-T, Lai C-L, Kew Yoon S, et al (Natl Cheng Kung Univ, Tainan, Taiwan, ROC; Queen Mary Hosp, Hong Kong, China; The Catholic Univ of Korea, Seoul; et al)

*Hepatology* 51:422-430, 2010

Sustained virologic suppression is a primary goal of therapy for chronic hepatitis B (CHB). In study entecavir (ETV)-022, 48 weeks of entecavir 0.5 mg was superior to lamivudine for virologic suppression for hepatitis B e antigen (HBeAg)-positive CHB. A total of 183 entecavir-treated patients from ETV-022 subsequently enrolled in study ETV-901. We present the results after up to 5 years (240 weeks) of continuous entecavir therapy. The entecavir long-term cohort consists of patients who received ≥1 year of entecavir 0.5 mg in ETV-022 and then entered ETV-901 with a treatment gap ≤35 days. In ETV-901 the entecavir dose was 1.0 mg daily. For patients with samples available at Year 5, proportions with hepatitis B virus (HBV) DNA <300 copies/mL, normal alanine aminotransferase (ALT) levels, HBeAg loss, and HBeAg seroconversion were determined. In all, 146 patients met criteria for inclusion in the entecavir long-term cohort. At Year 5, 94% (88/94) had HBV DNA <300 copies/mL and 80% (78/98) had normal ALT levels. In addition to patients who achieved serologic responses during study ETV-022, 23% (33/141) achieved HBeAg seroconversion and 1.4% (2/145) lost hepatitis B surface antigen (HBsAg) during study ETV-901. Through 5 years, entecavir resistance emerged in one patient. The safety profile of entecavir was consistent with previous reports.

*Conclusion.*—Extended therapy with entecavir through 5 years maintained or increased rates of HBV DNA suppression and ALT normalization. Additional patients also achieved HBeAg loss and seroconversion. Entecavir provides sustained viral suppression with minimal resistance during long-term treatment of HBeAg-positive CHB.

▶ Chronic hepatitis B (CHB) infection affects over 350 million people worldwide. Medications currently approved in the United States include standard interferon, pegylated interferon, lamivudine, adefovir dipivoxil, entecavir, telbivudine, and tenofovir disoproxil fumarate. Interferon therapies have been demonstrated to show a durable serologic response but are limited by the need for parenteral administration and their side effects. Lamivudine demonstrated efficacy initially, but resistance reaches 70% after 4 years of therapy. Current guidelines recommend avoidance of lamivudine as first-line therapy for this reason. Adefovir treatment for 48 weeks resulted in HB virus (HBV) DNA suppression in only 13% of HBe antigen (HBeAg)-positive patients and resistance in 20% of HBeAg patients after 5 years. Patients treated with telbivudine also demonstrated a virologic breakthrough in over 20% of HBeAg-positive patients treated for 2 years. Tenofovir treatment for HBeAg-positive patients with chronic HBV infection has been demonstrated in the past to achieve high levels of virologic suppression, but efficacy and resistance data were only reported through 2 years. Previously, entecavir demonstrated superior histologic and virologic benefit compared with lamivudine in nucleotide-naïve HBeAg-positive HBV-infected patients treated for 48 weeks. This study is an extension of this previous study with results up to 5 years of continuous entecavir therapy. At year 5, 94% of patients had HBV DNA $< 300$ IU/ml, and 80% had normal alanine transaminase (ALT) levels. Through 5 years, entecavir resistance emerged in only 1 patient. This study demonstrates a high level of sustained viral suppression, minimal resistance, and ALT normalization in patients treated with entecavir for CHB.

**D. M. Harnois, DO**

# 49 Miscellaneous

**Long-Term Outcome of Sacral Nerve Stimulation for Fecal Incontinence**

Altomare DF, Ratto C, Ganio E, et al (Univ of Bari, Italy; Catholic Univ, Rome, Italy; S. Rita Hosp, Vercelli, Italy; et al)

*Dis Colon Rectum* 52:11-17, 2009

*Purpose.*—Sacral nerve stimulation is a safe and effective procedure for fecal incontinence. We investigated whether its efficacy is maintained long term.

*Patients and Methods.*—Sixty patients with fecal incontinence underwent permanent sacral nerve stimulation. Patients' data were prospectively recorded in the national registry of the Italian Group of sacral nerve stimulation. The severity of fecal incontinence was evaluated by the Wexner score, and data were collected in a bowel function diary. Quality of life was evaluated by the Italian version of the Medical Outcomes Survey Short Form (SF-36) questionnaire.

*Results.*—Fifty-two patients were available for long-term follow-up lasting at least 5 years. Compared with baseline, the Wexner score decreased significantly after definitive implantation (from 15 ± 4 to 5 ± 5, $P < 0.001$). At least 50 percent improvement in continence was achieved in 74 percent of the patients, and at least 70 percent improvement (median value) was achieved in 50 percent. The mean number of solid/liquid incontinence episodes decreased significantly from 0.5 (±0.5) to 0.1 (±0.3) per day ($P = 0.004$). Quality of life improved in all domains. The overall mean improvement in SF-36 scores was 39.8 percent. Both mean resting and squeeze anal pressures increased significantly, and maximum volume tolerated decreased significantly.

*Conclusions.*—Sacral nerve stimulation maintains its efficacy long term, not only in regard to control of symptoms but also regarding quality of life.

► Fecal incontinence is a common referral in our gastrointestinal practice. Besides antimotility medications and a colostomy, we have not had much to offer these patients. Sacral nerve stimulation (SNS) has now been recognized as a safe and perhaps effective procedure for treating fecal incontinence. In this prospective study of 60 patients, the outcome of SNS was evaluated. Clinical improvement was noted in most patients with a follow-up period of 5 years. Given these and other published results I believe SNS should be tried in those patients in which antimotility agents have not helped and before performing a colostomy in most patients.

**J. S. Scolapio, MD**

# 50 Nutrition and Celiac Disease

---

**Indications for Percutaneous Endoscopic Gastrostomy and Procedure-related Outcome**

Srinivasan R, Irvine T, Dalzell M (Alder Hey Children's NHS Foundation Trust, Liverpool, UK)

*J Pediatr Gastroenterol Nutr* 49:584-588, 2009

---

*Objective.*—To describe the indications and practice of percutaneous endoscopic gastrostomy (PEG) device insertion for nutritional support and to ascertain procedure-related complications and outcome.

*Methods.*—Observational study with prospectively collected data on children who underwent PEG-related procedures (PEG insertion, removal, or change to low profile button devices [LPBD]) for a 5-year period (2002–2006) at our centre.

*Results.*—Six hundred one PEG-related procedures were performed during the study period (384 insertions, 165 conversions to LPBD, 49 permanent PEG removals, and 3 PEG reinsertions). The main indications for PEG insertion were feeding difficulties associated with neurodisability (160/384; 41.6%) and congenital heart disease (CHD 115/384; 30%). Children with CHD required feeding nutritional support at an earlier age than children with neurodisability regardless of underlying cardiac condition. The age of PEG insertion was significantly different between the 2 main groups (neurodisability 3.56 years vs CHD 0.39 years; $P < 0.001$ [$t$ test]). Fifty-nine patients were discharged on the same day as PEG insertion without complications (day case gastrostomy). The median time between PEG insertion to LPBD conversion was 0.83 year (0.12–3.86). Twenty-four of the 49 children having permanent PEG removal had CHD.

*Conclusions.*—Neurodisabilty and CHD were the main indications for PEG insertion, those with CHD requiring feeding support at an earlier age. Although CHD was an indication for PEG insertion in 30% of instances, a greater percentage of PEG removals (50%) were seen in this group indicating resolution of feeding difficulties.

▶ This is an excellent article reviewing the indications and outcome of percutaneous endoscopic gastrostomy (PEG)-related procedures in children. Neurodisability, specifically cerebral palsy, was the single most important indication for PEG placement in the 600 children studied. A low incidence of complications was noted in this group, despite being younger at the time of PEG placement. Infection was the most common complication following placement. Overall, this study would support that PEG placement in children is safe with a low procedure-related morbidity. For those gastrointestinal physicians who care for children, this would be an excellent article to review.

**J. S. Scolapio, MD**

**PART EIGHT**

# ENDOCRINOLOGY, DIABETES, AND METABOLISM

DEREK LEROITH, MD, PHD

# 51 Adrenal Cortex

---

**Late-night salivary cortisol for the diagnosis of Cushing syndrome: a meta-analysis**

Carroll T, Raff H, Findling JW (Med College of Wisconsin, Milwaukee)

*Endocr Pract* 15:335-342, 2009

---

*Objective.*—To report a meta-analysis of late-night salivary cortisol testing for the diagnosis of Cushing syndrome.

*Methods.*—MEDLINE and EMBASE computer databases were searched to identify relevant articles published between January 1950 and December 2007. The search strategy used the following medical subject headings and keywords: cortisol, Cushing or Cushing's, saliva, salivary, late-night, nocturnal, and nighttime. The results were limited to studies in humans older than 18 years. Titles and abstracts of all articles, as well as full text of relevant articles, were reviewed. Sensitivity, specificity, likelihood ratio positive, likelihood ratio negative, and diagnostic odds ratio were extracted by 2 authors. Discrepancies were resolved by mediation and discussion with a third author.

*Results.*—Seven articles contained sufficient information to be included in the analysis. A total of 947 patients (339 with Cushing syndrome) were identified. Pooled data from the 7 studies revealed a sensitivity of 92% (95% confidence interval [CI], 88%-94%), specificity of 96% (95% CI, 94%-97%), and diagnostic odds ratio of 311 (95% CI, 92-1059). Likelihood ratio positive was 21 (95% CI, 10-43), with a likelihood ratio negative of 0.08 (95% CI, 0.02-0.32). Inconsistencies for each of these results measured by the $I^2$ statistic ranged from moderate to high.

*Conclusion.*—This analysis demonstrates that late-night salivary cortisol has excellent diagnostic characteristics and as such, is a robust, convenient test for screening and diagnosis of Cushing syndrome.

► Correctly diagnosing mild Cushing syndrome often can be clinically difficult. Late-night salivary cortisol measurement is a simple and relatively inexpensive screening tool to detect hypercortisolemia and is potentially a very powerful test to diagnose diagnostically challenging cases of Cushing syndrome. Because of this, in the last several years, the use of late-night salivary cortisol measurements has become commonplace in the work up of Cushing syndrome. To address the question of whether late-night salivary cortisol measurements accurately diagnose Cushing syndrome and appropriately differentiate it from other ailments, such as generalized obesity, hypertension, diabetes, etc, Carroll et al performed a meta-analysis of articles published over a 57-year period

(1950–2007) and selected those articles that contained data describing the diagnostic accuracy of late-night salivary cortisol measurements. Nine hundred forty-seven patients (339 with Cushing syndrome) in 7 articles were identified. The authors determined that late-night salivary cortisol measurements have a sensitivity of 92% and a specificity of 96% and is therefore a powerful screening tool for the work-up of Cushing syndrome and has excellent diagnostic characteristics.

**W. H. Ludlam, MD, PhD**

**Specificity of Screening Tests for Cushing's Syndrome in an Overweight and Obese Population**

Baid SK, Rubino D, Sinaii N, et al (Natl Insts of Health, Bethesda, MD; The George Washington Univ Weight Management Program, DC)

*J Clin Endocrinol Metab* 94:3857-3864, 2009

*Context.*—Recent reports suggest a higher prevalence (1–5%) of Cushing's syndrome in certain patient populations with features of the disorder (*e.g.*, diabetes), but the prevalence in the over-weight and obese population is not known.

*Objective.*—The aim of the study was to evaluate the diagnostic performance of screening tests for Cushing's syndrome in overweight and obese subjects with at least two other features of the disorder.

*Design and Setting.*—We conducted a cross-sectional prospective study.

*Subjects and Methods.*—A total of 369 subjects (73% female) completed two or three tests: a 24-h urine cortisol, and/or late-night salivary cortisol, and/or 1 mg dexamethasone suppression test (DST). If any result was abnormal [based on laboratory reference range or cortisol after DST $\geq$1.8 $\mu$g/dl (50 nmol/liter)], tests were repeated and/or a dexamethasone-CRH test was performed. Subjects with abnormal DST results and a low dexamethasone level were asked to repeat the test with 2 mg of dexamethasone.

*Results.*—In addition to obesity, subjects had a mean of five to six features of Cushing's syndrome. None was found to have Cushing's syndrome. Test specificities to exclude Cushing's syndrome for subjects who completed three tests were: urine cortisol, 96% [95% confidence interval (CI), 93–98%]; DST, 90% (95% CI, 87–93%); salivary cortisol, 84% by RIA (95% CI, 79–89%) and 92% by liquid chromatography-tandem mass spectrometry (95% CI, 88–95%). The combined specificity (both tests normal) for all combinations of two tests was 84 to 90%, with overlapping CIs.

*Conclusion.*—These data do not support widespread screening of overweight and obese subjects for Cushing's syndrome; test results for such patients may be falsely abnormal.

► Patients who frequently appear to have Cushing's syndrome are frequently referred to specialized endocrine centers for evaluation. While the most severe cases can be easily diagnosed, borderline cases are much more challenging. The clinical manifestations of Cushing's syndrome involve nonspecific as well as specific symptoms and signs of hypercortisolism. Nonspecific findings include generalized obesity and hypertension, insulin-resistant diabetes mellitus, fatigue, irregular menses, hirsutism, irritability and depression, and all frequent comorbidities of obesity. The specific symptoms involve evidence of protein catabolism such as proximal muscle weakness, muscle atrophy, easy bruising, skin atrophy, atrophic striae, and osteopenia. Given the high prevalence of obesity and its comorbidities, the possibility of Cushing's syndrome should be considered and investigated by sensitive and specific diagnostic testing. This is what Baid et al have done in a series of 369 obese subjects attending a weight loss clinic who presented with at least 2 other features of Cushing's syndrome. In addition to obesity, these subjects had 5 to 6 features of Cushing's syndrome. Diagnostic studies included bedtime salivary cortisol, 24-hour urine cortisol, 1-mg dexamethasone suppression test, and Dex-CRH test. Some of these tests were repeated several times, and higher dose dexamethasone suppression was used in some cases. True Cushing's syndrome was rare. The conclusion of this elaborate study is that it did not support widespread screening of overweight and obese subjects for Cushing's syndrome. Results may be abnormal because of pseudo-Cushing's associated with obesity, a condition still not completely understood. The problem with the conclusion of this study is that patients with true Cushing's syndrome may not be diagnosed for at least 2 to 3 years and their symptoms were attributed to changes in eating habits, aging, hypothyroidism, depression, etc. I prefer to have a low threshold of suspicion and screen patients with at least a 2-hour urinary free cortisol and 1-mg dexamethasone suppression test. Patients can be quite miserable while they wait for a correct diagnosis and appropriate treatment.

**D. E. Schteingart, MD**

---

**Aldosterone Contributes to Blood Pressure Variance and to Likelihood of Hypertension in Normal-Weight and Overweight African Americans**

Kidambi S, Kotchen JM, Krishnaswami S, et al (Med College of Wisconsin, Milwaukee)

*Am J Hypertens* 22:1303-1308, 2009

---

*Background.*—Hypertension and obesity are highly prevalent among African Americans (AAs). We have previously reported that both plasma aldosterone (PA) and body mass index (BMI) are higher in hypertensive than in normotensive AAs. This study evaluates the relative contributions of adiposity and PA to hypertension in AAs.

*Methods.*—A total of 466 AAs (50% hypertensive, 51% women) were evaluated in a Clinical Research Center by stratifying them into three subgroups based on BMI (normal weight, overweight, and obese). Anthropometric measurements, ambulatory blood pressure (BP), fasting glucose, insulin, 24-h urine sodium and potassium, creatinine clearance, standing PA and plasma renin activity (PRA) were measured. Insulin resistance was estimated by the homeostasis model assessment.

*Results.*—Compared to normotensives, hypertensives had higher BMI, waist circumference (WC), and were more insulin resistant ($P \leq 0.01$). When stratified by BMI, hypertensives in each BMI strata had higher PA ($P \leq 0.05$) and lower PRA ($P \leq 0.01$) compared to normotensives. Compared to normotensives, WC was greater in overweight and obese hypertensives, but not in normal-weight hypertensives. In the overall sample, age, WC, PA, and PRA were the major contributors to BP variance and to hypertension. Among normal-weight subjects, PA and PRA significantly predicted BP and the odds ratio for hypertension, whereas WC had no predictive value.

*Conclusions.*—PA, but not WC, is associated with BP and likelihood of hypertension in normal-weight AAs, whereas both WC and PA are predictive of hypertension in overweight and obese individuals. This suggests that aldosterone antagonists may be useful for the treatment of hypertension among AAs, regardless of BMI.

▶ Continuing with the role of aldosterone in the hypertension of normal-weight and overweight African Americans (AA), the study by Kidambi et al in 466 AA shows a link between aldosterone levels and risk of hypertension in both normal-weight and overweight individuals. Waist circumference, a measure of visceral obesity, was a concurrent factor in obese AA individuals. Together with other reports in the literature, there is evidence that because aldosterone is associated with a risk for hypertension even in the absence of primary aldosteronism, treatment with aldosterone receptor antagonists (spironolactone and eplerenone) should be considered in these patients.

**D. E. Schteingart, MD**

---

**Aldosterone status associated with insulin resistance in patients with heart failure—data from the ALOFT study**

Freel EM, Tsorlalis IK, Lewsey JD, et al (Univ of Glasgow, UK; et al)

*Heart* 95:1920-1924, 2009

---

*Background.*—Aldosterone has a key role in the pathophysiology of heart failure. In around 50% of such patients, aldosterone "escapes" from inhibition by drugs that interrupt the renin-angiotensin axis; such patients have a worse clinical outcome. Insulin resistance is a risk factor in heart failure and cardiovascular disease. The relation between aldosterone status and insulin sensitivity was investigated in a cohort of heart failure patients.

*Methods.*—302 patients with New York Heart Association (NYHA) class II-IV heart failure on conventional therapy were randomised in the ALiskiren Observation of heart Failure Treatment study (ALOFT), designed to test the safety of a directly acting renin inhibitor. Plasma aldosterone and 24-hour urinary aldosterone excretion, as well as fasting insulin and homeostasis model assessment of insulin resistance (HOMA-IR) were measured. Subjects with aldosterone escape and high urinary aldosterone were identified according to previously accepted definitions.

*Results.*—20% of subjects demonstrated aldosterone escape and 34% had high urinary aldosterone levels. At baseline, there was a positive correlation between fasting insulin and plasma ($r = 0.22$ $p < 0.01$) and urinary aldosterone($r = 0.19$ $p < 0.03$). Aldosterone escape and high urinary aldosterone subjects both demonstrated higher levels of fasting insulin ($p < 0.008$, $p < 0.03$), HOMA-IR ($p < 0.06$, $p < 0.03$) and insulin-glucose ratios ($p < 0.006$, $p < 0.06$) when compared to low aldosterone counterparts. All associations remained significant when adjusted for potential confounders.

*Conclusions.*—This study demonstrates a novel direct relation between aldosterone status and insulin resistance in heart failure. This observation merits further study and may identify an additional mechanism that contributes to the adverse clinical outcome associated with aldosterone escape.

▶ Several articles over the past 10 years have emphasized the role of aldosterone in the pathogenesis of hypertension and cardiovascular and renal disease. The effect is not through the effect of aldosterone as a mineralocorticoid receptor agonist but a direct effect on myocardial and renal structure and function. Aldosterone antagonists, such as spironolactone and eplerenone have been suggested for the treatment of acute systolic and diastolic heart failure, refractory hypertension to antihypertensive drugs, hypertension in patients with abdominal/visceral obesity, prevention of cardiovascular events in patients with vascular disease and treatment, and prevention of cerebrovascular infarction. Significant increases in plasma aldosterone associated with decreases in plasma renin activity have been described in African Americans with hypertension and metabolic syndrome.[1] The study by Freel et al shows an association between aldosterone and insulin resistance. In a study of 302 patients with heart failure on conventional therapy randomized into the Aliskirin Observation of Heart Failure Treatment (ALOFT) trial, there was a direct correlation between aldosterone levels and insulin resistance as measured by homeostasis model assessment (HOMA). A relationship between aldosterone and glucose tolerance was first described by Jerome Conn in patients with primary aldosteronism. It was suggested then that hypokalemia impaired insulin secretion and caused a delay in insulin release following ingestion of glucose in a pattern similar to patients with type 2 diabetes mellitus. This glucose intolerance was observed in 50% of patients with primary aldosteronism and was reversible with potassium repletion. More recently, it was shown that these patients have diminished insulin sensitivity and that aldosterone decreases expression of insulin substrate[1] and induces insulin resistance at the vascular level via oxidative stress.[2,3] Another study showed higher prevalence of metabolic syndrome in primary aldosteronism than essential hypertension.[4]

**D. E. Schteingart, MD**

*References*

1. Kidambi S, Kotchen JM, Grim CE, et al. Association of adrenal steroids with hypertension and the metabolic syndrome in blacks. *Hypertension.* 2007;49:704.
2. Mosso LM, Carvajal CA, Maiz A, et al. A possible association between primary aldosteronism and a lower beta-cell function. *J Hypertens.* 2007;25:2125-2130.
3. Hitomi H, Kiyomoto H, Nishiyama A, et al. Aldosterone suppresses insulin signaling via the downregulation of insulin receptor substrate-1 in vascular smooth muscle cells. *Hypertension.* 2007;50:750.
4. Fallo F, Veglio F, Bertello C, et al. Prevalence and characteristics of the metabolic syndrome in primary aldosteronism. *J Clin Endocrinol Metab.* 2006;91:454.

# 52 Calcium and Bone Metabolism

**Denosumab in Men Receiving Androgen-Deprivation Therapy for Prostate Cancer**

Smith MR, for the Denosumab HALT Prostate Cancer Study Group (Massachusetts General Hosp Cancer Ctr, Boston, MA; et al)

*N Engl J Med* 361:745-755, 2009

*Background.*—Androgen-deprivation therapy is well-established for treating prostate cancer but is associated with bone loss and an increased risk of fracture. We investigated the effects of denosumab, a fully human monoclonal antibody against receptor activator of nuclear factor-κB ligand, on bone mineral density and fractures in men receiving androgen-deprivation therapy for nonmetastatic prostate cancer.

*Methods.*—In this double-blind, multicenter study, we randomly assigned patients to receive denosumab at a dose of 60 mg subcutaneously every 6 months or placebo (734 patients in each group). The primary end point was percent change in bone mineral density at the lumbar spine at 24 months. Key secondary end points included percent change in bone mineral densities at the femoral neck and total hip at 24 months and at all three sites at 36 months, as well as incidence of new vertebral fractures.

*Results.*—At 24 months, bone mineral density of the lumbar spine had increased by 5.6% in the denosumab group as compared with a loss of 1.0% in the placebo group ($P < 0.001$); significant differences between the two groups were seen at as early as 1 month and sustained through 36 months. Denosumab therapy was also associated with significant increases in bone mineral density at the total hip, femoral neck, and distal third of the radius at all time points. Patients who received denosumab had a decreased incidence of new vertebral fractures at 36 months (1.5%, vs. 3.9% with placebo) (relative risk, 0.38; 95% confidence interval, 0.19 to 0.78; $P = 0.006$). Rates of adverse events were similar between the two groups.

*Conclusions.*—Denosumab was associated with increased bone mineral density at all sites and a reduction in the incidence of new vertebral fractures among men receiving androgendeprivation therapy for nonmetastatic prostate cancer. (ClinicalTrials.gov number, NCT00089674.)

▶ Denosumab is an emerging treatment for bone disease that is being investigated for treatment of nonmetastatic prostate cancer. This drug is a fully human monoclonal antibody to the receptor activator of nuclear factor-κB ligand (RANKL) that blocks recruitment, activation, and survival of osteoclasts.[1,2] Denosumab primarily prevents bone loss, so it might help prevent bone loss in patients with prostate cancer treated with androgen-deprivation therapy. Androgen-deprivation therapy for prostate cancer causes hypogonadotropic hypogonadism, which is associated with bone loss and fractures.[3-7]

This clinical trial randomized 1468 men with nonmetastatic prostate cancer to receive either denosumab 60 mg by subcutaneous injection once every 6 months or placebo for 3 years. Subjects receiving denosumab experienced an increase in lumbar spine bone mineral density (BMD) of 5.6%, whereas subjects on placebo experienced a decrease of 1.0% over 2 years (Fig 2 in the original article). A difference in bone density between the 2 groups was seen as early as 1 month of treatment, and this difference persisted over 36 months. Denosumab was also associated with increased BMD at the total hip, femoral neck, and one-third distal radius across the duration of the study. Subjects receiving denosumab developed a cumulative incidence of new vertebral fractures of 1.5% over 3 years, whereas the placebo group experienced a cumulative incidence of 3.9%, for a reduction in new vertebral fractures of 62%. Adverse events were equally balanced between the denosumab and placebo groups.

This study demonstrates that denosumab is associated with increased BMD at the lumbar spine, hip, and wrist in men receiving androgen-deprivation therapy for prostate cancer. Denosumab also reduces new vertebral fractures in this population. These findings are important because androgen-deprivation therapy used in men with prostate cancer is associated with bone loss and fractures. Denosumab prevents bone loss and vertebral fractures in men with nonmetastatic prostate cancer receiving androgen-deprivation therapy.

**B. L. Clarke, MD**

*References*


1. Kearns AE, Khosla S, Kostenuik PJ. Receptor activator of nuclear factor kappaB ligand and osteoprotegerin regulation of bone remodeling in health and disease. *Endocr Rev.* 2008;29:155-192.
2. Hofbauer LC, Schoppet M. Clinical implications of the osteoprotegerin/RANK/RANKL system for bone and vascular diseases. *JAMA.* 2004;292:490-495.
3. Loblaw DA, Virgo KS, Nam R, et al. Initial hormonal management of androgen-sensitive metastatic, recurrent, or progressive prostate cancer: 2006 update of an American Society of Clinical Oncology practice guideline. *J Clin Oncol.* 2007;25:1596-1605.
4. Sharifi N, Gulley JL, Dahut WL. Androgen deprivation therapy for prostate cancer. *JAMA.* 2005;294:238-244.
5. Bolla M, Collette L, Blank L, et al. Long-term results with immediate androgen suppression and external irradiation in patients with locally advanced prostate cancer (an EORTC study): a phase III randomised trial. *Lancet.* 2002;360:103-108.
6. Messing EM, Manola J, Sarosdy M, Wilding G, Crawford ED, Trump D. Immediate hormonal therapy compared with observation after radical prostatectomy and pelvic lymphadenectomy in men with node-positive prostate cancer. *New Engl J Med.* 1999;341:1781-1788.

7. Michaelson MD, Marujo RM, Smith MR. Contribution of androgen deprivation therapy to elevated osteoclast activity in men with metastatic prostate cancer. *Clin Cancer Res.*. 2004;10:2705-2708.

**Effect of Rosiglitazone, Metformin, and Glyburide on Bone Biomarkers in Patients with Type 2 Diabetes**

Zinman B, the A Diabetes Outcome Progression Trial Study Group (Mount Sinai Hosp and Univ of Toronto, Ontario, Canada; et al)

*J Clin Endocrinol Metab* 95:134-142, 2010

*Context.*—An increase in bone fractures has been observed in women taking thiazolidinediones.

*Objective.*—The objective of the study was to examine whether changes in circulating bone biomarkers provide insight into the underlying mechanisms responsible for the increase in bone fractures in female participants randomized to rosiglitazone in A Diabetes Outcome Progression Trial (ADOPT).

*Research Design and Methods.*—Paired stored baseline and 12-month serum samples were available from 1605 participants (689 women, 916 men) in ADOPT, a long-term clinical trial comparing the effects of rosiglitazone, glyburide, and metformin on glycemic control in patients with type 2 diabetes.

*Results.*—This subset was well matched to the total ADOPT study population. In women a marker of osteoclast activity, C-terminal telopeptide (for type 1 collagen), increased by 6.1% with rosiglitazone compared with reductions of 1.3% ($P = 0.03$ *vs.* rosiglitazone) and 3.3% ($P = 0.002$ *vs.* rosiglitazone) with metformin and glyburide, respectively. In men, C-terminal telopeptide was unchanged on rosiglitazone (−1.0%) and fell on metformin (−12.7%; $P < 0.001$) and glyburide (−4.3%, $P = \text{NS}$). Markers of osteoblast activity, procollagen type 1 N-propeptide (P1NP) and bone alkaline phosphatase, were reduced for women and men in almost all treatment groups, with the greatest changes in the metformin group (P1NP in females, −14.4%; P1NP in males, −19.3%), intermediate for rosiglitazone (P1NP in females,−4.4%; P1NP in males,−14.4%), and smallest for glyburide (P1NP in males, +0.2%; bone alkaline phosphatase in females, −11.6%).

*Conclusions.*—Commonly measured bone biomarkers suggest that changes in bone resorption may be partly responsible for the increased risk of fracture in women taking thiazolidinediones.

► Postmenopausal women with type 2 diabetes mellitus who take thiazolidenediones (TZDs) have been reported to be at increased risk of fracture, independent of the fracture risk associated with their diabetes. The fact that TZDs increase fracture risk was reported in A Diabetes Outcome Progression Trial (ADOPT).[1] ADOPT was a randomized, double-blind, prospective, controlled clinical trial comparing the effects of the TZDs rosiglitazone, metformin, and glyburide on glucose control in recently diagnosed drug-naïve type 2 diabetic patients.[2] Rosiglitazone was not only shown to cause more durable blood glucose control than metformin or glyburide, as assessed by fasting glucose and hemoglobin A1c levels, but was also shown to be associated with increased risk of upper and lower limb peripheral fractures in postmenopausal women.[2] Rosiglitazone was not associated with vertebral or hip fractures in postmenopausal women, however, and not associated with fractures in men. Shortly after the results of ADOPT were released, pioglitazone was also reported to be associated with increased fracture risk.[3]

The mechanisms by which TZDs might cause limb fractures are not well understood. Cell culture studies have demonstrated that TZDs stimulate differentiation of mesenchymal progenitor cells into adipocytes rather than osteoblasts[4] and that they may decrease osteoblast differentiation by reducing IGF-1 levels in bone.[5] Rodent studies have shown that TZDs cause bone loss in most studies by reducing bone formation[6] but in some studies by increasing bone resorption.[7] Previous studies of markers of bone turnover in postmenopausal women have shown that TZDs suppress bone formation, without changing bone resorption.[8,9]

This study evaluated paired baseline and 12-month serum markers of bone turnover in a subset of 689 postmenopausal women and 916 men in ADOPT. Serum C-terminal telopeptide of type I collagen (CTX), a marker of bone resorption, increased in the women receiving rosiglitazone but remained stable in men. This marker decreased mildly in women, and more significantly in men, receiving metformin or glyburide. Serum procollagen type 1 aminoN-terminal propeptide (P1NP) and bone alkaline phosphatase, markers of bone formation, decreased in both women and men regardless of the drug received, with the greatest decreases seen in subjects receiving metformin.

These findings suggest that rosiglitazone may affect bone remodeling by both decreasing bone formation and stimulating bone resorption. Limitations of this study include lack of a placebo arm, measurements made only on samples collected during the first year of this 4-year study, lack of systematic collection of samples, and lack of bone density information. Differences in fractures between the 3 study drugs did not occur until after the first year.[2] Nevertheless, this is the largest study to evaluate the effects of TZDs on bone metabolism. Further controlled long-term studies evaluating markers of bone turnover, bone mineral density, and fractures will be required to clearly establish the mechanisms behind TZD-induced fractures.

**B. L. Clarke, MD**

*References*

1. Kahn SE, Haffner SM, Heise MA, et al. ADOPT Study Group. Glycemic durability of rosiglitazone, metformin, or glyburide monotherapy. *N Engl J Med.* 2006;355: 2427-2443.
2. Kahn SE, Zinman B, Lachin JM, et al. Diabetes Outcome Progression Trial (ADOPT) Study Group. Rosiglitazone-associated fractures in type 2 diabetes: an analysis from A Diabetes Outcome Progression Trial (ADOPT). *Diabetes Care.* 2008;31:845-851.

3. Takeda Pharmaceuticals. Observation of an increased incidence of fractures in female patients who received long-term treatment with ACTOS (pioglitazone HCl) tablets for type 2 diabetes mellitus (letter to health care providers), 2007.
4. Ali AA, Weinstein RS, Stewart SA, Parfitt AM, Manolagas SC, Jilka RL. Rosiglitazone causes bone loss in mice by suppressing osteoblast differentiation and bone formation. *Endocrinology.* 2005;146:1226-1235.
5. Lecka-Czernik B, Ackert-Bicknell C, Adamo ML, et al. Activation of peroxisome proliferator-activated receptor γ (PPARγ) by rosiglitazone suppresses components of the insulin-like growth factor regulatory system in vitro and in vivo. *Endocrinology.* 2007;148:903-911.
6. Grey A. Skeletal consequences of thiazolidinedione therapy. *Osteoporos Int.* 2008; 19:129-137.
7. Lazarenko OP, Rzonka SO, Hogue WR, et al. Rosiglitazone induces decreases in bone mass and strength that are reminiscent of age bone. *Endocrinology.* 2007; 75:2669-2680.
8. Grey A, Bolland M, Gamble G, et al. The peroxisome proliferator-activated receptor- rosiglitazone decreases bone formation and bone mineral density in healthy postmenopausal women: a randomized, controlled trial. *J Clin Endocrinol Metab.* 2007;92:1305-1310.
9. Berberoglu Z, Gursoy A, Bayraktar N, et al. Rosiglitazone decreases serum bone specific alkaline phosphatase activity in postmenopausal diabetic women. *J Clin Endocrinol Metab.* 2007;92:3523-3530.


## Effects of Teriparatide in Postmenopausal Women with Osteoporosis on Prior Alendronate or Raloxifene: Differences between Stopping and Continuing the Antiresorptive Agent

Cosman F, Wermers RA, Recknor C, et al (Helen Hayes Hosp, West Haverstraw, NY; Mayo Clinic, Rochester, MN; United Osteoporosis Ctrs, Gainesville, GA; et al)

*J Clin Endocrinol Metab* 94:3772-3780, 2009


*Objective.*—The aim of the study was to assess adding *vs.* switching to teriparatide 20μg/d in patients on alendronate or raloxifene.

*Design.*—We conducted a randomized, open-label trial.

*Patients and Interventions.*—Postmenopausal women with osteoporosis on alendronate or raloxifene for at least 18 months added teriparatide (Add groups) or switched to teriparatide (Switch groups) for 18 months.

*Main Outcome Measures.*—We measured bone turnover markers (BTM) and bone mineral density (BMD).

*Results.*—In the alendronate stratum, increases in BTM were smaller in the Add *vs.* Switch group [6-month PINP (64 *vs.* 401%); bone ALP (15 *vs.* 71%); βCTX (27 *vs.* 250%); all $P < 0.001$]. However, at 6 months, total hip BMD increased more in the Add *vs.* Switch group (1.4 *vs.* −0.8%; $P = 0.002$). In the Add *vs.* Switch group, 18-month BMD increments were higher in lumbar spine (8.4 *vs.* 4.8%; $P = 0.003$) and total hip (3.2 *vs.* 0.9%; $P = 0.02$), but not in femoral neck (2.7 *vs.* 2.3%; $P = 0.75$). In the raloxifene stratum, increases in BTM were also smaller in the Add *vs.* Switch group [6-month PINP (131 *vs.* 259%; $P < 0.001$), bone

ALP (31 *vs.* 44%; $P = 0.035$), and βCTX (67 *vs.* 144%; $P = 0.001$)]. At 6 months, total hip BMD increase was greater in the Add *vs.* Switch group (1.8 *vs.* 0.5%; $P = 0.028$). At 18 months, increases in lumbar spine (9.2 *vs.* 8.1%), total hip (2.8 *vs.* 1.8%), and femoral neck (3.8 *vs.* 2.2%) were not significantly different between groups.

*Conclusions.*—In women with osteoporosis treated with antiresorptives, greater bone turnover increases were achieved by switching to teriparatide, whereas greater BMD increases were achieved by adding teriparatide.

▶ Treatment of postmenopausal osteoporosis with the anabolic agent teriparatide (human recombinant parathyroid hormone 1-34) stimulates bone formation and bone resorption, improves cortical and trabecular microarchitecture, improves bone mineral density (BMD), and decreases fractures.[1-4] This agent is approved for the treatment of osteoporosis in postmenopausal women and men at high risk of fracture, or those who have not responded or been able to tolerate other therapies.

There have been fewer studies of the effect of parathyroid hormone in combination with other antiresorptive agents. In postmenopausal osteoporotic women who had not previously been treated for osteoporosis, parathyroid hormone (PTH) 1-84 in combination with alendronate caused similar increases in lumbar spine BMD, but greater increases in total hip and radius BMD, than PTH 1-84 alone.[5] Similar findings were reported in postmenopausal osteoporotic women not previously treated for osteoporosis who were treated with the combination of teriparatide and raloxifene.[6]

The effect of teriparatide in patients who were previously treated with other osteoporotic drugs is less well understood. This study compared the BMD, bone turnover marker, and calcemic responses to teriparatide over 18 months in 198 postmenopausal osteoporotic women previously treated with alendronate 70 mg/wk or raloxifene 60 mg/d for at least 18 months. Subjects were randomized to continue their previous treatment and add teriparatide 20 μg/d, or to switch from their previous agent to teriparatide 20 μg/d. Subjects who added teriparatide to their previous antiresorptive therapy had greater increases in lumbar spine and hip BMD when previously treated with alendronate, and in hip BMD when previously treated with raloxifene. Subjects who switched to teriparatide had greater increases in their bone turnover markers than those who continued their previous therapy in combination with teriparatide.

This study demonstrated that postmenopausal osteoporotic women previously treated with alendronate or raloxifene for at least 18 months, who added teriparatide for another 18 months, had significant further improvement in BMD at their lumbar spine and hip. Postmenopausal women previously treated with alendronate or raloxifene for at least 18 months, who switched to teriparatide for another 18 months, had mildly increased lumbar spine BMD, but stable hip BMD. In spite of these changes in BMD, the changes in markers of turnover were greater when subjects switched to teriparatide. These findings demonstrate the complexity of skeletal response that may be seen in patients treated sequentially with monotherapy followed by combination therapy, or who are switched to new monotherapy after previous monotherapy with a different agent, and give insight into the variations in response that might be seen with different permutations and combinations of osteoporosis therapies.

**B. L. Clarke, MD**

*References*


1. Neer RM, Arnaud CD, Zanchetta JR, et al. Effect of parathyroid hormone (1-34) on fractures and bone mineral density in postmenopausal women with osteoporosis. *N Engl J Med.* 2001;344:1434-1441.
2. Lindsay R, Zhou H, Cosman F, Nieves J, Dempster DW, Hodsman AB. Effects of a one-month treatment with PTH (1-34) on bone formation on cancellous, endocortical, and periosteal surfaces of the human ilium. *J Bone Miner Res.* 2007;22: 495-502.
3. McClung MR, San Martin J, Miller PD, et al. Opposite bone remodeling effects of teriparatide and alendronate in increasing bone mass. *Arch Int Med.* 2005;165: 1762-1768.
4. Jiang Y, Zhao JJ, Mitlak BH, Wang O, Genant HK, Eriksen EF. Recombinant human parathyroid hormone (1-34) [teriparatide] improves both cortical and cancellous bone structure. *J Bone Miner Res.* 2003;18:1932-1941.
5. Black DM, Greenspan SL, Ensrud KE, et al. PaTH Study Investigators. The effects of parathyroid hormone and alendronate alone or in combination in postmenopausal osteoporosis. *N Engl J Med.* 2003;349:1207-1215.
6. Deal C, Omizo M, Schwartz EN, et al. Combination teriparatide and raloxifene therapy for postmenopausal osteoporosis: results from a 6-month double-blind placebo-controlled trial. *J Bone Miner Res.* 2005;20:1905-1911.


---

## Thiazolidenedione Use and the Longitudinal Risk of Fractures in Patients with Type 2 Diabetes Mellitus

Habib ZA, Havstad SL, Wells K, et al (Henry Ford Hosp, Detroit, MI)
*J Clin Endocrinol Metab* 95:592-600, 2010

---


*Context.*—Thiazolidinedione (TZD) use has recently been associated with an increased risk of fractures.

*Objective.*—The aim of this study was to determine the time-dependent relationship between TZD use and fracture risk.

*Design.*—We conducted a retrospective cohort study in a large health system in southeast Michigan.

*Patients.*—Patients who received care from the health system were included if they were at least 18 yr of age, had a diagnosis of diabetes, and had at least one prescription for an oral diabetes medication. These criteria identified 19,070 individuals (9,620 women and 9,450 men).

*Intervention.*—This study compared patients treated with TZDs to patients without TZD treatment. Cox proportional hazard models were used to assess the relationship between exposure and outcomes.

*Main Outcome Measures.*—The primary outcome was the time to fracture. Secondary analyses examined the risk of fractures in subgroups defined by sex and age.

*Results.*—TZD use was associated with an increased risk of fracture in the cohort overall [adjusted hazard ratio (aHR), 1.35; 95% confidence interval (CI), 1.05–1.71] and in women (aHR, 1.57; 95% CI, 1.16–2.14), but not in men (aHR, 1.05; 95% CI, 0.70–1.58). Women more than 65 yr of age appeared to be at greatest risk for fracture (aHR, 1.72; 95% CI, 1.17–2.52). Among women, the increased fracture risk was not apparent until after 1 yr of TZD treatment.

*Conclusions.*—TZD use was associated with an increased risk for fractures in women, particularly at ages above 65 yr. Clinicians should be aware of this association when considering TZD therapy so as to appropriately manage and counsel their patients.

▶ Thiazolidenediones (TZDs) are effective in improving insulin resistance in patients with type 2 diabetes mellitus.[1] This category of drug is among the most commonly prescribed oral agent for treatment of type 2 diabetes mellitus in the United States. Several studies have reported an increased risk of bone loss and fractures in diabetic subjects taking TZDs.[2-6] The risk of bone loss and fractures associated with TZD use appears to be independent of the effect of the more rapid bone loss and increased fracture risk associated with type 2 diabetes mellitus.[7-9] Insulin use itself has been reported to be associated with increased fracture risk in patients with diabetes.[10] Other factors, including decreased visual acuity and peripheral neuropathy due to diabetes, may increase fall risk, and diabetic nephropathy also increases bone loss and fractures. Most studies reporting increased fracture risk associated with TZD use in type 2 diabetes are based on adverse event reports in large randomized controlled trials, small observational studies, a single case-control study, and one meta-analysis. One randomized controlled trial evaluated the effect of rosiglitazone on markers of bone turnover, but not fractures. Another longitudinal observational study evaluated fracture risk due to TZDs in older adults compared with other oral agent therapies. This study reports an increased risk of fracture in 9620 women, but not 9450 men, aged 18 years or older, who had type 2 diabetes mellitus followed for at least 7 years. The adjusted hazard ratio for fracture for women treated with TZDs was 1.35 (95% CI, 1.05-1.71). Postmenopausal women over age 65 years were at greatest risk of fracture, with an adjusted hazard ratio of 1.72 (95% CI, 1.17-2.52). The increased risk of fracture in these women took 1 year of TZD treatment to become evident (Fig 2 in the original article). Fractures seen in the women in this cohort were primarily in the upper and distal lower extremities, as reported in other clinical studies. These findings provide additional support that TZDs may increase fracture risk in older postmenopausal women. The mechanisms by which TZDs affect fracture risk are still not completely elucidated, although available bone marker data suggest that TZDs acting as PPAR$\gamma$ agonists stimulate the differentiation of bone marrow mesenchymal stem cells into adipocytes and not osteoblasts. In addition, TZDs appear to suppress osteoblast function and bone formation while stimulating osteoclast differentiation. Further studies are needed to clarify the mechanisms of bone loss associated with TZD use, and whether fracture risk is increased throughout the skeleton and not just the upper and distal lower extremities.

**B. L. Clarke, MD**

*References*


1. Yki-Järvinen H. Thiazolidenediones. *N Engl J Med.* 2004;351:1106-1118.
2. Schwartz AV, Sellmeyer DE, Vittinghoff E, et al. Thiazolidenedione use and bone loss in older diabetic patients. *J Clin Endocrinol Metab.* 2006;91:3349-3354.
3. Kahn SE, Haffner SM, Heise MA, et al. ADOPT Study Group. Glycemic durability of rosiglitazone, metformin, or glyburide monotherapy. *N Engl J Med.* 2006;355:2427-2443.
4. Dormandy J, Bhattacharya M, van Troostenburg de Bruyn AR, PRO active investigators. Safety and tolerability of pioglitazone in high-risk patients with type 2 diabetes: an overview of data from PROactive. *Drug Saf.* 2009;32:187-202.
5. Home PD, Pocock SJ, Beck-Nielsen H, et al. RECORD Study Team. Rosiglitazone evaluated for cardiovascular outcomes in oral agent combination therapy for type 2 diabetes (RECORD): a multicenter, randomised, open-label trial. *Lancet.* 2009;373:2125-2135.
6. Loke YK, Singh S, Furberg CD. Long-term use of thiazolidenediones and fractures in type 2 diabetes mellitus: a meta-analysis. *CMAJ.* 2009;180:32-39.
7. Schwartz AV, Sellmeyer DE, Strotmeyer ES, et al. Health ABC Study. Diabetes and bone loss at the hip in older black and white adults. *J Bone Miner Res.* 2005;20:596-603.
8. Bonds DE, Larson JC, Schwartz AV, et al. Risk of fracture in women with type 2 diabetes mellitus: the Women's Health Initiative Observational Study. *J Clin Endocrinol Metab.* 2006;91:3404-3410.
9. Leslie WD, Lix LM, Prior HJ, Derksen S, Metge C, O'Neil J. Biphasic fracture risk in diabetes: a population-based study. *Bone.* 2007;40:1595-1601.
10. Ivers RQ, Cumming RG, Mitchell P, Peduto AJ, Blue Mountains Eye Study. Diabetes and risk of fracture: the Blue Mountains Eye Study. *Diabetes Care.* 2001; 24:1198-1203.


---

**Zoledronic acid and risedronate in the prevention and treatment of glucocorticoid-induced osteoporosis (HORIZON): a multicentre, double-blind, double-dummy, randomised controlled trial**

Reid DM, for the HORIZON investigators (Univ of Aberdeen, UK; et al)

*Lancet* 373:1253-1263, 2009

---

*Background.*—Persistent use of glucocorticoid drugs is associated with bone loss and increased fracture risk. Concurrent oral bisphosphonates increase bone mineral density and reduce frequency of vertebral fractures, but are associated with poor compliance and adherence. We aimed to assess whether one intravenous infusion of zoledronic acid was non-inferior to daily oral risedronate for prevention and treatment of glucocorticoid-induced osteoporosis.

*Methods.*—This 1-year randomised, double-blind, double-dummy, non-inferiority study of 54 centres in 12 European countries, Australia, Hong

Kong, Israel, and the USA, tested the effectiveness of 5 mg intravenous infusion of zoledronic acid versus 5 mg oral risedronate for prevention and treatment of glucocorticoid-induced osteoporosis. 833 patients were randomised 1:1 to receive zoledronic acid (n=416) or risedronate (n=417). Patients were stratified by sex, and allocated to prevention or treatment subgroups dependent on duration of glucocorticoid use immediately preceding the study. The treatment subgroup consisted of those treated for more than 3 months (272 patients on zoledronic acid and 273 on risedronate), and the prevention subgroup of those treated for less than 3 months (144 patients on each drug). 62 patients did not complete the study because of adverse events, withdrawal of consent, loss to follow-up, death, misrandomisation, or protocol deviation. The primary endpoint was percentage change from baseline in lumbar spine bone mineral density. Drug efficacy was assessed on a modified intention-to-treat basis and safety was assessed on an intention-to-treat basis. This trial is registered with ClinicalTrials.gov, number NCT00100620.

*Findings.*—Zoledronic acid was non-inferior and superior to risedronate for increase of lumbar spine bone mineral density in both the treatment (least-squares mean 4·06% [SE 0·28] *vs* 2·71% [SE 0·28], mean difference 1·36% [95% CI 0·67–2·05], p=0·0001) and prevention (2·60% [0·45] *vs* 0·64% [0·46], 1·96% [1·04–2·88], p<0·0001) subgroups at 12 months. Adverse events were more frequent in patients given zoledronic acid than in those on risedronate, largely as a result of transient symptoms during the first 3 days after infusion. Serious adverse events were worsening rheumatoid arthritis for the treatment subgroup and pyrexia for the prevention subgroup.

*Interpretation.*—A single 5 mg intravenous infusion of zoledronic acid is non-inferior, possibly more effective, and more acceptable to patients than is 5 mg of oral risedronate daily for prevention and treatment of bone loss that is associated with glucocorticoid use (Fig 2).

▶ Persistent use of glucocorticoid therapy may suppress bone formation and result in increased bone loss and fractures.[1-3] Most studies have shown that the magnitude of the bone loss and increased fracture risk depends on the dose and duration of therapy with glucocorticoids.[4] Oral alendronate and risedronate have been shown to prevent bone loss in patients taking oral glucocorticoid therapy,[5-7] but these placebo-controlled studies were not powered to show fracture reduction.

Zoledronic acid is a potent, long-lasting, intravenous bisphosphonate used to treat postmenopausal osteoporosis and prevent fractures in subjects not taking glucocorticoids.[8,9] This noninferiority study evaluated the effectiveness of zoledronic acid 5 mg given intravenously once a year to risedronate 5 mg orally each day for 1 year for the prevention and treatment of glucocorticoid-induced osteoporosis. The study randomized 833 subjects to receive zoledronic acid or risedronate, and further stratified participants by duration of glucocorticoid therapy. Subjects treated for more than 3 months with glucocorticoids were considered part of the treatment group, whereas subjects taking

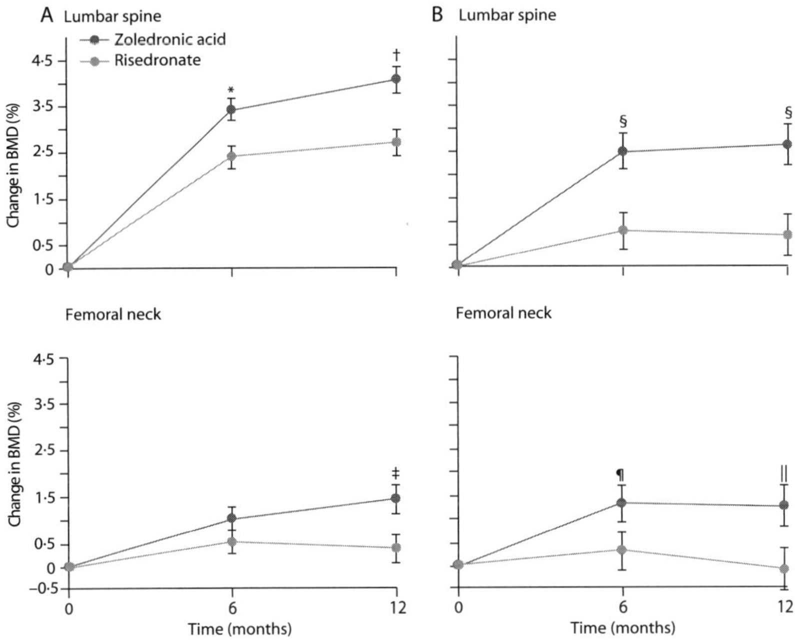


FIGURE 2.—Change in mean bone mineral density of lumbar spine and femoral neck for (A) treatment and (B) prevention subgroups (modified intention-to-treat group). Data are least-squares mean. Error bars=95% CI. BMD=bone mineral density. p values compare change in bone mineral density relative to baseline between drug groups, calculated from a three-way analysis of variance with adjustment for drug group, study region, and sex. *p=0·0005. †p=0·0001. ‡p=0·0050. §p<0·0001. ¶p=0·0156. ||p=0·0049. (Reprinted from Reid DM, for the HORIZON investigators. Zoledronic acid and risedronate in the prevention and treatment of glucocorticoid-induced osteoporosis (HORIZON): a multicentre, double-blind, double-dummy, randomised controlled trial. *Lancet*. 2009;373:1253-1263, with permission from Elsevier.)

glucocorticoids for less than 3 months were categorized as part of the prevention group. Zoledronic acid was found to be noninferior and superior to risedronate with regard to lumbar spine bone density increase in both the treatment and prevention groups at 1 year (Fig 2). Adverse events were more common in the zoledronic acid group because of transient symptoms during the first 3 days after the infusion.

This study concluded that once yearly zoledronic acid is noninferior, and possibly more effective, than risedronate in the prevention and treatment of glucocorticoid-induced bone loss. Different bisphosphonates effectively prevent bone loss in subjects treated with glucocorticoids, but studies to date have not been powered to show fracture prevention. This is the first study to compare the effects of two different bisphosphonate therapies head-to-head in patients treated with glucocorticoid-induced osteoporosis.

**B. L. Clarke, MD**

*References*


1. van Staa TP, Leufkens HG, Abenhaim L, Zhang B, Cooper C. Use of oral corticosteroids and risk of fractures. *J Bone Miner Res.* 2000;15:993-1000.
2. van Staa TP, Leufkens HG, Abenhaim L, Zhang B, Cooper C. Oral corticosteroids and fracture risk: relationship to daily and cumulative doses. *Rheumatology (Oxf).* 2000;39:1383-1389.
3. van Staa TP, Leufkens HG, Cooper C. The epidemiology of corticosteroid-induced osteoporosis: a meta-analysis. *Osteoporos Int.* 2002;13:777-787.
4. American College of Rheumatology Ad Hoc Committee on Glucocorticoid-Induced Osteoporosis. Recommendations for the prevention and treatment of glucocorticoid-induced osteoporosis: 2001 update. *Arthritis Rheum.* 2001;44: 1496-1503.
5. Cohen S, Levy RM, Keller M, et al. Risedronate therapy prevents corticosteroid-induced bone loss: a twelve-month, multicenter, randomized, double-blind, placebo-controlled, parallel-group study. *Arthritis Rheum.* 1999;42:2309-2318.
6. Reid DM, Hughes RA, Laan RF, et al. Efficacy and safety of daily risedronate in the treatment of corticosteroid-induced osteoporosis in men and women: a randomized trial. European Corticosteroid-Induced Osteoporosis Treatment Study. *J Bone Miner Res.* 2000;15:1006-1013.
7. Saag KG, Emkey R, Schnitzer TJ, et al. Alendronate for the prevention and treatment of glucocorticoid-induced osteoporosis. Glucocorticoid-Induced Osteoporosis Intervention Study Group. *N Engl J Med.* 1998;339:292-299.
8. Black DM, Cummings SR, Karpf DB, et al. HORIZON Pivotal Fracture Trial. Once-yearly zoledronic acid for treatment of postmenopausal osteoporosis. *N Engl J Med.* 2007;356:1809-1822.
9. Lyles KW, Colon-Emeric CS, Magaziner JS, et al. HORIZON Recurrent Fracture Trial. Zoledronic acid and clinical fractures and mortality after hip fracture. *N Engl J Med.* 2007;357:1799-1809.


---

## Bone Mineralization Defects and Vitamin D Deficiency: Histomorphometric Analysis of Iliac Crest Bone Biopsies and Circulating 25-Hydroxyvitamin D in 675 Patients

Priemel M, von Domarus C, Klatte TO, et al (Univ Med Ctr Hamburg-Eppendorf, Germany)

*J Bone Miner Res* 25:305-312, 2010

---

Parathyroid hormone (PTH) is only one measurable index of skeletal health, and we reasoned that a histomorphometric analysis of iliac crest biopsies would be another and even more direct approach to assess bone health and address the required minimum 25-Hydroxyvitamin D [25(OH)D] level. A cohort from the northern European population with its known high prevalence of vitamin D deficiency therefore would be ideal to answer the latter question. We examined 675 iliac crest biopsies from male and female individuals, excluding all patients who showed any signs of secondary bone diseases at autopsy. Structural histomorphometric parameters, including osteoid indices, were quantified using the Osteomeasure System according to ASBMR standards, and serum 25(OH)D levels were measured for all patients. Statistical analysis was performed by Student's $t$ test. The histologic results demonstrate an unexpected high prevalence of mineralization defects, that is, a pathologic increase in osteoid. Indeed, 36.15% of the analyzed patients presented with an osteoid surface per bone surface (OS/BS) of more than 20%. Based on the most conservative threshold that defines osteomalacia at the histomorphometric level with a pathologic increase in osteoid volume per bone volume (OV/BV) greater than 2% manifest mineralization defects were present in 25.63% of the patients. The latter were found independent of bone volume per trabecular volume (BV/TV) throughout all ages and affected both sexes equally. While we could not establish a minimum 25(OH)D level that was inevitably associated with mineralization defects, we did not find pathologic accumulation of osteoid in any patient with circulating 25(OH)D above 75 nmol/L. Our data demonstrate that pathologic mineralization defects of bone occur in patients with a serum 25(OH)D below 75 nmol/L and strongly argue that in conjunction with a sufficient calcium intake, the dose of vitamin D supplementation should ensure that circulating levels of 25(OH)D reach this minimum threshold (75 nmol/L or 30 ng/mL) to maintain skeletal health.

▶ Vitamin D and calcium are both important for maintenance of normal skeletal health. However, debate persists regarding the optimal amounts of vitamin D and calcium that older men and women require to protect their skeletal health.[1] It is widely agreed that vitamin D and calcium supplementation should be the first consideration in treatment regimens for osteoporosis.[2] Vitamin D and calcium supplementation helps offset low calcium intake or absorption that otherwise requires the skeleton to give up skeletal mineral to keep serum calcium levels in the normal range. Vitamin D and calcium together reduce increased skeletal bone turnover that results in increased bone fragility,[3] reduce fracture rates,[4] and improve neuromuscular function leading to decreased falls.[5]

It is generally agreed that serum 25-hydroxyvitamin D is the best measure of vitamin D status, but there is not yet a general consensus regarding the optimal vitamin D level for skeletal health. Recent studies have defined the optimal circulating serum 25-hydroxyvitamin D level to be the level required to maximally suppress parathyroid hormone secretion.[1] Multiple studies have shown that this threshold in adult humans is around a mean of 30 ng/mL, with a published range from 12 to 40 ng/mL.[6] Other indices of skeletal health could also be considered in helping to define the optimal serum 25-hydroxyvitamin D level, among them iliac crest bone histomorphometric mineralization.

The authors performed unlabeled iliac crest bone biopsies in 675 deceased male and female subjects at autopsy in one northern German city, excluding any subjects with obvious evidence of bone disease, and determined serum 25-hydroxyvitamin D levels in blood taken at the time of autopsy. Bone histomorphometry showed abnormally increased osteoid in 36.2% of subjects, with osteoid surface/bone surface greater than 20%. Osteoid volume/bone volume greater than 2% was found in 25.6% of subjects, regardless of age and sex. Pathological accumulation of osteoid or defective osteoid mineralization was not seen with serum 25-hydroxyvitamin D levels less than 30 ng/mL, although a lower threshold for serum 25-hydroxyvitamin D that was always associated with mineralization defects was not able to be determined.

This study concluded that serum 25-hydroxyvitamin D levels above 30 ng/mL were not associated with mineralization abnormalities on iliac crest bone biopsies but did not determine a lower threshold at which vitamin D prevented osteomalacia in all subjects. These findings suggest that the optimal serum 25-hydroxyvitamin D level required to prevent mineralization defects may be somewhat variable but that all subjects did well with serum 25-hydroxyvitamin D levels above 30 ng/mL. Unfortunately, serum parathyroid hormone levels were not measured on the same blood samples to see whether they also correlated with the bone histomorphometric findings.

**B. L. Clarke, MD**

*References*


1. Dawson-Hughes B, Heaney RP, Holick MF, Lips P, Meunier PJ, Vieth R. Estimates of optimal vitamin D status. *Osteoporos Int*. 2005;16:713-716.
2. Rizzoli R, Boonen S, Brandi ML, Burlet N, Delmas P, Reginster JY. The role of calcium and vitamin D in the management of osteoporosis. *Bone*. 2008;42: 246-249.
3. Dawson-Hughes B, Harris SS, Krall EA, Dallal GE. Effect of calcium and vitamin D supplementation on bone density in men and women 65 years or age or older. *N Engl J Med*. 1997;337:670-676.
4. Trivedi DP, Doll R, Khaw KT. Effect of four monthly oral vitamin D3 (cholecalciferol) supplementation on fractures and mortality in men and women living in the community: randomized, double-blind, controlled trial. *BMJ*. 2003;326:469.
5. Bischoff-Ferrari HA, Dawson-Hughes B, Willett WC, et al. Effect of vitamin D on falls: a meta-analysis. *JAMA*. 2004;291:1999-2006.
6. Chapuy MC, Pamphile R, Paris E, et al. Combined calcium and vitamin D3 supplementation in elderly women: confirmation of reversal of secondary hyperparathyroidism and hip fracture risk: the Decalyos II study. *Osteoporos Int*. 2002;13:257-264.

# 53 Diabetes

**Post-Challenge Hyperglycemia in Older Adults Is Associated with Increased Cardiovascular Risk Profile**

Crandall JP, Shamoon H, Cohen HW, et al (Albert Einstein College of Medicine, Bronx, NY)

*J Clin Endocrinol Metab* 94:1595-1601, 2009

*Context.*—Post-challenge hyperglycemia (PCH) is common in older adults and is associated with increased cardiovascular disease (CVD) risk and total mortality. However, PCH is rarely recognized in clinical settings, and the glycemic exposure and CVD risk profile of elderly individuals with PCH has not been defined.

*Objective.*—The aim of the study was to characterize metabolic and CVD risk profile of elderly subjects with PCH and to determine the effect of acute postprandial metabolic changes on vascular biomarkers.

*Design.*—We conducted a cross-sectional study with a standard meal challenge protocol.

*Participants.*—Older adults with normal glucose tolerance ($n = 30$) or PCH (fasting glucose <126 mg/dl and 2-h glucose ≥170 mg/dl; $n = 28$) participated in the study.

*Main Outcome Measures.*—We assessed fasting and postprandial levels of glucose, insulin, lipids, high sensitivity C-reactive protein, plasminogen activator inhibitor-1, and adiponectin and endothelial function using reactive hyperemia peripheral arterial tonometry.

*Results.*—Normal glucose tolerance and PCH subjects were matched for age, sex, body mass index, and ethnicity. Fasting glucose (102 ± 3 *vs.* 93 ± 2 mg/dl; $P < 0.001$) and glycosylated hemoglobin (5.7 vs. 5.4%; $P = 0.01$) were modestly higher in the PCH group, which was also more insulin resistant (homeostasis model assessment for insulin resistance, 7.0 ± 1.3 *vs.* 4.1 ± 0.6; $P = 0.03$). Fasting high sensitivity C-reactive protein was higher (2.6 ± 0.5 *vs.* 1.3 ± 0.2 mg/dl; $P = 0.05$), and adiponectin was lower (11.6 ± 1.6 *vs.* 14.0 ± 1.3 μg/ml; $P = 0.03$) in subjects with PCH. Peak and 6-h postprandial area under the curve glucose, insulin, and lipids were higher in PCH subjects, who also had higher fasting and postprandial levels of plasminogen activator inhibitor-1. Reactive hyperemia peripheral arterial tonometry declined postprandially only in PCH.

*Conclusions.*—Older adults with PCH experience significant fasting and postprandial metabolic dysregulation, which is accompanied by a proatherosclerotic and prothrombotic vascular profile.

▶ While it is clear that diabetes mellitus is a major risk factor for cardiovascular disease, there is ongoing debate on the contribution of impaired glucose tolerance (IGT) and impaired fasting glucose (IFG) to cardiovascular risk.

From a number of large-scale studies and meta-analyses there is evidence that IFG and IGT increase cardiovascular risk.[1-3] Probably the largest meta-analysis was performed by Coutinho and colleagues in 1999 and included a cumulative number of more than 100 000 patients.[1] The main outcome was an increased cardiovascular risk when the fasting plasma glucose was above 110 mg/dL.

In this study, Crandell and colleagues asked whether postchallenge hyperglycemia is associated with cardiovascular risk. They included patients with IGT and matched them to control subjects. Both groups were not diabetic by definition, but patients with IGT had a slightly higher glycosylated hemoglobin (HbA1c) (5.7% vs 5.4%) and fasting glucose (102 mg/dL vs 93 mg/dL). Patients with IGT had elevated, though subdiabetic, blood glucose values 2 hours after an oral glucose tolerance test (193 mg/dL). The patients in both groups were relatively old (71.4 years). The end point after a standard meal challenge was mainly reactive hyperemia peripheral arterial tonometry as a measure of endothelial function. As the main outcome, the authors found patients with IGT to have impaired endothelial function in response to a meal challenge.

The strengths of the study are the good clinical characterization of the patients and the physiologic stimulus (meal challenge). The end points are somehow indirect, but it is difficult to assess true clinical end points in that setting.

The article touches an interesting clinical topic and underlines the problem with defining cutoff values to determine the diagnosis of diabetes mellitus. In that context, it is interesting to take into account that the current diagnostic thresholds for diabetes derive from data from microvascular end points (retinopathy and nephropathy). Still it is conceivable but not clear whether macrovascular damage begins at blood glucose levels below the current diagnostic cutoff for diabetes mellitus.

**S. Schinner, MD, PhD**

*References*

1. Coutinho M, Gerstein HC, Wang Y, Yusuf S. The relationship between glucose and incident cardiovascular events. A metaregression analysis of published data from 20 studies of 95 783 individuals followed for 12.4 years. *Diabetes Care.* 1999;22:233-240.
2. Sorkin JD, Muller DC, Fleg JL, Andres R. The relation of fasting and 2-h postchallenge plasma glucose concentrations to mortality: data from the Baltimore Longitudinal Study of Aging with a critical review of the literature. *Diabetes Care.* 2005; 28:2626-2632.

3. Levitzky YS, Pencina MJ, D'Agostino RB, et al. Impact of impaired fasting glucose on cardiovascular disease: the Framingham Heart Study. *J Am Coll Cardiol.* 2008; 51:264-270.

**Intensive Glucose-Lowering Therapy Reduces Cardiovascular Disease Events in Veterans Affairs Diabetes Trial Participants With Lower Calcified Coronary Atherosclerosis**

Reaven PD, for the Veterans Affairs Diabetes Trial (Phoenix Veterans Affairs Health Care System, AZ; et al)

*Diabetes* 58:2642-2648, 2009

*Objective.*—This study investigated the hypothesis that baseline calcified coronary atherosclerosis may determine cardiovascular disease events in response to intensive glycemic control within the Veterans Affairs Diabetes Trial (VADT).

*Research Design and Methods.*—At baseline, 301 type 2 diabetic participants in the VADT, a randomized trial comparing the effects of intensive versus standard glucose lowering on cardiovascular events, had baseline coronary atherosclerosis assessed by coronary artery calcium (CAC) measured by computed tomography. Participants were followed over the 7.5-year study for development of cardiovascular end points.

*Results.*—During a median follow-up duration of 5.2 years, 89 cardiovascular events occurred. Although intensive glucose-lowering therapy did not significantly reduce cardiovascular events in the substudy cohort as a whole, there was evidence that the response was modified by baseline CAC, as indicated by significant *P* values for treatment by log(CAC + 1) interaction terms in unadjusted and multivariable-adjusted models (0.01 and 0.03, respectively). Multivariable-adjusted hazard ratios (HRs) for the effect of treatment indicated a progressive diminution of benefit with increasing CAC. Subgroup analyses were also conducted for clinically relevant CAC categories: those above and below an Agatston score of 100. Among those randomized to intensive treatment, for the subgroup with CAC > 100, 11 of 62 individuals had events, while only 1 of 52 individuals with CAC ≤ 100 had an event. The multivariable HR for intensive treatment for those with CAC > 100 was 0.74 (95% CI 0.46–1.20; $P = 0.21$), while for the subgroup with CAC ≤ 100, the corresponding HR was 0.08 (0.008–0.77; $P = 0.03$), with event rates of 39 and 4 per 1,000 person-years, respectively.

*Conclusions.*—These data indicate that intensive glucose lowering reduces cardiovascular events in those with less extensive calcified coronary atherosclerosis.

▶ The data and results presented here are a part of an important sub study of the Veteran Affairs Diabetes Trial (VADT) and the Risk Factors, Atherosclerosis, and Clinical Events in Diabetes (RACED) trial. The VADT was a large (n = 1490) randomized trial comparing the effects of intensive versus standard glucose lowering on the cardiovascular event rates and outcomes of patients with type 2 diabetes and known coronary artery disease (CAD). After a little more than 5 years of follow-up, the group receiving intensive glycemic control experienced no significant reduction in cardiovascular events despite an average A1c 1.5% lower, throughout the trial.

The RACED sub study examined coronary artery calcium (CAC) in a subset (n = 301) of the VADT participants and tried to determine whether the effect of intensive glycemic control on cardiovascular disease (CVD) depended on the initial extent of underlying atherosclerosis as estimated by vascular calcium.

Although a relatively small study, the results of this study are very reassuring and give guidance to those who believe that controlling blood glucose intensively is important from a CVD perspective, despite the recent findings of the Action to Control Cardiovascular Risk in Diabetes (ACCORD), Action in Diabetes and Vascular Disease: Preterax and Diamicron Modified Release Controlled Evaluation (ADVANCE), and Bypass Angioplasty Revascularization Investigation 2 Diabetes (BARI-2D) studies. Furthermore, it gives guidance to those designing future studies in this area, supporting the concept that intensive glucose lowering therapy may be most effective in reducing CVD in those with less extensive coronary atherosclerosis.

**F. Ovalle, MD**

## Metformin Associated With Lower Cancer Mortality in Type 2 Diabetes: ZODIAC-16

Landman GWD, Kleefstra N, van Hateren KJJ, et al (Isala Clinics, Zwolle, the Netherlands; et al)

*Diabetes Care* 33:322-326, 2010

*Objective.*—Several studies have suggested an association between specific diabetes treatment and cancer mortality. We studied the association between metformin use and cancer mortality in a prospectively followed cohort.

*Research Design and Methods.*—In 1998 and 1999, 1,353 patients with type 2 diabetes were enrolled in the Zwolle Outpatient Diabetes project Integrating Available Care (ZODIAC) study in the Netherlands. Vital status was assessed in January 2009. Cancer mortality rate was evaluated using standardized mortality ratios (SMRs), and the association between metformin use and cancer mortality was evaluated with a Cox proportional hazards model, taking possible confounders into account.

*Results.*—Median follow-up time was 9.6 years, average age at baseline was 68 years, and average A1C was 7.5%. Of the patients, 570 died, of which 122 died of malignancies. The SMR for cancer mortality was 1.47 (95% CI 1.22–1.76). In patients taking metformin compared with patients not taking metformin at baseline, the adjusted hazard ratio

(HR) for cancer mortality was 0.43 (95% CI 0.23–0.80), and the HR with every increase of 1 g of metformin was 0.58 (95% CI 0.36–0.93).

*Conclusions.*—In general, patients with type 2 diabetes are at increased risk for cancer mortality. In our group, metformin use was associated with lower cancer mortality compared with nonuse of metformin. Although the design cannot provide a conclusion about causality, our results suggest a protective effect of metformin on cancer mortality.

▶ Diabetes is known to be associated with an increased risk of cancer, and most recently, the use of the insulin analog glargine was linked to an increased risk of cancer also, although this remains to be proven. A study designed to try to study further the association between insulin use and cancer concluded that it is possible that some of the apparent increased rates of cancer seen associated with insulin use in comparison with other drugs to treat diabetes was rather possibly, at least in part, the result of a decrease in the risk of cancer associated with metformin use in many of those patients not taking insulin.[1]

This study followed 1353 subjects with type 2 diabetes for approximately 10 years, and it is the first observational study with a prospective design to show an association between metformin use and lower cancer mortality risk. The group of subjects taking metformin in this study had, at the end, a cancer mortality risk comparable with that of the nondiabetic population. In other words, metformin seems to take away the excess risk of cancer mortality known to be associated with diabetes.

While the evidence for this association is growing stronger, a cause and effect relationship remains to be proven. Nonetheless, as the authors state, this finding further strengthens the position of metformin as the first-line therapy for type 2 diabetes.

**F. Ovalle, MD**

*Reference*

1. Currie CJ, Poole CD, Gale EA. The influence of glucose-lowering therapies on cancer risk in type 2 diabetes. *Diabetologia*. 2009;52:1766-1777.

---

**Hyperglycemia–related mortality in critically ill patients varies with admission diagnosis**

Falciglia M, Freyberg RW, Almenoff PL, et al (Univ of Cincinnati College of Medicine, OH)

*Crit Care Med* 37:3001-3009, 2009

---

*Objective.*—Hyperglycemia during critical illness is common and is associated with increased mortality. Intensive insulin therapy has improved outcomes in some, but not all, intervention trials. It is unclear whether the benefits of treatment differ among specific patient populations. The purpose of the study was to determine the association between hyperglycemia and risk–adjusted mortality in critically ill patients and in separate groups stratified by admission diagnosis. A secondary purpose was to determine whether mortality risk from hyperglycemia varies with intensive care unit type, length of stay, or diagnosed diabetes.

*Design.*—Retrospective cohort study.

*Setting.*—One hundred seventy-three U.S. medical, surgical, and cardiac intensive care units.

*Patients.*—Two hundred fifty-nine thousand and forty admissions from October 2002 to September 2005; unadjusted mortality rate, 11.2%.

*Interventions.*—None.

*Measurements and Main Results.*—A two–level logistic regression model determined the relationship between glycemia and mortality. Age, diagnosis, comorbidities, and laboratory variables were used to calculate a predicted mortality rate, which was then analyzed with mean glucose to determine the association of hyperglycemia with hospital mortality. Hyperglycemia was associated with increased mortality independent of illness severity. Compared with normoglycemic individuals (70–110 mg/dL), adjusted odds of mortality (odds ratio, [95% confidence interval]) for mean glucose 111–145, 146–199, 200–300, and >300 mg/dL was 1.31 (1.26–1.36), 1.82 (1.74–1.90), 2.13 (2.03–2.25), and 2.85 (2.58–3.14), respectively. Furthermore, the adjusted odds of mortality related to hyperglycemia varied with admission diagnosis, demonstrating a clear association in some patients (acute myocardial infarction, arrhythmia, unstable angina, pulmonary embolism) and little or no association in others. Hyperglycemia was associated with increased mortality independent of intensive care unit type, length of stay, and diabetes.

*Conclusions.*—The association between hyperglycemia and mortality implicates hyperglycemia as a potentially harmful and correctable abnormality in critically ill patients. The finding that hyperglycemia–related risk varied with admission diagnosis suggests differences in the interaction between specific medical conditions and injury from hyperglycemia. The design and interpretation of future trials should consider the primary disease states of patients and the balance of medical conditions in the intensive care unit studied.

▶ This is a massive retrospective cohort study designed to determine the association between hyperglycemia and mortality in critically ill patients. It was possible because of the integrated VA electronic medical record system throughout the United States.

If there was any doubt in anyone's mind about the association between hyperglycemia and mortality in the critically ill, this should put those questions to rest.

Most importantly, this large and powerful study helped identify several important trends in the strength of the association between hyperglycemia and mortality according to the admission diagnosis. Particularly interesting and thought-provoking is the magnitude of the association between cerebrovascular accidents (CVA) and hyperglycemia. Alternatively, the relatively weak associations between coronary artery bypass grafting (CABG), pulmonary veno-occlusive disease (PVOD), and amputations and hyperglycemia is interesting too.

This study should serve to help generate and support the hypothesis, and it should help guide the design of future studies. However, it clearly does not prove a cause and effect. So, whether we should treat our critically ill patients with hyperglycemia aggressively, with the goal of near-normoglycemia, remains an unanswered question.

**F. Ovalle, MD**

### Hypoglycemia and Outcome in Critically Ill Patients

Egi M, Bellomo R, Stachowski E, et al (Okayama Univ Hosp, Japan; Austin Hosp, Melbourne, Victoria, Australia; Westmead Hosp, Sydney, New South Wales, Australia; et al)

*Mayo Clin Proc* 85:217-224, 2010

*Objective.*—To determine whether mild or moderate hypoglycemia that occurs in critically ill patients is independently associated with an increased risk of death.

*Patients and Methods.*—Of patients admitted to 2 hospital intensive care units (ICUs) in Melbourne and Sydney, Australia, from January 1, 2000, to October 14, 2004, we analyzed all those who had at least 1 episode of hypoglycemia (glucose concentration, <81 mg/dL). The independent association between hypoglycemia and outcome was statistically assessed.

*Results.*—Of 4946 patients admitted to the ICUs, a cohort of 1109 had at least 1 episode of hypoglycemia (blood glucose level, <81 mg/dL). Of these 1109 patients (22.4% of all admissions to the intensive care unit), hospital mortality was 36.6% compared with 19.7% in the 3837 nonhypoglycemic control patients ($P<.001$). Even patients with a minimum blood glucose concentration between 72 and 81 mg/dL had a greater unadjusted mortality rate than did control patients (25.9% vs 19.7%; unadjusted odds ratio, 1.42; 95% confidence interval, 1.12-1.80; $P=.004$.) Mortality increased significantly with increasing severity of hypoglycemia ($P<.001$). After adjustment for insulin therapy, hypoglycemia was independently associated with increased risk of death, cardiovascular death, and death due to infectious disease.

*Conclusion.*—In critically ill patients, an association exists between even mild or moderate hypoglycemia and mortality. Even after adjustment for insulin therapy or timing of hypoglycemic episode, the more severe the hypoglycemia, the greater the risk of death.

▶ This is a retrospective study conducted at 2 major teaching institutions in Australia. They enrolled 4946 patients admitted to their intensive care units (ICUs) over a period of 4 years and sought to determine whether mild to moderate hypoglycemia in the critically ill patient is associated with an increased risk of death. In summary, hypoglycemia was indeed independently associated with an increased risk of death, cardiovascular death, and death due to an infectious disease.

This study is another piece of the puzzle that has been rapidly progressing over the last few years. Not long ago, we all assumed that treating hyperglycemia intensively in the critically ill patient was a good idea, despite the well known increased risk of hypoglycemia, and many ICUs implemented protocols to achieve this. However, most recently, there have been several reports highlighting the increased risk of hypoglycemia with these protocols and the associated morbidity and mortality. It was not until the NICE-SUGAR study was published last year,[1] when all of a sudden the general attitude toward the treatment of hyperglycemia in the ICU suddenly changed. The NICE-SUGAR study found an increased 90-day mortality in the intensive insulin therapy group compared with the conventionally treated subjects.

At this point, further studies are needed to understand the pathophysiology of hypoglycemia in the critically ill individual and to find better ways to prevent it. As the authors point out, future studies will need to use continuous glucose monitoring systems (CGMS) to better document the glucose trends as well as the hyperglycemic and hypoglycemic events.

**F. Ovalle, MD**

*Reference*

1. NICE-SUGAR Study Investigators, Finfer S, Chittock DR, et al. Intensive versus conventional glucose control in critically ill patients. *N Engl J Med.* 2009;360: 1283-1297.

---

**10-year follow-up of diabetes incidence and weight loss in the Diabetes Prevention Program Outcomes Study**

Diabetes Prevention Program Research Group (Pennington Biomed Res Ctr, Baton Rouge, LA; et al)

*Lancet* 374:1677-1686, 2009

---

*Background.*—In the 2·8 years of the Diabetes Prevention Program (DPP) randomised clinical trial, diabetes incidence in high-risk adults was reduced by 58% with intensive lifestyle intervention and by 31% with metformin, compared with placebo. We investigated the persistence of these effects in the long term.

*Methods.*—All active DPP participants were eligible for continued follow-up. 2766 of 3150 (88%) enrolled for a median additional follow-up of 5·7 years (IQR 5·5–5·8). 910 participants were from the lifestyle, 924 from the metformin, and 932 were from the original placebo groups. On the basis of the benefits from the intensive lifestyle intervention in the DPP, all three groups were offered group-implemented lifestyle intervention. Metformin treatment was continued in the original metformin group (850 mg twice daily as tolerated), with participants unmasked to assignment, and the original lifestyle intervention group was offered additional lifestyle support. The primary outcome was development of diabetes according to American Diabetes Association criteria. Analysis was by intention-to-treat. This study is registered with ClinicalTrials.gov, number NCT00038727.

*Findings.*—During the 10·0-year (IQR 9·0–10·5) follow-up since randomisation to DPP, the original lifestyle group lost, then partly regained weight. The modest weight loss with metformin was maintained. Diabetes incidence rates during the DPP were 4·8 cases per 100 person-years (95% CI 4·1–5·7) in the intensive lifestyle intervention group, 7·8 (6·8–8·8) in the metformin group, and 11·0 (9·8–12·3) in the placebo group. Diabetes incidence rates in this follow-up study were similar between treatment groups: 5·9 per 100 person-years (5·1–6·8) for lifestyle, 4·9 (4·2–5·7) for metformin, and 5·6 (4·8–6·5) for placebo. Diabetes incidence in the 10 years since DPP randomisation was reduced by 34% (24–42) in the lifestyle group and 18% (7–28) in the metformin group compared with placebo.

*Interpretation.*—During follow-up after DPP, incidences in the former placebo and metformin groups fell to equal those in the former lifestyle group, but the cumulative incidence of diabetes remained lowest in the lifestyle group. Prevention or delay of diabetes with lifestyle intervention or metformin can persist for at least 10 years.

▶ This study, the Diabetes Prevention Program Outcomes Study (DPPOC), is the observational follow-up study of the participants in the Diabetes Prevention Program (DPP).

It was designed to determine whether the lower rates of diabetes observed in the lifestyle and metformin arms of the DPP were sustained. In other words, did the intervention help prevent, delay, or mask the onset of diabetes?

After an additional 5.7 years of follow-up (10 years after the randomization to DPP), those subjects who were originally assigned to the lifestyle intervention group gained back a good proportion of the weight they had lost during the DPP; those on the metformin arm maintained the weight they had lost; and those assigned to placebo maintained their original weight.

During the follow-up phase, the incidence rates of diabetes for the former placebo and metformin groups fell to levels similar to the former lifestyle group. However, the cumulative incidence of diabetes remained the lowest in the lifestyle group.

These results are consistent with those of most recent diabetes follow-up studies (eg, DCCT, EDIC, and UKPDS), demonstrating what some call a legacy effect or metabolic memory. This study demonstrates once again that early and aggressive treatment of diabetes and its comorbidities, pays off. Furthermore, it definitively shows that the lower rates of diabetes seen during the randomized phase of the DPP were not just the results of masking but rather represent evidence of true prevention of diabetes.

**F. Ovalle, MD**

# 54 Lipoproteins and Atherosclerosis

**Effects of Increasing High-Density Lipoprotein Cholesterol and Decreasing Low-Density Lipoprotein Cholesterol on the Incidence of First Acute Coronary Events (from the Air Force/Texas Coronary Atherosclerosis Prevention Study)**

Cui Y, Watson DJ, Girman CJ, et al (Merck & Company, Incorported, Whitehouse Station, NJ; et al)

*Am J Cardiol* 104:829-834, 2009

Reducing low-density lipoprotein (LDL) cholesterol with statins reduces cardiovascular risk, but the associations between increases in high-density lipoprotein (HDL) cholesterol and cardiovascular risk at different LDL levels have been less well characterized. To evaluate the associations between the 1-year changes in HDL cholesterol and LDL cholesterol with lovastatin and subsequent acute major coronary events (AMCEs), we studied 2,928 patients in the lovastatin arm who were followed for 5.2 years in a post-hoc analysis of the Air Force/Texas Coronary Atherosclerosis Prevention Study (AFCAPS/TexCAPS). The percentage of HDL cholesterol increase and apolipoproteins at year 1 and the incidence of AMCEs thereafter were assessed stratified by the LDL cholesterol levels. With lovastatin, LDL cholesterol was reduced by 25% on average to 115 mg/dl at year 1, and HDL cholesterol increased 6.0%. Patients with both an increase in HDL cholesterol of ≥7.5% and LDL cholesterol of <115 mg/dl at year 1 had the lowest event rate (3.53/1,000 person-years; $p = 0.028$). Similar results were found for an increase in HDL cholesterol of ≥7.5% and a decrease in LDL cholesterol of >25%, as well as for apolipoproteins A-I and B. The 1-year percent increase in HDL cholesterol appeared to be associated with a reduction in AMCEs in subsequent follow-up ($p = 0.07$ with the percentage of HDL cholesterol increase analyzed continuously). Patients with an HDL cholesterol increase of ≥7.5% had an AMCE rate of 5.18 compared with 7.66/1,000 person-years in patients with a lower HDL cholesterol increase ($p = 0.08$). In conclusion, lovastatin therapy was associated with a greater risk reduction of AMCEs when LDL cholesterol was substantially reduced and the HDL cholesterol increased by ≥7.5% (Fig 1).

▶ The Air Force/Texas Coronary Atherosclerosis Prevention Study (AFCAPS/TexCAPS) was the first clinical trial to demonstrate that treatment with a statin

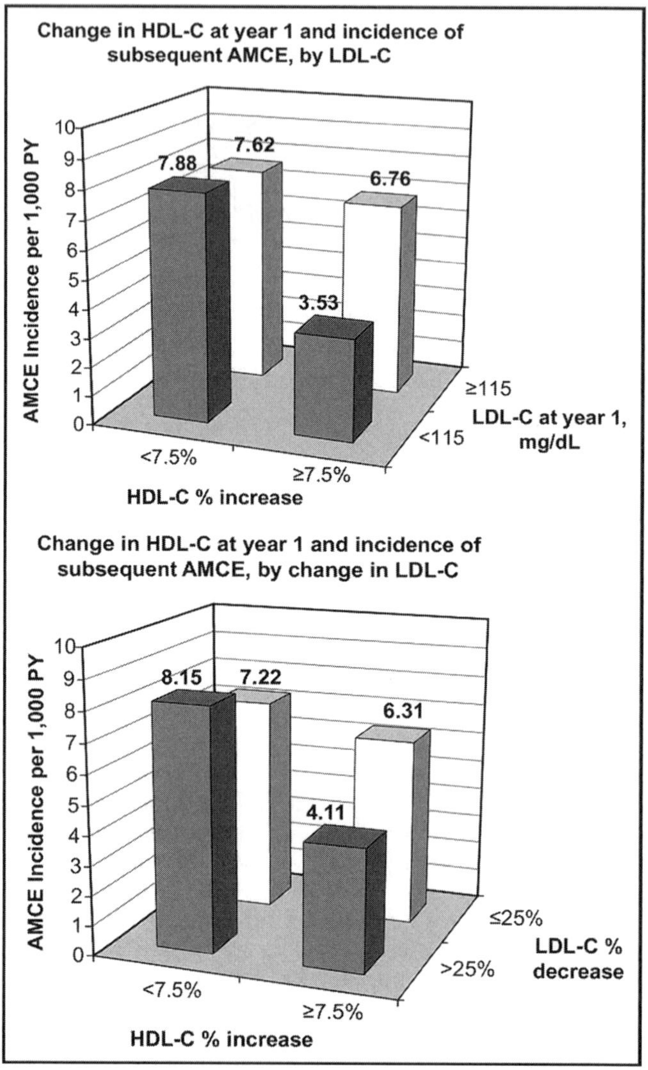


FIGURE 1.—HDL cholesterol percent change and incidence of AMCEs by LDL cholesterol. (*Top*) LDL cholesterol at year 1. (*Bottom*) LDL percent change. (Reprinted from Cui Y, Watson DJ, Girman CJ, et al. Effects of increasing high-density lipoprotein cholesterol and decreasing low-density lipoprotein cholesterol on the incidence of first acute coronary events (from the Air Force/Texas Coronary Atherosclerosis Prevention Study). *Am J Cardiol.* 2009;104:829-834, with permission from Elsevier Inc.)

significantly reduced the risk for cardiovascular morbidity and mortality among men and women without a history of coronary artery disease. The subjects in this trial had average levels of low-density lipoprotein cholesterol (LDL-C) (155 mg/dL), triglycerides(165 mg/dL), and low levels of high-density lipoprotein cholesterol (HDL-C) (mean 37 mg/dL). In a previous analysis, it was shown that the patients with baseline HDL-C <40 mg/dL derived 3 times more benefit in the primary composite end point of the trial than did those subjects with baseline HDL-C >40 mg/dL (45% vs 15%).[1] In this additional post hoc analysis, the investigators probe whether or not an HDL-C elevation on statin therapy >7.5% coupled with LDL-C reduction <115 mg/dL provides incremental risk reduction. Subjects with both an increase in HDL-C level of >7.5% and LDL-C level of <115 mg/dL at year 1 had the lowest event rate (3.53/1000 person-years; $P = .028$) compared to subjects with lower levels of HDL elevation or LDL-C reduction (Fig 1). Those subjects with HDL-C elevation >7.5% and a >25% reduction in LDL-C also did better compared with groups not achieving these changes in lipoprotein levels.

It has long been assumed that the primary benefit incurred by statin therapy is attributable to the reduction of atherogenic lipoprotein burden, especially LDL-C. Much skepticism surrounds the value of raising HDL-C and whether or not the modest increases in HDL-C stimulated by statin therapy contribute to overall risk reduction. This issue is complicated by the fact that, apart from using an infusible HDL mimetic, all currently available lipid-modifying therapies that increase HDL-C (statins, niacin, fibrates, and thiazolidinediones) impact serum levels of all components of the lipid profile, thereby necessitating multivariate regression analysis. A number of meta-analyses have shown that event rate reduction[2] and coronary atheromatous plaque regression based on intravascular ultrasonography[3] or quantitative coronary angiography[4] are a consequence of both aggressive LDL-C reduction and HDL-C elevation. This makes some sense on mechanistic grounds. Aggressive LDL-C reduction would be expected to provide less substrate for inducing endothelial cell dysfunction and promoting foam cell formation in the subendothelial space. Aggressive HDL raising may be associated with increased capacity for reverse cholesterol transport and other atheroprotective functions attributed to HDL particles.[5] Although a target for HDL-C elevation cannot be discerned from currently available clinical trials, this study provides important additional data supporting the importance of HDL-C elevation in patients with low baseline HDL-C levels. HDL-C elevation appears to contribute to cardiovascular risk reduction among patients with dyslipidemia treated with statin therapy. Consistent with other analyses, even a 2- to 3-mg/dL rise in HDL-C level appears to impact the risk for acute coronary events significantly.

**P. P. Toth, MD, PhD**

*References*

1. Downs JR, Clearfield M, Weis S, et al. Primary prevention of acute coronary events with lovastatin in men and women with average cholesterol levels: results of AFCAPS/TexCAPS. Air Force/Texas Coronary Atherosclerosis Prevention Study. *JAMA.* 1998;279:1615-1622.
2. Brown B, Zhao X, Cheung M. Should both HDL-C and LDL-C be targets for lipid therapy? A review of current evidence. *J Clin Lipidol.* 2007;1:88-94.
3. Nicholls SJ, Tuzcu EM, Sipahi I, et al. Statins, high-density lipoprotein cholesterol, and regression of coronary atherosclerosis. *JAMA.* 2007;297:499-508.
4. Ballantyne CM, Raichlen JS, Nicholls SJ, et al. for the ASTEROID Investigators. Effect of rosuvastatin therapy on coronary artery stenoses assessed by quantitative coronary angiography: a study to evaluate the effect of rosuvastatin on

intravascular ultrasound-derived coronary atheroma burden. *Circulation*. 2008; 117:2458-2466.
5. Toth PP. High-density lipoprotein: epidemiology, metabolism, and antiatherogenic effects. *Dis Mon*. 2001;47:365-416.

**Incidence and predictors of silent myocardial infarction in type 2 diabetes and the effect of fenofibrate: an analysis from the Fenofibrate Intervention and Event Lowering in Diabetes (FIELD) study**

Burgess DC, Hunt D, Li L, et al (Univ of Sydney, Camperdown, Australia; Royal Melbourne Hosp, Victoria, Australia; et al)
*Eur Heart J* 31:92-99, 2010

*Aims.*—To determine the incidence and predictors of, and effects of fenofibrate on silent myocardial infarction (MI) in a large contemporary cohort of patients with type 2 diabetes in the Fenofibrate Intervention and Event Lowering in Diabetes (FIELD) study.

*Methods and Results.*—Routine electrocardiograms taken throughout the study were assessed by Minnesota-code criteria for the presence of new Q-waves without clinical presentation and analysed with blinding to treatment allocation and clinical outcome. Of all MIs, 36.8 were silent. Being male, older age, longer diabetes duration, prior cardiovascular disease (CVD), neuropathy, higher $HbA_{1c}$, albuminuria, high serum creatinine, and insulin use all significantly predicted risk of clinical or silent MI. Fenofibrate reduced MI (clinical or silent) by 19 [hazard ratio (HR) 0.81, 95 confidence interval (CI) 0.69–0.94; $P = 0.006$], non-fatal clinical MI by 24 ($P = 0.01$), and silent MI by 16 ($P = 0.16$). Among those having silent MI, fenofibrate reduced subsequent clinical CVD events by 78 (HR 0.22, 95 CI 0.08–0.65; $P = 0.003$).

*Conclusion.*—Silent and clinical MI have similar risk factors and increase the risk of future CVD events. Fenofibrate reduces the risk of a first MI and substantially reduces the risk of further clinical CVD events after silent MI, supporting its use in type 2 diabetes (Fig 3).

▶ Silent myocardial infarction (MI) is a serious complication of coronary artery disease (CAD). Patients with diabetes have increased risk for silent MI due to cardiac autonomic neuropathy stemming from chronic exposure to hyperglycemia. In this intriguing analysis of data from the Fenofibrate Intervention and Event Lowering in Diabetes (FIELD) study, the impact of fenofibrate therapy on risk for fatal/nonfatal and silent Q wave MI was explored. Despite a high drop-in rate of statin therapy in the placebo- and fenofibrate-treated groups, the investigators were able to show reductions in total, nonfatal, and silent MIs of 19%, 24%, and a statistically nonsignifcant 16%, respectively. However, among patients with silent MI by the end of year 2 (evaluated with sequential EKGs during the course of the trial), the risk for cardiovascular events was reduced significantly by 78% in the fenofibrate group relative to placebo

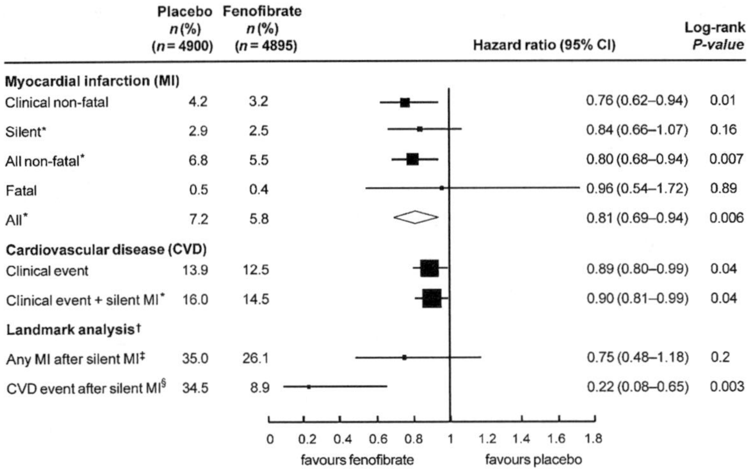


FIGURE 3.—Effects of fenofibrate treatment on myocardial infarction and cardiovascular events. *Interval-censored proportional-hazards methods were used. †Analyses were landmarked at 2 years (see methods for details). ‡Placebo group, 48 events, $n = 137$; fenofibrate group, 30 events, $n = 115$. §Placebo group, 20 events, $n = 58$; fenofibrate group, 4 events, $n = 45$. (Reprinted from Burgess DC, Hunt D, Li L, et al. Incidence and predictors of silent myocardial infarction in type 2 diabetes and the effect of fenofibrate: An analysis from the Fenofibrate Intervention and Event Lowering in Diabetes (FIELD) study. *Eur Heart J.* 2010;31:92-99, with permission from The European Society of Cardiology.)

(Fig 3). Thirty-seven percent of all MIs in this study were silent. This is a high incidence of MI that neither the patient nor the physician would have been aware of had the scheduled follow-up EKGs not been performed. The true incidence of MI may have been underestimated because non-Q wave MIs were not included in this analysis. This study emphasizes the importance of periodic screening for silent ischemia and perhaps stress testing in patients with diabetes mellitus, even if they have no perceptible symptoms of myocardial ischemia. This analysis also suggests that diabetic patients with a history of silent MI may benefit significantly from the addition of fenofibrate to their background pharmacologic therapy.

**P. P. Toth, MD, PhD**

## Cardiovascular Benefit of Magnitude of Low-Density Lipoprotein Cholesterol Reduction: A Comparison of Subgroups by Age

Rahilly-Tierney CR, Lawler EV, Scranton RE, et al (Massachusetts Veterans Epidemiology and Res Information Ctr, Boston, MA; et al)

*Circulation* 120:1491-1497, 2009

*Background.*—We examined the effect of the magnitude of low-density lipoprotein cholesterol (LDL-C) reduction across subjects of various ages in a retrospective cohort study.

*Methods and Results.*—We selected 20 132 male veterans at high risk for an acute cardiovascular event and who had 2 or more LDL-C measurements before their first documented acute myocardial infarction, revascularization, death, or censoring date. LDL-C reduction was categorized as no reduction (<10 mg/dL; reference), small reduction (between 10 and 40 mg/dL), moderate reduction (between 40 and 70 mg/dL), or large reduction (≥70 mg/dL). The primary outcome was combined acute myocardial infarction or revascularization. The first and last LDL-C levels in the databases were used to calculate the LDL-C reduction in patients who experienced no outcome or who died. Within each age quartile and in a subgroup of patients ≥80 years of age, a Cox proportional hazards model was used to determine hazard ratios for each category of LDL-C reduction compared with the reference category, with adjustment for age, body mass index, current smoking status, medications, and comorbidities. In all age groups, the magnitude of LDL-C reduction was proportional to the magnitude of cardiovascular risk reduction. Risk reduction for the combined outcome in patients who achieved a large LDL-C reduction was similar in all age quartiles, with multivariate-adjusted hazard ratios of approximately 0.30.

*Conclusions.*—In a cohort of veterans at high risk for cardiovascular events, patients of all ages, including those 80 years or older, benefitted the most from large reductions in LDL-C (Table 4).

▶ Questions that continue to be asked frequently are whether or not older patients derive as much benefit from lipid lowering as younger patients, and is there an "older limit" above which you should not treat patients for their dyslipidemia. The Pravastatin in Elderly Individuals at Risk of Vascular Disease (PROSPER)[1] trial, post hoc evaluations of data from the Heart Protection Study[2] (HPS), and the Long-Term Intervention with Pravastatin in Ischaemic Disease (LIPID)[3,4] trial all showed that older patients (>70 years) experience significant reductions in risk for acute cardiovascular events when treated with statin therapy. The issue concerning an upper limit on age appears best left to one's judgment. If a patient is 80 or 85 years old, is functional, and wants to reduce risk for myocardial infarction (MI) and stroke, then there should be little reluctance to start appropriate lipid-lowering therapy in the setting of dyslipidemia. If, on the other hand, the patient is demented or poorly functional, then decision making will be significantly influenced by the patient's comorbidities.

This retrospective cohort study by Rahilly-Tierney and coworkers lends important support to the conclusion reached by the PROSPER, LIPID, and HPS investigators, namely that lipid-lowering therapy confers just as much benefit to older high-risk patients as it does for younger ones. These investigators included 20 132 high-risk men who had been receiving care within the Veteran's Affairs health system. Within each age quartile, the percentage of patients with acute cardiovascular events (MI or revascularization) decreased with increasing magnitude of low-density lipoprotein-cholesterol (LDL-C) reduction. In all age quartiles, patients who achieved an LDL-C reduction of >70 mg/dL had the lowest event rates. The unadjusted and multivariate-adjusted hazard ratios for

**TABLE 4.**—Unadjusted and Multivariate-Adjusted* HRs (95% CI) for Each Category of LDL-C Reduction, by Age Quartile

| Category of LDL-C Reduction | <61.1 y | 61.1 to 69.3 y | 69.3 to 75.3 y | ≥75.3 y |
|---|---|---|---|---|
| Small: 10–40 mg/dL | | | | |
| Unadjusted | 0.87 (0.76–1.00) | 0.69 (0.59–0.79) | 0.77 (0.66–0.90) | 0.72 (0.61–0.85) |
| Multivariate adjusted | 0.73 (0.64–0.84) | 0.67 (0.58–0.78) | 0.70 (0.60–0.82) | 0.64 (0.54–0.76) |
| Moderate: 40–70 mg/dL | | | | |
| Unadjusted | 0.68 (0.59–0.79) | 0.57 (0.48–0.67) | 0.65 (0.55–0.77) | 0.73 (0.60–0.87) |
| Multivariate adjusted | 0.50 (0.43–0.58) | 0.45 (0.37–0.52) | 0.45 (0.39–0.56) | 0.53 (0.44–0.64) |
| Large: ≥70 mg/dL | | | | |
| Unadjusted | 0.73 (0.61–0.87) | 0.57 (0.47–0.68) | 0.53 (0.42–0.66) | 0.54 (0.42–0.70) |
| Multivariate adjusted | 0.37 (0.31–0.45) | 0.29 (0.24–0.37) | 0.26 (0.20–0.34) | 0.38 (0.30–0.49) |

*Adjusted for age, gender, current smoking status, body mass index, statin use, nonstatin cholesterol-modifying therapy use, hypertension, cerebrovascular disease, thyroid disease, and renal disease.

a given intensity of LDL-C reduction compared with the reference within each age quartile are shown in Table 4. After adjustment for age, body mass index (BMI), current smoking status, angiotensin-converting enzyme inhibitor use, aspirin use, beta-blocker use, and comorbidities, any LDL-C reduction was associated with a decreased risk for the combined outcome. The magnitude of benefit increased as the magnitude of LDL-C reduction increased. Interestingly, additional adjustment for either statin or nonstatin cholesterol-modifying therapy did not change the results. Among the patients > 75years, a 70 mg/dL reduction in serum LDL-C was associated with an approximately 70% reduction in risk for MI and need for revascularization, an effect size identical to that seen for younger patients.

Clearly, lipid lowering in high-risk patients is beneficial irrespective of age. Lipid-lowering therapy should not be withheld from patients at risk for cardiovascular events based on age alone. One limitation of these data is that women were not included in this study. However, given the fact that both HPS and Justification for the Use of Statins in Primary Prevention: An Intervention Trial Evaluating Rosuvastatin trials (JUPITER)[5] showed that women derive as much benefit from statin therapy as do men, it would be unreasonable to not treat older high-risk women with lipid-lowering therapy.

**P. P. Toth, MD, PhD**

*References*

1. Shepherd J, Blauw GJ, Murphy MB, et al. Pravastatin in elderly individuals at risk of vascular disease (PROSPER): a randomised controlled trial. *Lancet*. 2002;360: 1623-1630.
2. Heart Protection Study Collaborative G. MRC/BHF Heart Protection Study of cholesterol lowering with simvastatin in 20,536 high-risk individuals: a randomised placebo-controlled trial [see comment][summary for patients in Curr Cardiol Rep. 2002 Nov;4(6):486-7; PMID: 12379169]. *Lancet*. 2002;360:7-22.
3. Prevention of cardiovascular events and death with pravastatin in patients with coronary heart disease and a broad range of initial cholesterol levels. The

Long-Term Intervention with Pravastatin in Ischaemic Disease (LIPID) Study Group. *N Engl J Med.* 1998;339:1349-1357.
4. Hunt D, Young P, Simes J, et al. Benefits of pravastatin on cardiovascular events and mortality in older patients with coronary heart disease are equal to or exceed those seen in younger patients: results from the LIPID trial. *Ann Intern Med.* 2001; 134:931-940.
5. Ridker PM, Danielson E, Fonseca FA, et al. Reduction in C-reactive protein and LDL cholesterol and cardiovascular event rates after initiation of rosuvastatin: a prospective study of the JUPITER trial. *Lancet.* 2009;373:1175-1182.

## Impact of Prior Statin Therapy on Arrhythmic Events in Patients With Acute Coronary Syndromes (from the Global Registry of Acute Coronary Events [GRACE])

Vedre A, for the GRACE Investigators (Univ of Michigan, Ann Arbor; et al)
*Am J Cardiol* 104:1613-1617, 2009

Animal models of myocardial ischemia have demonstrated reduction in arrhythmias using statins. It was hypothesized that previous statin therapy before hospitalization might be associated with reductions of in-hospital arrhythmic events in patients with acute coronary syndromes. In this multinational, prospective, observational study (the Global Registry of Acute Coronary Events [GRACE]), data from 64,679 patients hospitalized for suspected acute coronary syndromes (from 1999 to 2007) were analyzed. The primary outcome of interest was in-hospital arrhythmic events in previous statin users compared with nonusers. The 2 primary end points were atrial fibrillation and the composite end point of ventricular tachycardia, ventricular fibrillation, and/or cardiac arrest. In-hospital death was also examined. Of the 64,679 patients, 17,636 (27%) had received previous statin therapy. Those taking statins had higher crude rates of histories of angina (69% vs 46%), diabetes (34% vs 22%), heart failure (15% vs 8.4%), hypertension (74% vs 58%), atrial fibrillation (9.3% vs 7.0%), and dyslipidemia (85% vs 35%). Patients previously taking statins were less likely to have in-hospital arrhythmias. In propensity-adjusted multivariable models, previous statin use was associated with a lower risk for ventricular tachycardia, ventricular fibrillation, or cardiac arrest (odds ratio 0.81, 95% confidence interval 0.72 to 0.96, $p = 0.002$); atrial fibrillation (odds ratio 0.81, 95% confidence interval 0.73 to 0.89, $p < 0.0001$); and death (odds ratio 0.82, 95% confidence interval 0.70 to 0.95, $p = 0.010$). In conclusion, patients previously taking statins had a lower incidence of in-hospital arrhythmic events after acute coronary syndrome than those not previously taking statins. Our study suggests another possible benefit from appropriate primary and secondary prevention therapy with statins (Fig 3, Table 3).

▶ In recent years, a number of studies have been published suggesting that statin therapy is associated with a lower frequency of new onset or recurrent

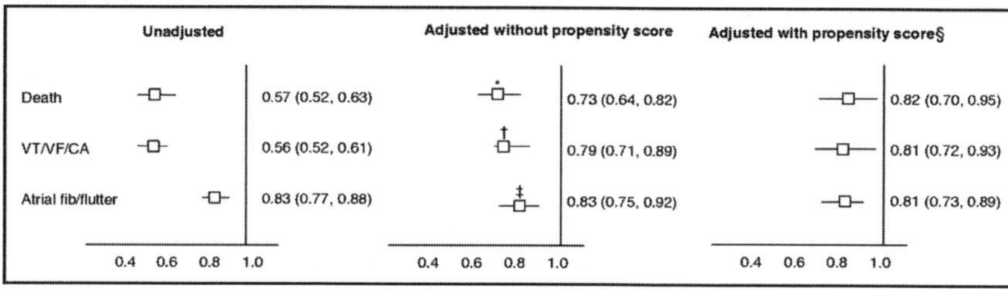


FIGURE 3.—Unadjusted and adjusted odds ratios (95% confidence intervals) for in-hospital outcomes (previous statin users vs nonusers). Unadjusted: n = 64,650 for death; n = 64,043 for VT, VF, and/or CA; and n = 64,277 for AF or atrial flutter. *Adjusted for country, GRACE risk score variables (age, Killip class, CA, systolic blood pressure, pulse, creatinine concentration, ST-segment change, positive initial cardiac biomarkers) (n = 39,844). †Adjusted for age, female gender, country, Killip class, systolic blood pressure, pulse, creatinine concentration, ST-segment change, positive initial cardiac biomarkers, previous therapy (aspirin, amiodarone, or digoxin), and medical history (percutaneous coronary intervention, angina, major bleeding, or stress test) (n = 39,306). ‡Adjusted for age, female gender, country, Killip class, systolic blood pressure, pulse, creatinine concentration, ST-segment change, positive initial cardiac biomarkers, previous therapy (aspirin, warfarin, digoxin, amiodarone, or thienopyridines), and medical history (hypertension, myocardial infarction, dyslipidemia, coronary artery bypass grafting, transient ischemic attack or stroke, smoking, or stress test) (n = 39,462). §Each outcome is adjusted for the same variables as the corresponding outcomes to the left plus propensity score. Corresponding samples sizes are equal. (Reprinted from Vedre A, for the GRACE Investigators. Impact of prior statin therapy on arrhythmic events in patients with acute coronary syndromes (from the Global Registry of Acute Coronary Events [GRACE]). *Am J Cardiol.* 2009;104:1613-1617, with permission from Elsevier.)

TABLE 3.—In-Hospital Outcomes According to Previous Statin Use

| Variable | Previous Statin Use (n = 17,636) | No Previous Statin Use (n = 47,043) | p Value |
|---|---|---|---|
| Death | 560 (3.2%) | 2,563 (5.5%) | <0.0001 |
| Heart failure or pulmonary edema | 1,967 (11%) | 6,727 (14%) | <0.0001 |
| Cardiogenic shock | 453 (2.6%) | 2,180 (4.7%) | <0.0001 |
| CA or VF | 517 (3.0%) | 2,553 (5.5%) | <0.0001 |
| Sustained VT | 754 (4.3%) | 3,448 (7.4%) | <0.0001 |
| AF or atrial flutter | 1,203 (6.9%) | 3,830 (8.2%) | <0.0001 |
| Renal failure | 685 (3.9%) | 1,868 (4.0%) | 0.60 |
| Myocardial infarction >24 hours after hospitalization or reinfarction* | 263 (2.3%) | 616 (2.5%) | 0.36 |

*For myocardial infarction >24 hours after hospitalization or reinfarction, n = 879 for previous statin use and n = 35,680 for no previous statin use.

atrial fibrillation in a variety of settings, including the postoperative period following coronary artery bypass grafting,[1] cardioversion for atrial fibrillation,[2] and in patients with left ventricular systolic dysfunction.[3] The precise mechanism(s) for this protective effect awaits more basic scientific investigation. Among the hypotheses entertained are: (1) reduction in small vessel disease potentially preserving pacemaking activity in both the sinoatrial and atrioventricular nodes; (2) reduction in adverse remodeling and abnormal intercellular matrix deposition; and (3) maintenance of appropriate ion channel activity and transmembrane ion fluxes, among others.

The Global Registry of Acute Coronary Events (GRACE) is a multinational (14 nations), prospective, observational cohort study of patients hospitalized for suspected acute coronary syndromes (ACSs). In this study, risk for developing cardiac arrhythmias among 64 679 patients admitted for ACS (unstable angina, non ST segment elevating myocardial infarction [NSTEMI], or ST segment elevating MI [STEMI]) was analyzed. The comparison groups were comprised of patients who were or were not taking statin therapy at the time of admission. Statin therapy before admission was associated with statistically significant reductions in mortality, heart failure and pulmonary edema, cardiogenic shock, cardiac arrest, sustained ventricular tachycardia, ventricular fibrillation, as well as atrial fibrillation and atrial flutter (Table 3). In propensity adjusted multivariable models (performed to adjust for bias potentially arising from the nonrandom observational design of the study), previous statin use is associated with a 19% lower risk for atrial fibrillation, ventricular tachycardia, ventricular fibrillation, and cardiac arrest and an 18% lower risk for death (Fig 3).

Statin administration in the setting of an ACS and in secondary prevention, in general, is well established and considered to be the standard of care. The development of cardiac arrhythmias in the setting of an ACS is associated with increased morbidity and mortality. Moreover, new onset arrhythmias may also require chronic treatment with anticoagulation and/or antiarrhythmic agents, which increase expense and risk for adverse side effects. This evaluation from the GRACE study suggests that statins beneficially impact risk for both atrial and ventricular arrhythmogenesis in a population highly vulnerable to these complications, and accentuates the critical importance of early and sustained statin therapy in these patients, irrespective of baseline lipid profile. Data from a committed, adequately powered, prospective randomized study using arrhythmia suppression as a prespecified end point would provide more definitive evidence for this benefit from statin therapy. However, in the current climate of severe funding constraints, such a trial is unlikely to see the light of day.

**P. P. Toth, MD, PhD**

*References*


1. Marin F, Pascual DA, Roldan V, et al. Statins and postoperative risk of atrial fibrillation following coronary artery bypass grafting. *Am J Cardiol.* 2006;97:55-60.
2. Ozaydin M, Varol E, Aslan SM, et al. Effect of atorvastatin on the recurrence rates of atrial fibrillation after electrical cardioversion. *Am J Cardiol.* 2006;97:1490-1493.
3. Hanna IR, Heeke B, Bush H, et al. Lipid-lowering drug use is associated with reduced prevalence of atrial fibrillation in patients with left ventricular systolic dysfunction. *Heart Rhythm.* 2006;3:881-886.

**Statin use is associated with lower risk of atrial fibrillation in women with coronary disease: the HERS trial**

Pellegrini CN, Vittinghoff E, Lin F, et al (Univ of California, San Francisco)
*Heart* 95:704-708, 2009

*Objective.*—To determine the efficacy of statin treatment in atrial fibrillation (AF) prevention in women.

*Design.*—Cohort study using data obtained in the Heart and Estrogen/Progestin Replacement Study (HERS).

*Setting.*—Secondary analysis of a multicentre, randomised controlled clinical trial.

*Patients.*—2673 Postmenopausal women with coronary disease.

*Main outcome measures.*—AF prevalence at baseline and incident AF over a mean follow-up of 4.1 years.

*Results.*—88 Women with AF were identified: 29 at baseline and 59 during follow-up. Women with AF were significantly less likely to be taking a statin at study enrolment than those without AF (22% vs 37%, $p = 0.003$). Baseline statin use was associated with a 65% lower odds of having AF at baseline after controlling for age, race, history of myocardial infarction or revascularisation and history of heart failure (odds ratio 0.35, 95% confidence interval (CI) 0.13 to 0.93, $p = 0.04$). The risk of developing AF during the study among those free from AF at baseline, adjusted for the same covariates, was 55% less for those receiving statin treatment (hazard ratio 0.45, 95% CI 0.26 to 0.78, $p = 0.004$).

*Conclusions.*—Statin treatment is associated with a lower prevalence and incidence of AF after adjustment for potential confounders in postmenopausal women with coronary disease (Fig 2).

▶ The Heart and Estrogen/Progestin Replacement Study (HERS) demonstrated that combination estrogen/progesterone supplementation therapy in

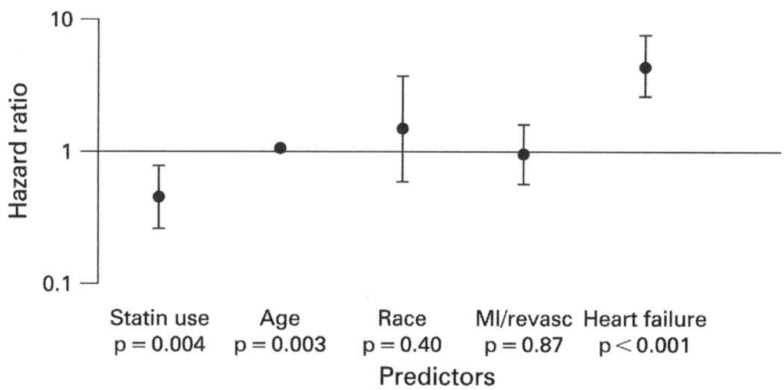


FIGURE 2.—Incidence of atrial fibrillation at follow-up based on presence of predictors. Points display hazard ratios, with adjustment for potential confounders. Bars represent 95% confidence intervals. Age, 10-year increase in age; race, Causcasian compared with all others; MI/revasc, history of myocardial infarction or revascularisation. (Reprinted from Pellegrini CN, Vittinghoff E, Lin F, et al. Statin use is associated with lower risk of atrial fibrillation in women with coronary disease: the HERS trial. *Heart.* 2009;95:704-708, with permission from the BMJ Publishing Group, Ltd.)

postmenopausal women with coronary heart disease (CHD) offered no benefit for reducing primary or secondary cardiovascular end points compared with placebo.[1] In this post hoc analysis from HERS, the impact of statin therapy on risk for atrial fibrillation (AF) in women with CHD was evaluated. After adjusting for confounders, statin usage was associated with lower baseline rates of AF at time of randomization (65%) as well as incident AF (55%) during the course of the trial (Fig 2). The data were adjusted for a variety of confounders, including antiarrhythmic agent usage. This is the only study of its kind done in a population of women, and lends additional confirmation of the relationship between statin usage in patients with CHD and reduction in risk for AF. At minimum, this study reinforces the need to treat women with CHD with statin therapy.

**P. P. Toth, MD, PhD**

*Reference*

1. Hulley S, Grady D, Bush T, et al. Randomized trial of estrogen plus progestin for secondary prevention of coronary heart disease in postmenopausal women. Heart and Estrogen/progestin Replacement Study (HERS) Research Group. *JAMA*. 1998;280:605-613.

---

**Arterial Structure and Function After Recovery From the Metabolic Syndrome: The Cardiovascular Risk in Young Finns Study**

Koskinen J, Magnussen CG, Taittonen L, et al (Univ of Turku, Finland; Vaasa Central Hosp and Univ of Oulu, Finland; et al)

*Circulation* 121:392-400, 2010

---

*Background.*—The reversibility of ultrasonographic vascular changes associated with the metabolic syndrome (MetS) recovery is unknown. We examined whether spontaneous recovery from MetS (according to the International Diabetes Federation definition) has a favorable effect on vascular properties and evaluated the associations between lifestyle factors and MetS recovery.

*Methods and Results.*—We measured carotid artery intima-media thickness, distensibility, and brachial low-mediated dilatation by ultrasound in 1673 subjects of the Young Finns Study cohort (age, 31.5 ± 5.0 years in 2001) who participated in follow-up studies in 2001 and 2007. At baseline, no differences in intima-media thickness, carotid artery distensibility, or flow-mediated dilatation were observed between the recovery group (baseline-only MetS) and those with incident (only at follow-up) or persistent (both at baseline and follow-up) MetS. After 6 years, the recovery group had smaller intima-media thickness (mean ± SEM, 0.62 ± 0.01 versus 0.68 ± 0.01 mm; $P = 0.0009$) and higher carotid artery distensibility (1.98 ± 0.07%/mm Hg versus 1.56 ± 0.04%/mm Hg; $P = 0.001$) compared with the persistent group and higher flow-mediated dilatation compared with the control group (9.91 ± 0.51% versus 8.57 ± 0.12%;

$P = 0.03$). The recovery group had reduced intima-media thickness progression compared with the persistent group (0.036 ± 0.005 versus 0.079 ± 0.010 mm; $P = 0.001$) and reduced carotid artery distensibility change compared with the incident group (−0.12 ± 0.05%/mm Hg versus −0.38 ± 0.10%/mm Hg; $P = 0.03$) over the 6-year follow-up. Differences in carotid artery distensibility levels were attenuated ($P = 0.11$) after the inclusion of weight change in the models. MetS recovery was paralleled with significant reductions in waist circumference that independently correlated with increased physical activity and increased attention paid to health habits during the follow-up.

*Conclusion.*—Recovery from the MetS was associated with positive effects on vascular properties during a 6-year follow-up period of young adults.

▶ Metabolic syndrome (MS) is highly prevalent throughout the world. Hypertriglyceridemia, hyperinsulinemia, hyperglycemia, hypertension, obesity, and low levels of high-density lipoprotein-cholesterol (HDL-C) are defining features of MS. The MS is associated with premature, accelerated atherogenesis, loss of vascular compliance, and endothelial dysfunction with compromised vasoreactivity. The insulin resistance that is etiologic for MS is a consequence of obesity, dysregulated/dysfunctional adipose tissue, and the formation of ectopic steatosis in skeletal, the liver, and epicardium. MS is an important precursor to diabetes mellitus and acute cardiovascular events. The various metabolic features of insulin resistance can be normalized through lifestyle modification, weight loss, smoking cessation, and dietary revision.

In this analysis of follow-up data from the Young Finns Study cohort (1673 patients, mean age 31.5 years at time of baseline measurements) the investigators demonstrate that patients who recover from MS through exercise, dietary modification, and weight loss also experience important changes in metabolic features as well as carotid arterial histology and physiology. In the recovery group, weight, serum insulin, glucose, and triglycerides, all decreased significantly. There was also a trend toward slight reduction in systolic blood pressure. HDL-C increased significantly. In the group persistent for MS, metabolic parameters continued to deteriorate over the 6 years of follow-up. In parallel with these changes, the recovery group experienced a significant decrease in carotid intima media thickness (CIMT) and an increase in carotid distensibility compared with baseline. In contrast, the patients with persistent MS had a higher rate of progression of CIMT and a greater rate of loss of carotid distensibility.

This study confirms that accelerated and adverse forms of carotid arterial remodeling occur in young patients with MS. It also demonstrates that CIMT can be reversed and carotid distensibility improved by relieving insulin resistance through lifestyle modification alone. These results extend findings from previous investigations supporting the front line role of lifestyle modification when managing insulin resistance and cardiometabolic risk.[1] It remains particularly important to intercept this process in younger patients.

**P. P. Toth, MD, PhD**

*Reference*

1. Tuomilehto J, Lindstrom J, Eriksson JG, et al. Prevention of type 2 diabetes mellitus by changes in lifestyle among subjects with impaired glucose tolerance. *N Engl J Med.* 2001;344:1343-1350.

# 55 Neuroendocrinology

**Growth Hormone Deficiency after Treatment of Acromegaly: A Randomized, Placebo-Controlled Study of Growth Hormone Replacement**

Miller KK, Wexler T, Fazeli P, et al (Massachusetts General Hosp and Harvard Med School, Boston)

*J Clin Endocrinol Metab* 95:567-577, 2010

*Context.*—The effects of GH replacement therapy in patients who develop GH deficiency (GHD) after cure of acromegaly have not been established in a placebo-controlled study.

*Objective.*—The objective of the study was to determine whether GH replacement improves body composition, cardiovascular risk markers and quality of life in patients with GHD and prior acromegaly.

*Design.*—This was a 6-month, randomized, placebo-controlled study.

*Setting.*—The study was conducted at a clinical translational science center.

*Study Participants.*—Participants included 30 subjects with prior acromegaly and current GHD.

*Intervention.*—Interventions included GH or placebo.

*Main Outcome Measures.*—Body composition (dual-energy x-ray absorptiometry and cross-sectional computed tomography at L4), cardiovascular risk markers (high-sensitivity C-reactive protein (hsCRP), total, high-density lipoprotein and low-density lipoprotein cholesterol, fibrinogen, and carotid intimal-medial thickness), and quality of life were measured.

*Results.*—The mean GH dose at 6 months was 0.58 ± 0.26 mg/d. Total fat mass, visceral adipose tissue (−15.3 ± 18.6 *vs.* 1.3 ± 12.5%, $P = 0.01$), and total abdominal fat decreased, and fat-free mass increased, in the GH *vs.* placebo group. Mean hsCRP levels decreased, but there was no GH effect on other cardiovascular risk markers. There was no change in glycosylated hemoglobin or homeostasis model assessment insulin resistance index. Quality of life improved with GH. Side effects were minimal.

*Conclusions.*—This is the first randomized, placebo-controlled study of the effects of GH replacement therapy on body composition and cardiovascular end points in patients who have developed GH deficiency after treatment for acromegaly, a disease complicated by metabolic and body composition alterations and increased cardiovascular risk. GH replacement decreased visceral adipose tissue, increased fat-free mass, decreased hsCRP, and improved quality of life in patients with GHD after cure of acromegaly, with minimal side effects and without an increase in insulin resistance.

► Growth hormone deficiency (GHD) can sometimes occur in patients with a history of acromegaly, either as a result of the destructive mass effects of the somatotroph tumor crushing the pituitary gland or as a consequence of pituitary damage from surgery or irradiation to the pituitary tumor. These patients can develop severe symptoms of GHD. The effects of GH replacement in this patient population have not been established. To address this issue, Miller et al performed a 6-month, randomized, placebo-controlled study to access body composition, cardiovascular risk markers, and quality of life. These authors noted an improvement in each of these areas in the GH-treated group and noted very little adverse effects of GH treatment. They conclude that acromegalic patients that subsequently develop GHD may benefit from a trial of GH replacement. These data suggest that patients with GHD who once had a history of acromegaly may benefit from GH treatment and that there are no risks of treatment specific to the acromegaly population.

**W. H. Ludlam, MD, PhD**

---

**Prevalence of pituitary adenomas: a community-based, cross-sectional study in Banbury (Oxfordshire, UK)**

Fernandez A, Karavitaki N, Wass JAH (Churchill Hosp, Oxford, UK)

*Clin Endocrinol* 72:377-382, 2010

---

*Background.*—Pituitary adenomas (PAs) are associated with increased morbidity and mortality. The optimal delivery of services and the provision of care for patients with PAs require distribution of the resources proportionate to the impact of these conditions on the community. Currently, the resource allocation for PAs in the health care system is lacking a reliable and an up-to-date epidemiological background that would reflect the recent advances in the diagnostic technologies, leading to the earlier recognition of these tumours.

*Objectives.*—To determine the prevalence, the diagnostic delay and the characteristics of patients with PA in a well-defined geographical area of the UK (Banbury, Oxfordshire).

*Patients and Methods.*—Sixteen general practitioner (GP) surgeries covering the area of Banbury and a total population of 89 334 inhabitants were asked to participate in the study (data confirmed on 31 July 2006). Fourteen surgeries with a total of 81,449 inhabitants (91% of the study population) agreed to take part. All cases of PAs were found following an exhaustive computer database search of agreed terms by the staff of each Practice and data on age, gender, presenting manifestations and their duration, imaging features at diagnosis, history of multiple endocrine neoplasia type 1 and family history of PA were collected.

*Results.*—A total of 63 patients with PA were identified amongst the study population of 81,149, with a prevalence of 77·6 PA cases/100,000 inhabitants (prolactinomas; PRLoma: 44·4, nonfunctioning PAs: 22·2, acromegaly; ACRO: 8·6, corticotroph adenoma: 1·2 and unknown functional status; UFS: 1·2/100,000 inhabitants). The distribution of each PA subtype was for PRLoma 57%, nonfunctioning PAs 28%, ACRO 11%, corticotroph adenoma 2% and UFS 2%. The median age at diagnosis and the duration of symptoms until diagnosis (in years) were for PRLoma 32·0 and 1·5, nonfunctioning PAs 51·5 and 0·8, ACRO 47 and 4·5 and corticotroph adenoma 57 and 7, respectively. PRLoma was the most frequent PA diagnosed up to the age of 60 years (0–20 years: 75% and 20–60 years: 61% of PAs) and nonfunctioning PA after the age of 60 years (60% of PAs). Nonfunctioning PAs dominated in men (57% of all men with PA) and PRLoma in women (76% of all women with PA). Five patients (7·9%) presented with classical pituitary apoplexy, with a prevalence of 6·2 cases/100,000 inhabitants.

*Conclusions.*—Based on a well-defined population in Banbury (Oxfordshire, UK), we have shown that PAs have a fourfold increased prevalence than previously thought; our data confirm that PAs have a higher burden on the Health Care System and optimal resource distribution for both clinical care and research activities aiming to improve the outcome of these patients are needed.

▶ The estimated prevalence of pituitary adenomas in the general population has been reported to be as low as 25 cases per 100 000 people. There can be significant morbidity and mortality associated with undiagnosed pituitary tumors, and once identified, these patients often require substantial medical resources to manage their disease. For this reason, it is important to obtain an accurate assessment of the true incidence and diagnostic characteristics of pituitary tumors in the general population. To address this need, Fernandez et al performed a review of patients with pituitary adenomas in a well-defined region of nearly 90 000 inhabitants in the United Kingdom. Ninety-one percent of this population was successfully analyzed in the study. These authors identified 63 patients (of the final study population of just over 80 000 people), which resulted in a prevalence of 77.6 cases per 100 000 people. The proportion of pituitary tumor types identified was as follows: 57% prolactinomas, 28% nonfunctional, 11% somatotroph, 2% corticotroph, and 2% other. These authors conclude that the prevalence of pituitary tumors is significantly higher than previously thought and that there needs to be optimization of medical resources to better manage this patient population.

**W. H. Ludlam, MD, PhD**

# 56 Obesity

**Eating Slowly Increases the Postprandial Response of the Anorexigenic Gut Hormones, Peptide YY And Glucagon-Like Peptide-1**

Kokkinos A, Le Roux CW, Alexiadou K, et al (Athens Univ Med School, Athens, Greece; Hammersmith Hosp, London, UK)

*J Clin Endocrinol Metab* 95:333-337, 2010

*Context.*—The rate at which people eat has been suggested to be positively associated with obesity, although appetite and related gut hormones have not been measured.

*Objective.*—The objective of the study was to determine whether eating the same meal at varying speeds elicits different postprandial gut peptide responses.

*Design and Setting.*—This was a crossover study at a clinical research facility.

*Study Participants.*—Seventeen healthy adult male volunteers participated in the study.

*Intervention.*—A test meal consisting of 300 ml ice cream (675 kcal) was consumed in random order on two different sessions by each subject: meal duration took either 5 or 30 min.

*Main Outcome Measures.*—The postprandial response of the orexigenic hormone ghrelin and the anorexigenic peptides peptide YY and glucagon-like peptide-1 over 210 min was assessed. Visual analog scales for the subjective feelings of hunger and fullness were completed throughout each session.

*Results.*—Peptide YY area under the curve (AUC) was higher after the 30-min meal than after the 5-min meal (mean ± SEM AUC 5 min meal: 4133 ± 324, AUC 30 min meal: 5250 ± 330 pmol/liter · min, $P = 0.004$), as was glucagon-like peptide-1 AUC (mean ± SEM AUC 5 min meal: 6219 ± 256, AUC 30 min meal: 8794 ± 656 pmol/liter · min, $P = 0.001$). There was a trend for higher visual analog scale fullness ratings immediately after the end of the 30-min meal compared with immediately after the 5-min meal. There were no differences in ghrelin response.

*Conclusions.*—Eating at a physiologically moderate pace leads to a more pronounced anorexigenic gut peptide response than eating very fast.

▶ The increased prevalence of obesity is best explained by a positive caloric balance. Dieters are advised to eat slowly, using strategies such as prolonged chewing and putting down the fork between bites. Whether these recommendations indeed increase satiety and whether there is a scientific explanation behind these popular strategies was investigated in the above study.

Kokkinos et al conducted a prospective study to evaluate whether eating a test meal consisting of 300 ml of ice cream (675 kcal, 59% of kcal fat, 33% carbohydrates, 8% protein) consumed quickly (within 5 minutes) or slowly (within 30 minutes) would impact satiety (subjective feel of hunger and fullness) and the secretion of orexigenic (ghrelin) and anorexigenic (peptide YY and glucagon-like-peptide-1) gut hormones. Seventeen healthy males were recruited. Blood samples were withdrawn before the meal and every 30 minutes for 210 minutes. Visual assessment of the subjective feelings of hunger and fullness were completed at the meal and thereafter for every 30 minutes. There was a trend toward higher fullness after the 30-minute meal compared with the 5-minute meal but no difference in hunger at the same point (Fig 1 in the original article). The areas under the curve (AUC) for PYY and GLP-1 over 210 minutes were significantly greater after the 30-minute meal (Fig 2 in the original article). Ghrelin levels were not significantly different among groups. Insulin and glucose levels were also similar in both groups.

This interesting study is the first to evaluate the physiological mechanism behind eating slowly. A rise in the anorexigenic peptides PYY and GLP-1 may explain part of the mechanism associated with increased satiety when eating slowly. It is important to evaluate whether the same effect will be reproduced in female subjects and in obese individuals. Nevertheless, now we have some physiological base for the beneficial effect of eating slowly.

**R. Ness-Abramof, MD**

---

**Effect of Moderate Diet-Induced Weight Loss and Weight Regain on Cardiovascular Structure and Function**

de las Fuentes L, Waggoner AD, Mohammed BS, et al (Washington Univ School of Medicine, St Louis, MO; et al)

*J Am Coll Cardiol* 54:2376-2381, 2009

---

*Objectives.*—The objective of this prospective, single-site, 2-year dietary intervention study was to evaluate the effects of moderate weight reduction and subsequent partial weight regain on cardiovascular structure and function.

*Background.*—Obesity is associated with adverse cardiac and vascular structural and functional alterations.

*Methods.*—Sixty obese subjects (age 46 ± 10 years, body mass index 37 ± 3 kg/m$^2$) were evaluated during their participation in a weight loss study. Cardiac and vascular ultrasound studies were performed at baseline and at 3, 6, 12, and 24 months after start of intervention.

*Results.*—Forty-seven subjects (78%) completed the entire 2-year follow-up. Average weight loss was 7.3 ± 4.0%, 9.2 ± 5.6%,

7.8 ± 6.6%, and 3.8 ± 7.9% at 3, 6, 12, and 24 months, respectively. Age- and sex-adjusted mixed linear models revealed that the follow-up time was significantly associated with decreases in weight ($p < 0.0001$), left ventricular (LV) mass ($p = 0.001$), and carotid intima-media thickness ($p < 0.0001$); there was also significant improvement in LV diastolic ($p \leq 0.0001$) and systolic ($p = 0.001$) function. Partial weight regain diminished the maximal observed beneficial effects of weight loss, however cardiovascular parameters measured at 2 years still showed a net benefit compared with baseline.

*Conclusions.*—Diet-induced moderate weight loss in obese subjects is associated with beneficial changes in cardiovascular structure and function. Subsequent weight regain is associated with partial loss of these beneficial effects. (The Safety and Effectiveness of Low and High Carbohydrate Diets; NCT00079547) (Fig 1).

▶ This study examines the effect of weight loss on cardiovascular structure and function, and whether this effect is sustained in patients who regain weight. Several abnormalities in cardiovascular structure and function have been associated with obesity, including left ventricular (LV) hypertrophy and LV systolic and diastolic dysfunction, all of which are known to be independent risk factors for development of heart failure.[1-3] Previous work has demonstrated that weight loss promotes cardiac remodeling and improves related measures of cardiac function.[4,5] However, most of the available data come from studies in class III obese patients undergoing bariatric surgery who experience considerable weight loss following surgery (often > 20% body weight) and often show resolution of underlying medical diseases known to increase cardiovascular risk, such as diabetes mellitus or hypertension. Therefore, improvements in cardiac function in patients following bariatric surgery may not be applicable to patients with more modest degrees of weight loss.

This prospective study follows a cohort of 60 patients randomly assigned to follow 1 of 2 calorie-restricted diets (low-carbohydrate or low-fat diet) over a 2-year period. Subjects also participated in weekly group counseling sessions and were encouraged to begin walking regularly. There were no significant differences between diet treatment groups in terms of baseline characteristics, weight loss, or primary outcome measures, and therefore data analyses were performed on the entire pooled sample. Patients lost an average of about 5% to 10% of their initial body weight during the study, with maximal weight loss occurring at 6 months and weight regain noted at 12 and 24 months, although mean weight at completion remained below baseline levels. In Fig 1, authors show that weight loss was significantly correlated with improvements in LV diastolic relaxation (E′ [early diastolic myocardial velocity]) at 6, 12, and 24 months, improvement in LV systolic function (S′ [systolic myocardial velocity]) at 24 months, decreased LV mass ($LVM/Ht^{2.7}$ [LVM indexed to height$^{2.7}$]) at 3, 6, and 12 months, and decreased carotid intima-media wall thickness at 6, 12, and 24 months. These favorable changes in cardiac structure and function appear to lag behind achievement of maximal weight loss by about 3 to 6 months. Subsequent weight regain was associated with worsening

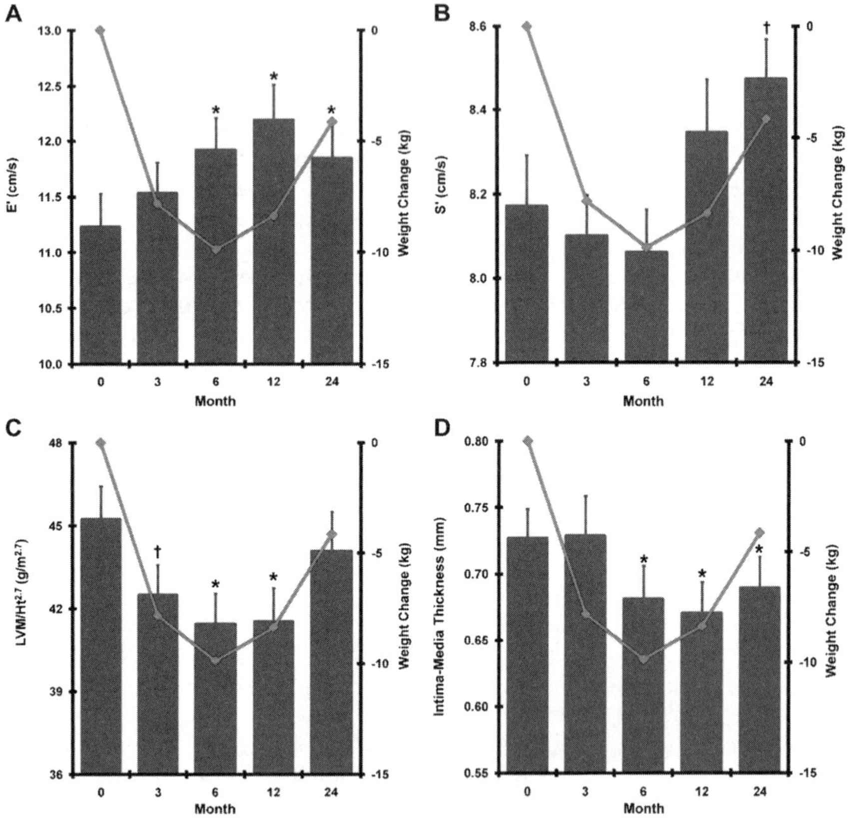


**FIGURE 1.**—Cardiovascular structure-function response to weight loss. Mean ( ± SEM) change in (**A**) early diastolic myocardial velocity (E'), (**B**) systolic myocardial velocity (S'), (**C**) left ventricular mass indexed to height$^{2.7}$ (LVM/Ht$^{2.7}$), and (**D**) carotid intima-media thickness in the combined cohort (**blue bars**) with weight change (**red line**) shown for reference. The combined group had 60 subjects at baseline and 3 months, 56 subjects at 6 months, and 47 subjects at 12 and 24 months. There was no significant difference between diet groups for any of these phenotypes. *Adjusted $p \leq 0.005$; †adjusted $p \leq 0.05$ versus baseline. For interpretation of the references to color in this figure legend, the reader is referred to web version of this article. (Reprinted form de las Fuentes L, Waggoner AD, Mohammed BS, et al. Effect of moderate diet-induced weight loss and weight regain on cardiovascular structure and function. *J Am Coll Cardiol*. 2009;54:2376-2381, with permission from the American College of Cardiology Foundation.)

of LVM, diastolic function, and vascular hypertrophy, although improvements in LV systolic function persisted at 24 months.

It is impossible to know whether these effects would last if an additional 3 to 6 months of time passed or if patients were followed after returning to their baseline weight. Another limitation of this study is that patients were encouraged, but not required, to participate in cardiovascular exercise, such as regular walking, and because patient exercise was neither supervised nor recorded in this study, its role as a confounding factor on outcomes cannot be accounted for. It would be premature to conclude that the improvements in cardiovascular function and structure can be attributed to weight loss alone. Additionally, it is unclear whether transient improvements in cardiac function associated with modest weight loss will show any sustained benefit and/or translate into meaningful improvements in clinical outcomes (eg, decreased hospitalizations for heart failure) over time. What is encouraging about this study is that the authors have shown that with modest weight loss (5%-10% of baseline weight), many of the changes seen in cardiomyopathy of obesity can be reversed. Weight regain attenuates the maximal observed benefit of these effects, although improvements in cardiac outcomes persist well beyond this period. Further studies to investigate the long-term effects of weight loss and gain on improvements in cardiovascular structure and function and the specific mechanisms underlying these changes are warranted.

**A. M. Port, MD**

*References*


1. Wong CY, O'Moore-Sullivan T, Leano R, Byrne N, Beller E, Marwick TH. Alterations of left ventricular myocardial characteristics associated with obesity. *Circulation.* 2004;110:3081-3087.
2. Alpert MA. Obesity cardiomyopathy: pathophysiology and evolution of the clinical syndrome. *Am J Med Sci.* 2001;321:225-236.
3. Kenchaiah S, Evans JC, Levy D, et al. Obesity and the risk of heart failure. *N Engl J Med.* 2002;347:305-313.
4. Alpert MA, Terry B, Lambert CR, et al. Factors influencing left ventricular systolic function in nonhypertensive morbidly obese patients, and effect of weight loss induced by gastroplasty. *Am J Cardiol.* 1993;71:733-737.
5. Ippisch HM, Inge TH, Daniels SR, Wang B, Khoury PR, Witt SA. Reversibility of cardiac abnormalities in morbidly obese adolescents. *J Am Coll Cardiol.* 2008;51:1342-1348.


### Cold-Activated Brown Adipose Tissue in Healthy Men

van Marken Lichtenbelt WD, Vanhommerig JW, Smulders NM, et al (Maastricht Univ Med Ctr, the Netherlands)
*N Engl J Med* 360:1500-1508, 2009

*Background.*—Studies in animals indicate that brown adipose tissue is important in the regulation of body weight, and it is possible that individual variation in adaptive thermogenesis can be attributed to variations in the amount or activity of brown adipose tissue. Until recently, the presence of brown adipose tissue was thought to be relevant only in small mammals and infants, with negligible physiologic relevance in adult humans. We performed a systematic examination of the presence, distribution, and activity of brown adipose tissue in lean and obese men during exposure to cold temperature. Brown-adipose-tissue activity was studied in relation to body composition and energy metabolism.

*Methods.*—We studied 24 healthy men — 10 who were lean (body-mass index [BMI] [the weight in kilograms divided by the square of the height in meters], <25) and 14 who were overweight or obese (BMI, ≥25) — under thermoneutral conditions (22°C) and during mild cold exposure (16°C). Putative brown-adipose-tissue activity was determined with the use of integrated $^{18}$F-fluorodeoxyglucose positron-emission tomography and computed tomography. Body composition and energy expenditure were measured with the use of dual-energy x-ray absorptiometry and indirect calorimetry.

*Results.*—Brown-adipose-tissue activity was observed in 23 of the 24 subjects (96%) during cold exposure but not under thermoneutral conditions. The activity was significantly lower in the overweight or obese subjects than in the lean subjects ($P = 0.007$). BMI and percentage of body fat both had significant negative correlations with brown adipose tissue, whereas resting metabolic rate had a significant positive correlation.

*Conclusions.*—The percentage of young men with brown adipose tissue is high, but its activity is reduced in men who are overweight or obese. Brown adipose tissue may be metabolically important in men, and the fact that it is reduced yet present in most overweight or obese subjects may make it a target for the treatment of obesity.

▶ Brown adipose tissue (BAT) is a metabolically active fat depot characterized by a high concentration of mitochondria. Uncoupling protein-1 (UCP-1) is an established marker of BAT and resides in the inner mitochondrial membrane.[1] In response to sympathetic nervous stimulation, typically due to cold temperatures, UCP-1 induces a leak in the inner mitochondrial membrane that causes energy to be released as heat.[2] The role of BAT in this nonshivering thermogenesis process has been well established in small mammals and infant humans.[1] For several years, researchers postulated that BAT is present in adult humans and that by manipulating this organ, we may be able to positively affect energy regulation in overweight and obese humans. van Marken Lichtenbelt et al present one of the first studies to demonstrate that BAT is present and metabolically active in adult humans and that BAT activity is associated with body-mass index (BMI) (Fig 1 in the original article). With the use of fluorodeoxyglucose (FDG)-positron emission tomography (PET)/X-ray computed tomography (CT) scan, van Marken Lichtenbelt et al identified BAT throughout the body, but the major depot was concentrated in the supraclavicular region in healthy adult males (Fig 1 in the original article). There was a marked increase in FDG uptake with cold exposure, suggesting that a standardized cold temperature exposure may be necessary to adequately quantify BAT activity in humans. The authors also demonstrated that there was significantly higher BAT tissue volume and activity in cold-exposed lean (BMI 21.3-24.5 kg/m$^2$) relative to overweight or obese (BMI 25.4-38.7 kg/m$^2$) individuals (Fig 1 in the original article). BMI and percent body fat determined by dual energy X-ray absorptiometry (DXA) were negatively correlated with BAT activity. Moreover, the authors provide some of the first evidence that BAT may contribute to whole body energy expenditure. Although this study provides strong support for the presence of a BAT in adults and that the activity of this BAT is influenced by cold temperatures and BMI, the study was limited by its smaller size (N = 24) and select population, young (18-30 years) healthy adult males. There is evidence to suggest that BAT activity may decrease with age,[3] indicating that further investigation is warranted in the aging population. This study, as well as 3 others[3-5] printed simultaneously, provide formidable evidence that there are marked quantities of active BAT in adult humans and that it likely contributes to body weight regulation. These studies present BAT as a novel target for development of therapeutic strategies to regulate adiposity and body weight. Future research should be directed at delineating the mechanisms and physiology of BAT as it relates to whole body energy expenditure.

**M. Ruth, PhD**

*References*

1. Porter RK. A new look at UCP-1. *Biochimica et Biophysica Acta*. 2006;1757: 446-448.
2. Celi FS. Brown adipose tissue? When it pays to be inefficient. *N Engl J Med*. 2009; 360:1553.
3. Saito M, Okamatsu-Ogura Y, Matsushita M, et al. High incidence of metabolically active brown adipose tissue in healthy adult humans. *Diabetes*. 2009;58: 1526-1531.
4. Cypess AM, Lehman S, Williams G, et al. Identification and importance of brown adipose tissue in adult humans. *N Engl J Med*. 2009;360:1509-1517.
5. Virtanen KA, Lidell ME, Orava J, et al. Functional brown adipose tissue in healthy adults. *N Engl J Med*. 2009;360:1518-1525.

### The Impact of Exercise Training Compared to Caloric Restriction on Hepatic and Peripheral Insulin Resistance in Obesity

Coker RH, Williams RH, Yeo SE, et al (Univ of Arkansas for Med Sciences, Little Rock)

*J Clin Endocrinol Metab* 94:4258-4266, 2009

*Context.*—It has been difficult to distinguish the independent effects of caloric restriction versus exercise training on insulin resistance.

*Objective.*—Utilizing metabolic feeding and supervised exercise training, we examined the influence of caloric restriction *vs.* exercise training with and without weight loss on hepatic and peripheral insulin resistance.

*Design, Participants, and Intervention.*—Thirty-four obese, older subjects were randomized to: caloric restriction with weight loss (CR), exercise training with weight loss (EWL), exercise training without weight loss (EX), or controls. Based on an equivalent caloric deficit in EWL and CR, we induced matched weight loss. Subjects in the EX group received caloric compensation. Combined with [6,6$^2H_2$]glucose, an octreotide, glucagon, multistage insulin infusion was performed to determine suppression of glucose production (SGP) and insulin-stimulated glucose disposal

(ISGD). Computed tomography scans were performed to assess changes in fat distribution.

*Results.*—Body weight decreased similarly in EWL and CR, and did not change in EX and controls. The reduction in visceral fat was significantly greater in EWL ($-71 \pm 15$ cm$^2$) compared to CR and EX. The increase in SGP was also almost 3-fold greater ($27 \pm 2\%$) in EWL. EWL and CR promoted similar improvements in ISGD [$+2.5 \pm 0.4$ and $2.4 \pm 0.9$ mg $\cdot$ kg fat-free mass (FFM)$^{-1} \cdot$ min$^{-1}$], respectively.

*Conclusions.*—EWL promoted the most significant reduction in visceral fat and the greatest improvement in SGP. Equivalent increases in ISGD were noted in EWL and CR, whereas EX provided a modest improvement. Based on our results, EWL promoted the optimal intervention-based changes in body fat distribution and systemic insulin resistance.

▶ The increased caloric intake and reduced physical activity are the main culprits for the obesity epidemic. Obesity is the most common cause of insulin resistance carrying a higher risk to develop type 2 diabetes mellitus and cardiovascular disease. Diabetes was shown to be delayed or prevented by lifestyle changes, including weight loss and exercise. The Diabetes Prevention Program (DPP) enrolled 3232 patients with impaired glucose tolerance to metformin, lifestyle changes, or control group.[1] Patients on lifestyle modification program had a goal to lose at least 7% of basal weight and to exercise at least 150 minutes per week. The incidence of diabetes was reduced by 58% in the lifestyle change group and by 31% on the metformin group compared with the placebo group. A 10-year follow-up of patients from the DPP trial still showed protective effect of lifestyle changes and metformin in the incidence of type 2 diabetes.[2]

Most weight loss programs combine dietary restriction and increased physical activity. Although an increase in physical activity would not promote a significant weight loss, it improves insulin sensitivity.[3] Coker et al designed a study to evaluate the effectiveness of weight loss through caloric restriction (CR), exercise training with weight loss (EWL), and exercise training without weight loss (EX) on hepatic and peripheral insulin resistance. They measured insulin-stimulated glucose disposal (ISGD) and determined the suppression of glucose production (SGP) in 34 obese patients. Weight decreased in both the CR and EWL group and remained unchanged in the EX and control group. The EWL group had the greatest reduction in visceral fat as assessed by computed tomography. The SGP was higher in the EWL group and ISGD was similar in the EWL and CR group. According to this study, EWL promoted the highest reduction in visceral fat and improvement in hepatic insulin resistance. EWL and CR both increased peripheral insulin sensitivity, whereas EX alone provided just a modest improvement.

The improvement in hepatic insulin sensitivity in this study was higher than that found with CR only, a finding that needs to be revalidated.

**R. Ness-Abramof, MD**

*References*

1. Diabetes Prevention Program Research, G. Reduction in the incidence of type 2 diabetes with lifestyle intervention or metformin. *N Engl J Med.* 2002;346: 393-403.
2. Diabetes Prevention Program Research, G. 10-year follow-up of diabetes incidence and weight loss in the Diabetes Prevention Program Outcomes Study. *Lancet.* 2009;374:1677-1686.
3. O'Gorman DJ, Krook A. Exercise and the treatment of diabetes and obesity. *Endocrinol Metab Clin North Am.* 2008;37:887-903.

# 57 Pediatric Endocrinology

---

**Maternal Vitamin D Status Determines Bone Variables in the Newborn**

Viljakainen HT, Saarnio E, Hytinantti T, et al (Univ of Helsinki, Finland; Helsinki Univ Central Hosp, Finland; et al)

*J Clin Endocrinol Metab* 95:1749-1757, 2010

---

*Context.*—Vitamin D regulates 3% of the human genome, including effects on bone health throughout life. Maternal vitamin D status may program neonatal skeletal development. The objective here was to determine the association of mothers' vitamin D status with bone variables of their newborns.

*Subjects and Methods.*—In a birth hospital, pregnant women (n = 125) participated in a cross-sectional study with a longitudinal follow-up of the pregnancy. The mean (SD) values for age, body mass index before pregnancy, pregnancy weight gain, and total vitamin D intake in mothers were 31 (4) yr, 23.5 (3.7) kg/m$^2$, 13.1 (4.3) kg, and 14.3 (5.8) $\mu$g, respectively. All newborns were full-term, 99% were appropriate for gestational age, and 53% were boys. Blood samples were collected from mothers during the first trimester and 2 d postpartum and from umbilical cords at birth for analysis of serum 25-hydroxyvitamin D (S-25-OHD), PTH, and bone remodeling markers. Bone variables were measured by pQCT at the 20% site of the newborn tibia on an average of 10 (11) d postpartum. Bone contour was analyzed with a single threshold of 180 mg/mm$^3$ for the detection of total bone mineral density (BMD), bone mineral content (BMC), and cross-sectional area (CSA).

*Results.*—Mean S-25-OHD was 41.0 (13.6), 45.1 (11.9), and 50.7 (14.9) nmol/liter during the first trimester, postpartum, and in the umbilical cord, respectively. The median value of the individual means for first trimester and the 2-d postpartum S-25-OHD was 42.6 nmol/liter, which was used as cutoff to define two equal-sized groups. Groups are called below median and above median in the text. Newborns below median were heavier ($P = 0.05$), and 60% were boys. Tibia bone mineral content was 0.047 (95% confidence interval, 0.011–0.082) g/cm higher ($P = 0.01$), and cross-sectional area was 12.3 (95% confidence interval, 2.0–22.6) mm$^2$ larger ($P = 0.02$), but no difference in bone mineral density was observed, above median compared with below median group. These results were adjusted for newborn Z-score birth weight, maternal height, and newborn age at the measurement. A positive, significant correlation was observed between remodeling markers in mothers at different time points and above median group in the cord.

*Conclusions.*—Although the mean total intake of vitamin D among mothers met current Nordic recommendations, 71% of women and 15% of newborns were vitamin D deficient during the pregnancy. Our results suggest that maternal vitamin D status affects bone mineral accrual during the intrauterine period and influences bone size. More efforts should be made to revise current nutrition recommendations for pregnant women that may have permanent effects on the well-being of children.

▶ This interesting study is a useful reminder that the establishment of an individual's risk and resilience factors for human disease begins not at birth, but during prenatal life. As the first investigation of the relationship between maternal vitamin D status and fetal bone development, this study represents a significant contribution to current understanding of intrauterine bone biology and growth. As seen in Fig 2 in the original article, infants born to mothers with above median 25-hydroxyvitamin D levels had higher tibial bone mineral content and cross-sectional area than those with maternal below mean 25, OHD concentrations, although no differences in bone mineral density were seen. Importantly, these results persisted after adjustment for Z-score birth weight. One of the most striking findings of the study was that > 95% of the mothers were deemed vitamin D deficient or insufficient during the first trimester as well as in the postpartum period, despite the fact that 80% were getting the recommended daily supplement of vitamin D for pregnant women. Since a linear relationship between maternal and cord blood vitamin D concentration was seen, this suggests that the recommended daily intake of vitamin D for Nordic women during pregnancy should be drastically revised. While maternal vitamin D status appears to directly impact fetal bone variables, to what extent it influences skeletal programming is less clear. Similarly, how postnatal factors might modulate the effect of intrauterine vitamin D exposure remains to be elucidated.

**E. Eugster, MD, PhD**

**Pediatric thyroid fine-needle aspiration cytology: a meta-analysis**

Stevens C, Lee JKP, Sadatsafavi M, et al (Univ of British Columbia, Vancouver, Canada)

*J Pediatr Surg* 44:2184-2191, 2009

*Background.*—There is conflicting evidence in the current literature regarding the use of fine-needle aspiration (FNA) biopsy in the diagnosis of a thyroid nodule in the pediatric population. There are numerous studies that look at the sensitivity and specificity of this test with varying results. A meta-analysis will provide further insight into this topic.

*Purpose.*—Our objective was to investigate the diagnostic parameters of FNA biopsy in the diagnosis of a thyroid nodule in the pediatric population, specifically, to determine the sensitivity, specificity, accuracy, positive predictive value (PPV), and negative predictive value (NPV) of the test in differentiating malignant vs benign tumors.

*Material and Methods.*—We performed a literature search of Medline, Embase, and evidence based medicine (EBM) reviews for English studies that looked at FNA biopsy in thyroid nodules in the pediatric population, in which diagnostic values were present or could be calculated and where FNA results were compared to an acceptable reference standard. Two reviewers independently selected all abstracts, and from these, studies to review. Two reviewers also independently checked diagnostic values in the studies or calculated them from data available. A meta-analysis was performed, and pooled diagnostic test values were calculated using a random-effects, bivariate meta-regression model. Studies were also assessed for quality using the quality assessment for diagnostic accuracy studies tool.

*Results.*—Twelve studies were included for review. The quality of the studies in general was good. The pooled estimate of sensitivity and specificity were 94% (95% confidence interval [CI], 86%-100%) and 81% (95% CI, 72%-91%), respectively. Assuming 20% of nodules are malignant, the accuracy, PPV, and NPV were 83.6%, 55.3%, and 98.2%, respectively.

*Conclusion.*—This meta-analysis provides good evidence that FNA biopsy of thyroid nodules is a sensitive test in the pediatric population and may be a useful tool for excluding malignancy in young patients. Future prospective studies are needed to evaluate this further.

▶ Unlike in adults, thyroid nodules in children and adolescents are rare. Due to the established higher incidence of thyroid cancer in isolated pediatric versus adult thyroid nodules, these lesions are also considered to be far more worrisome than in the adult population. Therefore, many pediatric endocrinologists have traditionally followed the practice of routinely referring such patients to an ENT specialist or pediatric surgeon to have a hemithyroidectomy or thyroidectomy performed. However, thyroid surgery is not without risks, which include laryngeal nerve damage and hypoparathyroidism, which may be permanent. Thus, the ability to accurately differentiate benign nodules from thyroid cancer would prevent unnecessary thyroid surgeries and enhance clinical care. A major strength of this meta-analysis is the stringent criteria used for including studies. Given the scarcity of reports of using fine-needle aspiration (FNA) in the diagnostic evaluation of pediatric thyroid nodules, combining the results of existing studies to derive the sensitivity and specificity of this tool in children makes intuitive sense. Nonetheless, it should be noted that all studies were retrospective and not all of them used ultrasound-guided FNA, which would be considered standard of care at most institutions. The take-home message of the authors' findings is that FNA of thyroid nodules in children does appear to be quite sensitive in excluding malignancy, and is undoubtedly underused as a diagnostic tool. It would behoove pediatric endocrinologists to identify the appropriate personnel to perform this procedure in their own institution, and to consider it in the evaluation of select patients. Additional guidelines regarding whether and when to repeat FNA, the significance of nodule size in predicting pathology, and how to deal with equivocal results are also needed.

**E. Eugster, MD, PhD**

# 58 Reproductive Endocrinology

---

**Relation between Serum Testosterone, Serum Estradiol, Sex Hormone-Binding Globulin, and Geometrical Measures of Adult Male Proximal Femur Strength**

Travison TG, Araujo AB, Beck TJ, et al (New England Res Insts, Watertown, MA; Johns Hopkins Univ School of Medicine, Baltimore, MD; et al)

*J Clin Endocrinol Metab* 94:853-860, 2009

---

*Context.*—Although previous studies have indicated associations between circulating testosterone (T) or estradiol (E2) concentrations and bone mineral density, the relationship between gonadal steroids and skeletal geometry is not well defined.

*Objective.*—Our objective was to uncover the relation between circulating T or E2 and proximal femur geometry in a diverse sample of men.

*Design.*—We used data on 808 men enrolled in the Boston Area Community Health/Bone Study. Serum concentrations of total and calculated free T and E2 were obtained via early-morning blood sampling. The geometry of the proximal femur at three sites (the narrow neck, intertrochanter, and shaft) was obtained using the Hip Structural Analysis technology. Analyses adjusted for subjects' age, height, total body lean mass and fat mass, and level of physical activity were performed.

*Setting.*—In-home interviews accompanied by subject visits to the General Clinical Research Center at Boston University School of Medicine were performed.

*Study Participants.*—A randomly selected cohort of men living in Boston, MA (ages 30–79 yr) was included in the study.

*Interventions.*—These were not applicable.

*Main Outcome Measures.*—Bone mineral density and bone outer diameter, cross-sectional area (measuring bone material), and section modulus (an index of bending strength) were calculated.

*Results.*—In age-adjusted models, E2 was positively associated with hip strength parameters, whereas T was not. Adjustment for age and other parameters resulted in substantial reductions in, but not complete elimination of, associations between E2 and hip strength parameters.

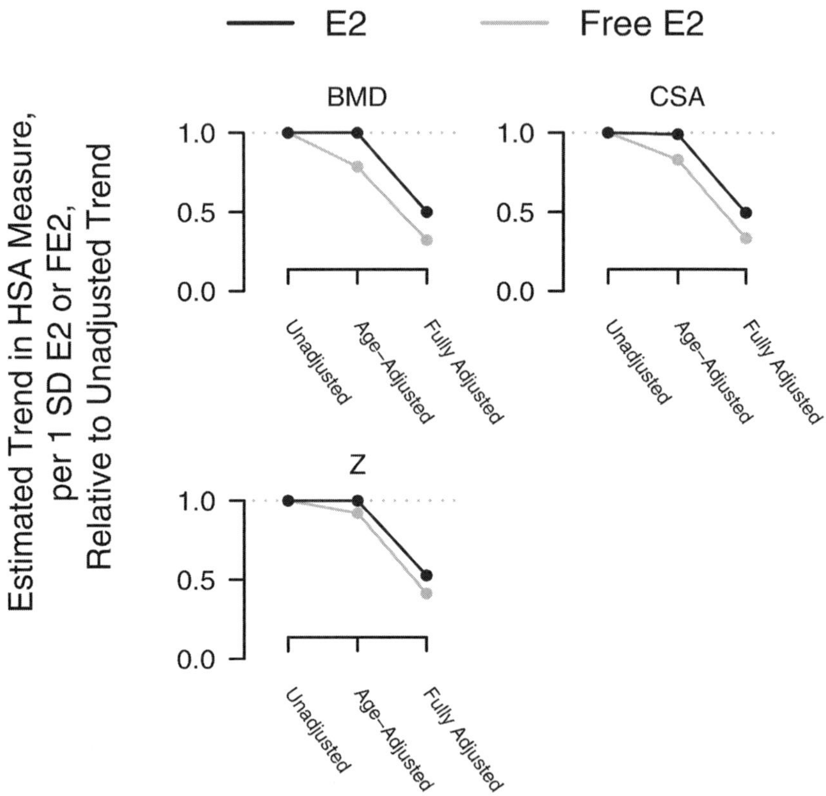


FIGURE 2.—Reduction in the magnitude of the association between E2 and NN hip geometry accompanying control for other parameters in a multivariate regression model. Points corresponding to "Age-adjusted" and "Fully Adjusted" models express the cross-sectional change in proximal femur strength indices accompanying a 1 SD increase in E2 or FE2, controlling for age and other parameters (LM, FM, PASE, and height). These differences are scaled to the crude difference observed when no other covariates are considered ("Unadjusted"). (Reprinted from Travison TG, Araujo AB, Beck TJ, et al. Relation between serum testosterone, serum estradiol, sex hormone-binding globulin, and geometrical measures of adult male proximal femur strength. *J Clin Endocrinol Metab*. 2009;94:853-860, with permission from The Endocrine Society.)

*Conclusion.*—Circulating E2 is strongly associated with proximal femur strength, an association that is partially mediated by body composition (Fig 2).

► Sex steroids are known to affect bone mineral density (BMD), and in men, aging is associated with alterations in sex steroid concentrations that might adversely affect BMD and predispose to fractures. Cross-sectional and longitudinal studies have shown a positive relationship between serum testosterone and estradiol concentrations and BMD with estradiol showing the stronger association. There are other factors besides sex steroids that affect bone fractures, and BMD is not directly associated with bone strength. In the study by Travison et al, 808 men were enrolled in a study to determine whether circulating sex steroids showed a relationship to proximal femur geometry in men aged 30 to 79 years. Results that estradiol but not testosterone was positively associated with hip strength parameters are consistent with other studies in elderly men that show stronger association serum estradiol concentrations than testosterone. Body composition also influences proximal femur strength. In studies of bone strength, the measurements are imperfect, and longitudinal studies are needed rather than cross-sectional studies.

**A. W. Meikle, MD**

### Effects of Testosterone on Muscle Strength, Physical Function, Body Composition, and Quality of Life in Intermediate-Frail and Frail Elderly Men: A Randomized, Double-Blind, Placebo-Controlled Study

Srinivas-Shankar U, Roberts SA, Connolly MJ, et al (Univ of Manchester, UK; Univ of Auckland, New Zealand)
*J Clin Endocrinol Metab* 95:639-650, 2010

*Context.*—Physical frailty is associated with reduced muscle strength, impaired physical function, and quality of life. Testosterone (T) increases muscle mass and strength in hypogonadal patients. It is unclear whether T has similar effects in intermediate-frail and frail elderly men with low to borderline-low T.

*Objective.*—Our objective was to determine the effects of 6 months T treatment in intermediate-frail and frail elderly men, on muscle mass and strength, physical function, and quality of life.

*Design and Setting.*—We conducted a randomized, double-blind, placebo-controlled, parallel-group, single-center study.

*Participants.*—Participants were community-dwelling intermediate-frail and frail elderly men at least 65 yr of age with a total T at or below 12 nmol/liter or free T at or below 250 pmol/liter.

*Methods.*—Two hundred seventy-four participants were randomized to transdermal T (50 mg/d) or placebo gel for 6 months. Outcome measures included muscle strength, lean and fat mass, physical function, and self-reported quality of life.

*Results.*—Isometric knee extension peak torque improved in the T group (*vs.* placebo at 6 months), adjusted difference was 8.6 (95% confidence interval, 1.3–16.0; $P = 0.02$) Newton-meters. Lean body mass increased and fat mass decreased significantly in the T group by 1.08 ± 1.8 and 0.9 ± 1.6 kg, respectively. Physical function improved among older and frailer men. Somatic and sexual symptom scores decreased with T treatment; adjusted difference was −1.2 (−2.4 to −0.04) and −1.3 (−2.5 to −0.2), respectively.

*Conclusions.*—T treatment in intermediate-frail and frail elderly men with low to borderline-low T for 6 months may prevent age-associated loss of lower limb muscle strength and improve body composition, quality of life, and physical function. Further investigations are warranted to extend these results.

▶ Physical frailty affects many organ systems, and aging is associated with a decline in muscle mass and strength, which is then associated with falls, disability, hospitalizations, and death. Hypogonadism, with a decline particularly in free testosterone, increases as men age and is deemed related to frailty of aging men. Some investigators have demonstrated improvement in muscle function with testosterone treatment of aging men, but other studies have failed to confirm that finding. The strength of the study by Srinivas-Shanker et al was that it was a single-center study and was a double-blind placebo-controlled study of the effect of testosterone therapy on muscle strength, physical function, and quality of life in intermediate-frail and frail elderly men. Men qualified for the study if their total testosterone was below 12 nmol/L (345 ng/dL) or a free testosterone of <250 pg/L (72 pg/mL). Treatment was either placebo or transdermal testosterone gel of 50 mg/d. Compared with placebo, men treated with testosterone had improved isometric knee extension peak torque and were physically functional. Lean body mass improved and fat mass decreased, as did somatic and sexual symptoms scores. The study was only for 6 months, which was not long enough to answer questions of the long-term benefits and safety of testosterone therapy in aging frail men. Adverse event increases were restricted to some rise in prostate-specific antigen (PSA) and hematocrit in the treated group, and serious adverse events listed did not appear to be testosterone related.

**A. W. Meikle, MD**

---

**Testosterone and Growth Hormone Improve Body Composition and Muscle Performance in Older Men**

Sattler FR, Castaneda-Sceppa C, Binder EF, et al (Univ of Southern California, Los Angeles; Tufts Univ, Boston, MA; Washington Univ, St. Louis, MO)

*J Clin Endocrinol Metab* 94:1991-2001, 2009

---

*Context.*—Impairments in the pituitary-gonadal axis with aging are associated with loss of muscle mass and function and accumulation of upper body fat.

*Objectives.*—We tested the hypothesis that physiological supplementation with testosterone and GH together improves body composition and muscle performance in older men.

*Design, Setting, and Participants.*—One hundred twenty-two community-dwelling men 70.8 ± 4.2 yr of age with body mass index of 27.4 ± 3.4 kg/m$^2$, testosterone of 550 ng/dl or less, and IGF-I in lower adult tertile (≤167 ng/dl) were randomized to receive transdermal testosterone (5 or 10 g/d) during a Leydig cell clamp plus GH (0, 3, or 5 μg/kg · d) for 16 wk.

*Main Outcome Measures.*—Body composition by dual-energy x-ray absorptiometry, muscle performance, and safety tests were conducted.

*Results.*—Total lean body mass increased (1.0 ± 1.7 to 3.0 ± 2.2 kg) as did appendicular lean tissue (0.4 ± 1.4 to 1.5 ± 1.3 kg), whereas total fat mass decreased by 0.4 ± 0.9 to 2.3 ± 1.7 kg as did trunk fat (0.5 ± 0.9 to 1.5 ± 1.0 kg) across the six treatment groups and by dose levels for each parameter ($P \leq 0.0004$ for linear trend). Composite maximum voluntary strength of upper and lower body muscles increased by 14 ± 34 to 35 ± 31% ($P < 0.003$ in the three highest dose groups) that correlated with changes in appendicular lean mass. Aerobic endurance increased in

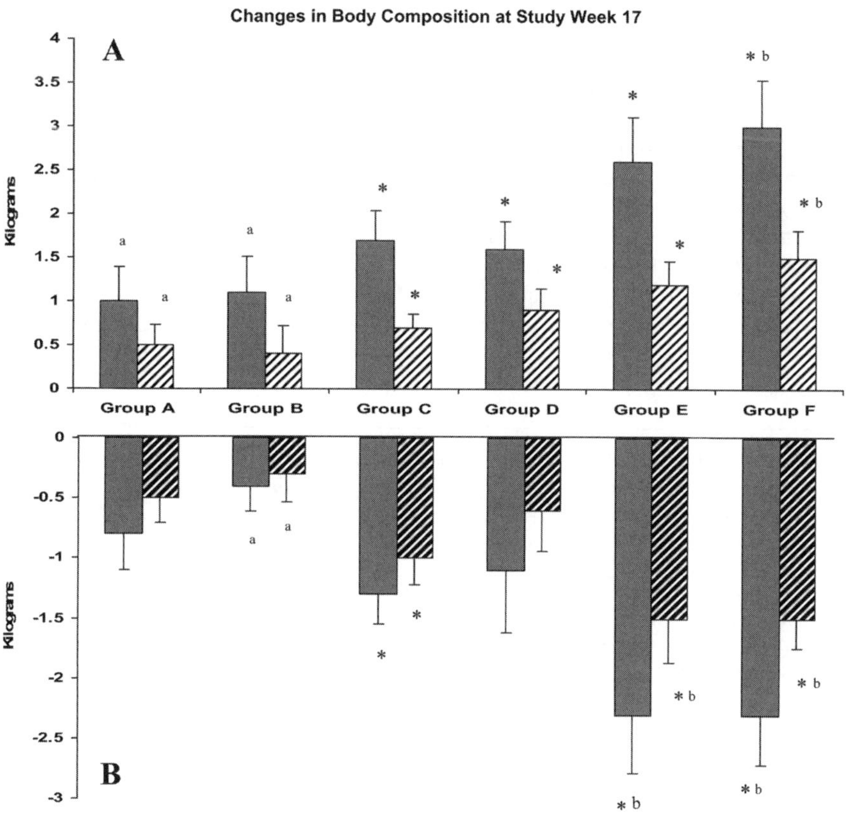


FIGURE 3.—DEXA-derived changes (mean ± 1 SE) in LBM and fat mass for each treatment group from baseline to wk 17. A, Increases in total LBM (*solid bars*) and appendicular lean mass (*hatched bars*). Changes across groups are significant for linear trend for total lean mass ($P = 0.0002$) and appendicular lean ($P = 0.0002$). B, Decreases in total body fat mass (*solid bars*) and trunk fat (*hatched bars*). Changes across groups are significant for linear trend for total fat mass ($P = 0.0004$) and trunk fat ($P = 0.0003$). *, Bonferoni adjusted within group changes ($P < 0.008$). Pairs of treatment groups with *different letters* (e.g. a *vs.* b) are significantly different by one-way ANCOVA with pairwise comparison (Tukey adjusted; $P < 0.05$). (Reprinted from Sattler FR, Castaneda-Sceppa C, Binder EF, et al. Testosterone and growth hormone improve body composition and muscle performance in older men. *J Clin Endocrinol Metab.* 2009;94:1991-2001, with permission from The Endocrine Society.)

all six groups (average 96 ± 137 sec longer). Systolic and diastolic blood pressure increased similarly in each group with mean increases of 12 ± 14 and 8 ± 8 mm Hg, respectively. Other predictable adverse events were modest and reversible.

*Conclusions.*—Supplemental testosterone produced significant gains in total and appendicular lean mass, muscle strength, and aerobic endurance with significant reductions in whole-body and trunk fat. Outcomes appeared to be further enhanced with GH supplementation (Fig 3).

▶ Aging men have impairment of gonadal function and a reduction in growth hormone secretion, which are associated with sarcopenia, decreased muscle strength, and increased body fat. The metabolic alterations have been shown to be reversible with testosterone therapy, and growth hormone has been shown to increase lean body mass and decrease body fat. The combination of therapy with testosterone and growth hormone has not been studied extensively in aging men. In the study by Sattler et al, the average age of the men was about 71 years and the men were randomized to receive various doses of testosterone with or without growth hormone. As might be expected, total and appendicular lean mass, muscle strength, and aerobic capacity improved significantly, and body fat and truck fat decreased. Growth hormone enhanced the response to testosterone. While these results are informative, this was a short-term study and long-term safety issues must be established for such intervention.

**A. W. Meikle, MD**

## Metabolic and Reproductive Features before and during Puberty in Daughters of Women with Polycystic Ovary Syndrome

Sir-Petermann T, Codner E, Pérez V, et al (Univ of Chile, Santiago; et al)
*J Clin Endocrinol Metab* 94:1923-1930, 2009

*Context.*—A significant proportion of the first-degree female relatives of women with polycystic ovary syndrome (PCOS) may be at risk for developing PCOS. However, it is not known at which stage of pubertal development the hormonal and metabolic abnormalities ensue in PCOS.

*Objective.*—The aim of the study was to assess the reproductive and metabolic profiles of daughters of women with PCOS (PCOSd) during the peripubertal period, a stage during which the gonadal axis is activated and PCOS may become clinically manifest.

*Design.*—Ninety-nine PCOSd [30 prepubertal and 69 pubertal (Tanner II-V)] and 84 daughters of control women (Cd) (20 prepubertal and 64 pubertal) were studied. An oral glucose tolerance test, a GnRH agonist test (leuprolide acetate, 10 μg/kg sc), and a transabdominal ultrasound were performed. Gonadotropins, sex steroids, SHBG, glucose, insulin, and lipids were determined.

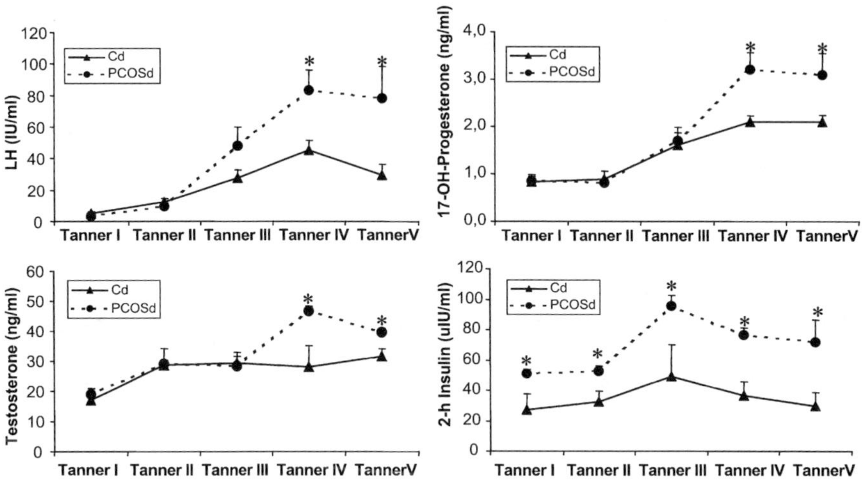


FIGURE 2.—LH, 17-OHP, and testosterone (LC-MS/MS) levels after stimulation with leuprolide acetate and the insulin levels after the glucose load (2-h) in PCOSd and Cd. Values are expressed as mean ± SEM. *, $P < 0.05$. (Reprinted from Sir-Petermann T, Codner E, Pérez V, et al. Metabolic and reproductive features before and during puberty in daughters of women with polycystic ovary syndrome. *J Clin Endocrinol Metab.* 2009;94:1923-1930, with permission from The Endocrine Society.)

*Results.*—Both groups had similar chronological ages and body mass index SD scores according to Tanner stage distribution. Ovarian volume and 2-h insulin were significantly higher in PCOSd compared to Cd at all Tanner stages. In Tanner stages IV and V, basal testosterone and post-stimulated LH, testosterone, and 17-hydroxyprogesterone concentrations were significantly higher in PCOSd compared to Cd.

*Conclusions.*—Hyperinsulinemia and an increased ovarian volume are present in PCOSd before the onset of puberty and persist during pubertal development. The biochemical abnormalities of PCOS appear during late puberty. Considering the early onset and the nature of the alterations, PCOSd constitute a high-risk group for metabolic and reproductive derangements (Fig 2).

▶ Polycystic ovary syndrome (PCOS) affects 5% to 10% of adult women, and is characterized by chronic anovulation and hyperandrogenism. Most of them have insulin resistance and are at high risk for type II diabetes mellitus and the metabolic syndrome. In most girls the clinical features begin after adolescence, but in some, clinical features can be recognized during the peripubertally. PCOS has a strong hereditary component. In the study by Sir-Petermann et al, daughters of women with PCOS were evaluated for their metabolic and hormonal abnormalities. High serum insulin concentrations and increased ovarian volume were observed before the onset of puberty and hormonal abnormalities characteristic of PCOS, such as increased luteinizing hormone (LH), testosterone, and 17 hydroxyprogesterone serum concentrations, were observed in late puberty. The clinical features of hyperandrogenism may not become apparent during early puberty because the effects of androgen excess may be delayed. They propose that the hyperinsulinemia may increase follicle-stimulating hormone (FSH) response to increase the number of ovarian follicles and increase the LH response on thecal cells of the ovary to increase testosterone production. Sensitive and specific measurements of sex steroids were critical for making the observations in these adolescents.

**A. W. Meikle, MD**

## Role of vitamin D treatment in glucose metabolism in polycystic ovary syndrome

Kotsa K, Yavropoulou MP, Anastasiou O, et al (Aristotle Univ of Thessaloniki, Greece)

*Fertil Steril* 92:1053-1058, 2009

*Objective.*—To determine the effect of treatment with vitamin $D_3$ analogue in the parameters of glucose metabolism in obese women with polycystic ovary syndrome (PCOS).

*Design.*—Observational study.

*Setting.*—Obese women with PCOS in an academic research environment.

*Patient(s).*—Fifteen obese women (mean age 28 ± 1.3 years, mean body mass index 32.55 ± 0.43) with documented chronic anovulation and hyperandrogenism were recruited into the study.

*Intervention(s).*—Alphacalcidol (1-α-hydroxyvitamin $D_3$) was administered orally 1 μg/day for 3 months. All subjects underwent a frequently sampled IV glucose tolerance test after a 10- to 12-hour overnight fast during a spontaneous bleeding episode before and after treatment with alphacalcidol.

*Main Outcome Measure(s).*—Peripheral insulin resistance and insulin effectiveness were estimated with minimal model.

*Result(s).*—The first phase of insulin secretion was significantly increased after treatment with alphacalcidol. A favorable statistically significant change also was observed in the lipid profile.

*Conclusion(s).*—Treatment with the vitamin $D_3$ analogue (alphacalcidol) could be of value in the management of PCOS (Fig 1).

▶ Vitamin D deficiency has been associated with many diseases in recent years in addition to its well-known influence on bone disease. Low concentrations of vitamin D 25 OH in cross sectional studies have been implicated in overall mortality, heart disease, hypertension, diabetes, autoimmune diseases, and some cancers. Both polycystic ovary syndrome (PCOS) and vitamin D 25 OH deficiency are very common. PCOS affects more than 6% of women, and vitamin D deficiency is even more common. In PCOS women, androgen excess and insulin resistance with high serum insulin concentrations are characteristic

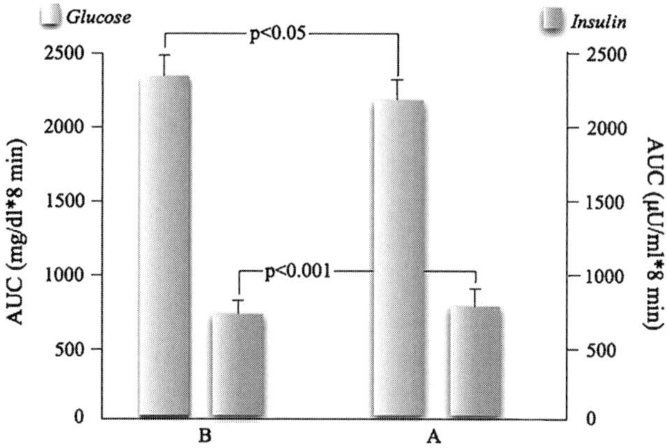


FIGURE 1.—Changes in glucose and insulin concentration during the first phase of insulin secretion ($AUC_{1-8}$) before and after treatment with alphacalcidol. Values are mean + SE. B = before treatment; A = after treatment. (Reprinted from Kotsa K, Yavropoulou MP, Anastasiou O, et al. Role of vitamin D treatment in glucose metabolism in polycystic ovary syndrome. *Fertil Steril.* 2009;92:1053-1058, with permission from the American Society for Reproductive Medicine.)

features. Vitamin D deficiency has been associated with impaired glucose tolerance and insulin secretion in both humans and experimental animals. Kotsa investigated the effect of alphacalcidol (1-α-hydroxyvitamin $D_3$) on peripheral insulin resistance and effectiveness in women with documented PCOS. They observed that the first phase of insulin secretion and the lipid profile were significantly improved after treatment with the vitamin $D_3$ analog. Vitamin D deficiency is more common in obesity compared with normal weight persons. Additional studies in diabetics without PCOS would be informative about the influence of vitamin D on insulin secretion and action.

**A. W. Meikle, MD**

# 59 Thyroid

---

**Evidence for a Specific Defect in Hippocampal Memory in Overt and Subclinical Hypothyroidism**

Correia N, Mullally S, Cooke G, et al (Adelaide and Meath Hosp, Tallaght, Dublin, Ireland; Trinity College Inst of Neuroscience, Dublin, Ireland)

*J Clin Endocrinol Metab* 94:3789-3797, 2009

---

*Context.*—Declarative memory largely depends upon normal functioning temporal lobes (hippocampal complex) and prefrontal cortex. Animal studies suggest abnormal hippocampal function in hypothyroidism.

*Objective.*—The aim of the study was to assess declarative memory in overt and subclinical (SCH) hypothyroid patients before and after L-$T_4$ (LT4) replacement and in matched normal subjects.

*Design and Setting.*—A prospective, open-labeled interventional study was conducted at a teaching hospital.

*Participants and Intervention.*—Hypothyroid (n = 21) and SCH (n = 17) patients underwent neuropsychological tests at baseline and 3 and 6 months after LT4 replacement. Normal subjects were studied at the same time-points.

*Main Outcome.*—Tests of spatial, verbal, associative, and working memory; attention; and response inhibition and the Hospital Anxiety and Depression Scale were administered.

*Results.*—Baseline deficits in spatial, associative, and verbal memory, which rely upon the integrity of the hippocampal and frontal areas, were identified in patients with overt hypothyroidism. Spatial and verbal memory were impaired in SCH patients ($P < 0.05$). TSH levels correlated negatively ($P < 0.05$) with these deficits. After LT4 replacement, verbal memory normalized. Spatial memory normalized in the SCH group but remained impaired in the hypothyroid group. Associative memory deficits persisted in the overt hypothyroid group. Hospital Anxiety and Depression Scale scores did not correlate with cognitive function. Measures of attention and response inhibition did not differ from control subjects.

*Conclusion.*—Cognitive impairment occurs in SCH and more markedly in overt hypothyroidism. These impairments appear predominantly mnemonic in nature, suggesting that the etiology is not indicative of general cognitive slowing. We propose that these deficits may reflect an underlying disruption of normal hippocampal function and/or connectivity.

▶ For a long time, it has been known that the cognitive function in overt hypothyroidism is impaired. Some studies have reported general cognitive slowing,[1] whereas others suggest a more specific mnemonic deficit.[2] Deficits in hippocampal-dependent memory tasks that are reversible with thyroid hormone replacement are apparent in animal models of hypothyroidism, whereas studies in hypothyroid rats have demonstrated impaired hippocampal neurogenesis, providing a potential mechanistic explanation for these mnemonic deficits. To date, it is not known whether similar mnemonic deficits occur in humans.

It is also not known whether the neurocognitive deficits associated with overt hypothyroidism occur in patients with subclinical hypothyroidism (SCH), which is defined as persistently raised serum thyroid-stimulating hormone (TSH) level in the presence of normal free $T_4$ (FT4) and which occurs in 4% to 10% of the adult population. Although some studies suggest impairment of cognitive function in SCH, there remain inconsistencies in the range and degree of these deficits. The authors of this article hypothesized that specific impairments in hippocampal and, possibly, frontally driven memory processes could be demonstrated in subjects with overt hypothyroidism and to a lesser degree in SCH, and these deficits would improve after L-$T_4$ (LT4) replacement. This can now be demonstrated. Summarized data are shown in Fig 3 in the original article. One major drawback of this study is the limited number of patients enrolled. Nonetheless, the data are convincing and should force doctors to prescribe thyroid hormone already at the level of subclinical hypothyroidism with elevated TSH levels.

**M. Schott, MD, PhD**

*References*

1. Constant EL, Adam S, Seron X, Bruyer R, Seghers A, Daumerie C. Anxiety and depression, attention, and executive functions in hypothyroidism. *J Int Neuropsychol Soc.* 2005;11:535-544.
2. Miller KJ, Parsons TD, Whybrow PC, et al. Memory improvement with treatment of hypothyroidism. *Int J Neurosci.* 2006;116:895-906.

---

**Genetic Predisposition to Elevated Serum Thyrotropin is Associated with Exceptional Longevity**

Atzmon G, Barzilai N, Surks MI, et al (Albert Einstein College of Medicine, Bronx, NY)

*J Clin Endocrinol Metab* 94:4768-4775, 2009

---

*Context.*—Exceptional longevity is associated with raised serum TSH.

*Objective.*—The aim of this study was to examine whether offspring of people with exceptional longevity have elevated serum TSH and whether specific single nucleotide polymorphisms (SNPs) in the *TSH*-B gene and *TSH* receptor (*TSHR*) gene are associated with this phenotype.

*Design/Setting/Patients.*—We measured serum TSH and free $T_4$ in Ashkenazi Jewish centenarians (n = 232; median age, 97 yr), their offspring (n = 366; median age, 69 yr), and age-matched controls without familial longevity (n = 163; median age, 70 yr). We determined TSH heritability, its distribution, and association with SNPs in the TSH-B and TSHR genes.

*Results.*—Offspring had higher median serum TSH [1.68 mIU/liter (97.5% confidence interval, 0.65 to 4.79 mIU/liter)], compared to controls [1.50 mIU/liter (97.5% confidence interval, 0.63 to 3.93 mIU/liter); $P = 0.02$], with estimated heritability of 0.33 ($P = 0.004$). Allele frequency of two SNPs in the promoter/enhancer region of *TSHR* gene, associated with increased serum TSH, was higher in centenarians and their offspring compared to controls (rs10149689 G allele frequency, 0.57 and 0.53 *vs.* 0.48; $P = 0.001$ and $P = 0.08$; odds ratio, 1.56 and 1.22, respectively; and rs12050077 A allele frequency, 0.57 and 0.53 *vs.* 0.46; $P = 0.0001$ and $P = 0.01$; odds ratio, 1.68 and 1.32, respectively). Linkage disequilibrium between the two SNPs was high ($r^2 = 0.95$), suggesting interaction between them. Furthermore, GA haplotype frequency was significantly higher among centenarians and offspring compared to controls (0.57 and 0.53 *vs.* 0.46; $P = 0.0001$ and $P = 0.01$, respectively).

*Conclusions.*—A heritable phenotype characterized by raised serum TSH is associated with human longevity. Carriers of rs12050077 and rs10149689 SNPs in the *TSHR* have higher serum TSH, possibly contributing to decreased thyroid function and longevity.

► The data presented by Atzmon et al show that offspring of the centenarian group have raised serum thyroid-stimulating hormone (TSH) concentrations compared with age-matched controls. Furthermore, offspring of the centenarian group who had elevated serum TSH levels also had higher TSH concentrations suggesting a heritable trait. After searching for genetic markers that could be associated with, and possibly responsible for, the raised serum TSH in centenarians and their offspring, the authors demonstrated for the first time that 2 single nucleotide polymorphisms (SNPs) (rs10149689 and rs12050077 of the thyroid-stimulating hormone receptor [TSHR]), located between enhancer regions and close to the promoter region, were significantly associated with raised TSH concentrations in the Ashkenazi Jewish centenarians and their offspring compared with controls, and showed strong linkage disequilibrium (Fig 5 in the original article). These results raise the possibility that these genetic changes exert an effect on TSHR gene expression that leads to increased TSH and may be, at least in part, transmitted from individuals with exceptional longevity to their offspring.

There are different reasons for the concordance between TSH levels and longevity. Thyroid hormone has profound impact on metabolic rate and body temperature by various mechanisms, including modulating mitochondrial activity, membrane composition and ion permeability, and substrate cycling.[1]

The relationship between longevity and hypothyroidism is considered to be due to lower levels of reactive oxygen species production and oxidative stress in response to changes in both obligate and facultative thermogenesis.[2]

A limitation of our study is that, at present, our findings and conclusions are restricted to the Ashkenazi Jewish population and cannot be generalized to other populations. Clearly, genetic studies in non-Ashkenazi populations in North America would be of great interest in this regard. Others have reported on serum TSH in individuals of exceptional longevity, some showing increased concentrations[3] and others showing decreased concentrations. None have reported on genetic changes as in the present work. Therefore, the authors suggest that those reported studies be interpreted cautiously because the study populations were small, have different genetic backgrounds from our study groups, and live in areas of variable iodine supply. Another limitation is that, because of lack of availability of serum in some individuals, the authors could not examine the relationship between free $T_4$ (FT4) and TSH in the entire control and offspring groups.

**M. Schott, MD, PhD**

*References*

1. Harper ME, Seifert EL. Thyroid hormone effects on mitochondrial energetics. *Thyroid*. 2008;18:145-156.
2. Hulbert AJ, Pamplona R, Buffenstein R, Buttemer WA. Life and death: metabolic rate, membrane composition, and life span of animals. *Physiol Rev*. 2007;87: 1175-1213.
3. Ravaglia G, Forti P, Maioli F, et al. Blood micronutrient and thyroid hormone concentrations in the oldest-old. *J Clin Endocrinol Metab*. 2000;85:2260-2265.

---

**Graves' Orbitopathy Activation after Radioactive Iodine Therapy with and without Steroid Prophylaxis**

Vannucchi G, Campi I, Covelli D, et al (Univ of Milan, Italy; et al)
*J Clin Endocrinol Metab* 94:3381-3386, 2009

---

*Context.*—The reactivation of Graves' orbitopathy (GO) after radioiodine (RAI) for Graves' disease (GD) is a known effect, and its clinical relevance is controversial. Prevention of RAI-induced GO activation is possible in at-risk patients with oral glucocorticoids (OGC).

*Objectives.*—The aim of the study was to analyze the effects of RAI on GO with or without prophylactic steroids based on known risk factors and to compare the effectiveness of prophylaxis with iv glucocorticoids (IVGC) and OGC.

*Design.*—We conducted a retrospective study in which patients were assessed before and 1–12 months after RAI.

*Patients and Setting.*—A total of 113 patients were included in the study; 83 underwent RAI without prophylactic steroids for the absence of risk of activation, and 30 were treated with either OGC (n = 21) or IVGC (n = 9).

*Main Outcome Measures.*—We analyzed the prevalence of GO activation with or without steroid prophylaxis and the difference in the prevalence of GO activation after OGC or IVGC.

*Results.*—GO activation was observed in 7.2% of patients without and 33.3% of patients with steroid prophylaxis ($P < 0.0001$), for an overall prevalence of 14.6%. GO activation occurred in 47.6% of patients treated with OGC but in none of the nine patients treated with IVGC ($P = 0.0001$). Disease activation was more prevalent in males ($P < 0.02$) and in older patients ($P = 0.04$) with a shorter duration of GD ($P < 0.01$) and time from GO onset ($P < 0.01$).

*Conclusions.*—GO may occur after RAI in approximately 15% of patients also in the absence of signs of active GO. Prophylactic OGC did not prevent GO activation in a large proportion of patients, compared to IVGC.

▶ The aim of the study by Vannucchi et al was to analyze the effects of radioiodine (RAI) on Graves' orbitopathy (GO) with or without prophylactic steroids based on known risk factors and to compare the effectiveness of prophylaxis with intravenous glucocorticoids (IVGC) and oral glucocorticoids (OGC). This work shows that GO may occur after RAI therapy in approximately 15% of patients with Graves' disease (GD) and also in the absence of signs of GO or of significantly active GO. Although these findings are obtained from a retrospective study, their significance relies on the fact that all patients were studied with the same approach in a standardized method before and after RAI therapy, according to the suggestions of a recent consensus statement (European Group on Graves'Orbitopathy [EUGOGO]).[1] GO activation after RAI therapy has been previously reported in about 15% to 20% of patients by several authors,[2,3] although in most studies patients with or without pre-existing signs of mild and/or minimally active eye disease were not clearly classified. Moreover, a definite assessment of the clinical activity of GO before and after RAI therapy has not been accurately performed.[4] The possibility of predicting, at the time of RAI therapy, which patients are at risk for the occurrence of GO has been a matter of controversy over the last few years. This is mostly due to the lack of controlled studies identifying plausible and consistent risk factors for de novo occurrence or relapse of active GO in GD patients with persistent hyperthyroidism treated with RAI therapy. Another major finding of this work is the observation that prophylactic treatment with OGC prevented GO activation in about 50% of patients compared with successful prevention in all patients with intravenous (IV) steroids (Fig 1 in the original article). Patients with signs of moderately active GO were more prevalent in the IVGC group, as shown by the significantly higher clinical activity score (CAS). Other clinical characteristics of the patients treated with the 2 modalities did not differ, that is, previous therapy for active GO, when present, and interval between such therapy and RAI. Therefore, it might be hypothesized that when given via IV route, steroids have a greater immunosuppressive effect on the thyroid and orbital autoimmune reactions involved in GO activation. In interpreting this finding, which should be confirmed in a randomized controlled study and on a larger series of patients, one also has to consider that patient compliance with OGC may not have been as adequate as with the IV administration route, because of the duration of therapy (up to 8 weeks) and the frequent appearance of side effects.

**M. Schott, MD, PhD**

*References*


1. Bartalena L, Baldeschi L, Dickinson A, et al. European Group on Graves' Orbitopathy (EUGOGO). Consensus statement of the European Group on Graves' orbitopathy (EUGOGO) on management of GO. *Eur J Endocrinol.* 2008;158: 273-285.
2. Rasmussen AK, Nygaard B, Feldt-Rasmussen U. (131)I and thyroid-associated ophthalmopathy. *Eur J Endocrinol.* 2000;143:155-160.
3. Bonnema SJ, Bartalena L, Toft AD, Hegedus L. Controversies in radioiodine therapy: relation to ophthalmopathy, the possible radioprotective effect of antithyroid drugs, and use in large goitres. *Eur J Endocrinol.* 2002;147:1-11.
4. Sisson JC, Schipper MJ, Nelson CC, Freitas JE, Frueh BR. Radioiodine therapy and Graves' ophthalmopathy. *J Nucl Med.* 2008;49:923-930.


## Follow-Up of Low-Risk Differentiated Thyroid Cancer Patients Who Underwent Radioiodine Ablation of Postsurgical Thyroid Remnants after Either Recombinant Human Thyrotropin or Thyroid Hormone Withdrawal

Elisei R, Schlumberger M, Driedger A, et al (Univ of Pisa, Italy; Univ of Paris-Sud XI, France; Univ of Western Ontario, London, Canada; et al)
*J Clin Endocrinol Metab* 94:4171-4179, 2009

*Background.*—We previously demonstrated comparable thyroid remnant ablation rates in postoperative low-risk thyroid cancer patients prepared for administration of 3.7GBq $^{131}$I (100 mCi) after recombinant human (rh) TSH during $T_4$ (L-T4) therapy *vs.* withholding L-T4 (euthyroid *vs.* hypothyroid groups). We now compared the outcomes of these patients 3.7 yr later.

*Patients and Methods.*—Fifty-one of the 63 original patients (28 euthyroid, 23 hypothyroid) participated. Forty-eight received rhTSH and serum thyroglobulin (Tg) sampling. A $^{131}$I whole-body scan was performed in 43 patients, and successful ablation was defined by criteria from the previous study. Based on the criterion of uptake less than 0.1% in thyroid bed, 100% (43 of 43) remained ablated. When no visible uptake instead was used, five patients (four euthyroid, one hypothyroid) had minimal visible activity. When the TSH-stimulated Tg criterion was used, only two of 45 (one euthyroid, one hypothyroid) had a stimulated Tg level greater than 2 ng/ml.

*Results.*—No patient in either group died, and no patient declared disease free had sustained tumor recurrence. Nine (four euthyroid, five hypothyroid) had received additional $^{131}$I between the original and current studies due to detectable Tg or imaging evidence of disease; with follow-up, all now had a negative rhTSH-stimulated whole-body scan and seven (three euthyroid, four hypothyroid) had a stimulated serum Tg less than 2 ng/ml.

*Conclusions.*—In conclusion, after a median 3.7 yr, low-risk thyroid cancer patients prepared for postoperative remnant ablation either with rhTSH or after L-T4 withdrawal were confirmed to have had their thyroid remnants ablated and to have comparable rates of tumor recurrence and persistence (Table 4).

▶ Ablation of postsurgical thyroid tissue is a key element in treatment for selected differentiated epithelial thyroid cancer (DTC) patients. Because postoperative thyroid remnant ablation requires TSH activation of tissue, the traditional approach of preparation for radioiodine therapy has been to withhold thyroid hormone therapy to induce an endogenous TSH rise.[1] Although this strategy is effective, it causes clinical hypothyroidism with unpleasant symptoms[2] and, in some settings, the need for longer hospitalization compared with patients prepared by recombinant human TSH (rhTSH).[3] In a previous prospective randomized trial,[4] comparable successful postsurgical $^{131}$I thyroid remnant ablation rates in 2 groups of low-risk DTC patients who were prepared for administration of 3.7 GBq $^{131}$I with either endogenous TSH stimulation induced by 4 or more weeks of thyroid hormone withdrawal or by rhTSH

**TABLE 4.**—Comparison of 8-Month and Current Study Result for Evaluable Patients

| | 8-Month Postablation Testing in Original Study | | 3- to 4-yr Postablation Testing in Current Study | |
|---|---|---|---|---|
| | Hypothyroid Group (n = 30) | Euthyroid Group (n = 33) | Former Hypothyroid Group (n = 21) | Former Euthyroid Group (n = 27) |
| Patients included in scan analysis/all original patients | 28/30 | 32/33 | 18/21 | 25/27 |
| Patients with no visible uptake or less than 0.1%/patients in scan analysis | 28/28 (100%) | 32/32 (100%) | 18/18 (100%) | 25/25 (100%) |
| Patients included in scan analysis/all original patients | 28/30 | 32/33 | 18/21 | 25/27 |
| Patients with no visible uptake/patients in scan analysis | 24/28 (86%) | 24/32 (75%) | 17/18 (94%) | 21/25 (84%) |
| Patients with serum Tg measured and no interfering TgAb/all original patients | 21/30 | 24/33 | 20/21 | 25/27 |
| Patients with serum Tg less than 2 ng/ml/all patients with Tg analyzed | 18/21 (86%) | 23/24 (96%) | 19/20 (95%) | 24/25 (96%) |
| Patients with serum Tg measured and no interfering TgAb/all original patients | 21/30 | 24/33 | 20/21 | 25/27 |
| Patients with serum Tg less than 1 ng/ml/all patients with Tg analyzed | 18/21 (86%) | 20/24 (83%) | 18/20 (90%) | 23/25 (92%) |

were demonstrated. Successful ablation was achieved in all patients in both groups, based on the primary prospectively defined criterion for thyroid remnant ablation: either no visible uptake or less than 0.1% thyroid bed uptake of the administered $^{131}I$ activity on imaging performed 8 months after therapy. Up to now, however, no study exists describing the outcome of patients receiving rhTSH. In this study by Elisei et al. there were no differences between the two approaches in eliminating thyroid remnants or in instances of residual disease detected (results summarized in Table 4). These findings confirm that rhTSH is an effective and safe alternative to thyroid hormone withdrawal in preparing low-risk DTC patients for the postsurgical thyroid remnant ablation. This study also confirms that rhTSH-stimulated serum Tg measurement is a highly sensitive indicator of residual disease or normal tissue and one that is superior to radioiodine scanning. Finally, the study confirms the long-term safety of repeated rhTSH exposures.

**M. Schott, MD, PhD**
**S. Schinner, MD, PhD**

*References*

1. Mazzaferri EL, Robyn J. Postsurgical management of differentiated thyroid carcinoma. *Otolaryngol Clin North Am.* 1996;29:637-662.
2. Dow KH, Ferrell BR, Anello C. Quality-of-life changes in patients with thyroid cancer after withdrawal of thyroid hormone therapy. *Thyroid.* 1997;7:613-619.
3. Borget I, Remy H, Chevalier J, et al. Length and cost of hospital stay of radioiodine ablation in thyroid cancer patients: comparison between preparation with thyroid hormone withdrawal and thyrogen. *Eur J Nucl Med Mol Imaging.* 2008;35:1457-1463.
4. Pacini F, Ladenson PW, Schlumberger M, et al. Radioiodine ablation of thyroid remnants after preparation with recombinant human thyrotropin in differentiated thyroid carcinoma: results of an international, randomized, controlled study. *J Clin Endocrinol Metab.* 2006;91:926-932.

---

**Impact of Lithium on Efficacy of Radioactive Iodine for Graves' Disease: A Cohort Study on Cure Rate, Time to Cure, and Frequency of Increased Serum Thyroxine After Antithyroid Drug Withdrawal**

Bogazzi F, Giovannetti C, Fessehatsion R, et al (Univ of Pisa, Italy)
*J Clin Endocrinol Metab* 95:201-208, 2010

---

*Context.*—Radioactive iodine (RAI) is a common therapy for hyperthyroidism due to Graves' disease. A small but significant proportion of patients have recurrence of hyperthyroidism after RAI therapy. Lithium might increase RAI effectiveness by increasing RAI retention in the thyroid. However, whether lithium favorably affects the long-term outcome of RAI therapy is still a matter of argument.

*Objective.*—The objective of the study was to compare the efficacy of RAI given with or without concomitant lithium treatment.

*Design.*—This was a retrospective cohort study.

*Setting.*—The study was conducted at a tertiary university center.

*Patients.*—Six hundred fifty-one patients with newly diagnosed Graves' disease participated in the study.

*Intervention.*—Two hundred ninety-eight patients were treated with RAI plus lithium (900 mg/d for 12 d) and 353 with RAI alone.

*Main Outcome Measures.*—Proportion of cured patients and time to achieve cure of hyperthyroidism during 1 yr of follow-up was measured.

*Results.*—Patients treated with RAI plus lithium had a higher cure rate (91.0%) than those treated with RAI alone (85.0%, $P = 0.030$). In addition, patients treated with RAI plus lithium were cured more rapidly (median 60 d) than those treated with RAI alone (median 90 d, $P = 0.000$). Treatment with lithium prevented the serum free $T_4$ increase after methimazole withdrawal and RAI therapy. Side effects after RAI therapy occurred in a subset of patients and were mild, transient, and without differences in the two groups.

*Conclusions.*—RAI combined with lithium is safe and more effective than RAI alone in the cure of hyperthyroidism due to Graves' disease.

▶ Radioactive iodine (RAI) is widely used for hyperthyroidism due to Graves' disease either as a first-line treatment or when hyperthyroidism relapses after a course of antithyroid drug treatment.[1] The target of RAI therapy (cure of hyperthyroidism) is a stable restoration of euthyroidism or permanent hypothyroidism. To this purpose, several regimens have been proposed, including, for example, selection of patients and different schedules based on variable RAI doses.[2] Pretreatment with thionamides may reduce RAI efficacy as pointed out in a recent meta-analysis, irrespective of the type of drug and discontinuation protocol.[3] Studies reported variable percentage of failure after RAI therapy, depending on several variables, including $^{131}I$ dose, although a recent meta-analysis did not show difference in the outcome of calculated or fixed doses. Lithium accumulates in the thyroid and increases (radio)iodine retention without affecting thyroidal radioiodine uptake (RAIU). The addition of lithium to RAI has been associated with an increase in the radiation dose delivered to the thyroid.[4] Whether this results in a higher cure rate of hyperthyroidism is still a matter of argument. Conflicting results have been reported on this issue. Furthermore, the potential toxicity of lithium raised some concern about its use in combination with RAI for hyperthyroidism.[5] The objective of this study was to compare the efficacy of RAI given with or without concomitant lithium treatment. The protocol, which has been used in the study by Bogazzi et al is shown in Fig 1. It has a good design to avoid interference with antithyroid drugs, and to deliver lithium at the most favorable time. In this study, lithium was given for only 9 days, beginning 5 days before $^{131}I$ therapy was initiated, and maintained for 7 days thereafter. This is a shorter protocol (12 vs 19 days) than that of a previous pilot study by Bogazzi and associates[4] that found that the effect of lithium on serum thyroid hormone concentrations occurred 3 to 5 days after $^{131}I$ was administered. Although this is a retrospective study, the scrupulous statistical analysis takes into account the possibility of selection bias by adjusting for confounding variables. Multivariate analysis

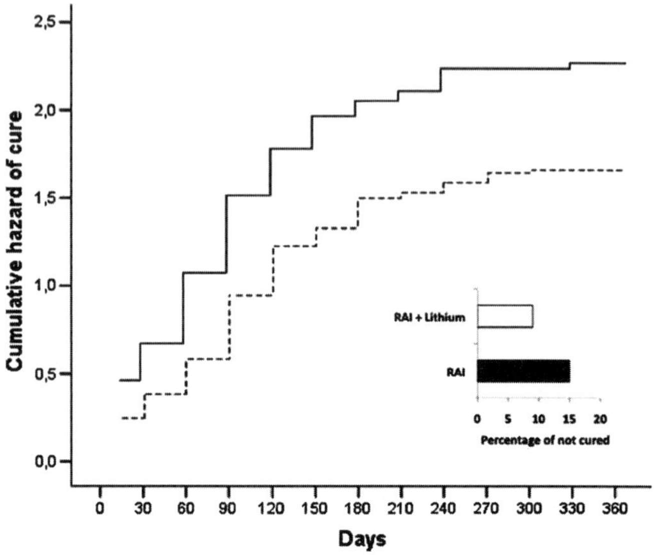


FIGURE 1.—Cumulative hazard of cured patients estimated by the Kaplan-Meier method. The two curves were compared by the log-rank test ($P = 0.000$). Difference in the cure rate at the end of the follow-up period was assessed by Fisher's exact test ($P = 0.030$). The outcome of patients treated with RAI and lithium is indicated by *solid line* and that of patients treated with RAI alone by *dotted line*. The cumulative hazard of cure is related to the cumulative proportion of patients not cured. The *insert figure* shows the percentage of patients not cured in the two groups. (Reprinted from Bogazzi F, Giovannetti C, Fessehatsion R, et al. Impact of lithium on efficacy of radioactive iodine for graves' disease: a cohort study on cure rate, time to cure, and frequency of increased serum thyroxine after antithyroid drug withdrawal. *J Clin Endocrinol Metab*. 2010;95:201-208, with permission from The Endrocrine Society.)

was performed using both the propensity score and significant covariates to control for possible bias from the nonrandomized assignment of patients to treatment. The main findings of the study were that patients treated with $^{131}$I plus lithium had a higher cure rate (91%) than those treated with $^{131}$I alone. Treatment with lithium also prevented an increase in serum free T4 and T3 levels after withdrawal of MMI, which had been given for 3 to 6 months before $^{131}$I therapy (Fig 2). Side effects of lithium were mild and transient and were not different in the 2 study groups with and without lithium pretreatment for $^{131}$I therapy. None of the patients had ophthalmopathy, and the thyroid volume decreased much more rapidly in the patients pretreated with lithium as compared with the group treated with $^{131}$I alone.

In summary, this study shows that lithium is of substantial benefit in the treatment of patients with Graves' hyperthyroidism. The authors suggest that a short course of lithium is safe and beneficial for patients treated with $^{131}$I, increasing the cure rate for hyperthyroidism and shortening the time for cure, and preventing an abrupt increase in thyroid hormone levels. It is highly likely that this important study will provide a strong impetus for a change in practice paradigms for patients with Graves' hyperthyroidism. It must be kept in mind, however, that all the positive effects of lithium found in this study rely upon

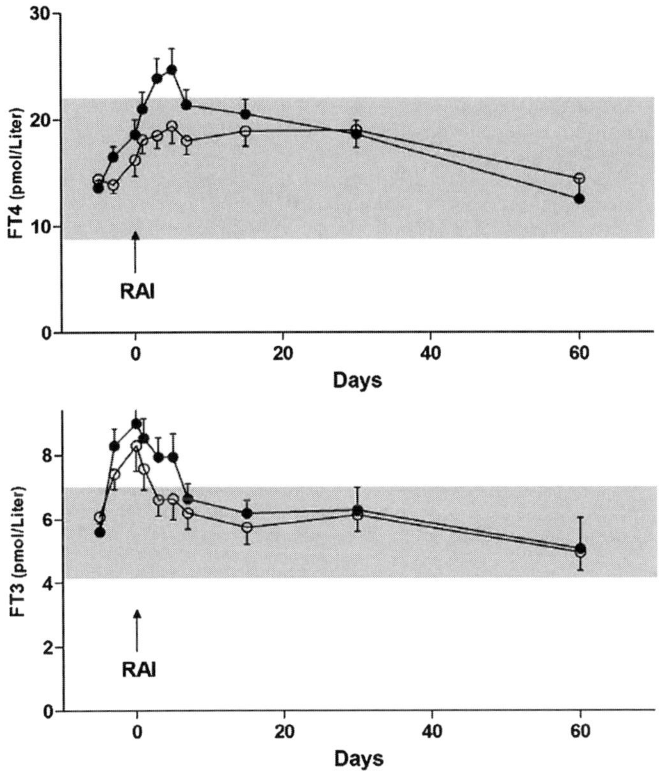


FIGURE 2.—Outcome of serum thyroid hormone concentrations. The *shaded area* shows the normal range for serum FT4 and FT3 levels. Outcome of mean serum FT4 and FT3 concentrations (±SE) in patients treated with RAI and lithium are shown by *white circles* and that in patients treated with RAI alone by *black circles*. Difference in the outcome of serum FT4 concentrations between the RAI plus lithium group and the RAI alone group were different at T + 3 and T + 5 ($P = 0.0139$ and $P = 0.0373$, respectively); on the contrary, mean serum FT3 concentrations, although lower in patients treated with RAI plus lithium, were not significantly different in the two treatment groups. (Reprinted from Bogazzi F, Giovannetti C, Fessehatsion R, et al. Impact of lithium on efficacy of radioactive iodine for graves' disease: a cohort study on cure rate, time to cure, and frequency of increased serum thyroxine after antithyroid drug withdrawal. *J Clin Endocrinol Metab.* 2010;95:201-208, with permission from The Endrocrine Society.)

careful adherence to a treatment protocol described in this article. Based on that, the present RAI treatment protocols will be changed in the near future.

**M. Schott, MD, PhD**

## *References*

1. Weetman AP. Radioiodine treatment for benign thyroid diseases. *Clin Endocrinol (Oxf).* 2007;66:757-764.
2. Allahabadia A, Daykin J, Sheppard MC, Gough SC, Franklyn JA. Radioiodine treatment of hyperthyroidism-prognostic factors for outcome. *J Clin Endocrinol Metab.* 2001;86:3611-3617.

3. Walter MA, Briel M, Christ-Crain M, et al. Effects of antithyroid drugs on radioiodine treatment: systematic review and meta-analysis of randomised controlled trials. *BMJ*. 2007;334:514.
4. Bogazzi F, Bartalena L, Campomori A, et al. Treatment with lithium prevents serum thyroid hormone increase after thionamide withdrawal and radioiodine therapy in patients with Graves' disease. *J Clin Endocrinol Metab*. 2002;87:4490-4495.
5. Dunkelmann S, Kunstner H, Nabavi E, Eberlein U, Groth P, Schumichen C. Lithium as an adjunct to radioiodine therapy in Graves' disease for prolonging the intrathyroidal effective half-life of radioiodine. Useful or not? *Nuklearmedizin*. 2006;45:213-218.

# Article Index

## Chapter 1: Osteoarthritis



## Chapter 2: Rheumatoid Arthritis



## Chapter 3: Genetics



## Chapter 4: Myopathies



## Chapter 5: Vasculitis

## Chapter 6: Sjögren's Syndrome



## Chapter 7: Miscellaneous



## Chapter 8: Bacterial Infections

## Chapter 9: Viral Infections



## Chapter 10: Tuberculosis



## Chapter 11: Fungal Infections

## Chapter 12: Nosocomial Infections



## Chapter 13: Vaccines



## Chapter 14: Breast Cancer

## Chapter 15: Central Nervous System



## Chapter 16: Chemotherapy: Mechanisms and Side Effects



## Chapter 17: Genitourinary



## Chapter 18: Gynecology

## Chapter 19: Hematologic Malignancies



## Chapter 20: Melanoma



## Chapter 21: Supportive Care



## Chapter 22: Thoracic Cancer



## Chapter 23: Miscellaneous



## Chapter 24: Metabolic Factors and Renal Disease Progression

## Chapter 25: Diabetes



## Chapter 26: Calcium, Phosphorus, and Bone



## Chapter 27: Chronic Renal Failure and Transplantation

## Chapter 28: Dialysis



## Chapter 29: Critical Care Medicine



## Chapter 30: Lung Cancer

## Chapter 31: Asthma and Cystic Fibrosis



## Chapter 32: Community-Acquired Pneumonia



## Chapter 33: Chronic Obstructive Pulmonary Disease



## Chapter 34: Lung Transplantation

## Chapter 35: Sleep Disorders



## Chapter 36: Pleural, Interstitial Lung, and Pulmonary Vascular Disease



## Chapter 37: Cardiac Arrhythmias, Conduction Disturbances, and Electrophysiology

## Chapter 38: Cardiac Surgery



## Chapter 39: Coronary Heart Disease

## Chapter 40: Hypertension



## Chapter 41: Non-Coronary Heart Disease in Adults



## Chapter 42: Pediatric Cardiovascular Disease



## Chapter 43: Esophagus

## Chapter 44: Gastrointestinal Cancers and Benign Polyps



## Chapter 45: Gastrointestinal Motility Disorders



## Chapter 46: Gastrointestinal Motility Disorders/Neurogastroenterology



## Chapter 47: Inflammatory Bowel Disease

## Chapter 48: Liver Disease



## Chapter 49: Miscellaneous



## Chapter 50: Nutrition and Celiac Disease



## Chapter 51: Adrenal Cortex

## Chapter 52: Calcium and Bone Metabolism



## Chapter 53: Diabetes



## Chapter 54: Lipoproteins and Atherosclerosis

## Chapter 55: Neuroendocrinology



## Chapter 56: Obesity



## Chapter 57: Pediatric Endocrinology



## Chapter 58: Reproductive Endocrinology

## Chapter 59: Thyroid

# Author Index

## N



## O



## P



## Q



## R

## Y



## Z